2705
g.d.15

D0721945

SECOND EDITION

NUTRITIONAL CONCERNS of WOMEN

CRC SERIES IN MODERN NUTRITION
Edited by Ira Wolinsky and James F. Hickson, Jr.

Published Titles

Manganese in Health and Disease, Dorothy J. Klimis-Zacas

Nutrition and AIDS: Effects and Treatments, Ronald R. Watson

Nutrition Care for HIV-Positive Persons: A Manual for Individuals and Their Caregivers,
Saroj M. Bahl and James F. Hickson, Jr.

Calcium and Phosphorus in Health and Disease, John J.B. Anderson and
Sanford C. Garner

Edited by Ira Wolinsky

Published Titles

Practical Handbook of Nutrition in Clinical Practice, Donald F. Kirby
and Stanley J. Dudrick

Handbook of Dairy Foods and Nutrition, Gregory D. Miller, Judith K. Jarvis,
and Lois D. McBean

Advanced Nutrition: Macronutrients, Carolyn D. Berdanier

Childhood Nutrition, Fima Lifschitz

Nutrition and Health: Topics and Controversies, Felix Bronner

Nutrition and Cancer Prevention, Ronald R. Watson and Siraj I. Mufti

Nutritional Concerns of Women, Second Edition, Ira Wolinsky
and Dorothy J. Klimis-Zacas

Nutrients and Gene Expression: Clinical Aspects, Carolyn D. Berdanier

Antioxidants and Disease Prevention, Harinda S. Garewal

Advanced Nutrition: Micronutrients, Carolyn D. Berdanier

Nutrition and Women's Cancers, Barbara Pence and Dale M. Dunn

Nutrients and Foods in AIDS, Ronald R. Watson

Nutrition: Chemistry and Biology, Second Edition, Julian E. Spallholz,
L. Mallory Boylan, and Judy A. Driskell

Melatonin in the Promotion of Health, Ronald R. Watson

Nutritional and Environmental Influences on the Eye, Allen Taylor

Laboratory Tests for the Assessment of Nutritional Status, Second Edition,
H.E. Sauberlich

Advanced Human Nutrition, Robert E.C. Wildman and Denis M. Medeiros

Handbook of Dairy Foods and Nutrition, Second Edition, Gregory D. Miller,
Judith K. Jarvis, and Lois D. McBean

Nutrition in Space Flight and Weightlessness Models, Helen W. Lane
and Dale A. Schoeller

Forthcoming Titles

SECOND EDITION

NUTRITIONAL CONCERNS
of
WOMEN

Edited by

Dorothy Klimis-Zacas
Ira Wolinsky

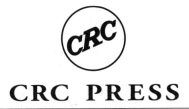

CRC PRESS

Boca Raton   London   New York   Washington, D.C.

Library of Congress Cataloging-in-Publication Data

Nutritional concerns of women / [editors] Dorothy Klimis-Zacas, Ira Wolinsky.--2nd ed.
    p. cm. -- (Modern nutrition)
Includes bibliographical references and index.
ISBN 0-8493-1337-6 (alk. paper)
1. Nutritionally induced diseases--Sex factors. 2. Women--Nutrition. 3.
Women--diseases. 4. Women-Health and Hygiene. I. Klimis-Zacas, Dorothy. II.
Wolinsky, Ira. III. Modern nutrition (Boca Raton, Fla.)

RC622.N8932 2003
616′.0082--dc21   2003051473

Visit the CRC Press Web site at www.crcpress.com

© 2004 by CRC Press LLC

No claim to original U.S. Government works
International Standard Book Number 0-8493-1337-6
Library of Congress Card Number 2003051473
Printed in the United States of America 1 2 3 4 5 6 7 8 9 0
Printed on acid-free paper

Dedication

To Miltiades, Mary Ann, Michael-John, Daniella and David

Series Preface for Modern Nutrition

The CRC Series in Modern Nutrition is dedicated to providing the widest possible coverage to topics in nutrition. Nutrition is an interdisciplinary, interprofessional field par excellence. It is noted for its broad range and diversity. We trust that the titles and authorship in this series will reflect that range and diversity.

Published for a scholarly audience, the volumes of the CRC Series in Modern Nutrition are designed to explain, review and explore present knowledge and recent trends, developments and advances in nutrition. As such, they will also appeal to the educated layman. The format for the series will vary with the needs of the author and the topic, including, but not limited to, edited volumes, monographs, handbooks and texts.

Dorothy Klimis-Zacas and I are most pleased to have had the opportunity of working together to bring you the second edition of *Nutritional Concerns of Women*.

Other books of interest to the reader in the CRC Series are *Nutrition and the Female Athlete; Nutrition and Women's Cancer; Gender Differences in Metabolism, Practical and Nutritional Implications; Eating Disorders in Women and Children, Prevention, Stress Management, and Treatment.*

Ira Wolinsky, Ph.D.
University of Houston

Preface

More than a decade ago, the U.S. National Institutes of Health (NIH), recognizing the lack of inclusion of women in health research and realizing that many diseases are unique to, more prevalent among or affect women differently from men, established the Office for Research in Women's Health (ORWH) with the goal to improve women's health status across the life span. Since that time, the ORWH, with the collaboration of the scientific community and different community groups, has worked diligently to increase awareness of the uniqueness of women's risk factors to different diseases and the need for women's inclusion in research studies. Their efforts culminated in the Institute of Medicine's 2001 report Exploring the Biological Contribution to Human Health: Does Sex Matter? This report outlined a plethora of sex differences in the prevention, manifestation and treatment of disease, which, in turn, necessitated and encouraged research in the above areas.

For the 21st century, the NIH National Research Agenda has expanded to include not only biomedical but also behavioral and psychosocial research. Since determinants of health include physical, mental, social and spiritual (such as education, economic status, housing, environmental and discrimination based on culture and ethnic background), the NIH 21st-century agenda focuses on women's diversity with respect to race or ethnicity, age, ability or disability, socioeconomic class, education and sexual orientation.

The second edition of *Nutritional Concerns of Women* is a product of recent advances in women's nutrition as it relates to health. New chapters on subjects unique to women, such as menopause, and prevalent among women, such as rheumatic disease and diseases of the thyroid, have been included. Additionally, a chapter on the role that gender and culture play on nutrition has been added.

The first edition was very well received indeed and used by a wide range of nutritionists and interested laymen. We were especially happy that the first edition found use as a text for university courses on women's nutrition. In this expanded second edition, we have again assembled an excellent team of writers, acknowledged experts in their fields, and we, the editors, are proud to appear alongside them. We have tried to be as comprehensive as possible in the selection of topics and trust that this volume will help facilitate nutrition recommendations for women and will formulate principles for them to follow in everyday life. Updated Dietary Reference Intakes (DRIs) can be found in the Appendix.

Dorothy Klimis-Zacas, Ph.D.
University of Maine, Orono

Ira Wolinsky, Ph.D.
University of Houston, Texas

Editors

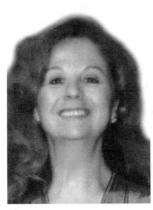

Dorothy Klimis-Zacas, Ph.D., is professor of Clinical Nutrition in the Food Science and Human Nutrition Department at the University of Maine, Orono, and cooperating professor of Nutrition and Dietetics at Harokopio University, Athens, Greece. Dr. Klimis-Zacas received her undergraduate training in Biology at Arcadia University, Glenside, Pennsylvania. She obtained her M.S. in Human Physiology and Ph.D. in Nutrition at the Pennsylvania State University.

Dr. Klimis-Zacas is a member of the American Dietetic Association, the American Society for Clinical Nutrition, the American Society for Nutritional Sciences, the Hellenic Dietetic Association and the International Atherosclerosis Society, among other scientific organizations.

Her current research interests relate to the role of trace minerals and functional foods on cardiovascular disease. She has contributed to international research through applied investigations on the nutritional status of populations in the Mediterranean region. She received a Senior Fulbright Fellowship to the National School of Public Health, Athens, Greece (1995).

Dr. Klimis-Zacas is the author of numerous research articles and the editor of the CRC books *Manganese in Health and Disease* and *Nutritional Concerns for Women* (1st edition). She is also the editor of McGraw-Hill/Dushkin's *Annual Editions in Nutrition 2001/2002, 2002/2003* and *2003/2004.*

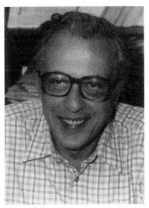

Ira Wolinsky, Ph.D., is Professor of Nutrition at the University of Houston. He received his B.S. degree in Chemistry from the City College of New York and his M.S. and Ph.D. degrees in Biochemistry from the University of Kansas. He has served in research and teaching positions at the Hebrew University, the University of Missouri and The Pennsylvania State University, as well as conducting basic research in NASA life sciences facilities and abroad.

Dr. Wolinsky is a member of the American Society for Nutritional Sciences, among other honorary and scientific organizations. He has contributed numerous nutrition research papers in the open literature. His major research interests relate to the nutrition of bone and calcium and trace elements, and to sports nutrition. He has been the recipient of research grants from both public and private sources and of several international research fellowships and consultantships to the former Soviet Union, Bulgaria, Hungary and India. He merited a Fulbright Senior Scholar Fellowship to Greece (Harokopio University, Athens) in 1999–2000.

Dr. Wolinsky has coauthored a book on the history of the science of nutrition, *Nutrition and Nutritional Diseases*. He coedited *Sports Nutrition: Vitamins and Trace Elements*; *Macroelements, Water, and Electrolytes in Sports Nutrition*; *Energy-Yielding Macronutrients and Energy Metabolism in Sports Nutrition*; *Nutritional Applications in Exercise and Sport*, and *Nutritional Assessment of Athletes*, all with Judy Driskell. Additionally, he coedited the first edition of *Nutritional Concerns of Women* with Dorothy Klimis-Tavantzis and *The Mediterranean Diet: Constituents and Health Promotion* with his colleagues from Harokopio University, Athens, Greece. He edited three editions of *Nutrition in Exercise and Sport*, and also served as the editor or coeditor for the CRC Series *Nutrition in Exercise and Sport*; *Modern Nutrition*; *Methods in Nutrition Research* and *Exercise Physiology*.

Acknowledgments

We wish to acknowledge with thanks the expert contribution of each and every chapter author. We learned a great deal from them.

Contributors

John J.B. Anderson, Ph.D.
Department of Nutrition
University of North Carolina
School of Public Health and Medicine
Chapel Hill, NC
Email: jjb_anderson@unc.edu

E. Wayne Askew, Ph.D.
Division of Foods and Nutrition
University of Utah
Salt Lake City, UT
Email: Wayne.Askew@health.utah.edu

Carol J. Baker-Fulco, M.S., R.D.
Military Nutrition Division
United States Army Research Institute
  of Environmental Medicine
Natick, MA
Email: Carol.Baker-
  Fulco@na.amedd.army.mil

Carolyn Berdanier, Ph.D.
Food and Nutrition at Family Consumer
  Services
Professor of Nutrition
University of Georgia
Athens, GA
Email: cberdan@fcs.uga.edu

Lisa Bodnar, M.P.H., R.D.
Magee-Women's Research Institute
Pittsburgh, PA
Email: lbodnar@email.unc.edu or
  bodnar@mwri.magee.edu

Timothy P. Carr, Ph.D.
Department of Nutrition Science and
  Dietetics
University of Nebraska
Lincoln, NE
Email: tcarr2@unl.edu

Yolanda Cartwright, M.S., R.D.
School of Public Health
University of Minnesota
Minneapolis, MN
Email:
  yolandacartwright@sbcglobal.net

Mary E. Cogswell, Dr.Ph., R.N.
Maternal and Child Nutrition Branch
Division of Nutrition and Physical
  Activity
Centers for Disease Control and
  Prevention
Atlanta, GA
Email: meco@cdc.gov

Cristanna M. Cook, Ph.D.
Husson College
Bangor, ME
Email: cookctank@aol.com

Richard A. Cook, Ph.D.
Dept of Food Science and Human
  Nutrition
University of Maine
Orono, ME
Email, racook@unmenfa.maine.edu

Nancy B. Cummings, M.D.
National Institute of Diabetes and
  Digestive and Kidney Diseases
National Institute of Health
Bethesda, MD
Email: drnbcummings@aol.com

Patricia A. Dyett, M.S.
Department of Nutrition
Loma Linda University
Loma Linda, CA
Email: pdyett03p@sph.llu.edu

Janet Friedmann, Ph.D., R.D.
Vanderbilt Center for Human Nutrition
Vanderbilt UniversityMedical Center
Nashville, TN
Email:
  janet.friedmann@mcmail.vanderbilt.edu

L. Gaetke, Ph.D., R.D.
Department of Food Science and
  Human Nutrition
University of KentuckyMedical Center
Lexington, KY
Email: lgaetke@uky.edu

Michael Hamilton, M.D.
Pennington Biomedical Research
Louisiana State University
Baton Rouge, LA
Email: hamiltma@pbrc.edu

Rachel Hayes-Bohn, B.S.
Division of Epidemiology
University of Minnesota
Minneapolis, MN
Email: haye0154@tc.umn.edu

Daniell B. Hill, M.D.
Department of Internal Medicine
University of Louisville School of
  Medicine
Louisville, KY
Email: daniell.hill@louisville.edu

Kelly K. Hill, M.D.
Department of Psychiatry
University of Kentucky
College of Medicine
Lexington, KY
Email: khill1@uky.edu or
  daniell.hill@louisville.edu

Catherine G.R. Jackson, Ph.D.
Department of Kinesiology
California State University, Fresno
Fresno, CA
Email: cgrjack@csufresno.edu

Gordon Jensen, M.D., Ph.D.
Vanderbilt Center for Human Nutrition
Vanderbilt University Medical Center
Nashville, TN
Email:
  gordon.jensen@mcmail.vanderbilt.edu

Anastasia Z. Kalea, B.S.
Department of Food Science and
  Human Nutrition
University of Maine
Orono, ME
Email:
  Anastasia_Kalea@umit.maine.edu

Nancy King, Ph.D., R.D.
Division of Sciences, Mathematics and
  Health Technology
Department of Biology
Prince George's Community College
Largo, MD
Email: kingnx@pg.cc.md.us

Dorothy Klimis-Zacas, Ph.D.
Department of Food Science and
  Human Nutrition
University of Maine
Orono, ME
Email:
  Dorothy_Klimis@umenfa.maine.edu

Jenny H. Ledikwe, Ph.D.
Department of Nutrition
The Pennsylvania State University
University Park, PA
Email: mvh111@psu.edu

Jennifer C. Lovejoy, Ph.D.
Pennington Biomedical Research
 Center
Louisiana State University
Baton Rouge, LA
Email: lovejoy@pbrc.edu

Priscille G. Massé, Ph.D.
Ecole de Nutrition et d'Etudes
 Familiales
Université de Moncton
Moncton, NB
E-mail: massep@umoncton.ca

Craig J. McClain, M.D.
University of Louisville
School of Medicine
Department of Gastroenterology
Louisville, KY
E-mail: craig.mcclain@louisville.edu

Marion P. McClain, M.S.
University of Louisville
School of Medicine
Department of Gastroenterology
E-mail:
 mpmccl01@gwise.louisville.edu

Susan H. Mitmesser, Ph.D.
Department of Nutritional Science and
 Dietetics
University of Nebraska
Lincoln, NE
Email: susanhazels@hotmail.com

Ellen Parham, Ph.D., R.D., L.D., LCPC
Department of Nutrition, Dietetics and
 Hospitality Administration
Northern Illinois University
School of Family and Consumer
 Nutrition Sciences
De Kalb, IL
Email: eparham@niu.edu

Barbara C. Pence, Ph.D.
Department of Pathology
Texas Technical Health Science Center
Lubbock, TX
Email: barbara.pence@ttuhsc.edu or
 dawn.bender@ttuhsc.edu

Sujatha Rajaram, Ph.D.
Department of Nutrition
School of Public Health
Loma Linda University
Loma Linda, CA
Email: srajaram@sph.llu.edu

Jaime S. Ruud, M.S., R.D.
Sports Nutrition Consultant
Lincoln, NE
Email: jruud1841@aol.com

Joan Sabate, M.D., Dr.Ph.
School of Public Health
Loma Linda University
Loma Linda, CA
Email: jsabate@sph.llu.edu

Kelly S. Scanlon, Ph.D., R.D.
Maternal and Child Nutrition Branch
Division of Nutrition and Physical
 Activity
Center for Disease Control and
 Prevention
Atlanta, GA
Email: kxs5@cdc.gov

Helen Smiciklas-Wright, Ph.D.
Department of Nutrition
Pennsylvania State University
University Park, PA
Email: hsw@psu.edu

Jamie S. Stang, Ph.D., R.D.
University of Minnesota
Division of Epidemiology
Minneapolis, MN
Email: Stang@epi.umn.edu

Mary Story, Ph.D., R.D.
Division of Epidemiology
University of Minnesota
Minneapolis, MN
Email: story@epi.umn.edu

Bonnie Taub-Dix, M.A., R.D., C.D.N.
BTD Nutrition Consultants
Woodmere, NY
Email: eatsmart@aol.com

Caroll C. Tranchant, Ph.D.
Ecole de Nutrition et d'Etudes
  Familiales
Université de Moncton
Moncton, NB
Email: tranch@umoncton.ca

Tammy O. Utset, M.D., M.P.H.
University of Chicago
Section of Rheumatology
Chicago, IL
Email:
  tutset@medicine.bsd.Uchicago.edu

Adrienne A. White, Ph.D., L.D.
Department of Food Science and
  Nutrition
University of Maine
Orono, ME
Email: Awhite@umenfa.maine.edu

Ira Wolinsky, Ph.D.
Department of Health and Human
  Performance
University of Houston (6020)
Houston, TX
Email: Iwolinsky@UH.edu

Contents

1 Women's Health, Nutrition and Research

Nancy B. Cummings

CONTENTS

I. INTRODUCTION

With an increasing focus on women's rights, starting in the 1970s in the United States,[1] came a concern about women's health. The practice of medicine had been primarily a male-dominated one, so many of major concerns for women's health and nutrition appeared to have been neglected. Women were not included in major clinical trials. Research tended to be conducted on male animal models because of stated concerns that the variations in the menstrual cycle would make interpretation of experimental results difficult.

The number of women going into medicine has increased markedly, which affects the interests and consequent emphases on women's health issues. In the 1980s, a number of efforts to evaluate the place of women and their health in research, treatment and prevention of disease were spearheaded by the U.S. government. The Assistant Secretary for Health of the Department of Health and Human Services appointed a Task Force on Women's Health Issues. When the report of this task force was issued, responsibilities for implementation were delegated to the government agencies in accord with their mandates. The National Institutes of Health (NIH) developed an Advisory Committee on Women's Health Issues. The Government Accounting Office conducted a study of the inclusion of women in clinical trials issued in 1990. With NIH support, the Institute of Medicine of the National Academy of Science convened a Planning Panel for Including Women in Clinical Trials. The United States Public Health Service (USPHS) developed an Action Plan for Women's Health. The NIH developed and Congress called for establishment of an Office of Research on Women's Health. The Director of the National Institutes of Health announced The Women's Health Initiative, a clinical trial of major proportions, which would address significant women's health issues involving morbidity and mortality in postmenopausal women: cardiovascular disease, breast and colon cancer and osteoporosis, along with risk factors such as obesity, poor nutrition and tobacco use that affect these diseases. Dramatically, on July 9, 2002 the NIH Women's Health Initiative (WHI) sent letters to the 16,000 women enrolled in the Hormone Replacement Trial (HRT) limb of the study to notify them that the preliminary analysis of the data showed that the risks of this portion of the trial outweighed the benefits.[2,3]

Women's health research has become a major commitment of the NIH, the Public Health Service and, more broadly, the United States Congress. Congress passed the NIH Revitalization Act in 1993 that emphasized its concerns about the inclusion of women in health research. The panoply of initiatives addressing women's health concerns is both welcome and exciting. There is complexity in the interaction between the people and the government, especially when there are broad concerns about such a significant issue as the interface among medicine, nutrition and women's health research.

After the report of the Task Force on Women's Health Issues[4] was published in 1985, the NIH organized an Advisory Committee on Women's Health Issues. This committee assessed NIH's involvement in women's health research and made recommendations for implementation or expansion of this research. Within 2 months of the committee's inception, a recommendation was made that women be included in clinical trials. The NIH and most of its institutes, centers and divisions support a great deal of research devoted to diseases that affect only women, women primarily and both sexes. Women were not included in significant clinical studies for a prolonged period of time for two reasons: (1) concerns about the hazards of experimentation for women during the reproductive years and (2) difficulties in interpretation of variations in results because of hormonal effects. In fact, most laboratory research on mammals was conducted on male rats.

II. INCIDENCE AND PREVALENCE OF DISEASES IN WOMEN

A brief survey of data about incidence and prevalence from the U.S. National Center for Health Statistics provides an objective picture of the diseases and risk factors women encounter. These data address the five leading causes of death and some risk factors. The data come from 29 tables of morbidity and mortality derived from several different National Center for Health Statistics sources.

Of the five leading causes of death for males and females, both white and black, rates of death from heart disease led all other causes for all groups, with malignant neoplasms a close second. Lesser death rates are observed for cerebrovascular disease, accidents, chronic obstructive pulmonary disease, pneumonia and diabetes mellitus, for which rates differ between the groups.

For black women ages 25 to 85+ years, heart disease, cerebrovascular disease and malignant neoplasms are the leading causes of death. Other prominent causes among the top five for specified age groups include accidents and liver disease. In a comparison of death rates for ischemic heart disease and acute myocardial infarction in all females, white females and black females, deaths for black females are low throughout all age groupings. Deaths from heart failure for all females and white females are almost the same.

Breast cancer rates for all women, white women and black women are comparable throughout age groups. The age-adjusted death rates per 100,000 population for those countries for which data are available show a linear correlation with dietary intake of fat in grams/day. As Japanese women aged 50 to 59 years have increased their fat intake in the years between 1955 and 1975, their breast cancer death rate has also increased.[5]

Women have three major risk factors: obesity, cigarette smoking and alcohol. While 25 to 45% of all women aged 20 to 74 are overweight, black women are significantly more overweight in every age group. About 60% of black women from ages 45 to 54 are overweight. More than 25% of women over 18 years of age smoke cigarettes. Five percent more black than white women in the aged 25- to 44-year group are smokers.

The National Center for Health Statistics Health Interview Survey reported that 45% of women said they abstained from alcohol, 35% were light drinkers, 15% were moderate drinkers and 4% were heavier drinkers. Due to reticence to admit drinking habits, percentages for light/moderate/heavy drinking are apt to be artificially low.

III. HEALTH MAINTENANCE: WHO'S "ESSENTIAL ELEMENTS"

In addition to considering disease, it is vitally important to view health maintenance as a potential means for decreasing the occurrence and morbidity of disease. Americans, especially health professionals, tend to focus on treatment of illness rather than on disease prevention. In the United States, as well as worldwide, women usually are responsible not only for their own health care but also for that of their family. Hence, emphasis is on primary health care, of which nutrition and nutrition education should be major components. In the late 1970s, the following eight essential elements for primary health care were delineated by the World Health Organization (WHO):[6]

1. Education concerning primary health problems and methods of preventing and controlling them
2. Promotion of food supply and proper nutrition
3. Adequate supply of safe water and basic sanitation
4. Maternal and child health care, including family planning
5. Immunization against major infectious diseases
6. Prevention and control of locally endemic diseases
7. Appropriate treatment of common diseases and injuries
8. Provision of essential drugs

IV. THE UNITED STATES PUBLIC HEALTH SERVICE

A. TASK FORCE ON WOMEN'S HEALTH ISSUES (1983–1985)

In 1983, the Assistant Secretary for Health charged the Task Force on Women's Health Issues with assessment of problems of women's health in the context of contemporary American women's lives. After identification of women's health issues of contemporary societal significance, these issues were integrated with Public Health Service priorities. Recommendations of the task force[7] were organized as follows:

1. Promotion of a safe, healthful physical and social environment
2. Provision of services for prevention and treatment of disease
3. Research and evaluation
4. Recruitment and training of health care personnel
5. Public education and dissemination of research information
6. Design of guidelines for legislative and regulatory measures

Fifteen subcategories were designated under these six recommendations. Three major recommendations, of which two were for conduct of research and evaluation, were:

1. Expansion of biomedical and behavioral research with emphasis on conditions and diseases unique to or more prevalent in women in all age groups
2 Expansion of research and development for more effective, acceptable and safe contraceptive methods for both men and women
3. Expansion of studies of causes, prevention, improved diagnosis and treatment of debilitating diseases such as breast and other reproductive-system cancers, sexually transmitted diseases, arthritic diseases including systemic lupus erythematosus, osteoporosis, and certain mental disorders

The following other research categories were included under the recommendations for research and evaluation: baseline data, diagnostic methods, nutritional requirements, care settings, psychosocial factors, pharmacokinetics, chronic conditions, safety and efficacy of estrogen and other therapies for treatment of menopausal and post-menopausal symptoms and osteoporosis, mental illnesses, risk factors, socioeconomic issues affecting women and especially older women and the effects of gender differences on longevity. Emphasis throughout the report was on the impact of societal changes on women's lives and the effect on health and disease of human behavior as shaped by cultural and social values.

Following publication of the task force report and its summary, a National Conference on Women's Health (June, 1986)[5] was sponsored by the Public Health Service (PHS) Coordinating Committee on Women's Health Issues and the Food and Drug Administration (FDA). The main topics of this conference were:

- Women's health (a course of action, nutrition, issues in mental health, alcoholism and substance abuse, pregnancy and childbirth)
- Older women's health (contemporary and emerging health issues)[*]
- Taking charge (how to make a difference, cancer, menstrual cycle, osteoporosis)
- Women and their health care providers (a matter of communication).

B. NIH ADVISORY COMMITTEE ON WOMEN'S HEALTH ISSUES

The USPHS Task Force mandate included establishment of groups within each agency to implement the recommendations according to their appropriate responsibilities. The Advisory Committee on Women's Health Issues, established in 1985, has produced two reports on the NIH support of research related to women's health and disease, identified the limited inclusion of women in clinical trials and recommended policies to correct this shortage. These policies were published in the NIH Guide to Grants and Contracts.[8]

C. GOVERNMENT ACCOUNTING OFFICE STUDY

Many congressional hearings focused on various aspects of women's health. Congress also has formed a Women's Health Caucus. Typical of the concerns about exclusion of women from clinical trials was the National Institute of Aging's (NIA) Baltimore Longitudinal Study,[9] which did not add women until 20 years after its inception in 1958.

Three members of Congress requested a study by the Government Accounting Office (GAO) to address the concerns about failure to include women in most of the major clinical trials. Special concerns were voiced about exclusion of women from long-term trials, such as the Multiple Risk Factor Intervention Trial (MRFIT)[10] and the Harvard Physicians Trials,[11] that focused on cardiovascular diseases. The GAO report was presented at a hearing in June, 1990. At this time, NIH reemphasized its policy of commitment to and emphasis on research pertinent to women and their illnesses. This policy requires research grant applicants to justify exclusion or under-representation of women in clinical trials.

---

[*] 1995-women: 59% if over 65 and 72% if over 85 (U.S. Bureau of the Census) U.S. population in estimates by age, sex and race, 1993–2005

In 1991, the Nurses' Health Study had been started to compensate for the exclusion of women in the Harvard Physicians Trials. The study, which included 87,000 registered nurses who were followed for 6 years, was an observational study of women. Women who took 1 to 6 aspirin per week had a 25% lower incidence of heart attacks than those who took no aspirin.

D. OFFICE OF RESEARCH ON WOMEN'S HEALTH

Creation of the Office of Research on Women's Health was announced by the acting director of NIH in September 1990 at an NIH hearing. The director, National Institute of General Medical Sciences, who had chaired the Task Force on Women's Health, was appointed acting director of this new office and immediately organized a public hearing about women's health (June, 1991). Public testimony from 62 organizations interested in both women's health and the need for research on women's health was accepted. Written testimony was received from an additional 30 organizations.

A workshop entitled Opportunities for Research on Women's Health: What We Know and What Needs to Be Done, was held in September, 1991. The first director of the Office of Research on Women's Health was appointed. The workshop set a scientific agenda for women's health across the life span: birth to young adulthood, young adulthood to perimenopausal years, perimenopausal to mature years and mature years. The agenda also included cross-cutting disciplinary areas of science: reproductive biology, early developmental biology, cardiovascular diseases, malignant neoplasms, immune and infectious diseases and aging. The workshop addressed the current status of research on women's health and gaps in research, identified biomedical research opportunities and recommended approaches and options for research on women's health.

With NIH support, an Institute of Medicine Planning Panel for Including Women in Clinical Trials[12] was convened in March 1991. The goal of this panel was to determine whether a study to develop policies allowing orderly progress toward inclusion of women in clinical research was needed, timely, feasible and suited to the capabilities of the Institute of Medicine. The panel included experts in relevant areas of science and clinical trials methodology, as well as persons knowledgeable about ethics, law, Institutional Review Boards, the Food and Drug Administration and concerns of women and minorities. The report of this 2-day meeting distills the major issues of women's health research. Inadequate representation of women in clinical research had been highlighted by the GAO, some segments of the research community, the media and women's advocacy groups, among others. Major studies were cited that failed to include women: the Physicians Health Study,[8] Multiple Risk Factor Intervention Trials,[7] the Baltimore Longitudinal Study[10] and trials of AIDS therapy, as well as other drug trials.[11]

Six reasons for exclusion of women from the study populations of some trials or for the failure to include gender analyses in publications were identified. These were:

1. Cyclical hormonal changes occurring in women.
2. Inclusion of women with men would make the study population less homogeneous.

3. Significant increase in cost of trials if the study population were enlarged enough to allow testing gender hypotheses or subgroup analyses.
4. Increase in cost and accrual burdens of the trial if representative numbers of women were included in the trial for conditions in which the incidence is lower in women than in men.
5. Ethical reasons to avoid exposing existing, or potential, fetuses to harm.
6. Legal and financial consequences if the fetus or child were harmed as a result of the mother's participation in a clinical trial.

The panel voiced a major concern about the need to use funds efficiently by targeting priority areas for data analysis by gender, testing gender-specific hypotheses and identifying research areas critical for women's health.

The relative neglect of concerns pertinent to the health of women in clinical research included:

- A pervasive sense in the research community that women's issues are of secondary importance and that the need for fetal protection overrides other values such as women's autonomous decision making
- The overwhelming proportion of men in biomedical science whose perspectives may be different from those of women
- The longer lifespan of women and their lesser or later representation in some major diseases, leading to the perception that women are healthier and less in need of study
- Attitudinal stances that must be altered if gender equity in research is to be achieved

Three questions raised were:

1. When are gender-specific hypotheses relevant?
2. When is women's reproductive health likely to be affected?
3. What subgroup analyses pertinent to gender are needed?

The panel study concluded that three fundamental questions persist:

1. Are there problems in the use of women in clinical trials and in the design of trials that are retarding the contribution of biomedical science to the health of women?
2. If problems are identified, are they amenable to solution?
3. Are there agencies, institutions or groups whose policies and activities have an effect on the ways in which relevant research is conducted and to whom a study would address its recommendations?

The panel identified other questions related to barriers to inclusion of women in research and proposed two general investigations: (1) examination of the language commonly used to discuss women as research subjects and (2) examination of the political factors that influence science policy. This study viewed its audience as broad and the groups that should provide answers to the questions as numerous.

The Director of NIH gave women's health research a high priority. In her testimony before the U.S. House of Representatives' Committee on Energy and Commerce, Subcommittee on Health and Environment, a month after her (1991) confirmation hearing, The director emphasized her "deep personal commitment to research on women's health ... and that [she was] encouraged that the critical issues related to research on women's health [were] receiving the spirited consideration of Congress." She announced[12] a "far-reaching Women's Health Study that would take a comprehensive approach to the three major sources of morbidity and mortality in women of all socioeconomic strata: cancer, cardiovascular diseases and disorders such as osteoporosis, which leads to fractures and severe musculoskeletal frailty in aging women."

E. USPHS ACTION PLAN FOR WOMEN'S HEALTH

The USPHS Action Plan for Women's Health (September, 1991)provided a sweeping proposal for improvement of women's health through prevention, research, treatment, services, education, information and policy. The plan established substantive goals that reflected the USPHS commitment to maintain and forward the health and quality of life of American women and to implement these goals within the limited resources available. All USPHS agencies and program offices, in line with their respective missions, have established goals and action steps addressing the breadth of women's health issues across age, biology and sociocultural issues. The Office of Women's Health, Office of Assistant Secretary for Health, bears the responsibility for monitoring implementation of the action plan using annual progress reports that identify accomplishments, barriers, modifications and other related USPHS initiatives, as well as utilizing a computerized system to track the status of specific goals and actions by intervention categories, priority health issues and target populations. Each of the 12 agencies and offices is responsible for one to five of the 38 goals.

The Healthy People 2000 (HP 2000) — National Health Promotion and Disease Prevention Objectives[13] campaign has the goal of developing a national strategy to improve significantly the health of the nation over the coming decade by addressing the prevention of major chronic illnesses, injuries and infectious diseases. Among objectives and targets are: physical activity and obesity; tobacco and heart disease; lung cancer; cigarette smoking; breast cancer and mammography; maternal, child health and prenatal care.

Healthy People 2010 (HP 2010) continued in the paths of Healthy People 1999 and HP 2000 with the hope of improving health in the first decade of the 21st century. The HP2010 consortium brought together over 350 organizations and 250 state public health, mental health and substance abuse and environmental agencies and held three national meetings along with teams of experts from federal agencies under the direction of the Secretary of Health and current and past Assistant Secretaries of Health. This consortium operated with the underlying premise that "the health of an individual is almost inseparable from the health of the larger community and that the health of every community in every state and territory determines the overall health status of the Nation." The major task resulted in identification of two overarching goals: (1) increase quality and years of healthy life and (2) eliminate health disparities, as well as focus 28 areas that included 467 objectives. While all aspects of HP2010 are applicable to all Americans, of especial note for women and nutrition are two foci: number 19, Nutrition and Overweight and number 22, Physical Fitness and Activity, along with number 9, Family Planning and number 16, Maternal, Infant and Child Health. Focus number 19 deals with one of the three behavioral patterns (physical activity, overweight and obesity and tobacco use) that influence chronic disease; its goal is to "promote health and reduce chronic disease associated with diet and weight." HP 2010 states that "women[14,15] are generally less active than men at all ages." Obesity[16] is especially prevalent in low-income women and commoner in African American and Mexican American women. Total costs, both medical and lost productivity, attributed to obesity alone, were estimated at $99 billion in 1995.

F. FOOD AND DRUG ADMINISTRATION

Women are recipients of about 70% of prescriptions and frequently hold health responsibilities for children and spouses so that women's understanding and health information are important for the majority of people. Under the HP 2000[13] Initiative of the Department of Health and Human Services, the FDA has the lead responsibility for increasing communications between primary care providers and elderly patients. The implementation of this plan is multifaceted and includes work with private groups such as the National Council on Patient Information and Education, presentations to both professional and consumer organizations and publication of relevant articles. This initiative focuses on a team approach and recognizes the unique position of pharmacists in the health care-provider relationship.

Under the Omnibus Budget Reconciliation Act of 1990,[17] a Drug Use Review Program was mandated that requires states to provide counseling for all Medicaid patients and a drug use review program to assure that prescriptions are appropriate, medically necessary and unlikely to produce adverse effects.

A Campaign on Women and Medicines whose purpose was to ensure safer and more effective use of medicines through improved communication among women and health care providers (e.g., doctors, pharmacists, nurses), was initiated by the FDA. Women use more medicines than do men and serve as "medicine managers" for other family members.[18] The interaction of foods, alcohol and medicines, timing of medications, side effects and adverse actions of medications are important informational aspects of this campaign. While it focuses on all women's concerns, it is directed especially toward concerns of pregnant and lactating women, menopausal women and special populations such as minorities and the elderly. The National Council on Patient Information and Education, which cooperates with the FDA in its educational mission, has published information[15] about women and medicines, counseling women about medicines and diseases and conditions common to women.

V. OFFICE OF RESEARCH ON WOMEN'S HEALTH

The Office of Research on Women's Health (ORWH) is responsible for assuring that research conducted and supported by NIH adequately addresses issues regarding women's health and that there is appropriate participation of women in clinical research, especially in clinical trials. The three main ORWH goals are:

1. To strengthen and enhance NIH efforts to improve prevention, diagnosis and treatment of illness in women
2. To ensure that research conducted and supported by the NIH addresses issues regarding women's health appropriately
3. To ensure appropriate participation of women in clinical studies

The ORWH also has the charge to set the NIH research agenda for women's health and provide the relevant NIH tracking system, monitor recruitment, retention, promotion and follow-up of women in science and of women in biomedical research, involve the scientific community and include medical, legal and ethical issues.

The codification of the requirement to include women in clinical trials has been announced in the NIH Guide to Grants and Contracts. It specifies that:[16]

- Adequate numbers of women proportional to their prevalence of the condition under study shall be included in clinical studies.
- Failure to include an adequate number of women without compelling justification will be considered to affect the investigator's ability to answer the scientific question being posed.
- Any justification for excluding women in such studies will be evaluated by the peer review group and factored into the relative level of merit given the proposal.
- No application or proposal for any application excluding women will be approved for funding unless compelling justification has been provided.

After Congress mandated the creation of the ORWH, it replaced the Advisory Committee of Women's Health Issues with the Coordinating Committee on Women's Health Activities. The activities of ORWH in the past year have expanded markedly. Beginning in 1991, the ORWH provided administrative supplements to ongoing clinical studies that enhanced the number of women or provided for inclusion of women in these studies. After its inception, 20 supplemental grants totaling over $800,000 were awarded and more than half of the principal investigators on these grants in 1991 were women.

The ORWH produced an Agenda for Research on Women's Health in the 21st Century, a six-volume report resulting from four scientific meetings and public hearings convened to establish this agenda.

A. WOMEN'S HEALTH INITIATIVE

The WHI addresses the three leading causes of death and disability among American women over 45 years of age: cardiovascular diseases, cancer and osteoporosis.

The three study components are epidemiological surveillance, a clinical trial and a community prevention trial. The Clinical Trial's Coordinating Center in Seattle was selected for the WHI. The 16 Vanguard Centers were chosen and another 30 centers followed within a year. The NIH Women's Health Initiative provides an integrated multidisciplinary approach to the prevention of some of the most common causes of disability, mortality and death in postmenopausal women. Clinical trials, observational studies and community trials will be used. These address evaluation of benefit and risk in prevention as well as adverse effects. There is a paucity of research on conditions and treatments unique to or of greater concern for women. No preventive clinical trials have assessed the effect of dietary change on prevention of breast and colon cancer or of coronary heart disease using these diseases as endpoints. Clinical trials of hormone replacement therapy using coronary heart disease, stroke and osteoporosis as endpoints had been lacking. There is a paucity of longitudinal data on predictors and markers of disease development in women, yet a considerable gap exists between the established value of healthy behavior and adoption of these behaviors, especially among minorities and the medically underserved.

A WHI Oversight Committee is monitoring the progress of the entire program. Three important considerations for the WHI are that proposed studies build on other studies and do not supplant or compete with them. Measurements, especially clinical outcomes, will be comparable to those in similar studies, and opportunities exist for ancillary studies that could use the unique opportunity provided by this large cohort of women.

The Clinical Trials, in three integrated trials, are evaluating hormone replacement therapy (HRT), calcium and vitamin D and dietary modification of fat and fiber. Harbingers of the July9, 2002 announcement discontinuing the Hormone Replacement Trial were evident in the preliminary 2000 data from NIH that indicated doubts that hormones prevent heart disease and the American Heart Association advice that women with heart disease should not start HRT. The recent NIH/WHI announcement reported that while the risk (0.4%) for an individual woman might appear low, if six million women were on HRT, 25,000 cases of life-threatening side effects, e.g., breast cancer, heart attacks, strokes and blood clots would occur. The incidence of side effects increases with the length of time on treatment. The *New York Times* reporter noted, as "head of NIH (Dr. Healy) was able to see the neglect of gender in medical research when others in her position had not, and she was motivated to fix it."

The Community Trials will implement known interventions in over 30,000 residents. Postmenopausal women, aged 50 to 79, will be invited to participate in either the clinical trial or the observational study. The clinical trial is a large randomized control trial of women that involves 45 clinics, one coordinating center, two to three central laboratories and a drug distribution center.

It is anticipated that the benefit of the WHI will exceed the risks. The clinical outcomes expected on HRT were a decrease in coronary heart disease and in fractures, which will be greater than the possible increase in breast and endometrial cancers. Dietary modification will decrease breast and colorectal cancer, diabetes and coronary heart disease. The potential of calcium and vitamin D to decrease fractures and colorectal cancer is anticipated to be greater than that to increase the incidence of renal calculi. Total mortality, quality of life and side effects will be evaluated.

B. COMMUNITY RANDOMIZED TRIAL

The purpose of the Community Randomized Trial is to evaluate strategies to achieve healthful behaviors, including improved diet, nutritional supplementation, smoking prevention and cessation, increased physical activity and early disease detection for women of all races, ethnic groups and socioeconomic strata. Selection for the Community Randomized Trial will be from geopolitical regions of 30,000 or more adult residents of both sexes where the intervention must be able to reach an inclusive sample of the population. At least 20% of the Community Randomized Trial participants will be minority or "underserved" persons. The observational studies will provide estimates of risk factors and disease prevalence and incidence for comparison with the clinical trial cohort, as well as for women of those age cohorts in general. Community Randomized Trial evaluation strategies include cross-sectional samples, an estimated 500 women per sample per community, comparison of the first and last samples and use of a middle sample for intervention corrections. The approach to the communities will involve community participation established or modified, or new community channels and potential channels including health care providers, worksites and organizations, public education, food services and media.

There is an acute awareness of the need to address the issue of minority representation, since health maintenance and disease prevention are particularly important in these groups, which have a statistically higher morbidity and mortality. It is recognized that some of this morbidity and mortality may be related to the fact that in 1993 some 40.9 million nonelderly Americans had no health coverage[17] and a similar number have inadequate coverage. Further, psychosocial and behavioral aspects will be assessed since they are potential predictors of both compliance and future disease and disability.

VI. SUMMARY

There is continued excitement and vibrancy in the area of women's health. Not only is it an idea whose time has come, but it is a concept of vital importance to more than half of the American population and to the rest of the population who need and are dependent on women. Of major significance is the recognition of the importance of prevention and of health maintenance, both modalities for which good nutrition is of major importance.

Under the leadership of the USPHS and with the recommendations included in its action plan, all of its agencies and offices are moving to encourage interventions that include prevention, research, treatment and services, education, information and policy.

The accomplishments in women's health and in relevant research that we will see in the next decades will be dramatic. The anticipated cooperative efforts across health care disciplines and among the many organizations concerned with women's health give promise of great advances.

REFERENCES

1. Cummings, M.C., Jr. and D. Wise, *Democracy Under Pressure,* 7th ed., 1993, Fort Worth, TX, Thomson/Wadsworth, 126, 136–142.
2. Hormone replacement study: A shock to the medical system, G. Kolata and M. Petersen, *NYTimes*, A1, 7/10/02.
3. Study is halted over rise in cancer risk: Hormone replacement is called into doubt, G. Kolata, *NYTimes*, A1, 7/9/02.
4. Women's Health, Report of the Public Health Service Task Force on Women's Health Issues, Volume I, 100: 73–106, Washington, D.C., U.S. Government Printing Office, 461–1950: 37708, Washington, D.C., 1985.
5. Personal Communication, National Cancer Institute.
6. Mahler, H., Blueprint for Health for All. *WHO Chron.* 31: 491–498, 1980.
7. Women's Health, *J. U.S. Public Health Service*, Supplement to July–August Issue, 1986. PHS 86-50193 (USPHS 324-990), DHHS, Washington, D.C.
8. NIH Guide to Grants & Contracts, 1986: 86-50193(USPHS 324-990), 1987, 1988, 1991 (20:102).
9. Hallfrisch, J., D. Muller, D. Drinkwater, J. Tobin and R. Andres, Continuing diet trends in men: The Baltimore Longitudinal Study of Aging (1961–1987), *J. Geront.* 45: M186–191.
10. Multiple risk factor intervention trial: Risk factor changes and mortality results, *JAMA* 248: 1465–1477, 1982.
11. Steering Committee of the Physicians' Health Study Research Group, Final Report of the Aspirin Component of the Ongoing Physicians' Health Study, *N Eng J Med* 321: 129–135, 1989.
12. Institute of Medicine, Planning panel for Including Women in Clinical Trials, 1991 (March), Washington, D.C.
13. Healthy People 2000, National Health Promotion and Disease Prevention Objectives, U.S. Department of Health and Human Services, DHHS Publication No. (PHS) 91-50213, USA Government Printing Office, Washington, D.C.
14. NCHS, Healthy People 2000 Review, 1998–99, 1999, Hyattsville, MD, DHHS.
15. NCHS, Health, United States, 1999, Hyattsville, MD, DHHS.
16. NCHS, Healthy People 2000 Review, 1998–1999, Hyattsville, MD, HHS.
17. NIH, Statistics Related to Overweight and Obesity, 86-50193 (USPHS 324-990), DHHS, Washington, D.C.; Obesity, 1996, Bethesda, MD, National Institute of Diabetes and Digestive and Kidney Diseases.
18. Public Law (P.L.) 101–508, Paragraph 4401 (g), Omnibus Reconciliation Act of 1990.
19. Talk about Prescriptions Month, October 1991, pp.4–6.

2 Major Diet-Related Risk Factors for Women*

Susan H. Mitmesser and Timothy P. Carr

CONTENTS

I. INTRODUCTION

Women and men share many of the same nutritional concerns; however, women are more predisposed to certain diseases than men simply due to physiological differences. While both genders possess some of the same concerns regarding cancers (esophageal, stomach, colon, lung, pancreatic, bladder), heart disease and Alzhe-

---

* Adapted and expanded from the first edition (1996) chapter, written by the late Carolyn K. Clifford.

imer's disease, other diseases such as breast cancer, anemia and osteoporosis are greater concerns for women. Nutritional concerns for women may be magnified because, in their lifespan, women go through several major hormonal changes, such as menarche, pregnancy, lactation and menopause. For example, nutritional needs during pregnancy and lactation greatly increase for most of the nutrients, while the risk of osteoporosis tends to parallel the hormonal changes that occur throughout the lifespan.

Health statistics related to women were not recorded in any regular or standardized manner prior to the 20th century. Discussions of women's health centered almost exclusively on childbearing capabilities and complications. Many of these early attitudes have not been easily abandoned. Recently, however, nutrition concerns for women have taken a front seat in many research arenas because women have demanded recognition of the need for and action toward equal status for female health considerations and biomedical research. Because women are now breadwinners as well as child-bearers, women's nutritional well being has begun to attract attention, rightfully so.

II. SOCIETY'S IMPACT ON NUTRITION

Extensive changes in eating patterns, food choices and methods of food preparation have occurred over the last 50 years. Women also now contribute a significant number to the work force. Where women once traditionally did not extend their work outside the home, more than half of the U.S. work force is now female. This has led to decreased amount of time spent on food preparation in the home as well as an increased number of people dining out; hence, the demand for convenience and "fast" foods has increased.[1] The food industry has shifted its focus to convenient food items that require little preparation, for instance, ready-to-serve bagged salad, frozen entrees and deli preparations. Convenient foods such as these can be found in many aspects of the food industry. Additionally, fast-food chains have become a booming industry. The demand for quick, inexpensive food has the food industry seeking new means to satisfy consumers. Fast food, for the most part, is calorically dense and the portion sizes are well over the recommended size. This is one contributor to the increased incidence of obesity observed in the United States. In fact, Popkin has observed a shift from a whole-grain, unprocessed diet including heavy physical activity to a diet low in fiber, high in fat and very little physical activity. These findings are consistent with the rapid changes in child and adult obesity.[2]

III. NUTRITION CONSIDERATIONS FOR WOMEN

A normal diet should "… supply all essential nutrients in adequate amounts; supply a physiologic quantity of bulk and fluids, be easily digestible and confer a feeling of satiety; it should be readily available from the standpoint of both supply and cost; it should live up to the gustatory expectations of the prospective consumer and conform to the gastronomic customs of the group."[3] Consuming a variety of foods will supply the body with essential nutrients needed to maintain proper growth and development throughout the course of a lifetime. However, nutritional requirements are different depending on age, gender, pregnancy or lactation. For example, women have different requirements than men for calcium and iron depending on menarche, menopause, pregnancy or lactation.[4,5] All four of these stages in a female's life cycle are accompanied by physiological, psychological and biochemical changes that require an alteration in the daily intake of nutrients.[4] For example, a decrease in circulating estrogen after menopause can lead to an increased rate of bone loss and affect overall calcium balance.[5]

Dietary factors are associated with five of the 10 leading causes of death for both men and women: coronary heart disease, cancer, stroke, non-insulin-dependent diabetes mellitus and atherosclerosis.[6] However, women may be more at risk for some of these diseases or may be affected differently from men.[7] Therefore, more women than men will face the health problems that accompany advanced age.

IV. DIET–DISEASE RELATIONSHIPS

Extensive scientific evidence highlights the associations between foods or eating patterns and health maintenance or chronic disease. Of the $666 billion in national health care costs, 30% are related to an inappropriate diet.[6] Of the many disease states that cause metabolic, physiologic and psychologic trauma to women, five have a scientific-based connection to the diet: anemia, osteoporosis, heart disease, non-insulin-dependent diabetes mellitus and some types of cancer.

A. ANEMIA

The word "anemia" basically refers to a deficiency of whole blood volume or of the number or quality of the red blood cells. The three primary types of anemia are: iron deficiency, pernicious and macrocytic anemia. All three types are caused by a deficiency in a vitamin or mineral. Based on the definition of anemia, a deficiency in a vitamin or mineral can cause a decline in whole blood volume.

1. Iron Deficiency Anemia

Iron deficiency anemia is the most common type of anemia. Most of the iron in the body is a component of hemoglobin and myoglobin, which help carry or hold oxygen. In the case of anemia, the red blood cells contain too little hemoglobin; therefore, they deliver too little oxygen to the tissues. Symptoms of this type of anemia consist of fatigue, apathy and the tendency to feel cold. The current iron recommendation for women is 15 mg/day (10 mg/day if >50 y).[8] According to the latest National Health and Nutrition Examination Surveys (NHANES) study, the average American woman consumes 11mg/day of iron daily, which is well below the recommendation. Frith-Terhune and colleagues found that Mexican-American women are more prone to iron deficiency anemia than nonHispanic white women, 6.2% versus 2.3%, respectively.[9]

2. Pernicious Anemia

Pernicious anemia is caused by vitamin B_{12} deficiency or malabsorption. This anemia is characterized by large, immature red blood cells, which could lead to damage of the nervous system. This type of anemia is many times undetected by blood tests. Because vitamin B_{12} is found only in animal tissues, vegetarians are susceptible to pernicious anemia. The recommendation for vitamin B_{12} is 1.8 µg/day for females9 to 13 y and 2.4 µg/day for women >14 y.[8] During pregnancy and lactation, the recommended intake of vitamin B_{12} is 2.6 µg/day and 2.8 µg/day, respectively.

3. Macrocytic Anemia

Macrocytic anemia is caused by a deficiency in folate. Folate is required for the manufacturing of new cells. A deficiency could be the result of inadequate intake, malabsorption, increased excretion or an increased metabolic need. Folate works closely with vitamin B_{12}, making a diagnosis between pernicious and macrocytic anemia a difficult task. Many times, a deficiency in one of these vitamins is masked by the other, leading to a mistake in treatment. The current folate recommendation for females 9 to 13 y and >14 y is 300 µg/day and 400 µg/day, respectively. During pregnancy and lactation, the recommendation is increased to 600 µg/day and 500 µg/day.[8]

B. Osteoporosis

Osteoporosis is defined as a condition in which the bone is excessively fragile. Often termed as the "silent epidemic," osteoporosis is believed to affect half of women in the U.S. over the age of 50 years. After menopause, a woman increases her chance of sustaining a vertebral fracture by 32%, a hip fracture by 16% and a wrist fracture by 15%.[10] Many conditions, such as celiac disease, hormone insensitivity syndromes, increased body mass and vitamin metabolism and mutations in type I collagen, contribute to a predisposition to osteoporosis.[11]

The prevention of osteoporosis involves diet and physical activity. Weight-bearing activities at all stages of life have been shown to reduce the onset of bone mineral loss. Nutritionally speaking, calcium, vitamin D, magnesium, copper, zinc and vitamin C are the primary dietary influences on bone loss.

The average calcium intake of women >20 y is 500 mg/day, compared with the recommendation of 1,300 mg/day for 9 to 18 y, 1,000 mg/day for 19 to 50 y and 1,200 mg/day for >51 y.[8,12] In the 5 years following menopause, an intake of 800 mg/day of calcium is not able to inhibit the already rapid loss of skeletal mass.[13] Additionally, poor vitamin D intake can contribute to increased bone loss in the >50 age group. Micronutrients, such as zinc and copper, have recently been recognized as important determinants of bone mass.[14] In addition to zinc and copper, an insufficient dietary supply of magnesium can result in a reduction of bone growth in children.[14] Similarly, vitamin C is required for the synthesis of type I collagen, the main component of bone. Vitamin C allows the formation of collagen cross-links to occur. Therefore, a vitamin C deficiency could contribute to the development of osteoporosis.

Circulating levels of estrogen in the female body assist in skeletal stability. Once naturally occurring hormone levels decrease after menopause, the risk of osteoporosis increases dramatically. The mechanism of estrogen is also influenced by dietary components such as protein, fat, carbohydrate and fiber. A diet high in protein and fat and low in carbohydrate and fiber will lead to higher plasma levels of biologically active sex hormones and lower sex hormone-binding globulin. The mechanism by which low estrogen levels cause a decrease in bone formation does not require a prior reduction in bone resorption.[13] Interestingly enough, isoflavones have been investigated to simulate the effect of estrogen in the body. According to Cassidy, 60 g of textured soy protein can mimic the functions of circulating estrogen in the body and decrease the effects of menopausal bone resorption.[15] Isoflavones offer promise as an alternative to hormone replacement therapy (HRT) for women during menopause.

C. HEART DISEASE

Cardiovascular disease refers to any disease of the heart and circulatory system. Coronary heart disease (CHD), one form of cardiovascular disease, is a chronic disease that accounts for about 20% of all deaths in the United States,[16] where 58 million Americans have one or more forms of cardiovascular disease. Cardiovascular disease is the leading cause of death in American women today. One in eight women 45 years and older has had a myocardial infarction or stroke. By the age of 40 to 45 years, the formation of atherosclerotic lesions in the intimal region of the artery have increased. Unlike men, women of all ages have greater lesion involvement in the aorta than in the carotid or coronary arteries.[17] The incidence of CHD begins to rise around menopause and then rapidly increases after age 65. In the past, CHD in women has been taken less seriously and treated less aggressively than in men. Compared with men, women are more likely to have a recurrent heart attack and die from the disease during the recovery period.[16] Due to the lack of invasiveness in the diagnoses and treatment of women with CHD, it is critical to promote any and all heart disease prevention techniques necessary for optimal health for women, as well as for men.

Many risk factors, including sedentary lifestyle, non-insulin-dependent diabetes mellitus, high blood pressure, obesity, elevated serum cholesterol and low fiber intake, are associated with CHD. The primary dietary risk factors involved in the cause or prevention of this disease include dietary antioxidants, dietary fiber and fat (amount and type of fat).[18,19]

1. Antioxidant Status

Extensive research has explored the relationship between oxidative damage and CHD. The oxidation of low-density lipoproteins (LDL) in the artery wall is postulated to play an important role in the development of atherosclerotic lesions. It is hypothesized that dietary antioxidants have the ability to protect LDL from oxidation and, therefore, prevent the onset of atherosclerosis. Examples of antioxidants include vitamins C, A (or β-carotene) and E. The current Dietary Reference Intakes (DRI) for these vitamins are: 60 mg vitamin C for women >15 years of age and 50 mg for women <14 years old, 800 RE vitamin A for women of all ages and 8 mg vitamin E for women of all ages.[8] Women reportedly consumed 147% and 114% of the DRI for vitamins C and A.[20] According to the NHANES III survey, the median daily intake for vitamin E was 6.3 mg, which is almost 2 mg less than the recommendation. Similarly, the Continuing Survey of Food Intake by Individuals reported that women >20 y consumed only 87% of the DRI for vitamin E.[20]

2.   Dietary Fiber

Dietary fiber, which is a constituent of dietary carbohydrate, serves many functions in the body. Fiber has the ability to affect circulating blood glucose, reduce the incidence of constipation and diverticulosis and affect serum lipids.[18,21,22] Fiber has the ability to bind bile acids in the intestine, which stimulates the liver to increase production of bile acids.[18] Bile acids and cholesterol form mixed micelles, which are important in the solubilization of ingested fats. Specifically, bile is the vehicle for the excretion of cholesterol. The National Cancer Institute's recommendation for dietary fiber is 20 to 30 g/day.[23] Unfortunately, women are not meeting the National Cancer Institute's recommendation, with an average intake of 12 g/day.[24]

3.   Fat

The link between fat intake and CHD in normal individuals has been extensively studied. One of the primary problems with an increased fat consumption is that it leads to obesity. More than half of white women over age 50 and 60% of black and Mexican women are overweight (BMI >27.3).[25] The incidence of overweight appears to be highest in younger women. Thirty-seven percent of U.S. women age 25 to 40 y gained 5 to 15% of their body weight over a 10-year period.[26] Not only is the addition of body fat critical in the development of CHD, distribution of the added fat is also predictive of risk. Abdominal obesity, which is commonly observed in postmenopausal women, is associated with a worsening lipoprotein profile and glucose metabolism.[27] According to Haarbo and colleagues,[28] HRT (combined estrogen/progesterone) can prevent abdominal obesity in postmenopausal women.

The amount and type of fat in the diet can be an indicator of CHD risk. It has long been known that saturated fat intake can increase blood cholesterol concentration, which is a well-established risk factor for CHD.[19,29] The consumption of *trans* fatty acids has been suggested as a reason for the rise in LDL and the drop in high density lipoprotein (HDL).[30] To address the "fat" issue, the American Heart Association recommends <30% of total calories come from fat and <10% from saturated fat.[5] Based on the recommended LDL levels, 27% of all women and 50% of women 55 to 74 y need diet intervention for hypercholesterolemia.[31] Additionally, women with higher triglyceride levels (>400 mg/dL) in combination with low HDL (<50 mg/dL) have a higher rate of developing cardiovascular disease, according to the Framingham study.[19] The extent to which a high fat diet will exacerbate the risk in women with normal lipid levels is uncertain.

D. Non-Insulin-Dependent Diabetes Mellitus

Characterized by elevated blood glucose concentrations, non-insulin-dependent diabetes mellitus (Type 2 diabetes) can lead to kidney failure, blindness, nerve degeneration and circulatory disorders.[21] Ninety percent of all diabetes cases are attributed to Type 2 diabetes. The mechanism responsible for elevated glucose in Type 2 diabetes is an insensitivity to insulin by the cells, which are no longer able to bring insulin inside the cell.[21] A decreased insulin production may also occur. Factors that influence Type 2 diabetes include lack of physical activity, aging and obesity. Dietary changes, such as increasing dietary fiber and decreasing dietary fat, have proven to be effective means of improving insulin sensitivity and blood glucose concentrations.[21,22]

E. Cancer

The top five cancers causing death among women are lung, colon, breast, ovarian and uterine. Women's dietary concerns with regard to the development of cancer may differ from men's. Moreover, one-third of all human cancers can be directly linked to diet.[29]While dietary fat is considered to be one of the main risk factors in some cancers (breast and colon), it is not the only dietary component to consider.

1. Lung

Lung cancer is the leading cause of cancer death among U.S. women and men. Research has proven that lung cancer is directly correlated to cigarette smoking. However, lung cancer is also associated with diet. In a study of 282 female lung cancer victims, a significant association was observed between lung cancer risk and the consumption of red meat and poultry, while an inverse association was observed with the intake of vegetables. Additionally, coffee consumption was inversely association with lung cancer risk.[32] Smoking still remains the primary risk factor involved in the development of lung cancer; however, dietary influences may contribute.

2. Breast

Breast cancer is the second leading cause of cancer death among females in the United States and other developed countries.[33] Certain dietary components, including alcohol, red meat, sugar and fat, have been widely implemented as risks for developing breast cancer.[34–38] Dietary components that tend to decrease breast cancer risk include fruit and vegetables, low-fat dairy products, fish and tea. [36–41]

Dietary fat intake has been linked to an increase in breast cancer risk, although the type and amount of fat in the diet remains a controversial issue. A strong association with breast cancer was found with fatty foods such as fried meat.[42] The mean fat intake for women >20 y is 60.2 g/day and the mean calorie intake for the same group of women is 1556 Kcal/day. This calculates to an average of 34% of total energy coming from fat.[20] Recall that the current recommendation of the American Heart Association is less than 30% of total calories from fat. Additionally, a body mass index (BMI) greater than 28 to 30 was associated with an increased risk for breast cancer, according to epidemiological studies.[43]

According to the World Cancer Research Fund and the American Institute for Cancer Research, fiber and carotenoids show potential for decreasing breast cancer risk.[44] Additionally, carrots, spinach and supplements containing vitamin A show modest protective effects against breast cancer.[45] Phytoestrogens, such as isoflavonoids and lignans, have begun to gain considerable attention regarding their anticarcinogenic affects. The role of phytochemicals in breast cancer development is a new and important area of research that has yet to be fully explored.

3. Colon

Colon cancer is the third leading cause of cancer death in the United States. A connection between high consumption of meat, protein and fat, in combination with a low consumption of fiber, increases the risk for colon cancer.[46] Additionally, a high intake of triacylglycerol and alcohol has been implicated in colon cancer.[47] Consumption of red meat and cured meats containing nitrates can lead to the formation of nitroso compounds, which are associated with an increased risk of colorectal cancer.[48] On the other hand, vegetables, dietary fiber and physical activity have been linked to a reduction in the risk of colon cancer.[49] Cruciferous vegetables may be especially effective.[44,50]

4. Ovary

Ovarian cancer is the fourth leading cause of cancer death among U.S. women. Approximately 24,000 new cases of ovarian cancer are documented each year.[51] Unfortunately, most tumors are advanced at the time of diagnosis due to the lack of early warning signs or diagnostic screening.[51] Epidemiological studies support a relationship between saturated fat consumption and ovarian cancer.[52–54] Mono- and polyunsaturated fats have displayed an inverse association with the disease.[52]

V. DIETARY REFERENCE INTAKES

Numerous health organizations have actively endorsed good nutrition as an integral part of healthy development and maintenance of the body. In 1943, The Food and Nutrition Board of the National Research Council developed the recommended dietary allowances (RDAs). The RDAs represent safe and adequate intakes of energy and nutrients designed for the maintenance of good nutrition for healthy people in the United States.[55] The last edition of the RDAs, published in 1989, represented an estimated standard for protein, 11 vitamins and 7 minerals, which was meant to meet the known nutritional needs for males and females of different ages.[55] Recently, experts in the field of nutrition have argued that the RDAs should also reflect the role of nutrients in reducing the risk of chronic diseases. This discussion has led to the current set of dietary standards, called Dietary Reference Intakes (DRIs). All DRI values, like the RDAs, are specific for age and gender, which reflect differences in nutrient requirements. The DRIs are usually higher for men than women, with the exception of during pregnancy and lactation. The primary difference from the RDAs is that the DRIs now take into account research that has shown safe and effective reduction in disease risk, such as cancer and CHD.

The difficulty that arises is the ability to translate the DRIs into a practical eating pattern that remains satisfying and enjoyable to individuals and meets all nutritional needs at the same time. To address this dilemma, many federal agencies and private health organizations have developed dietary recommendations and guidelines for individuals. The U.S. Department of Agriculture (USDA) and U.S. Department of Health and Human Services established one such set of guidelines, the Dietary Guidelines for Americans.[20,56] The USDA set forth these guidelines as a basis for all Americans to follow to promote a healthy lifestyle. These guidelines are:

- Aim for a healthy weight.
- Be physically active each day.
- Let the pyramid guide your food choices.
- Choose a variety of grains daily.
- Choose a variety of fruits and vegetables daily.
- Keep food safe to eat.
- Choose a diet that is low in saturated fat and cholesterol and moderate in total fat.
- Choose beverages and foods to moderate your intake of sugar.
- Choose and prepare foods with less salt.
- If you drink alcoholic beverages, do so in moderation.[20,56]

VI. WOMEN'S HEALTH AS A RESEARCH FOCUS

Policies to improve health, in underdeveloped countries as well as developed, require evaluation and integration of nutrition needs with regard to economic growth and development, agriculture and food production, processing, marketing, health care and education, changing lifestyles and food choices. An increase in research support is needed to achieve national health goals with an emphasis on better overall nutrition for women. Furthermore, a decrease in the occurrence and duration of chronic diseases will reduce the cost of health care and allow the resources to benefit a country as a whole.[6]

Most biomedical knowledge about the causes, expression and treatment of diseases such as CHD and cancer is derived from studies performed on men and subsequently applied to women, with the supposition that there are no differences between men and women. To the contrary, there are many differences — body mass, body composition, hormone levels, blood volume and basic physiology. In response to the need for more direct research for women, the Office of Research on Women's Health (ORWH) was established at the National Institutes of Health (NIH) in 1990.[4] The primary goal of the ORWH was to strengthen and enhance research related to diseases, disorders and conditions that affect women. Additionally, the ORWH was to ensure that women were appropriately represented in biomedical and biobehavorial research studies.

In 1993, the NIH Revitalization Act added new policies for the inclusion of women and minorities in clinical research funded by the NIH.[57] Following the NIH footsteps, other studies around the world began to focus on women's health issues. Within the last 10 years, many epidemiology studies have taken this new focus. The

Women's Health Study is currently monitoring the effects of vitamin E and aspirin on the development of cardiovascular disease and cancer.[58] Similarly, the New York Women's Health Study is investigating sex hormones, diet and breast cancer development.[59]The Iowa Women's Health Study is monitoring women 55 to 69 years of age currently on HRT and the incidence of cancer.[60] Some epidemiology studies are now focusing on females of different age groups. For example, the Penn State Young Women's Health Study is monitoring the dietary patterns of 12 to 18-y girls in the U.S.[61] Additionally, the Women's Health and Aging Study is conducting an investigation on disabled women 65 y and older in the Balmier, Maryland area.[62] It is important to note that countries other than the U.S. are also investigating women's health issues. The European Community Multicentre Study on Antioxidants, Myocardial Infarction and Cancer of the Breast (EURAMIC) investigated fruit, vegetable and folate intake in connection with breast cancer risk.[63] Similarly, the UK Women's Cohort Study focused on the eating patterns of women 35 to 69 y, thus identifying "healthy" and "unhealthy" diets among women.[64]

VIII. SUMMARY

The interrelationships among nutrition, health promotion and disease prevention are evident throughout an individual's lifespan. Clearly, women have specific nutritional needs and concerns that are different from those of men. The chapters in this volume demonstrate that nutritional status is an integral part of a woman's overall health status at every age and contributes to many aspects of her life. The roles of diet and nutrition in major life events such as menarche, contraception, pregnancy, lactation, menopause and aging, as well as chronic diseases including cardiovascular diseases, cancer, non-insulin-dependent diabetes mellitus and osteoporosis, are discussed. Nutrition is also explored as a component of self-image, body weight, eating disorders and physical fitness. Though an optimal diet is difficult to define for every individual, more concerted strategies are needed to assist women in modifying their eating habits to achieve dietary patterns that are consistent with the dietary guidelines for improving health and have the potential for reducing the morbidity and mortality of several diet-related chronic diseases. The public health implications are not limited to women alone, but will likely improve the health of their families and the nation.

REFERENCES

1. Smith, R.E., Food demands of the emerging consumer: The role of modern food technology in meeting that challenge, *Am J Clin Nutr,* 58 (suppl.), 307S, 1993.
2. Popkin, B.M., The nutrition transition and obesity in the developing world, *J Nutr,* 131, 871, 2001.
3. Burton, B.T., *Human Nutrition,* a Blakiston Publication, The McGraw-Hill Companies, New York, 153, 1976.
4. U.S. Department of Health and Human Services, The Surgeon General's Report on Nutrition and Health, NIH Publ. No. 88-50210, Public Health Service, U.S. Government Printing Office, Washington, D.C., 539, 1988.

5. National Academy of Sciences, National Research Council, Commission on Life Sciences, Food and Nutrition Board, Diet and Health, Implications for Reducing Chronic Disease Risk, National Academy Press, Washington, D.C., 615, 1989.

6. Bidlack, W.R., Interrelationships of food, nutrition, diet and health: The national association of state universities and land grant colleges white paper, *J Am Coll Nutr*, 15, 422, 1996.

7. Pinn, V.W., Women's health issues: a U.S. perspective, *Can J Obst Gynecol Women's Hlth Care*, 6, 671, 1994.

8. Barr, S.I., Murphy, S.P. and Poos, M.I. Interpreting and using the dietary references intakes in dietary assessment of individuals and groups, *J Am Diet Assoc*, 102, 780, 2002.

9. Frith-Terhune, A.L., Cogswell, M.E., Khan, L.K., Will, J.C. and Ramakrishnan, U., Iron deficiency anemia: Higher prevalence in Mexican American than in nonHispanic white females in the third National Health and Nutrition Examination Survey, 188–1994, *Am J Clin Nutr*, 72, 963, 2000.

10. Christensen, R.H., Biochemical marker of bone metabolism: An overview, *Clin Biochem*, 30, 573, 1997.

11. Mora, S., Barera, G., Beccio, S., Proverbio, M.C., Weber, G., Bianchi, C. and Chiumello, G., Bone density and the bone metabolism are normal after long-term gluten-free diet in young celiac patients, *Am J Gastroenter*, 94, 398, 1999.

12. Carroll, M.D., Abraham, S. and Dresser, C.M., Dietary intake source data: US, 1979-80. Washington, D.C.: Government Printing Office, Vital and Health Statistics Serv, 11-NO231, DHHS, Publication no. 83-PHS, 1983.

13. Ogawa, S., Hosoi, T., Shiraki, M., Orimo, H., Emi, M., Muramatsu, M., Ouchi, Y. and Inoue, S., Association of estrogen receptor beta gene polymorphism with bone mineral density, *Biochem Biophys Res Commun*, 269, 537, 2000.

14. Saltman, P. and Strause, L., The role of trace minerals in osteoporosis, *J Am Coll Nutr*,11, 599, 1992.

15. Cassidy, A., Bingham, S. and Setchell, K.D.R., Biological effect of isoflavones present in soy in premenopausal women: Implications for the prevention of breast cancer, *Am J Clin Nutr*, 60, 333, 1994.

16. Massachusetts Medical Society, Coronary heart disease incidence, by sex — United States, 1971–1987, *MMWR*, 41, 526, 1992.

17. Blankenhorn, D.H. and Hodis, H.H., Arterial imagery and atherosclerosis reversal, *Arterioscler Thromb*, 14, 177, 1994.

18. Schneeman, B.O. and Tietyen, J., Dietary Fiber, In: *Modern Nutrition in Health and Disease*, Shils, M.E., Olson, J.A., Shike, M., Eds., 8th ed., Philadelphia, PA, Lea & Febiger, 89, 1994.

19. Bass, K.M., Newschaffer, C.J., Klag, M.J. and Bush, T.L., Plasma lipoprotein levels as predictors of cardiovascular death in women, *Arch Intern Med*,153, 2209, 1993.

20. U.S. Department of Agriculture, Agriculture Research Service, Food and nutrient intakes by individuals in the United States, 1 Day, 1989–1991. Continuing survey of food intake by individuals, 1989–1991, *NFS Report*, 91, 1994.

21. Vinik, A.I. and Jenkins, D.J.A., Dietary fiber in the management of diabetes, *Diabetes Care*, 11, 160, 1988.

22. Snustad, D., Lee, V. and Abraham, I., Dietary fiber in hospitalized geriatric patients: Too soft a solution for too hard a problem, *J Nutr Elderly*, 10, 49, 1991.

23. National Cancer Institute. A.P. John Institute for Cancer Research, Connecticut, 2000.

24. Human Nutrition Information Service CSFII, Nationwide food consumption survey, U.S. Department of Agriculture, Washington, D.C., 1985.

25. Kuczmarski, R.J., Flegal, K.M., Campbell, S.M. and Johnson, C.L., Increasing prevalence of overweight among US adults, *J Amer Med Assoc*, 272, 2205, 1994.

26. Williamson, D.F., Descriptive epidemiology of body weight and weight change in U.S. adults, *Ann Intern Med*, 119, 646, 1993.

27. Soler, J.T., Folsom, A.R., Kushi, L.H., Prineas, R.J. and Seal, U.S., Association of body fat distribution with plasma lipids, lipoproteins, apolipoproteins AI and B in postmenopausal women, *J Clin Epidemiol*, 41, 1075, 1988.

28. Haarbo, J., Marslew, U., Gotfredsen, A. and Christiansen, C., Postmenopausal hormone replacement therapy prevents central distribution of body fat after menopause, *Metabolism*, 40, 1323, 1991.

29. Doll, R. and Peto, R, The causes of cancer: Quantitative estimates of avoidable risks of cancer in the United States today, *J Natl Cancer Inst*, 66, 1191, 1981.

30. Tinajas Ruiz, A., Cardiovascular health and trans fatty acid consumption, *Alimentaria*, 35, 75, 1998.

31. Sempos, C.T., Cleeman, J.I. and Carroll, M.D., Prevalence of high blood cholesterol among US adults, *J Amer Med Assoc*, 269, 3009, 1993.

32. Kubik, A., Zatloukal, P., Tomasek, L., Kriz, J., Petruzelka, L. and Plesko, I., Diet and the risk of lung cancer among women. A hospital-based case-control study, *Neoplasma*, 48, 262, 2001.

33. Parkin, D.M., Pisani, P. and Ferlay, J., Estimates of the worldwide incidence of 25 major cancers in 1990, *Int J Cancer*, 80, 827, 1999.

34. Willett, W.C., Diet and breast cancer, *J Intern Med*, 249, 395, 2001.

35. Toniolo, P., Riboli, E., Shore, R.E. and Pasternack, B.S., Consumption of meat, animal products, protein and fat and risk of breast cancer: A prospective cohort study in New York, *Epidemiology*, 5, 391, 1994.

36. Witte, J.S., Ursin, G., Siemiatrycki, J., Thompson, W.D., Paganini-Hill, A. and Haile, R.W., Diet and premenopausal bilateral breast cancer: A case-control study, *Breast Cancer Res Treat*, 42, 243, 1997.

37. Favero, A., Parpinel, M. and Franceschi, S., Diet and risk of breast cancer: Major finds from an Italian case-control study, *Biomed Pharmacother*, 52, 109, 1998.

38. Hunter, D.J. and Willett, W.C., Nutrition and breast cancer, *Cancer Causes Control*, 7, 56, 1996.

39. Gandini, S., Merzenich, H., Robertson, C. and Boyle, P, Meta-analysis of studies on breast cancer risk and diet: The role of fruit and vegetable consumption and the intake of associated micronutrients, *Eur J Cancer*, 36, 636, 2000.

40. Braga, C., La Vecchia, C., Negri, E., Franceshi, S. and Parpinel, M., Intake of selected foods and nutrients and breast cancer risk: An age- and menopause-specific analysis, *Nutr Cancer*, 28, 258, 1997.

41. Franceschi, S., Favero, A., La Vecchia, C., Negri, E., Dal Maso, L., Salvini, S., Decarli, A. and Giacose, A., Influence of food groups and food diversity on breast cancer risk in Italy, *Int J Cancer*, 63, 785, 1995.

42. DeStefani, D., Ronco, A., Mendilahasu, M., Guidobobo, M. and Deneo-Pellegrini, H., Meat intake, heterocyclic amines and risk of breast cncer: a case-control study in Uruguay, *Cancer Epid Biom Prevent*, 6, 573, 1997.

43. Wynder, E.L., Cohen, A.L., Muscat, J.E., Winters, B., Dwyer, J.T. and Blackburn, G., Breast cancer: Weighing the evidence for a promotion role of dietary fat, *J Nat Cancer Inst*, 89, 766, 1997.

44. World Cancer Research Fund and American Institute for Cancer Research, Food, nutrition and the prevention of cancer: A global perspective, Washington, D.C., American Institute for Cancer Research, 1997.

45. Longnecker, M.P., Newcomb, P.A., Mittendorf, R., Greenberg, E.R. and Willett, W.C., Intake of carrots, spinach and supplements containing vitamin A in relation to risk of breast cancer, *Cancer Epid, Biom and Prevent*, 6, 887, 1997.
46. Levi, F., Pasche, C., La Vecchia, C., Lucchini, F. and Franceschi, S., Food groups and colorectal cancer risk, *Brit J Cancer*, 79, 1283, 1999.
47. Manus, B., Adang, R.P., Ambergen, A.W., Bragelmann, R., Armbrecht, U. and Stockbrugger, R.W., The risk factor profile of rectosigmoid adenomas: aprospective screening study of 665 patients in a clinical rehabilitiation center, *Eur J Cancer*, 6, 38, 1997.
48. Knekt, P., Jarvinen, R., Dich, J. and Hakulinen, T., Risk of colorectal and other gastrointestinal cancers after exposure to nitrate, nitrite and N-nitroso compounds: a follow-up study, *Int J Cancer*, 80, 852, 1999.
49. Potter, J.D. and Steinmetz, K.A., Vegetables, fruit and phytoestrogens as preventive agents, In: *Principles of Chemoprevention*, Stewart, B.W., McGregor, D.B. and Kleihues, P., Eds., Lyon, France, International Agency for Research on Cancer, 61–90, 1996.
50. Wijnands, M.V., Appel, M.J., Hollanders, V.M. and Woutersen, R.A., A comparison of the effects of dietary cellulose and fermentable galacto oligosaccharide, in a rat model of colorectal carcinogensis: Fermentable confers greater protection than nonfermentable fiber in both high- and low-fat backgrounds, *Carcinogenesis*, 20, 651, 1999.
51. Marshall, J., Freudenheim, J., Graham, S. and Brasure, J. Diet in the epidemiology of ovarian cancer, *FASEB J*, 7, 65, 1993.
52. La Vecchia, C., Decarli, A. and Negri, E. Dietary factors and the risk of epithelial ovarian cancer, *J Natl Cancer Inst*, 79, 663, 1987.
53. Shu, X., Gao, Y., Yuan, J., Ziegler, R. and Brinton, L. Dietary factors and epithelial ovarian cancer, *Br J Cancer*, 59, 92, 1989.
54. Tzonou, A., Hsieh, C-C. and Polychronopoulou, A. Diet and ovarian cancer: A case-control study in Greece, *Int J Cancer*, 55, 411, 1993.
55. National Research Council, Recommended Dietary Allowances, 10th ed., National Academy Press, Washington, D.C., 1, 1989.
56. U.S. Department of Agriculture and U.S. Department of Health and Human Services, Dietary Guidelines for Americans, Washington, D.C., 1, 2000.
57. NIH guidelines on the inclusion of women and minorities as subjects in clinical research, *Fed Reg*, 59, 14509, 1994.
58. Liu, S., Manson, J., Lee, I., Cole, S., Hennekens, C., Willett, W. and Buring, J. Fruit and vegetable intake and risk of cardiovascular disease: The Women's Health Study, *Am J Clin Nutr*, 72, 922, 2000.
59. van Kappel, A., Steghens, J., Zeleniuch-Jacquotte, A., Chajes, V., Toniolo, P. and Riboli, E. Serum carotenoids as biomarkers of fruit and vegetable consumption in the New York Women's Health Study, *Public Hlth Nutr*, 4, 829, 2001.
60. Kasum, C., Nicodemus, K., Harnack, L., Jacobs, D. and Folsom, A. Whole grain intake and incident endometrial cancer : The Iowa Women's Health Study, *Nutr Cancer*, 39, 180, 2001.
61. Cusatis, D., Chinchilli, V., Johnson-Rollings, N., Kieselhorst, K., Stallings, V. and Lloyd, T. Longitudinal nutrient intake patterns of US adolescent women: The Penn State Yound Women's Health Study, *J Adolesc Hlth*, 26, 194, 2000.
62. Klesges, L., Pahor, M., Shorr, R., Wan, J., Williamson, J. and Guralnik, J. Financial difficulty in acquiring food among elderly disabled women: Results from the Women's Health and Aging Study, *Am J Pub Hlth*, 91, 68, 2001.

63. Thorand, B., Kohlmeier, L., Simonsen, N., Groghan, C. and Thamm, M. Intake of fruits, vegetables, folic acid and related nutrients and risk of breast cancer in post-menopausal women, *Pub Hlth Nutr*, 1, 147, 1998.

64. Cade, J., Upmeier, H., Calvert, C. and Greenwood, D. Costs of a healthy diet: Analysis from the UK Women's Cohort Study, *Pub Hlth Nutr*, 2, 505, 1999.

3 Gender, Culture and Nutrition

Cristanna M. Cook and Richard A. Cook

CONTENTS

I. INTRODUCTION

A. THE ELEMENTS OF CULTURE

While there are hundreds of definitions of culture, the elements of culture can be categorized as economic, social, world-view, political, aesthetic, and techno-logical.[1] Culture comprises the material and nonmaterial aspects of a group of people. The material culture is made up of the artifacts of the group that have been created from the nonmaterial rules that define the proper way to construct, distribute and consume the material artifacts. The nonmaterial rules also include the accepted world view, such as the appropriate religious norms, family kinship structure and inheritance, accepted social and political organizations, and the

beliefs and values of the group. While nonWestern cultures studied by Mali-
nowski, Boas, Mead and other famous anthropologists may have been quite
homogeneous, modern-day cultures are far more diverse and contain subcultures
with their own sets of norms regulating the elements of culture. The norms of
the group that define the elements of culture also regulate the role of women in
that culture or subculture.

B. Relationships of Gender, Culture and Nutrition

Nutritional concerns of women with respect to gender and culture are recognized
internationally, usually with different areas of concern existing in the developing
world vs. the developed world. There are, of course, nutritional concerns of American
women, as discussed throughout this book and in Part VII of this chapter. However,
the major issues that impact negatively on the nutrition of families through cultural
influences on women come from less developed nations.

Micronutrient and macronutrient undernutrition in developing countries is
especially an issue for woman and children. It is clear that nutrient deficiencies
affect intellectual development in children, limit physical growth and increase
child mortality.[2] We can model the causes of undernutrition in society starting
with potential resources that are available through the existing economic, political
and ideological, formal and nonformal structures in a society. Lack of resources
or inefficient use of resources can lead to inadequate access to food, inadequate
care for mothers and children, insufficient health services and an unhealthy
environment. Inadequate dietary intake and disease result, which in turn lead to
undernutrition and possibly death.[3] Access to resources is mediated by the culture
and subcultures of a society. Based on this resource model, the following factors
are impacted by the rules of the culture and subsequently influence common
nutrition problems:

- The interaction of women with income-generating opportunities in pro-
  duction, distribution and consumption
- Women's access to technology
- Power relationships in the household
- Level of care provided women and children
- The education of women

Diverse nutrition problems affect women and children worldwide. Allen and
Gillespie[3] list five common nutrition problems in developing countries (particularly
Asian countries) that affect the nutrition of women and children:

- Low birthweight
- Early growth failure
- Iron deficiency
- Iodine deficiency
- Vitamin A deficiency

II. NUTRIENT PROBLEMS ACROSS
CULTURE AND GENDER

A. Low Birthweight

Undernutrition of the mother has a cumulative negative effect on the birthweight of babies.[3] Undernutrition that affects subsequent births can occur during pregnancy, childhood and adolescence.[3] In Asia, the prevalence of low birthweight (defined as < 2500 g) is high primarily because of the undernutrition of the mother before and during pregnancy.[4] Low birthweight is likely the main reason that more than 50% of the children in Southeast Asia are underweight.[3] Overall, 75% of all low-birth-weight babies are born in Asia (mostly South Central Asia, which includes Afghanistan, Bangladesh, India, Iran, Pakistan, Maldives, Sri Lanka and Tajikistan), 20% are in Africa and 5% are in Latin America.[4] Infants born in Subsaharan Africa, particularly Zaire, Angola, Guinea and The Gambia have the highest levels of low birthweight — greater than or equal to 15%. Other countries that have between 10 and 15% low birthweight are Tanzania, Rwanda, Niger, Nigeria, Togo and Guinea-Bissau.[4] At least 13.7 million babies in developing countries are already malnourished at birth each year, which represents 11% of all newborns in these countries.[4]

Low birthweight has impact on morbidity and mortality in developing countries.[5] Intrauterine growth retardation (IUGR) is associated most often in infants with low birthweights in developing countries. In affluent groups, low birthweight is associated with preterm pregnancies. IUGR is defined as birthweight >2 SD below the median for gestational age.[5] For infants weighing 2000 to 2499 g at birth, the risk of neonatal death is four times higher than for infants weighing 2500 to 2499 g and 10 times higher than for infants weighing 3000 to 3400 g. The risk of postneonatal death in term infants weighing 2000 to 2499g is estimated to be twice as high as for infants 2500 to 2499 g and four times higher than for infants weighing 3000 to 3400 g.[5]

There is a definite relationship between low birthweight and maternal undernutrition. A World Health Organization (WHO) study in 25 diverse cultural populations showed that being in the lowest quartile of prepregnancy weight carried an elevated risk of IUGR of 2.5 times.[6] One third of Asian Indian babies are born with low birthweight, which is attributed to maternal undernutrition, particularly of folate.[7] In fact, there is evidence that to enhance birthweight, micronutrients may have more effect on maternal weight gain than high-protein concentration.[8]

B. Early Childhood Growth Failure

During the first few years after birth, children in developing countries grow more slowly than children in wealthier regions of the world.[3] They may be stunted or have a height-for-age more than 2 SD below the median value of the NCHS/WHO International Growth Reference for height-for-age.[8] Underweight is defined as more than 2 SD below the NCHS/WHO international growth reference weight-for-age median. Wasting is defined as more than 2 SD below the NCHS/WHO international growth reference weight-for-height median.

In order of prevalence of stunting, East Africa is first with 48%, South Central Asia is next with 44%, then West Africa with 35%, North Africa with 20%, the Caribbean with 19% and South America with 13%.[9] The global prevalence of underweight is 26.7%. Cultural patterns associated with underweight are similar to those of stunting with 72% of underweight children in Asia.[9] South Central Asia with 15.4% and West Africa with 15.6% have the highest prevalence of wasting in the world.[9] The global prevalence is 9.4%.[9]

Poor growth of children in developing countries is caused by poor maternal nutrition before and during pregnancy, inadequate breast feeding, delayed or poor quality complementary feeding and poor absorption of nutrients due to infections or parasites in both mother and child.[3]

Poor growth (e.g., birthweight) is associated with increased risk of mortality. An analysis of 28 studies showed that about 45 to 65% of all child deaths in 12 Asian and Subsaharan African countries were due to undernutrition.[10] Higher energy availability, higher immunization rates, higher female literacy and higher gross national product seem to be the most important factors associated with lower prevalence of stunting and wasting.[11]

C. IRON DEFICIENCY ANEMIA

Parasites are a non-nutritional cause of anemia affecting men, women and children,[12] but women and children have a higher prevalence of nutritional anemia than men. Other micronutrients needed for hemoglobin absorption or synthesis are vitamins A and B_{12}, folic acid and riboflavin. Where there are problems with the availability of these micronutrients, anemia may be more common.[3] Iron deficiency is two to two-and-one-half times more prevalent than anemia.[3]

Asia has the highest rate of anemia in the world. Of the anemic women on the Indian subcontinent, 88% develop anemia during pregnancy.[9] A further complication is the high consumption of nonheme iron from mainly vegetarian diets. Although it is difficult to collect accurate figures on the prevalence of anemia in developing countries because the data come from small surveys or clinical records or from imprecise national or regional surveys, it appears that the rate of anemia in developing countries is about four times that of developed countries.[13]

Severe anemia during pregnancy has been associated with low birthweight and preterm delivery.[14] Anemia affects performance and productivity and, considering that women farmers produce the majority of food in parts of the world such as Subsaharan Africa, this is a major problem. In Indonesia, anemic women produced 5% less in factory work and 6.5 hours less housework per week.[15] Anemia is also associated with maternal mortality. Estimates of mortality ranged from 27 per 100,000 live births in India to 194 per 100,000 live births from a hospital-based study in Pakistan.[16]

D. IODINE DEFICIENCY

IDD or iodine deficiency disorders include goiter, problems with cognitive functioning, cretinism, limited growth, low birthweight, infant mortality and stillbirths.[3,17] It has been estimated that 130 out of 191 countries have had IDD problems.[9] Twelve percent of Southeast Asian people are affected by goiter and 41% are at risk of goiter (in total, 172 million people).[9] In Africa, 250 million people are at risk of IDD and 50 million have goiter.[17] Areas such as mountainous regions, where soils are leached by glaciation, floods or high rainfall will have high a prevalence of iodine deficiency.[18]

Many staple foods in the developing world contain cyanogenic glucosides that can liberate cyanide that is converted in the body to thiocyanate, which blocks the uptake of iodine in the thyroid.[18] The cyanogenic glucosides are located in the inedible parts of plants such as cassava, which is extensively eaten around the globe. Hence, cassava must be properly soaked to remove the substance. If cassava is not properly prepared, its consumption can be associated with goiter and cretinism, as found in Sarawak, Malaysia.[19]

Iron deficiency can impair iodine metabolism. A study in the Cote d'Ivoire showed that the prevalence of goiter was lower in children with adequate iron storage.[17]

E. VITAMIN A DEFICIENCY

Areas of the world most affected by vitamin A deficiency (VAD) are those in which there is a low consumption of animal products and fruits and vegetables rich in beta-carotene.[3] Pregnant and lactating women are especially affected. Low vitamin A status in pregnant women and subsequent low retinol content in breast milk is a risk factor for the onset of VAD in infants in Indonesia.[19] Breast feeding is also associated with lower levels of VAD in children.[19] Infant stores of retinol at birth are not highly affected by the vitamin A status of the mother.[3] However, there is value in vitamin A supplementation during pregnancy since it can prevent night blindness, which normally increases as pregnancy advances.[3] Night blindness is associated with a higher risk of maternal mortality and morbidity in Nepal, although the exact mechanism of how vitamin A is implicated in mortality is not clear.[20]

How is undernutrition affected by culture? The reason that many nutritional deficiencies exist, particularly among women and children in developing countries, can be partly attributed to the role of women in the culture.

III. CULTURAL DIFFERENCES THAT INFLUENCE INCOME-GENERATING OPPORTUNITIES, INCLUDING ACCESS TO TECHNOLOGY BY GENDER

We are interested in the impact of culture on women's roles because there is a direct relationship between the ability of women to generate income and to feed their families, particularly their children.[21,22] According to the Food and Agriculture Organization of the United Nations, women provide more than half of the labor required to produce the food consumed in developing countries, including about three fourths of the labor in Africa.[22] Women have a prominent role in agriculture and their efforts have a greater impact on household nutrition than that of men in the household.

Some countries and regions have decreased child undernutrition more than others, which is thought to be partly the result of the role of women as income generators.

Increasing the income-generating capacity of women would help decrease the 30% of all developing-country children under 5 years of age who are undernourished.[22] Although child undernutrition has decreased from 46.5% to 31% worldwide from 1970 to 1995, such undernutrition has been rising in SubSaharan Africa, where the prevalence has increased from 26% to 31%. The rates of underweight children have increased for 12 developing countries, declined for 35 developing countries and remained the same for 15 developing countries.[23]

There are immediate determinants of child nutritional status (dietary intake and health status); underlying determinants (food security, adequate care for mothers and children, a supportive health environment); and basic determinants (resources, access to technology, the quality of human resources and the political, economic and social factors such as the status of women that affect the availability and use of resources).[23] As a woman's status increases in a society, she is more likely to have access to the productive resources necessary to earn income. As this income is earned, it is returned to the family. The higher rate of child undernutrition in Southeast Asia may be the result of the lower status of women relative to their status in other parts of the world. The relative status of women as measured by the female-to-male life expectancy ratio has been declining in SubSaharan Africa.[23] This situation may be the reason for the increase in child undernutrition in that region. Women with lower status are not able to pursue economic opportunities.

While the child undernutrition prevalence is 50% in Southeast Asia, the rate in SubSaharan Africa is 31%. Although South Asia is economically better off than SubSaharan Africa, the rate of child undernutrition is much worse. South Asia is doing better in all the immediate, underlying and basic determinants of child nutrition than SubSaharan Africa except for women's relative status.[23] Other gender-related reasons for child nutrition problems are the cultural traditions that hinder breast feeding and the introduction of weaning foods.[24]

The lower relative status of women makes it difficult for them to have the necessary resources to increase efficiency, productivity and income. Compared with men, women have less land, capital, technology and access to agricultural information through agricultural extension programs.[21,22]

Women farmers have relatively low rates of adoption of new technologies such as high-yielding varieties and improved management systems.[25] Well-intentioned projects try to encourage women to adopt more efficient technology. However, it is not sufficient to simply take women into account when designing projects. Sometimes, agricultural projects that purport to include women end up reallocating resources more to men than to women. It is necessary to identify how roles will change and the what will be the ability of women to gather the fruits of their labor from such well-intentioned projects. Men often take over female farming activity when it is profitable to do so.[25] The effect of the introduction of any new technology must be viewed in terms of the effects of the reallocation of resources in the household. Why should a woman adopt a new technology if the income-generating result of that technology is removed from her control?

Studies on the efficiency of production between men and women show that women are as efficient as men when given appropriate inputs such as technology.[26] Cultural barriers that limit access of women to technology lead to productivity differences, as women must spend more of their time in raising children and caring for the household, as these roles are determined through cultural norms. Women often cannot devote as much time to agricultural activity because of their many other roles.

The adoption of technology is related to another vital input into the production process — land. If there is a secure land title, then the adoption of technology seems a wise investment. Men most often have the rights to land in most of the developing agricultural economies. Women may have access to land through marriage. Women may have access to land informally, but when land becomes titled, it is usually titled in the man's name. This factor may lead to the loss of control of land previously worked.[9] If technology is used that increases the productivity of land previously used by women, there must be some policy in place to retain a woman's right to access to and income from the land.[25]

Access to credit is necessary to buy the needed inputs to the agricultural process such as fertilizer and seed. Studies indicate that women have less access to credit than men.[25] In Zimbabwe, women who were small landholders had more trouble receiving credit because their small plots did not allow sufficiently large marketable surplus. As women are perceived as producers for family consumption only or to have small plots, they have a difficult time getting needed credit for expansion.[26,28]

It is necessary to implement programs that will provide women with the capital to purchase necessary inputs to increase their productive efficiency. In countries where the status of women is very low and women are discriminated against, such as Bangladesh, women have lower nutritional status and higher morbidity and mortality rates.[2,29] In such societies, it is necessary to provide access to technology through group-based programs rather than targeting women in individual households. Women organized in production where new technology is introduced have more control over their output and income.[2]

Even if women have access to capital to purchase technology, they may not have the informational resources available to them to allow efficient application of that technology. The problem is not only that women are not reached by extension services, but also that such services are more likely to be offered to women in male-headed households, thus biasing access to information to female-headed households.[30,31]

IV. CULTURAL VARIATION IN GOOD CARE PRACTICE FOR MOTHERS (INCLUDING FEEDING PRACTICES) AND THE IMPACT ON CHILD NUTRITION

According to the International Conference on Nutrition, care is defined as the provision of time, attention and support to meet the physical, mental and social needs of household members.[32,33] Good care practices are strong determinants of children's nutritional status and more so for children from poorer households and children of mothers with less than a secondary school education.[32]

There are six care practices that are important for the good nutrition status, growth and development of children.[3] These care practices, which, in many parts of the world, women are not able to apply are:

1. Support to women to make sure they receive adequate prenatal care and have equal access to education
2. Adequate food preparation resources
3. Good hygiene practice in the home
4. Ability to have a safe home and apply preventive health care
5. Good psychosocial care, including warmth
6. Verbal interaction
7. Encouragement of learning and good child feeding styles, including breast feeding[3]

Even when women lack the support and education they need, when good care practices are applied in the household there is nutritional improvement for children. In Accra, Ghana, almost three fourths of mothers in a household study of good care practices had less than a secondary education. But among this group, the height-for-weight z scores were the same level as that of children from wealthier families or of more educated mothers for those who practiced good care (appropriate child feeding practices and the use of health services for immunization and monitoring of growth).[32] Thus, the prevalence of stunting and underweight was significantly lower among children whose mothers scored the highest in good care practice. An interesting result of this study was that poor maternal schooling and low income were found to have a negative effect on children's height-for-weight z scores only if mothers were poor caregivers. So, good care practice could compensate for poor education and low income. The major implication of this study is that training in child feeding and the use of preventive health practices for poor households with mothers with low education can improve the nutrient well-being of children. Nutrition education should target the most efficient care practices such as breast feeding and attempt to modify the constraints that limit the adoption of good care practice.[34]

The strongest evidence of bias against women in nutritional care comes from South Asia.[35] It is the norm for families to pay men to marry their daughters. Daughters are more of a financial burden as a result and there is less nutritional care for female siblings in the household, possibly because of the dowry that must be paid for a husband. In SubSaharan Africa, daughters receive better nutritional care than sons since they bring in money to the household, as men must provide resources to acquire a wife.

V. THE ROLE OF THE MOTHER'S EDUCATION IN NUTRITION

The areas of the world that have achieved the most economic and social progress have also promoted equal educational achievements for men and women. Areas that have lagged in their economic growth have also lagged in their relative investments in women's education.[35] The relative returns for society of an additional year of schooling for a female are greater than for an additional year of schooling for a male. These returns are not just private, but are social as well, in the form of better child health, stature and schooling.[35] There are economic efficiencies when social investments are redirected toward the education of women.

Maternal education is important in the provision of good care practices to children and was the most important predictor of good care practices in the sample of households from Accra.[32] It is estimated that of all the underlying determinants of child nutritional status in developing countries, women's education is responsible for a reduction of 43% in child undernutrition.[36] Other major determinants are improvements in per capita food availability, improvements in health environments and improvements in women's status.[36] Female education increases knowledge and skills that enable income-generating activity. A higher income increases household food security. Female education makes it more likely that women will be able to provide good care practices to their children.

VI. FOOD SECURITY, HOUSEHOLD POWER IMBALANCES AND GENDER

It has been estimated that 800 million people in the developing world face food insecurity.[37] One way to help reduce this is to release the untapped potential of women in agriculture by reducing the bias against women in much of the developing world.[37] Women account for 70 to 80% of household food production in SubSaharan Africa, 65% in Asia and 45% in Latin America and the Caribbean.[37] This contribution by women is amazing, considering that women suffer from many biases, including limited access to credit and other inputs, insecure land tenure, lack of access to extension services, cultural norms prohibiting them from more intensive farming or income-generating activity and lower levels of education relative to men.

Food security would also be helped through increasing income-generating opportunities for women. Women are more likely to spend their income on household food than are men.[21,22,37] The reasons for this practice are possibly the social and cultural norms that make nurturing part of the woman's role and the fact that, since women's income comes in smaller amounts and more regularly, it is more likely to be spent on immediate consumption for the children.[37]

It is clear that women are a major factor in food security. It is also clear that household expenditure patterns are shaped by the relative power of different household members.[38] In standard economic theory, the household is viewed as a single decision-making unit, which is called the "unitary" theory of household expenditure allocation. However, different bargaining positions in the household call for a more realistic view of expenditure patterns. This latter view is called the "collective" model of household expenditure allocation. Expenditure patterns affect the nutritional consumption patterns and the nutritional distribution patterns in the household. There is a growing body of scientific evidence that expenditure allocation within the household and, thus, access to good nutrition, is a function of the relative bargaining positions of men and women in the household.[38,39]

Bargaining power is affected by several determinants such as control over resources, influence brought to bear on the household (perhaps from outside the household), mobilization of support networks and the attitudes of household members.[39] Resources are labor, assets brought into a marriage, unearned income, transfer payments and various kinds of welfare payments.[39] Influences can be relative education of household members, legal rights and bargaining skills.[39] Membership in organizations and access to relatives can alter the distribution of power between men and women in the household.[39] Women with attitudes such as self-esteem and self-confidence feel more adept at bargaining[39]

The empirical rejection of "unitary" models of the household means that programs that are designed to transfer resources to households must, in fact, address the issue of who is the household recipient of those resources. When women get resources, they are more likely to use those resources for the nutritional betterment of the household.

Among Malaysian Islamic women, those with more asset power have greater ability to purchase items that they prefer. Malaysian migrant daughters who work in the urban economy and send money home are more able to express preferences for the allocation of money. Women are thus able to increase their economic power with the help of their daughters.[38] As the opportunities for women increase in the workforce in Malaysia, the expenditures on food and schooling for household members should increase.

Contract farming in the Dominican Republic has redefined the roles of women in household power negotiations since it is impossible to fulfill a labor contract without the use of women's labor.[40] Women, thus, are able to claim a share of the economic rewards from contract farming. Since they are more likely than men to make decisions concerning food purchases, this extra influence allows them more resources for such purchases.

VII. AMERICAN CULTURE AND NUTRITION

The American culture is a blending of ancestry from many cultures, primarily of European heritage, but presently of increasing influences from many developing nations. Asians are an especially fast-growing ethnic group in America.[41] Thus, food habits vary from region to region in the country and, although hunger does exist in the United States, the American culture provides ready access to a wide variety of foodstuffs and incomes usually allow an ample selection of foods for nutrient intakes. The American environment provides many inexpensive high-calorie meal alternatives as well as ready access to nutrient supplements. Hence, it is the goal of many individuals to fill and over-fill energy (fat) reserves in the body and to bring nutrients to saturation levels in tissues as a preventive health care measure and for supposedly promoting longevity. In recognition of the danger of overconsumption due to combinations of supplements and foods, the new Dietary Reference Intakes (DRI) for the country now include proposed values for tolerable upper intake levels.[42]

Previously in this chapter, discussions were focused on the main nutrition problems worldwide (primarily in developing countries), which included lack of total calorie and protein needs in the diet and deficiencies of vitamin A, iodine and iron.

With respect to energy, American women are facing a major obesity crisis in this nation due to overconsumption of calories, accompanied by increased stresses in everyday life (at work and home), with decreased opportunities for exercise.[43,44] Obesity complicates most major health problems such as cardiovascular disease, risk of stroke, diabetes, kidney disease, cancer, high blood pressure and arthritis. Also, it can adversely affect a woman's pregnancy and menstrual cycle, and cause hirsutism. A problem with vitamin A would more likely involve overconsumption than underconsumption, with a danger of teratogenesis.[45] Iodine deficiency resulting in goiter (adult) or cretinism (fetus), although notable in some parts of the world, is rare in North America.[46] Protection is obtained from iodized salt and ample intakes of marine and dairy products, with no real danger of toxicity. Iron is a nutrient with stores often low in women from both developing and developed nations. Menstrual blood losses and high nonheme iron intakes (vegetarians) make women especially vulnerable to iron deficiency anemia. Maternal anemia places women in danger of premature delivery, low-birthweight offspring and perinatal infant mortality.[46]

Another nutrient of special concern for women of childbearing age in this country is folate. In 1998, a folic acid fortification program was initiated, putting folate in cereal and grain products to help in the prevention of neural tube defects during gestation.[47] National survey data indicating low natural food folate intakes among women capable of conceiving children[48] would suggest a regular additional intake of fortified food or supplements. Folate from these sources is absorbed about twice as readily as that from natural foods alone.[46]

Great interest has been generated in calcium and vitamin D needs of women, especially if Caucasian and living in northern areas of the country, due to a higher risk of osteoporosis.[49] Supplementation of both calcium and vitamin D with aging appears to be warranted to prevent more rapid deterioration of the skeleton from low bone mass accretion (calcium storage) during childhood and early adulthood, as well as poor ultraviolet light exposure (to produce vitamin D in the skin) in higher latitudes.

VIII. CONCLUSIONS

It is apparent that, worldwide, the role of women as providers of agricultural labor, good caregivers, generators of household income and providers of adequate nutrition for their children is intrinsically linked to their status in their society. Where that status has increased, there is an increase in household nutritional adequacy. It is necessary to change the legal, social and cultural institutions of a society to allow women to realize their full potential as pillars of food security worldwide.[37] The development of innovative projects that improve women's role as gatekeepers of food security can also help.[37] These projects should also be carefully administered when creating new household resources to allow women to have a share of any newly generated resource. Otherwise, simply increasing household income may not be translated into improved nutrition for all household members. Women in developed countries also have unique nutritional concerns. Major concerns of American women now include inadequate intakes of folate, calcium and vitamin D. Overuse of supplements and excess energy intakes combined with decreased exercise levels, leading to increased overweight and obesity at young ages, is another major issue. Cultural norms dictate similarities and differences but, overall, women are facing major nutritional challenges in the world today, with culture helping or hindering their resolution.

REFERENCES

1. Cateora, P.R. and Graham, J.L., *International Marketing*, McGraw-Hill/Irwin Co., Chicago, 2001.
2. Naved, R.T., Intrahoushold impact of the transfer of modern agricultural technology: A gender perspective, Food Consumption and Nutrition Division Paper No.85, International Food Policy Research Institute, 2000.
3. Allen, L. and Gillespie, S., What works? A review of the efficiency and effectiveness of nutrition interventions, Asian Development Bank, 2001.
4. de Onis, M., Blossner, M. and Villar, J., Levels and patterns of intrauterine growth and retardation in developing countries, *J Clin Nutr*, 52, S5, 1998.
5. Ashworth, A., Effects of intrauterine growth retardation in infants and young children, *Eur J Clin Nutr*, 52, S34, 1998.
6. World Health Organization, Maternal anthropometry and pregnancy outcomes: a WHO collaborative study, Bulletin, Supplement to Volume 73, 1995.
7. Rao, S., Yajnik, C.S., Kanade, A., Fall, C., Margetts, B.M., Jackson, A.A., Shier, R., Joshi, S., Rege, S., Lubree, H. and Desai, B., Intake of micronutrient-rich foods in rural Indian mothers is associated with the size of their babies at birth: Pune maternal nutrition study, *J Nutr*, 131, 1217, 2001.
8. Susser, M., Maternal weight gain, infant birth weight and diet: Causal sequences, *Amer J Clin Nutr*, 53, 1384, 1991.
9. World Health Organization, 1995 Physical statistics: The use and interpretation of anthropometry, Report Series No. 854, 1995.
10. The United Nation Administrative Committee on Coordination, Sub-committee on Nutrition, Fourth Report on the World Nutrition Situation, 2000.
11. Frongillo, E.A., de Onis, M. and Hansen, K., Socioeconomic and demographic factors are associated with worldwide patterns of stunting and wasting of children, *J Nutr*, 127, 2302, 1997.
12. Stoltzfus, R.J., Albnico, M., Chwaya, H.M., Tielsch, J.M., Schulze, K.J. and Savioli, L., Effects of the Zanzibar school-based deworming program on iron status of children, *Am J Clin Nutr*, 68, 179, 1998.
13. World Health Organization, Malnutrition, the Global Picture, 2000.
14. Rasmussen, K.M., Is there a causal relationship between iron deficiency or iron-deficiency anemia and weight at birth, length of gestation and perinatal mortality? *J Nutr*, 131, S590, 2001.
15. Scholz, B.D., Gross, R., Schultink, W. and Sastroamidjojo, S., Anaemia is associated with reduced productivity of women, *Br J Nutr*, 77, 47, 1997.
16. Brabin, B.J., Hakimi, M. and Pelletier, D., An analysis of anemia and pregnancy-related maternal mortality, *J Nutr*, 131, S604, 2001.
17. Zimmermann, M., Adou, P, Torresanai, T., Zeder, C. and Hurrell, R., Persistence of goiter despite oral iodine supplementation in goitrous children with iron deficiency anemia in Cote d'Ivoire, *Am J Clin Nutr*, 71, 88, 2000.
18. Maberly, G.F., Eastman, C.J., Waite, K.V., Corcoran, J. and Rashford, V., *The Role of Cassava: Current Problems in Thyroid Research*, Ui, N., Torizuka, K., Nagataki S. and Miyai, K., Eds., Excerpta Medica, Amsterdam, 1983.

19. Tarwotjo, I., Sommer, A., Soegiharto, T. and Susanto, D., Dietary practices and xerophthalmia among Indonesian children, *Am J Clin Nutr*, 35, 574, 1982.

20. Christian, P., West, K.P., Khatry, S.K., Katz, J., Shrestha, S.R., Pradham, E.K., LeClerq, S.C. and Pokhrel, R.P., Night blindness or pregnancy in rural Nepal-nutritional and health risks, *Int J Epidemiol*, 27, 231, 1998.

21. Quisumbing, A.R., Brown, L.R., Sims-Fieldstein, H., Haddad, L. and Peca, C., Women, the key to food security, Food Policy Statement No. 21, International Food Policy Research Institute, 1999.

22. Feeding the world 2020: What role will women play? 2020 Vision News and Views, International Food Policy Research Institute, 1995.

23. Smith, L. and Haddad, L., Explaining child malnutrition in developing countries: A cross-country analysis, Research Report 111, International Food Policy Research Institute, 2000.

24. Ramalingaswami, V., Johnson, U. and Rohde, J., The Asian enigma, in Progress of Nations, UN Children's Fund, New York, 1996.

25. Doss, C.R., Designing agricultural technology for African women farmers: Lessons from 25 years of experience, *World Development*, 29, 2075, 2001.

26. Quisumbing, A.R., Male-female differences in agricultural productivity: Methodological issues and empirical evidence, *World Development*, 24, 1579, 1996.

27. Lastarria-Cornheil, S., Impact of privatization on gender and property rights in Africa, *World Development*, 25, 1317, 1997.

28. Rohrbach, D.D., The Economics of Small Holder Maize Production in Zimbabwe: Implications for Food Security, Ph.D. thesis, Michigan State University, 1989.

29. Chen, L.C., Huq, E. and D'Souza, S., Sex bias in the family allocation of food and health care in rural Bangladesh, *Pop Dev Rev*, 7, 55, 1981.

30. Saito, K.A., Raising the productivity of women farmers in SubSaharan Africa, Discussion Paper No. 230, World Bank, 1994.

31. Alwary, J. and Siegal, P.B., Rural poverty in Zambia: An analysis of causes and policy recommendations, World Bank, 1994.

32. Ruel, M.T., Levin, C.E., Armar-Klemesu, M., Maxwell, D. and Morris, S.S., Good care practices can mitigate the effects of poverty and low maternal schooling on children's nutritional status: Evidence from Accra, Discussion Paper No. 62, International Food Policy Research Institute, 1999.

33. FAO, UN/WHO, International conference on nutrition, Rome, 1992.

34. Armar-Klemesu, M., Ruel, M.T., Maxwell, D.G., Levin, C.E. and Morris, S.S., The constraints to good child care practice in Accra: Implications for programs, Discussion Paper No. 81, International Food Policy Research Institute, 2000.

35. Schultz, T.P., Why governments should invest more to educate girls, *World Development*, 30, 202, 2002.

36. Smith, L. and Haddard, L., Overcoming child malnutrition in developing countries: past achievements and future choices, 2020 Brief No. 64, International Food Policy Research Institute, 2000.

37. Quisumbing, A.R., Brown, L.R., Sims-Feldstein, H., Haddad, L. and Peca, C., Women, the key to food security, Food Policy Statement No. 2, International Food Policy Research Institute, 1999.

38. Kusago, T. and Barhan, B.L., Preference heterogeneity, power and intra-household decision-making in rural Malaysia, *World Development*, 29, 1237, 2001.

39. Quisumbing, A.R. and Maluccio, J., Intra-household allocation and gender relations: New empirical evidence from four developing countries, Discussion Paper No .84, International Food Policy Research Institute, 2000.

40. Reynolds, L.T., Renegotiating gender and production relations in contract farming in the Dominican Republic, *World Development*, 30, 782, 2002.

41. Kittler, P.G. and Sucher, K.P., *Food and Culture*, 3rd ed., Wadsworth/Thomson Learning, 2001.

42. Monsen, E.R., New dietary reference intakes proposed to replace the recommended dietary allowances, *J Am Diet Assoc*, 96, 754, 1996.

43. Farley, T. and Cohen, D., Fixing a fat nation, The Washington Monthly Online, December 2001.

44. Mokdad, A.H., Ford, E.S., Bowman, B.A., Dietz, W.H., Vinicor, F., Bales, V.S. and Marks, J.S., Prevalence of obesity, diabetes and obesity-related health risk factors, 2001, *JAMA*, 289, 76, 2003.

45. Eckhoff, C. and Nan, H., Vitamin A supplementation increases levels of retinoic acid compounds in human plasma: Possible implications for teratogenesis, *Arch Toxicol*, 64, 502, 1990.

46. Food and Nutrition Board, Institute of Medicine, *Dietary Reference Intakes for Vitamin A, Vitamin K, Arsenic, Boron, Chromium, Copper, Iodine, Iron, Manganese, Molybdenum, Nickel, Silicon, Vanadium and Zinc,* National Academy Press, Washington, D.C., 2002.

47. Honein, M.A., Paulozzi, L.J., Mathews, T.J., Erickson, J.D. and Wang, L-Y.C., Impact of folic acid fortification of the US food supply on the occurrence of neural tube defects, *JAMA*, 285, 2981, 2001.

48. Gates, G.E. and Holmes, T.W., Folate intake and supplement use in women of childbearing age, *Fam Econ Nutr Rev*, 12, 14, 1999.

49. Sahyoun, N.R., Nutrition education for the healthy elderly population: Isn't it time? *J Nutr Educ Behav*, 34 (suppl. 1), S42, 2002.

4 Nutritional Needs of Female Adolescents

Jamie S. Stang and Rachel Hayes-Bohn

CONTENTS

I. INTRODUCTION

Adolescence is a time of remarkable physical, emotional and cognitive development. Due to the rapid rates of biological growth that occur during puberty, nutrient requirements are higher during adolescence than at any other time of life. Eating behaviors of female teens can influence their risk for immediate health consequences such as overweight, underweight, delayed sexual maturation, iron deficiency anemia, disordered eating, dental caries and suboptimal bone mineralization.[1,2] Nutritional status during adolescence may also affect adult health status. Suboptimal calcium intake during adolescence increases a female's lifelong risk of osteoporosis,[1] while overweight status increases the risk of adulthood obesity.[3-5] High intakes of total and saturated fat during the teenage years can promote the development of atherosclerotic plaque, thus increasing risk of cardiovascular disease later in life.[6] Low intakes of fruit, vegetables and whole grains have been suggested to increase a woman's lifetime risk of developing cardiovascular disease and some types of cancer.[7,8] Eating behaviors adopted during childhood and adolescence are likely to influence a female's adult eating habits, thus further affecting long-term risk of chronic disease occurrence.

Eating habits of adolescents may also affect cognitive and emotional development. After controlling for potential confounding factors, youths who skip breakfast have been shown to have decreased levels of concentration, reduced scores on math tests, poorer school performance in general and higher levels of disruptive behavior.[1,9,10] In addition, poor dietary habits among teens have been associated with other risk-taking behaviors such as smoking cigarettes.[11,12]

This chapter describes the nutritional needs of female adolescents, with emphasis on nutrients that are most likely to be underconsumed by teens. Information about common eating practices and how these affect immediate and long-term health are also included.

II. NORMAL PHYSICAL GROWTH AND DEVELOPMENT

Biological, emotional and cognitive transformations that begin during puberty and continue throughout the remainder of adolescence directly influence dietary intake and nutrient requirements. Adolescents undergo remarkable biological growth and development during puberty, which in turn substantially increases their need for energy, protein and many vitamins and minerals. Teenagers also undergo considerable transformations in their ability to analyze and decipher complex situations or information, as well as in their aspiration to become autonomous, independent individuals. Elevated requirements for energy and macro- and micronutrients, together with growing financial self-sufficiency, an increasing need for independence when making food choices and still-evolving cognitive capabilities, increase an adolescent's likelihood of developing nutritional deficiencies. Therefore, it is imperative that health care professionals develop a thorough knowledge of the role of adolescent physical and psychosocial growth and development on nutritional needs of teenage females.

Biological growth and development during adolescence is signified by the process of puberty, which is often defined as the physical transformation of a child into an adult. A multitude of biological transformations occur during puberty including sexual maturation; increases in height, weight and bone mineral content; completion of skeletal growth and alterations in body composition. The sequence of biological changes during puberty is generally consistent among adolescents; however, there may be a great deal of divergence in the age of inception, duration and velocity of these events between and within individual females. Thus, adolescents of comparable chronological age can differ significantly in physical appearance and nutrient requirements. A 13-year-old female who has experienced menarche and has all but completed the linear growth spurt will have very different energy and nutrient needs from a 13-year-old female who has not yet experienced menarche and has yet to experience the peak velocity of pubertal linear growth. As a result, sexual maturation, instead of chronological age, should be used to calculate the degree of biological growth and development and the beginning individual nutrient needs of adolescent females.

Sexual Maturation Rating (SMR), sometimes called Tanner Staging, is determined by a scale of secondary sexual characteristics that assist health professionals in gauging the extent of pubertal maturation that has occurred among adolescents, regardless of chronological age (Table 4.1). SMR is based on the presence and extent of pubic hair growth, the development of breasts and the occurrence of menarche among females. SMR stage 1 is consistent with prepubertal growth and development, while stages 2 to 5 indicate the advancement of puberty. SMR stage 5 signifies that sexual maturation has been completed. Sexual maturation parallels linear growth, changes in weight and body composition and hormonal changes remarkably well.

The linear growth spurt begins during SMR stage 2 in females between 9.5 and 14.5 years of age. Peak velocity of linear growth takes place toward the end of SMR stage 2 and during SMR stage 3, approximately 6 to 12 months prior to menarche (Figure 4.1).[13] The linear growth spurt is not completed until 16.5 to 17 years of age in most females, with relatively small increases in height occurring after menses. However, some female adolescents experience increases in height past age 18 years. An estimated 15 to 20% of final adult height among females is gained during the pubertal growth spurt. Linear growth may well be delayed or slowed among females with restricted energy, protein, fat or zinc intakes.

Almost half of final adult bone mass is accumulated during adolescence.[14] By 18 years of age, more than 90% of adult skeletal mass has been accumulated. Factors known to influence the accrual of bone mass include genetic predisposition,

TABLE 4.1
Sexual Maturity Rating in Girls

Breast Development	Stage	Pubic Hair Growth
Prepubertal; nipple elevation only	1	Prepubertal; no pubic hair
Small, raised breast bud	2	Sparse growth of hair along labia
General enlargement of raising of breast and areola	3	Pigmentation, coarsening and curling, with an increase in amount
Further enlargement with projection of areola and nipple as secondary mound	4	Hair resembles adult type, but not spread to medial thighs
Mature, adult contour, with areola in same contour as breast and only nipple projecting	5	Adult type and quantity, spread to medial thighs

Source: Story M., Stang J. (Eds.). *Nutrition and the Pregnant Adolescent: A Practical Reference Guide*, Minneapolis, MN: Center for Leadership, Education and Training in Maternal and Child Nutrition, University of Minnesota, 2000.

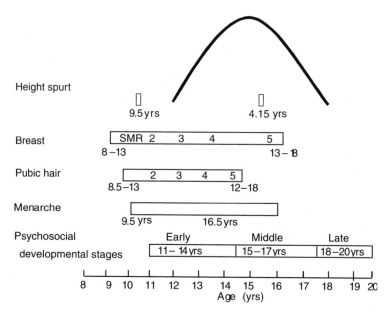

FIGURE 4.1 Sequence of physiological changes during puberty in females.

variability in hormone levels, weight-bearing exercise, cigarette smoking, alcohol consumption and dietary and supplemental intakes of vitamin D, calcium, phosphorous, boron and iron. Bone mineral content is thought to accrue in females at twice the usual rates during puberty compared with other developmental periods of life.[15] Once adult height is achieved, the accumulation of significant amounts of bone mass is unlikely.

A. CHANGES IN WEIGHT AND BODY COMPOSITION

On average, half of adult ideal body weight is gained during adolescence. The highest velocity of weight gain may precede the peak velocity of linear growth by 3 to 6 months in females. Average weight increases by 18.3 lbs. (8.3 kg) per year, with a mean gain of more than 30 lbs. (13.6 kg) during puberty among females.[16] The rate of weight gain slows around the onset of menses, but will persist into late adolescence. Female teens gain as much as 14 lbs (6.3 kg) during the later years of adolescence.

Typical lean body mass percentages of teen females fall from 82% to 74%, while mean body fat levels rise from 16% to 27% by early adulthood.[17,18] On average, teen females acquire approximately 2.5 lbs (1.14 kg) of fat mass each year during puberty. While the accretion of body fat is a biologically fundamental process, teens often view it with trepidation. Weight dissatisfaction is very prevalent among adolescent females, resulting in an increased risk of engaging in health-compromising behaviors such as chronic dieting, use of diet pills or laxatives, severe restriction of energy intake, body image distortions and disordered eating behaviors.

Table 4.2 illustrates body mass index percentile (BMI) cut points for determining appropriateness of weight-for-height among adolescent females. When weight-for-height is below the 5th percentile, biological growth and development may be

TABLE 4.2
BMI Percentile Cutpoints to Determine At-Risk of Overweight and Overweight Among Adolescent Females, By Age

Age (y)	85th percentile (At risk of overweight)	95th percentile (Overweight)
10	20	23
11	21	25
12	22	26
13	23	27
14	24	28
15	24	29
16	25	29
17	25	30
18	26	30
19	26	30

Source: Adapted from: Himes JH, Dietz WH. Guidelines for overweight in adolescent preventive services: recommendations from an expert committee. *Am J Clin Nutr* 59:307–316; 1994.

compromised. A thorough medical assessment should be completed to investigate the possibility of metabolic disorders or the prevalence of eating disorders. When weight for height is above the 85th percentile, but below the 95th percentile, an adolescent is considered to be at risk for overweight. Adolescents with a BMI at or above the 95th percentile are considered to be overweight. In both instances, teens should be referred for a complete medical examination to rule out potential medical complications such as hypertension, insulin resistance, hyperlipidemia, type 2 diabetes, orthopedic disorders, hypoventilation disorders or depression.

The broad chronological age range during which biological growth and development begins and advances can become a significant source of personal dissatisfaction for many adolescents as they struggle to conform to their peers. For females, early maturation is often associated with poor body image, poor self-esteem, frequent dieting and, possibly, disturbed or disordered eating behaviors.[19,20] Early menarche in females has been associated with increased risk of developing adolescent and adult obesity as well as associated medical complications.[4,18] Early maturing female teens are also at increased risk for engaging in health-compromising behaviors such as smoking, drinking alcohol and early sexual intercourse.[19,21]

III. NORMAL PSYCHOSOCIAL AND COGNITIVE DEVELOPMENT

Psychosocial and cognitive development is usually divided into three distinct developmental periods:

1. Early adolescence (11 to 14 years)
2. Middle adolescence (15 to 17 years)
3. Late adolescence (18 to 21 years) (see Figure 4.1).

Each developmental period is marked by the mastery of new emotional, cognitive and social skills that can affect food choices and preferences as well as nutrient needs. It is essential that health professionals who work with teens develop an appreciation for how psychosocial and cognitive development relate to biological growth and development and how these processes affect nutritional intake.

The initial stage of adolescence is a period of extensive cognitive advancement largely dominated by concrete thinking, egocentrism and impetuous behavior. The ability to utilize abstract reasoning skills is not substantially developed in most young adolescents, limiting their capability to grasp nutrition and health relationships. Young teens also lack the knowledge required to problem solve when trying to overcome obstacles to behavior change and are often unable to comprehend how present behaviors can affect future health status.

Biological growth and development is largely accomplished during early adolescence. The dramatic changes in body shape, size and composition that occur can lead to body image dissatisfaction among females. Peer acceptance becomes more important in adolescence than in previous developmental stages and the desire to "fit in" can exacerbate body image issues among young adolescents.

Mid-adolescence is distinguished by growth in emotional autonomy and emergent detachment from family. The majority of physical growth and development is accomplished during this phase, but body image issues may continue to be a source of anxiety, especially among females who have experienced a rapid transformation in body composition and size. Disagreements over personal food choices become increasingly common throughout this period of adolescence. Peer groups become more significant than family and their impact with regard to making food choices peaks. Concurrent with the increased importance of peer acceptance during middle adolescence is the initiation of health-compromising behaviors such as smoking, drinking alcohol, using street drugs and engaging in sexual activities. Teens in the middle adolescence phase may believe themselves to be indestructible and often exhibit impulsive behaviors.

Abstract reasoning abilities begin to become apparent during middle adolescence, but these skills may not be highly developed in many teens. Adolescents frequently revert to concrete thinking skills when confronted with strong emotions or difficult situations. Teenagers begin to grasp the relationship between current behaviors and future health conditions; however, their desire to fit in with peers may supersede their ability to make choices based on health rather than peer pressure.

The last stage of adolescent psychosocial development is characterized by the formation of a strong personal identity. Biological growth and development has concluded and body image concerns are less prevalent. Older teens are able to handle increasingly sophisticated social circumstances, are able to restrain impulsive behaviors and are less influenced by peer pressure. Monetary and emotional reliance upon family decreases, as do disagreements over personal issues, such as food choices. Relationships with specific individuals become more important than those with a group of peers and an innate sense of personal uniqueness emerges.

The development of abstract reasoning abilities continues during late adolescence, which aids in comprehending how present behaviors affect long-term health status. This is an especially critical skill for teen females who plan to have children or who become pregnant. Older teens are now able to learn problem-solving skills that can aid them in overcoming barriers to behavior change.

IV. HEALTH IMPLICATIONS OF COMMON EATING BEHAVIORS OF ADOLESCENT FEMALES

The eating behaviors of adolescent females are influenced by a myriad of factors that include peer pressure, taste preferences, food costs, convenience, cultural and moral beliefs, media messages and parental behaviors. Focus groups with adolescent females have shown that the most important influences on food choices of teens include cravings, preferences, preparation time and convenience.[22] Other factors that were reported as important influences on food choices included easy access to foods, parental influences, social situations (who they ate with or where they ate) and perceived health benefits. Reported barriers to improving dietary choices included the perception that dairy products, fruits and vegetables didn't taste as good as other foods; that eating establishments frequented by teens didn't offer healthy food choices; that healthful foods cost more; and that fruits and vegetables weren't as convenient as other food choices.[22]

Other barriers to making more healthful food choices are directly related to psychosocial development issues. One particularly common issue among young adolescents is the inability to comprehend the abstract relationship between eating habits and long-term health outcomes. Many teens feel that healthy eating habits are something they will need to worry about only later in life when chronic health problems become apparent. The increasing need for autonomy and independence that is central to adolescent psychosocial development also influences food choices of teen females. The consumption of "junk food" is seen as an integral part of being an adolescent; to stop eating "junk food" would be to give up part of one's emerging identity. Similar connotations exist for fast-food consumption among adolescents. Fast-food-restaurant visits by teens account for almost one third of all food eaten away from home.[23] In addition to fast foods' being associated with independence, fast-food restaurants are also major employers of teens, which increases their social acceptability.

A common eating behavior among adolescent females that has negative nutritional consequences is meal skipping. Breakfast is the most common meal skipped by teens. The frequency of skipping breakfast increases with age; while only 15% of 9- to 13-year-old girls skip breakfast, that number rises to 34% among 14- to 18-year-old females.[24] Lunch is the second most commonly skipped meal; almost one fourth of teens skip lunch.[24] Adolescents who skip meals, particularly breakfast, have been found to be two to five times more likely to have inadequate dietary intakes than teens who don't.[25] Teens who skip meals are at particularly high risk for inadequate intakes of calcium, folate and iron — three nutrients that are very important to short-term and long-term health. Fasting and restricting calories in an attempt to reduce weight are behaviors that are inextricably linked to meal skipping among female teens.

Snacking is another common eating behavior among adolescents. The proportion of energy and nutrients obtained from snacking has increased substantially during the past 30 years.[26] Snacks provide up to one-third of daily caloric intake among adolescents.[23] Surveys of teens have demonstrated that most consume between one and seven snacks per day, with most of the choices being high in fat or sugar and relatively low in micronutrients.[27,28] Teens cite lack of access to healthy food choices, cost, taste preference and convenience as factors that influence their snack choices.[22]

Restricting calories to lose weight, or dieting, is perhaps the most common eating behavior of adolescent females. Results of a national survey show that 59% of high school-aged females reported they had dieted while trying to lose weight during the month preceding the survey.[29] An alarming 19% of these young women had gone without food for 24 or more hours, 11% had used diet pills and 8% had taken laxatives or vomited to lose weight.[29] Dissatisfaction with body shape or size, which results from the rapid biological changes that occur during puberty, predisposes female teens to the development of food-restricting behaviors. As dieting behaviors become more drastic, as in the use of laxatives, diuretics and vomiting to lose weight, the risk of development of an eating disorder increases. Females who report severe dieting behaviors have been found to be at 18 times greater risk and those who are "moderate" dieters appear to be at five times greater risk for the development of eating disorders than teens who do not diet.[30] Dieting is considered the most important predictor of newly diagnosed cases of eating disorders among teens.

V. FOOD AND NUTRIENT INTAKE AND ADEQUACY AMONG ADOLESCENT FEMALES

Data on food intakes of U.S. adolescents indicate that many females do not consume diets consistent with the Dietary Guidelines for Americans, the Food Guide Pyramid, or the Healthy People 2010 recommendations.[7,8] National data suggest that only 1% of teens meet recommendations for all food groups in the Food Guide Pyramid;[31] a full 18% of female adolescents do not meet any of the Food Guide Pyramid recommendations. Of particular concern is the limited consumption of fruits, vegetables, dairy products and whole grains within this age group.

Few adolescents meet or exceed the Five-a-Day recommendations for fruit and vegetable consumption. Krebs-Smith and colleagues found that 64% of female teens consume less than one serving of fruit per day.[32] Fruit consumption also appears to decline with increasing age during adolescence.[31] Analyses of vegetable intake indicate that 13% of female adolescents consume less than one serving of vegetables per day. However, when French fries are excluded from analyses, the number doubles to 26%; french fries alone account for 23% of all vegetables consumed by adolescents.[32] Vegetable intake among youths increased slightly between the 1989–91 and 1994–96 CSFII surveys, resulting in a slight increase in total fruit and vegetable intake from 3.7 to 4.1 servings per day.[24]

Dairy product consumption by adolescents is declining, according to CSFII data. Mean daily consumption of milk and milk products dropped from 2.4 to 2.0 servings per day between the 1989–91 and 1994–95 surveys.[24,33] During that same time period, intake of soft drinks/soda increased from 1.0–1.4 servings per day while intake of fruit drinks increased from 0.5–0.8 servings per day.

Consumption of whole grain products by teens is also of concern. Although consumption of grain products by adolescents has increased overall, consumption of whole grains appears to be quite limited.[24]

Obviously, if minimum recommendations for food group intakes are not being met, specific nutrient recommendations are not being achieved. A few nutrients are of special concern within the adolescent female population due to the increased likelihood of underconsumption and increased risk of associated adverse health consequences. Statistics regarding calcium consumption are particularly troublesome; only 20% of female adolescents meet the recommended dietary intakes for calcium.[34] Iron is another nutrient of concern; approximately 40% of adolescent females actually meet the recommended dietary intake for iron.[34] Folate is a nutrient of paramount importance to females, particularly as they enter the childbearing years. Only about 17% of adolescent females consume recommended levels of folate each day.[34]

The implication from existing national data is that the average diet consumed by female adolescents is not adequate to promote optimal health or to reduce the risk of adult chronic diseases such as cancer, osteoporosis and cardiovascular disease. Clearly, adolescent females do not consume diets that comply with national nutrition recommendations or provide the recommended level of intakes for many food groups.

While intakes of many vital nutrients are suboptimal, consumption of fat and refined sugar surpass recommended maximum levels. Although fat intake as a percentage of calories has declined over time, absolute fat intakes have remained fairly stable and adolescent females continue to consume diets that surpass upper limits of recommended fat intakes.[24,33] National data suggest that adolescent females obtain approximately 33% of energy intake from fat, with 12% of energy derived from saturated fatty acids.[35] Approximately two thirds of adolescent females consume diets that exceed recommendations for total and saturated fat.[35] Consumption of refined sugars has increased among the adolescent population; this coincides with the surge in soft drink and other sweetened beverage popularity.[24,33] Soft drinks are a major source of added sweeteners in the diets of adolescents, accounting for as much as 15% of all energy consumed.[15] Research indicates that soft drinks are displacing milk in the diet; this creates a concern not only for increased sugar consumption, but also for decreased calcium intakes.[33,36]

VI. NUTRITIONAL REQUIREMENTS OF ADOLESCENT FEMALES

The Dietary Reference Intakes (DRIs) provide the best estimates of nutrient requirements for adolescent females (Table 4.3)[37] and can serve as a benchmark by which to assess the quality of an individual teen's dietary intake. However, it should be noted that most nutrient requirements for adolescents are not based on experimental data specific to teens. Rather, they are based on median intakes of energy and nutrients among cohorts of teenagers, or are extrapolated from adult experimental

TABLE 4.3
Dietary Reference Intakes for Adolescent Females

	FEMALES			PREGNANCY	
	9-13 y	14-18 y	10-30 y	≤ 18 y	19-30 y
Calcium (mg/d)	1,300*	1,300*	1,000*	1,300*	1,000*
Phosphorus (mg/d)	1,250	1,250	700	1,250	700
Magnesium (mg/d)	240	360	310	400	350
Vitamin D (μg/d)[a,b]	5*	5*	5*	5*	5*
Fluoride (mg/d)	2*	3*	3*	3*	3*
Thiamin (mg/d)	0.9	1.0	1.1	1.4	1.4
Riboflavin (mg/d)	0.9	1.0	1.1	1.4	1.4
Niacin (mg/d)[c]	12	14	14	18	18
Vitamin B_6 (mg/d)	1.0	1.2	1.3	1.9	1.9
Folate (μg/d)	300	400[e]	**400**[e]	600	600
Vitamin B_{12} (μg/d)	1.8	2.4	2.4	2.6	2.6
Pantothenic Acid (mg/d)	4*	5*	5*	6*	6*
Biotin (μg/d)	20*	25*	30*	30*	30*
Choline[d] (mg/d)	375*	400*	425*	450*	450*
Vitamin C (mg/d)	45	65	75	80	85
Vitamin E (mg/d)	11	15	15	15	15
Selenium (μg/d)	40	55	55	60	60

Note: This table presents Recommended Dietary Allowances (RDAs) in **bold type** and Adequate Intakes (AIs) in ordinary type followed by an asterisk (*). RDAs and AIs may both be used as goals for individual intake. RDAs are set to meet the needs of almost all (97 to 98%) individuals in a group. For healthy and breastfed infants, the AI is the mean intake. The AI for other life stage and gender groups is believed to cover needs of all individuals in the group, but lack of data or uncertainty in the data prevent being able to specify with confidence the percentage of individuals covered by this intake.

[a] As cholecalciferol. 1 μg cholecalciferol=40 IU vitamin D.

[b] In the absence of adequate exposure to sunlight.

[c] As niacin equivalents (NE). 1 mg of niacin = 60 mg tryptophan; 0–6 months = preformed niacin (not NE).

[d] Although AIs have been set for choline, there are few data to assess whether a dietary supplement of choline is needed at all stages of the life cycle and it may be that the choline requirement can be met by endogenous synthesis at some of these stages.

[e] In view of evidence linking folate intake with neural tube defects in the fetus, it is recommended that all women capable of becoming pregnant consume 400 μg from supplements or fortified food until their pregnancy is confirmed and they enter prenatal care, which ordinarily occurs after the end of the periconceptional period — the critical time for formation of the neural tube.

Source: Food and Nutrition Board, Institute of Medicine, National Academies. Dietary Reference Intakes: Recommended Intakes for Individuals. Washington, D.C.: National Academy Press, 2000.

data. In addition, the DRIs are categorized by chronological age as opposed to SMR, and need to be applied judiciously when assessing the diet of an individual adolescent. Clinical assessment of SMR will provide a better indication of the actual nutrient needs of a teen than will chronological age.

A. ENERGY

Energy needs of female teens are highest during the pubertal growth spurt (approximately 12 years of age), dropping to levels consistent with adult needs as biological growth is concluded. The assessment of individual energy requirements is often difficult due the variety of biological, environmental and metabolic factors that influence energy needs. The RDAs for energy for adolescent females (Table 4.3)[38] can be used as a reference point when assessing the adequacy of caloric intake; however, measures of growth and development should also be taken into account. Energy intakes of girls have been found to correlate well with stages of physiological development, but not with chronological age.[15] Therefore, the use of kcal per cm of height or kg of weight may serve as better predictors of individual energy needs than the RDAs for many females. Table 4.4 lists recommended energy needs based on the RDAs as well as those based on height and weight increments.

Growth can be used as a gross indicator of sufficiency of energy intake. When energy intake is insufficient to meet metabolic needs, weight loss occurs and growth and development will be retarded or delayed. When energy intake is in excess of that required for growth and development, increases in body fatness will occur and BMI will increase. It should be noted that transient increases in body fatness and BMI are common during puberty when the peak velocity of weight gain precedes or supersedes that of linear growth. If BMI percentile increases significantly prior to menarche during puberty and remains elevated for more than 8 to 12 months after menarche, excessive energy intake should be investigated.

B. PROTEIN

Protein needs are elevated during adolescence to support biological growth and development, with the highest requirements corresponding to peak rates of weight gain and linear growth (Table 4.4).[14,38] National dietary surveys suggest that, as a group, adolescent females consume adequate amounts of protein to support growth

---

TABLE 4.4
Estimated Energy and Protein Needs of Adolescent Females Based on Biological Growth Parameters

Age (yrs)	Energy		Protein
	Kcals/cm	Kcals/kg	G/cm
11-14	14.0	47	0.29
15-18	13.5	40	0.26
19-24	13.4	38	0.28

Source: Table compiled from Gong EJ, Heard FP. Diet, nutrition and adolescence. In: Shils ME, Olson JA, Shike M, Eds. *Modern Nutrition in Health and Disease.* 8th ed. Philadelphia, PA: Lea & Febiger; 1994:759–769 and *Recommended Dietary Allowances,* 10th ed. Washington, D.C.: National Research Council Subcommittee on the 10th edition of the RDAs, Food and Nutrition Board, Commission on Life Sciences, National Academy Press; 1989.

and development.[39,40] Subgroups of teens who may be at risk for poor protein intake include those living in food-insecure households or temporary housing, those that adhere to a vegan or macrobiotic vegetarian diet and those who severely restrict calories.

The rate of pubertal biological growth and development is sensitive to protein intake. When protein intakes fall below minimal requirements, weight gain and linear growth can be compromised. Sustained deficiencies in protein can result in reductions of lean body mass. Teens with a BMI at or below the fifth percentile should be referred for a medical evaluation to determine the presence of metabolic syndromes, eating disorders or indicators of protein malnutrition.

C. CARBOHYDRATES AND FIBER

Absolute recommendations for carbohydrate intake based on biological growth and development or chronological age have not been established. Current dietary guidance suggests that teens consume at least 50% of total calories from carbohydrate, with an emphasis on complex carbohydrates.[41] Complex forms of carbohydrate are major sources of dietary fiber for most teens. Using the "age plus five" rule for determining fiber intakes results in estimated fiber requirements for 12- to 21-year-old females of between 17 and 26 grams of fiber.[42]

National surveys suggest adolescents consume approximately 55% of total energy from carbohydrates and 13 grams of dietary fiber each day.[24] However, sweeteners and added sugars provide almost 20% of energy consumed by teens, with soft drinks and other sweetened beverages providing up to 15% of energy alone.[15] Consumption of complex carbohydrates — especially whole grain products, fruits and vegetables — among adolescent females falls below national recommendations, resulting in only 15 to 24% of teenaged females meeting or exceeding their daily fiber requirements.[24]

D. DIETARY FAT

Absolute requirements for dietary fat do not exist for adolescents. Instead, dietary guidance suggests that 20 to 30% of total energy consumed should come from dietary fat, with not more than 10% of total energy derived from saturated fats.[43,44] The lower limit of fat intake is meant to assure an adequate intake of essential fatty acids to support rapid rates of physiological growth and development during adolescence, while the upper limit is meant to reduce adult risk of cardiovascular disease. National survey data estimate that adolescent females derive 32% of daily energy intake from total fat and 11 to 12% from saturated fat.[24] Frequent consumption of fast-food meals and savory snacks is related to excess fat consumption among adolescents.

E. VITAMINS AND MINERALS

The DRIs for vitamins and minerals are listed in Table 4.3.[45] In general, adolescent females have poor intakes of calcium, iron, zinc, magnesium, folate and vitamins A and E.[46] Teens at highest risk for inadequate intakes of vitamins and minerals are those who restrict calories, those who cut out entire food groups (such as dairy products) and those who frequently skip meals. Common advice given to adolescents with poor dietary intake is to rely on vitamin and mineral supplements to supply missing nutrients, however, research suggests that teen females with poor diets are less likely to use these supplements than are those with more well-balanced diets.[46] Therefore, it is important to focus on dietary strategies to improve vitamin and mineral intakes of female adolescents.

F. CALCIUM

Calcium needs of females are higher during adolescence than at any other time in life due to the very rapid rates of bone mineralization that occur between 10 and 20 years of age. The Adequate Intake for calcium is 1300 mg/day for females 9 to 18 years old;[37] however, much debate exists over the adequacy of that level to meet the needs of growing teenaged females. The National Institute of Health, Consensus Development Conference Statement on Optimal Calcium Intake recommends an intake of 1200 to 1500 mg of calcium per day for 11- to 24-year-old females.[47]

Most adolescent females do not consume even marginally adequate levels of calcium. Population survey data suggest that teen females consume about half of the DRI for calcium each day.[24] Calcium intakes have decreased substantially during the past two decades as consumption of milk and dairy products has decreased.[24] In addition, calcium consumption decreases with age during adolescence. Survey data suggest that soft drinks and other sweetened beverages may displace milk in the diets of children and adolescents and that the frequency of this displacement increases with age.[24,36] In light of the decrease in fluid milk consumption, calcium-fortified foods are likely to become increasingly important sources of this nutrient. Survey data suggest that as many as half of teens reported drinking calcium-fortified juices and almost one third ate calcium-fortified cereals.[48] The fortification of breads, cereals, margarine, juices and other beverages with calcium may become an important public health strategy to improve bone health among youths and women.

G. IRON

Iron requirements are increased during adolescence in response to requirements to support linear growth as well as to replace losses that occur during menses. Daily iron needs are estimated at 15 mg/day for female teens during the peak growth spurt and at 13 to 15 mg/day after menarche.[49] Adolescent females typically consume between 10 and 12 mg of iron per day through dietary sources.[50] Research suggests that as many as half of female adolescents do not consume recommended levels of dietary iron.[24]

The failure to consume adequate dietary iron results in compromised iron stores, followed by the occurrence of iron deficiency anemia.[51] Table 4.5 lists indicators of iron status for 12- to 18-year-old females. Estimates of iron deficiency anemia suggest that 9 to 11% of adolescent females are iron deficient,[51,52] while as many as 25% demonstrate one or more clinical indicators of low iron stores.[50] Two to three percent of teenaged females meet the criteria for iron deficiency anemia.[51]

TABLE 4.5
Indicators of Iron Deficiency for 12- to 18-Year-Old Females

	Hemoglobin < g/dL	Hematocrit <%
12 to < 15 yrs	11.8	35.7
15 to < 18 yrs	12	35.9
≥ 18 yrs	12	35.7

Source: Data from Centers for Disease Control and Prevention. Recommendations to prevent and control iron deficiency in the United States. *Morb. Mortal. Wkly. Rep.* 47 (No. RR-3); 1998.

Iron deficiency has been associated with fatigue, impaired temperature regulation, decreased athletic performance, increased risk of infection and compromised growth during adolescence.[15,53] Halterman et al.[52] found that average math scores were lower among youths with iron deficiency, than in peers with adequate iron stores. Other researchers have demonstrated that supplementation of iron-deficient teen females resulted in increased verbal learning and memory abilities.[54]

H. ZINC

Zinc is required for RNA, DNA and protein synthesis. Inadequate intakes of zinc during childhood and adolescence have been shown to delay sexual development and retard growth. Supplementation of zinc appears to accelerate growth and sexual maturation in youths from developing countries who experience zinc deficiency. Data on zinc intakes of U.S. teens suggest that fewer than half of 14- to 18-year-old females meet the DRI for zinc (Table 4.3).[24] Serum zinc levels indicative of subclinical zinc deficiency have been reported to occur in 18 to 33% of female teens.[50] Adolescent females at highest risk for inadequate intakes of zinc include those who consume vegetarian diets, those who live in food-insecure homes or temporary housing and those who frequently skip meals or restrict energy intake.

I. FOLATE

Due to its role in RNA, DNA and protein synthesis, folate requirements are elevated during adolescence (Table 4.3).[37] While the DRIs suggest that folate requirements of 9- to 13-year-old females are 300 mcg/day and the needs of 14- to 18-year-old females are 400 mcg/day,[37] it is currently recommended that all females of childbearing age consume at least 400 mcg of folate each day.[55] This level of intake is believed to reduce the risk of neural tube defects among offspring in the event of pregnancy. Therefore, all adolescent females who have experienced menarche should be counseled to consume at least 400 mcg of folate daily, regardless of their chronological age. Daily intake of folate falls short of recommended levels for most teen females. National data suggest that 14- to 18-year-old females consume 54% of the DRI for folate, far short of levels suggested in national nutrition guidelines.[24] Teens who skip meals (especially breakfast), restrict energy intake, or have low intakes of fruit and vegetables are at highest risk for inadequate intakes of folate.

VII. IMPLICATIONS FOR NUTRITION INTERVENTION

Because adolescence is a time of tremendous psychosocial and cognitive development, nutrition interventions need to be tailored to the developmental level of each individual adolescent. Health professionals should allow adequate time during nutrition education sessions to determine their students' degree of biological maturity and level of cognitive development. These characteristics should be used to determine the individual nutritional needs and the type of educational messages given when counseling the adolescent.

Nutrition interventions for teens should focus on values that are important to adolescents, such as being attractive, having "a lot of energy," being a good student, becoming autonomous and "fitting in." When dietary changes are put into the context of meeting these values, adolescents are more likely to become engaged in learning and to adopt behavior changes. Because fast foods and snacking are seen as integral parts of adolescence by many teens, providing examples of healthy fast-food and snack choices will be more likely to result in behavior change than telling teenagers to stop eating fast foods or snacks.

Nutrition education messages need to be concrete in nature, providing very specific examples of suggested behavior changes. For instance, instead of advising an adolescent to "eat snacks that contain less fat," it is more useful to provide a list of lower fat snacks that would be acceptable to teens. Providing simple guidelines for making healthful choices is also useful. Advising a teen to choose only snack foods with 5 grams or less of fat per serving is much easier for an adolescent to comprehend than simply telling the teen to choose lower-fat foods.

VIII. CONCLUSIONS

Adolescence is a time of dramatic emotional, psychological and physiological changes. For this reason, nutritional needs of teenagers are best determined in relation to biological development instead of according to chronological age. Diets of teenaged females are, on average, inadequate in whole grains, dairy products, fruits and vegetables and are often high in total and saturated fat and sugars. Micronutrients likely to be lacking among adolescent females include calcium, iron, zinc, magnesium, folate and vitamins A and E. The lack of abstract reasoning skills, especially in early adolescence, results in the inability of many teens to comprehend relationships between dietary choices and health. Therefore, nutrition interventions need to focus on values that are important to teens, including physical appearance, energy and academic achievement.

ACKNOWLEDGMENTS

This manuscript was supported by Grant # 2MCJ 009118-11-0 from the Maternal and Child Health Bureau, Health Resources and Services Administration, U.S. Department of Health and Human Services.

REFERENCES

1. Centers for Disease Control and Prevention. Guidelines for school health programs to promote lifelong healthy eating. *Morb. Mortal. Wkly. Rep.* 45:1–37, 1996.

2. Stang J. Adolescent Nutrition: Conditions and Intervention. In: Brown J (Ed). *Nutrition Through the Lifecycle*, Belmont, CA: Wadsworth/Thomson Learning; 355–381, 2002.

3. Gortmaker SL, Must A, Perrin JM, Sobol AM and Dietz WH. Social and economic consequences of overweight in adolescence and young adulthood. *New Engl. J. Med.* 329:1008–1012, 1993.

4. Guo SS, Roche AF, Chumlea WC, Gardner JD and Siervogel RM. The predictive value of childhood body mass index values for overweight at age 35 y. *Am. J. Clin. Nutr.* 59:810–819, 1994.

5. Wright CM, Parker L, Lamont D and Craft AW. Implications of childhood obesity for adult health: findings from Thousand Families Cohort Study. *Br. Med. J.* 323:1280–1284, 2001.

6. Centers for Disease Control and Prevention. Guidelines for school and community programs to promote lifelong physical activity among young people. *Morb. Mortal. Wkly. Rep.* 46:1–36, 1997.

7. U.S. Department of Health and Human Services. Healthy People 2010: Conference Edition, Vol I. Washington, DC, 2000.

8. U.S. Department of Health and Human Services. Healthy People 2010: Conference Edition, Vol II. Washington, DC, 2000.

9. Murphy JM, Pagano ME, Nachmani J, Sperling P, Kane S and Kleinman RE. The relationship of school breakfast to psychosocial and academic functioning: cross-sectional and longitudinal observations in an inner-city school sample. *Arch. Pediatr. Adolesc. Med.* 152:899–907, 1998.

10. Kleinman RE, Hall S, Green H, Korsec-Ramirez D, Patten K, Pagano M and Murphy JM. Diet, breakfast and academic performance in children. *Ann. Nutr. Metab.*, in press.

11. Neumark-Sztainer D, Story M, Toporoff E, Himes JH, Resnick MD and Blum RW. Covariations of eating behaviors with other health-related behaviors among adolescents. *J. Adolesc. Health* 20:450–458, 1997.

12. Lytle L and Achterberg C. Changing the diet of America's children: What works and why? *J. Nutr. Educ.* 27:250–260, 1995.

13. Slap GB. Normal physiological and psychosocial growth in the adolescent. *J Adolesc Health Care* 7:13S-23S, 1986.

14. Gong EJ and Heard FP. Diet, nutrition, and adolescence. In: Shils ME, Olson JA and Shike M (Eds). *Modern Nutrition in Health and Disease*, 8th ed., Philadelphia, PA: Lead & Febiger; pp. 759–769, 1994.

15. Spear BA. Adolescent growth and development. *J. Am. Diet. Assoc.* 102:S23-29, 2002.

16. Barnes HV. Physical growth and development during puberty. *Med. Clin. North Am.* 59:1305–1317, 1975.

17. Frisch RE. Fatness, puberty and fertility: The effects of nutrition and physical training on menarche and ovulation. In: Brooks-Gunn J and Peterson AC (Eds.). *Girls at Puberty: Biological and Psychosocial Perspectives,* New York, NY: Plenum Press; pp. 29–49, 1983.

18. Frisch RE and McArthur JW. Menstrual cycles: fatness as a determinant of minimum weight for height necessary for their maintenance or onset. *Science* 185:949–951, 1974.

19. Killen JD, Hayward C, Litt I, Hammer LD, Wilson DM, Miner B, Taylor CB, Varady A and Shisslak C. Is puberty a risk factor for eating disorders? *Am. J. Dis. Child.* 146:323–325, 1992.

20. Attie I and Brooks-Gunn J. Development of eating problems in adolescent girls: A longitudinal study. *Dev. Psychol.* 25:70–79, 1989.

21. Wilson DM, Killen JD, Hayward C, Robinson TN, Hammer LD, Kraemer HC, Varady A and Taylor CB. Timing and rate of sexual maturation and the onset of cigarette and alcohol use among teenage girls. *Arch. Pediatr. Adolesc. Med.* 148:789–795, 1994.

22. Neumark-Sztainer D, Story M, Perry C and Casey MA. Factors influencing food choices of adolescents: findings from focus group discussions with adolescents. *J. Am. Diet. Assoc.* 99:929–937, 1999.

23. Story M and Stang J (Eds.). *Adolescent Nutrition Guidelines,* Minneapolis, MN: Center for Leadership, Education and Training in Maternal and Child Health, in press.

24. Gleason P and Suiter CW. Changes in children's diets: 1989–1991 to 1994–1996. U.S. Department of Agriculture Food and Nutrition Service, Alexandria, VA, 2001.

25. Nicklas TA, Myers L, Reger C, Beech B and Berenson GS. Impact of breakfast consumption on nutritional adequacy of the diets of young adults in Bogalusa, Louisiana: Ethnic and gender contrasts. *J. Am. Diet. Assoc.* 98:1432–1438, 1998.

26. Jahns L, Siega-Riz AM and Popkin BM. The increasing prevalence of snacking among U.S. children from 1977 to 1996. *J. Pediatr.* 138:493–498, 2001.

27. American School Health Association, Association for the Advancement of Health Education, Society for Public Health Education, The National Adolescent Student Health Survey. A report on the health of America's youth, Oakland, CA: Third Party Publication Co.; 1988.

28. Bigler-Doughten S and Jenkins RM. Adolescent snacks: Nutrient density and nutritional contribution to total intake. *J. Am. Diet. Assoc.* 87:1678–1679, 1987.

29. Kann L, Kinchen SA, Williams BI, Ross JG, Lowry R, Grunbaum JA and Kolbe LJ. Youth Risk Behavior Surveillance--United States, 1999. *Morb. Mortal. Wkly. Rep* 49:81, 2000.

30. Patton GC, Selzer R, Coffey C, Carlin JB and Wolfe R. Onset of adolescent eating disorders: population based cohort study over 3 years. *Br. Med. J.* 318:765–768, 1999.

31. Munoz KA, Krebs-Smith SM, Ballard-Barbash R and Cleveland LE. Food intakes of U.S. children and adolescents compared with recommendations [published erratum appears in *Pediatrics* 1998; 101(5):952–3]. *Pediatrics* 100:323–329, 1997.

32. Krebs-Smith SM, Cook A, Subar AF, Cleveland L, Friday J and Kahle LL. Fruit and vegetable intakes of children and adolescents in the United States. *Arch. Pediatr. Adolesc. Med.* 150:81–86, 1996.

33. Morton JF and Guthrie JF. Changes in children's total fat intakes and their food group sources of fat, 1989–91 versus 1994–95: Implications for diet quality. *Family Econ. Nutr. Rev.* 11:44–57, 1998.

34. Cavadini C, Siega-Riz AM and Popkin BM. U.S. adolescent food intake trends from 1965 to 1996. *Arch. Dis. Child.* 83:18–24, 2000.

35. Kennedy E and Powell R. Changing eating patterns of American children: a view from 1996. *J. Am. Coll. Nutr.* 16:524–529, 1997.

36. Harnack L, Stang J and Story M. Soft drink consumption among U.S. children and adolescents: nutritional consequences. *J. Am. Diet. Assoc.* 99:436–441, 1999.

37. Yates AA, Schlicker SA and Suitor CW. Dietary Reference Intakes: the new basis for recommendations for calcium and related nutrients, B vitamins, and choline. *J. Am. Diet. Assoc.* 98:699–706, 1998.

38. National Research Council Food and Nutrition Board, Commission on Life Sciences. *Recommended Dietary Allowances,* 10th ed., Washington, DC: National Academy Press; 1989.
39. Devaney BL, Gordon AR and Burghardt JA. Dietary intakes of students. *Am. J. Clin. Nutr.* 61:205S-212S, 1995.
40. Kennedy E and Goldberg J. What are American children eating? Implications for public policy. *Nutr. Rev.* 53:111–126, 1995.
41. U.S. Department of Agriculture, U.S. Department of Health and Human Services. *Nutrition and your Health: Dietary Guidelines for Americans,* 5th ed., Washington, D.C.; 2000.
42. Williams CL, Bollella M and Wynder EL. A new recommendation for dietary fiber in childhood. *Pediatrics* 96:985–988, 1995.
43. National Heart Lung, and Blood Institute, National Cholesterol Education Program. Report of the Expert Panel on Blood Cholesterol Levels in Children and Adolescents. Bethesda, MD, National Institutes of Health; 1991.
44. American Academy of Pediatrics Committee on Nutrition. Cholesterol in childhood. *Pediatrics* 101:141–147, 1998.
45. Institute of Medicine Food and Nutrition Board. Dietary Reference Intakes: Recommended Intakes for Individuals. Washington, DC, National Academy Press; 2000.
46. Stang J, Story MT, Harnack L and Neumark-Sztainer D. Relationships between vitamin and mineral supplement use, dietary intake, and dietary adequacy among adolescents. *J. Am. Diet. Assoc.* 100:905–910, 2000.
47. Consensus Development Conference Statement: Optimal Calcium Intake. Bethesda, MD: National Institutes of Health; 1994.
48. Harel Z, Riggs S, Vaz R, White L and Menzies G. Adolescents and calcium: what they do and do not know and how much they consume. *J. Adolesc. Hlth* 22:225–228, 1998.
49. Strasburger VC and Brown RT. *Adolescent Medicine: A Practical Guide* Little, Brown and Company, New York, NY, 1991.
50. Donovan UM and Gibson RS. Iron and zinc status of young women aged 14 to 19 years consuming vegetarian and omnivorous diets. *J. Am. Coll. Nutr.* 14:463–472, 1995.
51. Centers for Disease Control and Prevention. Recommendations to prevent and control iron deficiency in the U.S. *Morb. Mortal. Wkly. Rep.* 47:1–29, 1998.
52. Halterman JS, Kaczorowski JM, Aligne CA, Auinger P and Szilagyi PG. Iron deficiency and cognitive achievement among school-aged children and adolescents in the United States. *Pediatrics* 107:1381–1386, 2001.
53. Alton I. Iron deficiency anemia. In: Story M and Stang J (Eds). *Adolescent Nutrition Guidelines*, Minneapolis, MN: Center for Leadership, Education and Training in Maternal and Child Health, in press.
54. Bruner AB, Joffe A, Duggan AK, Casella JF and Brandt J. Randomised study of cognitive effects of iron supplementation in nonanaemic iron-deficient adolescent girls. *Lancet* 348:992–996, 1996.
55. Institute of Medicine. *Nutrition During Pregnancy: Part I, Weight Gain; Part II, Nutrient Supplements:* Washington, D.C., National Academy Press, 1990.

5 Premenstrual Syndrome: Nutritional Implications

Jaime S. Ruud and Bonnie Taub-Dix

CONTENTS

I. INTRODUCTION

Premenstrual syndrome (PMS) is a condition that has existed throughout history. Literary descriptions of premenstrual changes in women date as far back as 2600 years ago.[1] Accounts of rituals and beliefs surrounding premenstrual distress can also be found.

In recent years, a proliferation of interest and research on PMS has increased our knowledge of the diagnosis and management of this phenomenon. Many factors contribute to PMS and several nutritional, hormonal and psychosocial theories exist. Yet, PMS has not been clearly defined and the causes are still unknown.[2] In the meantime, PMS sufferers search for ways to cope with monthly physical and psychological symptoms.

II. DEFINITION

The symptom of what was originally known as "premenstrual tension" was first described by R.T. Frank in 1931.[3] He theorized that premenstrual tension was caused by high levels of female sex hormones in the blood. He used calcium lactate, either alone or in combination with caffeine preparations, to relieve symptoms.

In 1953, Greene and Dalton[4] changed the term to "premenstrual syndrome" because "tension is only one of the many components of the syndrome." They attributed symptoms of PMS to water retention caused by abnormal estrogen/progesterone ratios and treated the syndrome with progesterone.

Since that time, the definition and classification of PMS has been controversial. According to Reid,[5] PMS is "the cyclic recurrence in the late luteal phase of the menstrual cycle, of a combination of distressing physical, psychologic and/or behavioral changes of sufficient severity to result in deterioration of interpersonal relationships and/or interference with normal activities."

In 1994, the American Psychiatric Association (APA) concluded that severe PMS is actually a psychiatric disorder. It introduced a new definition, "premenstrual dysphoric disorder" (PMDD), to the appendix of the *Diagnostic and Statistical Manual of Mental Disorders*.[6] According to the APA's definition, the essential feature of PMDD is a pattern of clinically significant emotional and behavioral symptoms that occur during the last week of the luteal phase of the menstrual cycle and remit during the follicular phase. Diagnosis of PMDD is based on retrospective reports (past events and experiences). Two symptomatic cycles are needed to confirm the diagnosis. Preliminary data by Hurt et al.[7] indicated that between 14 and 45% of women with PMS in their study met the criteria for PMDD.

III. SYMPTOMS

PMS symptoms vary, ranging from mild to incapacitating. More than 150 symptoms have been attributed to PMS.[8–10] Smith and Schiff[11] categorized PMS symptoms into three groups: psychologic, physical and behavioral (Table 5.1). The most common complaints include abdominal bloating or pain, backache, headache, constipation, breast tenderness, food cravings (carbohydrates, sweets, chocolate, salt), fatigue, irritability and symptoms related to depression.

Bancroft and co-workers[12] studied four groups of women in terms of their perimenstrual complaints, menorrhagia (excessive bleeding) and dysmenorrhea (menstrual cramping) and found considerable overlap in a number of symptoms. However, the premenstrual group was significantly more depressed than the other two groups during the premenstrual phase. Other symptoms that stood out for the PMS group included food cravings and clumsiness. In another study, Siegel et al.,[13] evaluated symptoms in a group of women with severe PMS and reported two distinct clusters of emotional or behavioral symptoms, "withdrawn mood" and "anxious/tense mood." They noted two clusters of physical symptoms, as well, "physical discomfort" and "water retention."

TABLE 5.1
Criteria for Premenstrual Dysphoric Disorder

Feelings of sadness or hopelessness
Feelings of tension or anxiety
Mood swings marked by periods of teariness
Fatigue or low energy
Trouble concentrating
Change in appetite or binge eating
Insomnia or hypersomnia
Feeling out of control
Physical symptoms such as breast tenderness, swelling, headaches, joint or muscle pain
Symptoms seriously interfere with daily activity and/or relationships

Adapted from Stearns, S., PMS and PMDD in the domain of mental health nursing, *J. Psychosoc. Nurs. Mental Health Serv.*, 38, 16, 2001.

To further complicate matters, PMS complaints may also be the result of an underlying disease. Thyroid disease, hyperprolactinemia, diabetes mellitus and hypoglycemia can cause physical and psychological symptoms similar to PMS.[14]

IV. MENSTRUAL CYCLE

To better understand PMS, a review of the basic facts about menstruation is necessary. The average menstrual cycle lasts about 28 days, although cycles vary from woman to woman and even in the same woman at different times. The menstrual cycle can be divided into four phases: the menstrual phase (4 days beginning with the first day of menstruation); the follicular phase (the fifth day after menstruation to the periovulatory phase (4 days to the approximate time of ovulation); and the luteal phase (the days between the periovulatory phase and the day before the beginning of menstruation).[15]

During the follicular phase, estrogen and progesterone levels are low. The pituitary gland secretes follicle-stimulating hormone (FSH), which stimulates growth in one of the follicles in a woman's ovary. Toward the end of the follicular phase, estrogen levels increase, signaling the lining of the uterus to prepare for a fertilized egg. Rising estrogen levels stimulate the pituitary gland to secrete luteinizing hormone (LH), which causes the follicle to release the mature egg.

In the luteal phase, the follicle continues to secrete estrogen and the level of LH increases. This produces progesterone, the hormone responsible for changes in the uterine endometrium in the luteal phase of the menstrual cycle. If conception does not occur, hormone levels decrease and the lining of the uterus is shed by menstruation.

To be diagnosed with PMS, a woman's symptoms must correspond with the luteal phase and be absent during the follicular phase of the menstrual cycle. It is the timing of the appearance and disappearance of symptoms, rather than a specific symptom, that leads to the diagnosis of PMS. Two symptomatic cycles are needed and symptoms must be severe enough to disrupt normal daily activities.

V. PREVALENCE

The prevalence of PMS varies depending on the diagnostic tool used to measure symptoms. The Moos' Menstrual Distress Questionnaire (MDQ) is one of the most widely used self-rating instruments for diagnosis of PMS.[16] It requires women to rate 47 symptoms on a scale of one to six, with six being "acute or partially disabling." Woods et al.[17] administered the MDQ to a group of women and found 30% or more reported common PMS symptoms such as weight gain, cramps, anxiety, fatigue, painful breasts, mood swings or tension, although only 2 to 8% of women found these symptoms severe or disabling.

Fisher and colleagues[18] administered the Premenstrual Assessment Form (PAF) to 207 adolescent females. The PAF, developed by Halbreich et al.,[1] consists of 95 items describing premenstrual changes in mood, behavior and physical condition. Items are rated on a six-point scale, from "no change" to "extreme change."

Mortola et al.[20] developed a simple prospective inventory, the Calendar of Premenstrual Experiences, which includes the 10 most common physical and 12 most common behavioral (affective) symptoms of PMS. Each symptom is rated daily on a four-point Likert scale where symptom severity is based on interference with ability to perform daily activities. The calendar is a reliable and practical tool, applicable to some clinical and research settings.

Plouffe et al.[21] used the Calendar of Prospective Records to determine the number of women who met the criteria for PMS. A total of 43 women had previously been diagnosed as having PMS by other physicians. However, results showed that only 19 of those women were confirmed as having PMS. This study demonstrates the importance of appropriate prospective documentation.

In summary, there are several types of questionnaires used to rate PMS symptoms. Questionnaires can be retrospective, based on past events and experiences, or prospective, based on actual events as they occur. Although prospective measures are thought to underestimate symptom prevalences, retrospective measures may overestimate actual prevalence rates because of recall bias.[22]

VI. ETIOLOGY

The etiology of PMS is unknown, but the fact that PMS is a female disorder makes hormones a major suspect. Levels of estrogen and progesterone change dramatically the week before menstruation and thus can affect many psychological and physiological functions. This may explain why progesterone therapy is widely prescribed for PMS even though there are few well-controlled studies demonstrating its efficacy. Wyatt and co-workers[23] conducted a systematic review of published randomized placebo-controlled trials that assessed the efficacy of progesterone in the management of premenstrual syndrome. Their analysis showed no published evidence to support the use of progesterone in treating PMS.

Among American women, researchers have even speculated that symptoms of PMS are the result of learned attitudes and expectations. In a study by Ruble[24] in 1977, 44 women at Princeton University were told they were participating in a new technique for predicting the expected date of menstruation. Unknown to the subjects, the scheduled day of testing corresponded with the sixth or seventh day before her next period. Subjects were told they were either premenstrual (due in 1 or 2 days) or intermenstrual (due in 7 or 10 days). Women who were led to believe they were premenstrual reported a significantly higher degree of water retention, menstrual pain and changes in eating habits than did women who were led to believe they were intermenstrual. The results of this study demonstrate that psychosocial factors can influence self-reports of menstrual-related symptoms in some women.

Several other theories have been advanced for PMS including endogenous opiate withdrawal, prostaglandin deficiency, fluid retention and hypoglycemia.[11]

A. Serotonin Theory

There is increasing evidence that serotonin, the neurotransmitter synthesized from tryptophan, is important in the pathogenesis of PMS. Data have shown that, compared with a group of controls, PMS subjects had significantly lower serotonin blood levels during the last 10 days of the menstrual cycle,[25] which could account for some of the psychological symptoms of PMS such as depression, anxiety, sleeplessness, headaches and mental confusion. Low serotonin levels may also trigger early ovulation and a shift in estrogen and progesterone patterns, which could account for some of the physical symptoms of PMS such as breast tenderness, abdominal bloating, water retention, acne and food cravings.

Although it is not known exactly how a deficiency of serotonin relates to PMS symptoms, the amino acid tryptophan is involved. According to Fernstrom,[26] tryptophan and other large neutral amino acids such as valine, leucine and phenylalanine, compete for the same saturable carrier protein for transport across the blood–brain barrier. Data suggest that the ratio of plasma tryptophan to the sum of those competing amino acids predicts the level of tryptophan and thus serotonin levels in the brain.[26] Rapkin and co-workers[27] tested the hypothesis that diminution of central nervous system L-tryptophan uptake in women with PMS could account for the symptoms seen in the luteal phase of the menstrual cycle, although they found no significant differences between PMS and control subjects.

Tryptophan was a popular nutritional supplement for PMS, insomnia, depression and weight loss until it was linked to a blood disorder in 1989.[28] At that time, the Food and Administration (FDA) ordered a recall of all dietary supplements containing L-tryptophan because the rare blood disorder eosinophilia-myalgia syndrome was associated with the use of this amino acid.[28]

VII. NUTRITIONAL IMPLICATIONS

A. Vitamin B₆ Deficiency

Perhaps one of the most widely held nutritional theories regarding PMS is that it results from a deficiency of vitamin B_6 (Pyridoxine). As such, supplementation with vitamin B_6 has been a popular approach to treating PMS. Arguments for the use of vitamin B_6 are based on its role as a co-factor for several enzymes and its association with low levels of the neurotransmitter serotonin and depression.[29] Early studies[30,31] reported significant improvement in women receiving 100–250 mg of vitamin B_6/d compared with those receiving a placebo. More recent data shows that, while vitamin B_6 may be more effective than a placebo for treating the discomforts associated with PMS, there is not enough evidence to recommend its use.[32,33] Although the RDA for vitamin B_6 is 1.6 mg/d for women ages 19–50,[34] some women have been known to take 50–300 mg/d supplemented by a number of multivitamin preparations.[35] Because high intakes of vitamin B_6 (> 500 mg/d) can result in sensory neuropathy (nerve damage to the arms and legs),[36] caution is indicated and indiscriminate use is not advised. The Food and Nutrition Board of the Institute of Medicine has established an upper tolerable intake level (UL) for vitamin B_6 at 100 mg/d for all adults.[37] Vitamin B_6 is found in a wide variety of foods including fortified cereals, beans, meat, poultry, fish and some fruits and vegetables.

B. Vitamin E

Vitamin E (alpha-tocopherol) has also been implicated in PMS because of its effects on PMS symptoms through regulation of aberrant prostaglandin synthesis.[38] London and colleagues[38] conducted a double-blind study of 41 women with PMS and reported that daily treatment with 400 IU vitamin E per day was effective in reducing mood and physical symptoms, including breast tenderness. On the other hand, Chuong et al.[39] examined whether changes in vitamin E levels in the blood were associated with PMS symptoms and found no association.

Mira et al.[40] measured plasma levels of magnesium, zinc, vitamin A, and vitamin E in 38 women suffering from PMS and in a control group during the luteal phase and midfollicular phase. They found no evidence of nutritional deficiencies including vitamin E. They concluded that vitamin E supplementation can only be considered an empirical theory for PMS until further studies are conducted. The year 2000 RDA for vitamin E is 15 mg/d (22 IU) for women ages 19 and older.[41] Vegetable oils, nuts, fortified cereals, wheat germ and green leafy vegetables are the main dietary sources of vitamin E in the United States. The Institute of Medicine has set an upper tolerable intake level for vitamin E at 1000 mg (1,500 IU).[37]

C. Magnesium

Abraham and Lubran[42] theorized that a magnesium (Mg) deficiency may cause PMS. They reported significantly lower mean levels of serum magnesium in a group of PMS patients than in a control group. Magnesium is involved in the synthesis of dopamine and thus a deficiency may produce changes in behavior. Magnesium is also involved in the activity of serotonin, another pathway by which it may influence PMS.[33]

Magnesium supplementation has been reported successful in relieving pre-menstrual mood fluctuations in PMS sufferers. Facchinetti et al.[43] conducted a double-blind randomized study involving 28 women with confirmed PMS. For 2 months, magnesium carboxylate (360 mg) or a placebo was administered three times a day from the 15th day of the menstrual cycle to the onset of menstrual flow. Magnesium supplementation was shown to be more effective than the placebo in improvement of PMS mood, providing preliminary evidence that this nutrient may have pharmacologic benefits in instances of magnesium deficiency. Walker and colleagues[44] also studied the benefit of magnesium supplementation in a double-blind placebo-controlled crossover trial. Thirty-eight women with PMS received a daily supplement of 200 mg of magnesium or placebo for two cycles. No effects were reported at the end of the first month. However, the second month, there was a greater reduction in symptoms of swelling, breast tenderness and abdominal bloating. The study concluded that magnesium supplementation alleviates premenstrual symptoms of fluid retention.

Dietary intake of magnesium in the U.S. is generally lower than the RDA of 280 mg/d for women of reproductive age.[34] Alcohol abuse, vomiting, diarrhea, or endocrine disorders may contribute to a deficiency of magnesium. A balanced diet generally contains an adequate supply of magnesium. Good sources of magnesium include legumes, seeds, nuts and leafy green vegetables.

D. CALCIUM

The role of calcium in the treatment of PMS has been verified by Thys-Jacobs and colleagues.[45] They conducted a series of clinical trials to evaluate the treatment benefits of calcium supplementation.[46–48] Healthy premenopausal women aged 18–45 years with PMS were given either elemental calcium (1200 mg/d) in the form of calcium carbonate or placebo for three menstrual cycles. The calcium-treated group showed an overall 48% reduction in total symptom scores from baseline compared with an overall 30% reduction in the placebo group. The authors concluded that "calcium supplementation is a simple and effective treatment in PMS, resulting in a major reduction in overall luteal phase symptoms." Elemental calcium of 1200–1600 mg/d, unless contraindicated, is considered an appropriate treatment option in women who suffer from PMS.[49] The supplemental dose should not exceed the safe, tolerable maximum of 2500 mg/d and should complement a balanced diet containing the recommended 2 to 3 servings of dairy products a day.[49] Good sources of calcium include milk, cheese, yogurt, legumes, almonds, broccoli, calcium-fortified orange juice and some brands of tofu. The supplemental dose of calcium should also be adjusted downward in those individuals who routinely consume a lot of dairy products.[49]

E. CAFFEINE

Most dietary guidelines for PMS recommend avoiding caffeine even though it has not been shown to cause PMS. In most cases, this recommendation is based on personal experiences of some women with PMS who have reported improvements in symptoms with caffeine reduction. Rossignol et al.[50] found that consumption of caffeine-containing beverages affected the prevalence and severity of PMS. In women with more severe symptoms, the effect was higher, per amount of exposure, for consumers of tea and coffee than for soft drink consumers over the range of consumption studied (0–8 cups of soft drink and 0–3 cups of tea or coffee). The investigators suggested that women with PMS consider eliminating caffeine from their diets and then evaluate any changes in the severity of symptoms after several months.

Cann et al.[51] examined the association between alcohol and caffeine consumption and PMS and found no significant difference in total caffeine intake or in the individual caffeine-containing beverages consumed during the premenstrual period. PMS subjects were more likely to be heavy consumers of decaffeinated coffee or herbal tea than control subjects. While the average intake of alcohol was much greater in subjects with PMS compared with control subjects, this was true only during the postmenstrual period.

F. Food Cravings

Increased hunger and food cravings are symptoms frequently reported by women who suffer from PMS.[10,11] Cravings for sweet or salty foods are particularly strong. It has been proposed that these food cravings are related to abnormal serotonin activity in the brain that, in turn, may affect mood and appetite.[52] In the past, the treatment approach has been to reduce intake of refined carbohydrates, especially during the late luteal phase of the menstrual cycle. However, research now suggests exactly the opposite, that eating carbohydrates may actually relieve PMS symptoms and improve mood.

Cross et al.[53] examined changes in nutrient intake during the menstrual cycles in overweight women with PMS. One hundred forty-four women completed 4-day diet records pre- and post menstrually over two cycles. Results showed a significant increase in total energy and all macronutrients (protein, carbohydrates, fats) premenstrually when compared with nutrient intake postmenstrually. There was a preference for sweet high-carbohydrate, high-fat foods in the women with PMS.

VIII. TREATMENT FOR PMS

PMS symptoms can be physical, psychological or behavioral. Therefore, treatment must address all three areas. Women with mild symptoms may respond well to a combination of diet, exercise and lifestyle changes. However, for women with severe PMS symptoms, drug therapy and psychiatric counseling are probably necessary. Treatment depends on the individual and the severity of her symptoms.

A. Selective Serotonin-Reuptake Inhibitors

Selective serotonin-reuptake inhibitors (SSRIs) are increasingly being used as the first-line therapy for patients with primarily mood symptoms.[54] Examples of SSRI medications include fluoxetine (Sarafem), paroxetin (Paxil) and sertraline (Zoloft). In 1999, the FDA approved fluoxetine (Sarafem) for the treatment of PMDD. Fluoxetine was approved in 1987 under the name of Prozac for treating depression and has also been approved for treating obsessive-compulsive disorder and bulimia. A dose of 20 mg daily has been shown to be superior to placebo in improving the most common physical symptoms associated with PMDD.[55] Long-term studies have shown that fluoxetine is well tolerated and effective with continued use.[55]

TABLE 5.2
Psychological, Physical and Behavioral Symptoms of PMS

Psychological Symptoms

Anxiety-related	Depression-related	Other
Nervous tension	Anxious-depression	Insomnia
Mood swings	Crying	Forgetfulness
Irritability	Loneliness	Confusion
Restlessness	Low self-image	Reduced concentration
		Distractability

Physical Symptoms

Tension headaches	Generalized achiness	Dizziness
Migraine headaches	Weight gain	Nausea
Breast tenderness	Hot flashes	Heart pounding
Abdominal bloating	Faintness	Behavioral Symptoms
Peripheral edema	Abdominal cramps	Fatigue

Behavioral Symptoms

Increased appetite

Food cravings

Avoidance of social or work activities

Staying at home

Increased alcohol consumption

Increased or decreased libido

Adapted from Smith S. and Schiff, I., The premenstrual syndrome — diagnosis and management, *Fertil. Steril.*, 52, 527, 1989.

B. COMPLEMENTARY AND ALTERNATIVE THERAPIES

Practical experience shows that many women prefer not to use medication to treat PMS and therefore often seek alternative therapies such as dietary supplements, massage, hypnosis, herbal products (i.e., dong quai, vitex, agnus-castus), homeopathy and acupuncture. However, there is little scientific evidence to support their use. Stevinson and Ernst[56] conducted a systematic review of randomized controlled trials investigating complementary and alternative therapies in women with PMS. A total of 27 trials studying the effectiveness of homeopathy, dietary supplements, relaxation, massage, reflexology, chiropractic and biofeedback were reviewed. The authors concluded there is little scientific evidence to support the use of alternative therapies for treatment of PMS. However, one should not underestimate the power of the placebo. If a patient believes a supplement or remedy is effective, it actually can improve symptoms and if the supplement is taken away, systems can persist.

Health professionals who treat women with PMS need to provide support and encouragement to their patients. Many PMS clinics report that symptoms improve as a result of a caring relationship between the patient and health professional. A sense of hopefulness about a woman's situation may be one of the most important factors in the treatment of PMS.[21] That is one reason that self-help strategies can be

TABLE 5.3
Internet Resources for PMS and Women's Health

Academy of Family Physicians	http://www.familydoctor.org
Women's Health Information Center	http://www.ama-assn.org/special/womh/index.htm
Mayo Clinic	http://www.mayohealth.org
PMS Institute	http://www.pmsinst.com
Understanding PMS	http://www.conquerpms.com
The National Organization for	http://www.pms.org
Premenstrual Syndrome	

useful as part of the approach to coping with PMS.[57] Table 5.3 provides internet resources that patients and providers may find helpful.

C. DIETARY RECOMMENDATIONS

Most dietary recommendations include simple modifications such as limiting caffeine, salt and sugar. These recommendations, however, are empirically based and may not work for everyone.

A diet high in complex carbohydrates, such as whole grains, vegetables, breads, pasta and cereals is encouraged. These foods contain important vitamins and minerals such as vitamin B_6, and magnesium, as well as fiber, which helps prevent constipation. Eating carbohydrates may also reduce PMS symptoms by increasing serotonin levels in the brain.

D. EXERCISE

Regular exercise plays a therapeutic role in treating PMS. Studies show that women who are physically active tend to suffer less from PMS. Prior and colleagues[58] conducted a 3-month controlled study involving six sedentary women plus eight women who began an exercise training program. The exercising women reported significant decreases in breast tenderness and fluid retention after 3 months of gradual training. In another study, Steege and Blumenthal[59] found that women who participated in aerobic exercise for 60 minutes three times a week showed significant improvements in PMS symptoms, especially premenstrual depression. The most persuasive evidence linking exercise to PMS involves beta-endorphin, a chemical in the brain associated with emotion and behavior. One study showed that PMS subjects had lower levels of plasma beta-endorphin during the luteal phase of the menstrual cycle.[60] Because exercise stimulates endorphin production,[61] exercise may provide some relief from PMS symptoms. However, further research is needed to confirm this observation.

IX. CONCLUSIONS

PMS is a cyclic disorder that occurs during the luteal phase of the menstrual cycle, producing a number of physical and emotional changes. Commonly reported symptoms include abdominal bloating, backache, breast tenderness, food cravings, fatigue, irritability and symptoms related to depression. Research shows that it is the timing of the appearance and disappearance of symptoms, rather than a specific symptom, that leads to the diagnosis of PMS.

The direct cause of PMS is unknown. Numerous theories have been proposed and investigated, but none can be proven. The nutritional factors that have been studied are vitamin B_6, vitamin E, magnesium, calcium, caffeine and food cravings.

Some research suggests that low levels of the neurotransmitter serotonin may account for some of the physical as well as psychological symptoms of PMS. Increasing complex carbohydrates in the diet may relieve PMS symptoms by increasing serotonin levels in the brain.

At present, guidelines for PMS include a combination of diet, exercise and lifestyle changes. Most women prefer not to use medication. In addition, support and encouragement are important considerations in the treatment of PMS.

REFERENCES

1. Speroff, L., Historical and social perspectives, in *The Premenstrual Syndrome*, Keye, W.R., Ed., W.B.Sanders Company, Philadelphia, 1988, 3.
2. Rubinow, D.R., The premenstrual syndrome, *JAMA,* 268, 1908, 1992.
3. Frank, R.T., The hormonal causes of premenstrual tension, *Arch. Neurol. Psychiatr.,* 26, 1053, 1931.
4. Greene, R. and Dalton, K., The premenstrual syndrome, *Brit. Med. J.,* 1, 1007, 1953.
5. Reid, R.L., Premenstrual Syndrome, *New Eng. J. Med.,* 324, 1208, 1991.
6. American Psychiatric Association, *Diagnostic and Statistical Manual of Mental Disorders* — DSM — 4th ed., Washington, D.C. 1994.
7. Hurt, S.W., Schnurr, P.P., Severion, S.K., Freeman, E.W., Gise, L.H., Rivera-Tovar, A. and Steege, J.F., Late luteal phase dysphoric disorder in 670 women evaluated for premenstrual complaints, *Am. J. Psychiatr.,* 149, 525, 1992.
8. Reid, R.L., Premenstrual syndrome, *Curr. Probl. Obstet. Gynecol. Fertil.,* 8, 1, 1985.
9. Moos, R.H., Typology of menstrual cycle symptoms, *Am. J. Obstet. Gynecol.,* 103, 390, 1969.
10. Abraham, G.E., Nutritional factors in the etiology of the premenstrual tension syndromes, *J. Reprod. Med.,* 28, 446, 1983.
11. Smith S. and Schiff, I., The premenstrual syndrome — diagnosis and management, *Fertil. Steril.,* 52, 527, 1989.
12. Bancroft, J., Williamson, L., Warner, P., Rennie, D. and Smith, S.K., *Psychosom. Med.,* 55, 133, 1993.
13. Siegel, J.P., Myers, B.J., Dineen, M.K., Premenstrual tension syndrome symptom clusters, *J. Reprod. Med.,* 32, 395, 1987.
14. Chuong, C.J., Pearsall-Otey, L.R. and Rosenfeld, B.L., Revising treatments for premenstrual syndrome, *Cont. Ob. Gyn. ,*66, 1994.
15. Gong, E.J., Garrel, D., Calloway, D.H., Menstrual cycle and voluntary food intake, *Am. J. Clin. Nutr.,* 49, 252, 1989.
16. Moos, R.H., The development of menstrual distress questionnaire, *Psychosom. Med.,* 30, 853, 1968.
17. Woods, N.F., Most, A. and Dery, G.K., Prevalence of perimenstrual symptoms, *Am. J. Publ. Health,* 72, 1257, 1982.

18. Fisher, M., Trieller, K. and Napolitano, B., Premenstrual symptoms in adolescents, *J. Adoles. Health Care*, 10, 369, 1989.

19. Halbreich, V., Endicott, J., Schacht, S. and Nee, J., The diversity of premenstrual changes as reflected in the premenstrual assessment form, *Acta. Psychiatr. Scand.*, 65, 177, 1980.

20. Mortola, J.F., Girton, L., Beck, L. and Yen, S.S.C., Diagnosis of premenstrual syndrome by a simple, prospective and reliable instrument: The calendar of premenstrual experiences, *Obstet. Gynecol.*, 76, 302, 1990.

21. Plouffe, L., Stewart, K., Craft, K.S., Maddox, M.S. and Rausch, J.L., Diagnostic and treatment results from a southeastern academic center-based premenstrual syndrome clinic: The first year, *Am. J. Obstet. Gynecol.*, 169, 295, 1993.

22. Rubinow, D.R., Roy-Byrne, P., Hobban, M.C., Premenstrual mood changes: characteristic patterns in women with and without premenstrual syndrome, *J. Affective. Dis.* 10, 85, 1986.

23. Wyatt, K., Dimmock, P., Jones, P., Obhrai, M., O'Brien, S., Efficacy of progesterone and progestogens in management of premenstrual syndrome: Systemic review, *Brit. Med. J.* 323,776, 2001.

24. Ruble, D.K., Premenstrual symptoms: A reinterpretation, *Science,* 197, 291, 1977.

25. Rapkin, A.J., Edelmuth, E., Chang, L.C., Reading, A.E., McGuire, M.T. and Tung-Ping, Su., Whole-blood serotonin in premenstrual syndrome, *Obstet. Gynecol.*, 70, 533, 1987.

26. Fernstrom, J.D., Role of precursor availability in control of monoamine biosynthesis in brain, *Physiol. Rev.*, 63, 484, 1983.

27. Rapkin, A.J., Reading, A., Woo, S. and Goldman, L.M., Tryptophan and neutral amino acids in premenstrual syndrome, *Am. J. Obstet. Gynecol.*, 165, 1830, 1991.

28. Hertzman, P.A., Blevins, W.L., Mayer, J., Greenfield, B., Ting, M. and Gleich, G.J., Association of the eosinophilia-myalgia syndrome with the ingestion of tryptophan, *New Engl. J. Med.,* 322, 869, 1990.

29. Rose, D.P., The interactions between vitamin B_6 and hormones. *Vitamin Horm.,* 36, 53, 1978.

30. Williams, M.J., Taylor, M.L. and Dean, B.C., Controlled trial of pyridoxine in the premenstrual syndrome, *J. Int. Med. Res.*, 13, 174, 1985.

31. Berman, M.K., Taylor, M.L. and Freeman, E., Vitamin B_6 in premenstrual syndrome, *J. Am. Diet. Assoc.*, 90, 859, 1990.

32. Wyatt, K.M., Dimmock, P.W., Jones, P.W., O'Brien, S.Efficacy of vitamin B-6 in the treatment of premenstrual syndrome: Systematic review, *Brit. Med. J.* 318,1375, 1999.

33. Bendich, A.The potential for dietary supplements to reduce premenstrual syndrome (PMS) symptoms, *J. Am. College Nutr.*, 19, 3, 2000.

34. Food and Nutrition Board, *Recommended Dietary Allowances*, National Academy of Sciences, Washington, D.C., 1989.

35. Dalton, K., Pyridoxine overdose in premenstrual syndrome, *Lancet*, 1, 1168, 1985.

36. Schaumburg, H., Kaplan, J., Windebank, A., Nicholas, V., Rasmus, S., Pleasure, D. and Brown, M.J., Sensory neuropathy from pyridoxine abuse, *New Engl. J. Med.*, 309, 445, 1983.

37. Institute of Medicine: *Dietary Reference Intakes for Thiamin, Riboflavin, Niacin, Vitamin B_6, Folate, Vitamin B_{12}, Pantothenic Acid, Biotin and Choline.* Washington, D.C.: National Academy Press, 1998.

38. London, R.S., Murphy, L., Kitlowski, K E., Reynolds, M.A., Efficacy of alpha-tocopherol in the treatment of premenstrual syndrome, *J. Reprod. Med.*, 32, 400, 1987.

39. Chuong, C.J., Dawson, E.B. and Smith, E.R., Vitamin E levels in premenstrual syndrome, *Am. J. Obstet. Gynecol.*, 163, 1591, 1990.
40. Mira, M., Stewart, P.M. and Abraham, S.F., Vitamin and trace element status in premenstrual syndrome, *Am. J. Clin. Nutr.*, 47, 636, 1988.
41. Monsen, E.R.Dietary reference intakes for the antioxidant nutrients: Vitamin C, vitamin E, selenium and carotenoids. *J. Am. Diet. Assoc.*, 100, 637, 2000.
42. Abraham, G.E. and Lubran M.M., Serum and red cell magnesium levels in patients with premenstrual tension, *Am. J. Clin. Nutr.*, 34, 2364, 1981.
43. Facchinetti, F., Borella, P., Sances, G., Fioroni, L., Nappi, R.E. and Genazzani, A.R., Oral magnesium successfully relieves premenstrual mood changes, *Obstet. Gynecol.*, 78, 177, 1991.
44. Walker, A.F., De Souza, M.C., Vickers, M.F., Abeyasekera, S., Collins, M.L. and Trinca, L.A. Magnesium supplementation alleviates premenstrual symptoms of fluid retention, *J. Women's Health*, 7, 1157, 1998.
45. Thys-Jacobs, S. Micronutrients and the premenstrual syndrome: The case for calcium, *J. Amer. College Nutr.*, 19, 220, 2000.
46. Thys-Jacobs, S., Ceccarelli, S., Bierman, A., Weisman, H., Cohen, M.A., Alvir, M.J. Calcium supplementation in premenstrual syndrome: a randomized crossover trial, *J. Gen. Intern. Med.*, 4, 183, 1989.
47. Thys-Jacobs, S., Alvir, M.J., Calcium-regulating hormones across the menstrual cycle: Evidence of a secondary hyperparathyroidism in women with PMS, *J. Clin. Endocrinol. Metab.* 80, 2227, 1997.
48. Thys-Jacobs, S., Starkey, P., Bernstein, D. and Tian, J., Calcium carbonate and the premenstrual syndrome: Effects of premenstrual and menstrual symptoms.Premenstrual Syndrome Study Group, *Am. J. Obstet. Gynecol.*, 179, 444, 1998.
49. Ward, M.W. and Holimon, T.D., Calcium treatment for premenstrual syndrome, *Ann. Pharmacother.*, 33, 1356, 1999.
50. Rossignol, A.M. and Bonnlander, H., Caffeine-containing beverages, total fluid consumption and premenstrual syndrome, *Am. J. Public Health*, 80, 1106, 1990.
51. Cann, B., Duncan, D., Hiatt, R., Lewis, J., Chapman, J. and Armstrong, M.A., Association between alcoholic and caffeinated beverages and premenstrual syndrome, *J. Reprod. Med.*, 38, 630, 1993.
52. Wurtman, J.J., Brzezinski, A., Wurtman, R.J. and Laferrere, B., Effect of nutrient intake on premenstrual depression, *Am. J. Obstet. Gynecol.*, 161, 1228, 1989.
53. Cross, G.B., Marley, J., Miles, H. and Willson, K., Changes in nutrient intake during the menstrual cycle of overweight women with premenstrual syndrome, *Br. J. Nutr.*, 85, 475, 2001.
54. Frackiewicz, E.J. and Shiovitz, T.M., Evaluation and management of premenstrual syndrome and premenstrual dysphoric disorder. *J. Am. Pharm. Assoc.*, 41, 437, 2001.
55. Steiner, M., Steinberg, S., Stewart, D., Carter, D., Berger, C., Reid, R., Grover, D., Streiner, D., Fluoxetine in the treatment of premenstrual dysphoria, *New Engl. J. Med.*, 332, 1529, 1995.
56. Stevinson, C. and Ernst, E., Complementary/alternative therapies for premenstrual syndrome: A systematic review of randomized controlled trials, *Am. J. Obstet. Gynecol.*, 185, 227, 2001.
57. Stearns, S., PMS and PMDD in the domain of mental health nursing, *J. Psychosoc. Nurs. Mental Health Serv.*, 38, 16, 2001.
58. Prior, J.C., Vigna, Y. and Alojada, N., Conditioning exercise decreases premenstrual symptoms, *Eur. J. Appl. Physiol.*, 55, 349, 1986.

59. Steege, J.F. and Blumenthal, J.A., The effects of aerobic exercise on premenstrual symptoms in middle-aged women: A preliminary study, *J. Psych. Res.*, 37, 127, 1993.
60. Chuong, C.J., Coulam C.B., Kao, P.C., Neuropeptide levels in premenstrual syndrome, *Fertil. Steril.*, 44, 760, 1985.
61. Thoren, P., Floras, J.S., Hoffmann, P. and Seals, D.R., Endorphins and exercise: physiological mechanisms and clinical implications. *Med. Sci. Sports Exerc.*, 22, 417, 1990.

6 Nutritional Guidelines During Pregnancy and Lactation

Yolanda Cartwright and Mary Story

CONTENTS

I. INTRODUCTION

Pregnancy and lactation are critical periods during which good nutrition is a key factor influencing the health of both child and mother. A woman's dietary intake and nutritional status prior to conception and during pregnancy profoundly influence embryonic and fetal development, infant birthweight and health and the course and outcome of pregnancy. A woman's dietary intake after delivery affects lactational performance and postpartum recovery. Promoting good nutrition for women through-out the childbearing years could reduce infant morbidity and mortality and improve the health status of infants and mothers. This chapter reviews the major nutrition issues that are important before, during and after pregnancy.

II. PRECONCEPTIONAL NUTRITION ISSUES

While it was once believed that a woman's nutritional status during pregnancy was the most important determinant of positive pregnancy outcomes, it is now evident that health and nutrition status prior to pregnancy is equally as important. For example, maternal folate status prior to conception and during early pregnancy is critical for embryonic neural tube formation. A woman's weight status prior to pregnancy is a strong predictor of fetal growth and birthweight. Whether a woman smokes, consumes alcohol or uses illicit drugs prior to pregnancy has a significant influence on the health of the infant and mother. Women should be encouraged to consume nutritious diets and maintain healthy lifestyles throughout the childbearing years. Good health and adequate nutrient stores at the time a woman enters pregnancy will help to ensure normal embryonic and fetal development and optimal maternal health.

A. FOLATE STATUS

Folate is critically important for fetal development. A central feature of embryonic and fetal development is widespread cell division. Folate is required for cell division because of its role in DNA synthesis, and the need for folate increases during times of rapid tissue growth such as pregnancy.[1,2] Folate deficiency can occur during pregnancy because dietary folate intake is low or because the metabolic requirement for folate is increased. Folate insufficiency has been demonstrated to play a role in the etiology of first occurrence and recurrent neural tube defects (NTDs) (i.e., spina bifida, anencephaly, encephalocele).[3] Neural tube formation is completed during the 28 days after conception, often before a woman is aware of her pregnancy.[4] Hence, a woman's risk of having a fetus or infant with a neural tube defect can be reduced by the consumption of folic acid during the periconceptional period and the first 28 days after conception. The protective effects of folic acid were demonstrated by a Medical Research Council randomized study in the United Kingdom, where supplementation with 400 mcg of folate prior to and during early gestation was demonstrated to have a 71% protective effect against the recurrence of NTDs in the offspring of women who had a previously affected pregnancy.[5] Subsequently, Hungarian researchers showed that folate supplementation of 800 mcg/d for 1 month prior to conception can reduce the risk of first-time NTD occurrence.[3] More recently, periconceptional supplementation of 400 mcg of folic acid daily was found to reduce the risk of NTDs in areas of China with high rates of these defects.[6]

The U.S. Public Health Service (PHS) has recommended that all women who are capable of becoming pregnant consume 400 mcg of folate per day from dietary sources or through supplementation.[7] Most grain products (including enriched flour, breads, breakfast cereals, rice and pasta) are now fortified with folic acid. Yet, the amount of folic acid that women receive through their diet might not adequately meet the PHS recommendation of 400 mcg daily. Thus, women capable of becoming pregnant should review their dietary options, eat a diet that includes folate-rich foods including folic acid-fortified foods and take a folic acid-containing supplement.[8]

B. Weight Status

Maternal weight status, reflected by body mass index (BMI = wt/ht2) is a major predictor of fetal growth and birthweight.[9,10] Women who enter pregnancy underweight (BMI <19.8) are more likely than women of normal weight to deliver a low-birth-weight infant.[11] Birthweight has long been recognized as an important determinant of infant morbidity and mortality.[12] Low birthweight has recently been linked to a number of adulthood diseases, such as cardiovascular disease and diabetes.[51]

Women who enter pregnancy overweight (BMI>29.0) are at increased risk for maternal and fetal morbidity.[13] Overweight prior to pregnancy is a risk factor for gestational diabetes, hypertensive disorders of pregnancy, cesarean deliveries, complications during delivery and congenital defects.[13] Low apgar scores, macrosomia (large for gestational age) and neural tube defects are also more common in infants of overweight and obese mothers than in infants of normal weight mothers.[13] Achieving a healthy weight before pregnancy may enhance the ease of conception and improve pregnancy outcomes.[14] Weight change requires long-term effort. Hence, weight control efforts must begin long before pregnancy is planned.

C. Substance Use

Among women of reproductive age in the U.S., 29% smoke cigarettes, 20% are moderate to heavy drinkers and 10% use illicit drugs.[15] Women who use or abuse these substances prior to conception are more likely to enter pregnancy with a low BMI and depleted nutrient stores. Since substance use can retard fetal growth even among women who quit early in their pregnancies, counseling and support related to cessation of substance use should occur before conception.[16]

D. MEDICAL CONDITION

Maternal iron deficiency anemia is associated with increased risk of preterm delivery and subsequent low birthweight and may be related to low iron status during infancy.[17,18] These adverse outcomes have been observed when anemia occurred in the first trimester only, rather than later in pregnancy.[19] Currently, approximately 12% of women in industrialized countries including the U.S. enter pregnancy with anemia.[19] Blood volume expands substantially during the course of a normal healthy pregnancy. Hence, a woman who enters pregnancy with depleted iron stores might find it very difficult to replete her stores during pregnancy. Iron supplements have failed to replete iron stores fully for women who entered pregnancy with low iron stores in several studies.[20–23] Correction of anemia (hgb < 12.0) prior to conception is critical for lessening the risk of low birthweight and preterm delivery and for maintaining optimum maternal health throughout pregnancy.

The incidence of diabetes mellitus is increasing in the U.S. Consequently, more women are expected to enter pregnancy with preexisting diabetes. Elevated blood glucose levels in early pregnancy are associated with increased risk of congenital abnormalities, miscarriage and neonatal death.[24] The vast majority of women with diabetes do not plan their pregnancies, and enter pregnancy with inadequate blood glucose control.[25] Women with diabetes who plan to become pregnant should be encouraged to obtain preconceptional medical and nutritional care in order to gain optimal blood glucose control prior to conception.

Women who have been diagnosed with human immunodeficiency virus (HIV) may have a severely compromised nutritional status, including protein-calorie, malnutrition and deficiencies of vitamins and minerals such as zinc, calcium, vitamin A, vitamin C and vitamin B_6.[15] Poor maternal micronutrient status during HIV infection has been associated with adverse birth outcomes including fetal growth retardation and death.[26] HIV represents a very complex disease process and the reasons for malnutrition are multifactorial. Women who plan to become pregnant or who enter pregnancy with HIV are at very high nutritional risk. They should be counseled and treated to optimize their nutritional status and to prevent adverse pregnancy outcomes.

E. BREASTFEEDING PROMOTION

Most women make the decision to breastfeed prior to becoming pregnant. Health professionals in prenatal practice should educate women about the benefits of breastfeeding prior to pregnancy, before a decision about feeding method is reached.[27] Materials and counseling related to infant feeding should unequivocally support breastfeeding as the optimal feeding choice.[28]

TABLE 6.1
Indicators of Nutrition Risk

Risk Condition	Pre/Interpregnancy	Pregnancy	Lactation
Young maternal age	X	X	X
Poverty/homelessness	X	X	X
Complete vegetarianism	X	X	X
Anemia	X	X	X
HIV/AIDS	X	X	X
Gastrointestinal Disorders	X	X	X
Phenylketonuria	X	X	X
Diabetes	X	X	X
Gestational Diabetes		X	X
Eating Disorders	X	X	X
Rigid Dieting	X	X	X
Low/High BMI	X	X	X
Excessive/inadequate gestational weight gain		X	X
High parity/close-spaced pregnancies	X	X	X
Suspected IUGR		X	
Hyperemesis		X	
Long-term oral contraceptive use	X		
Excessive vitamin/mineral supplement use	X	X	X

F. NUTRITION SERVICES

The prenatal period represents a prime opportunity to educate women about the benefits of consuming a nutritious diet and maintaining a healthy lifestyle.[29] To assure optimal pregnancy outcomes, nutrition assessment and counseling for women of childbearing age should be a routine part of preventive health care. Risk conditions that warrant nutrition management are listed in Table 6.1.

III. PERICONCEPTIONAL NUTRITION ISSUES

A woman's nutritional intake and health status during pregnancy are critical for embryonic and fetal growth and development. Poor nutritional intake, uncontrolled medical conditions, inadequate weight gain and substance use during pregnancy can severely compromise the health of both the mother and developing fetus. Nutritional requirements for most nutrients increase during pregnancy due to an increase in metabolic demand. Hence, it is imperative that pregnant women meet these demands by consuming high-quality diets.

A. ENERGY

Pregnancy represents an anabolic state where adequate energy is required for developing fetal tissues and products of conception, maternal fat storage and an increase in basal metabolism to maintain new tissue. The energy demands of pregnancy are met by increasing food intake, decreasing energy expenditure or by mobilizing fat stores.[30] The combination of strategies used by pregnant women to meet the additional energy demands of pregnancy are influenced by her pre-pregnant BMI, body composition, stage of pregnancy, availability of food and physical activity level.[30] Hence, energy expenditure during pregnancy is quite variable among individuals, making it difficult to set standards for energy intake.[31] Nonetheless, the additional energy needs during pregnancy are approximately 300 kcal/d for adults and older adolescents and 500 kcal/d for younger adolescents (<14 years).[31,32] For some women, the additional energy need may be less than 300 kcal/d, especially among sedentary women.[33] Appropriate weight gain and appetite are better indicators of adequate energy intake than calories consumed.

B. PROTEIN

Additional protein is required during pregnancy for maternal, placental and fetal tissue synthesis. Approximately 8.5 g of additional protein per day is needed to support peak fetal growth. Assuming a 70% efficiency of utilization, the RDA for protein is 10 additional grams or a total of 60 g per day.[31] Higher intakes recommended previously were based on erroneous estimates of protein storage during pregnancy. Average U.S. dietary intakes of protein are approximately 75 to 110 g/day and inadequate intakes during pregnancy are rarely reported.[34] Complete vegetarians who exclude all animal products, or women with low energy intakes, as well as those with hyperemesis or eating disorders, may be at risk for low protein intake. High protein supplements could increase the risk of premature delivery and are not recommended during pregnancy.[12]

C. VITAMINS AND MINERALS

The demand for many vitamins and minerals is increased during pregnancy. Consequently, deficiencies often exist among pregnant women due to inadequate micronutrient intake, lack of knowledge about adequate prenatal nutrition or dietary taboos associated with pregnancy. Many women of childbearing age in the United States have inadequate dietary intake of vitamins and minerals before, during and after pregnancy. Studies on dietary intakes of U.S. women between the ages of 20 and 49 indicate that mean intakes of several vitamins and minerals are consistently below the RDAs, particularly vitamin B_6, folate, iron, zinc and calcium.[35] These nutrients are especially important during pregnancy, and deficiencies could result in adverse consequences for both mother and infant. Vitamin B_6 deficiency has been associated with preeclampsia, carbohydrate intolerance, hyperemesis gravidum and neurological disease of infants.[36] Vitamin B_6 concentrations decline during pregnancy due to increased blood volume and increased requirement for transport across the placenta. Hence the RDA for vitamin B_6 is 1.9 mg/d — 46% greater for pregnant than nonpregnant women.[31]

Folate requirements during pregnancy increase by 50% to build or maintain maternal stores and to meet the needs of rapidly growing maternal and fetal tissues. The current dietary reference intake (DRI) for folate during pregnancy is 600 mcg/d.[37] This amount can be consumed through diet or supplementation. Supplementation with folic acid during early gestation has been associated with a 72% protective effect against recurrent neural tube defects.[5] During pregnancy, low concentrations of folate are associated with increased risks of preterm delivery, infant low birthweight and fetal growth retardation.[38] The United States began fortification of grain products with folic acid in 1998, however, the concern that women will have inadequate intake remains. Good food sources of folic acid include fortified cereals, dried beans, orange juice, leafy greens, beets and broccoli.

Anemia due to iron deficiency is associated with maternal morbidity and mortality.[19] It is also associated with preterm delivery, low birthweight and low iron status during infancy.[17] Although iron absorption increases during pregnancy, a marked expansion of blood volume and red cell mass causes decreased hemoglobin and hematocrit concentrations. Consequently, iron deficiency anemia is relatively common during pregnancy. At highest risk are adolescents; African-Americans; Hispanics; women with high parity, short inter-pregnancy interval; multiple gestation and low dietary intake of meat or ascorbic acid.[12] The RDA for iron is 30 mg/d, 200% higher for pregnant than nonpregnant women.[31] Iron supplementation is necessary to achieve this level. However, pregnant women are also encouraged to consume iron-rich foods such as meats, dried beans and peas, dark green leafy vegetables, whole grain or enriched breads and fortified cereals. Iron absorption is enhanced by vitamin C-rich foods such as oranges and other citrus fruits and juices, broccoli, spinach, potatoes and tomatoes.

Zinc is essential for normal growth, as it is involved in nucleic acid metabolism and cell replication. Plasma zinc levels decline progressively during pregnancy due to inadequate dietary intake or very high amounts of copper or iron in the diet that compete with zinc at absorption sites.[39] Zinc requirements are highest during the third trimester when the fetus acquires two thirds of its zinc stores. Zinc deficiency has been associated with congenital abnormalities, abortion, intrauterine growth retardation and premature birth.[40] Those at highest risk for zinc deficiency follow diets very high in fiber or phytate such as vegan diets, have insufficient food intake, very high iron or folate intakes, inflammatory bowel disease or uncontrolled diabetes, or consume excess alcohol.[40] The RDA during pregnancy for zinc is 15 mg/d, 25% higher than the RDA for nonpregnant women.[31]

During pregnancy, approximately 25–30 g of calcium is transferred to the fetus.[41] The majority of deposition occurs during the third trimester, the period where fetal skeletal growth is highest. The DRI for calcium during pregnancy is 1000 mg/d for women ages 19–50 and 1300 mg/d for pregnant adolescents who are still increasing their bone mass.[41] The DRI is not increased above pre-pregnancy levels, as calcium absorption increases during pregnancy. Nonetheless, inadequate intake of calcium is common among women of childbearing age. Adequate dietary calcium intake is encouraged for all women. Approximately three fourths of calcium in the American diet comes from dairy products such as milk, yogurt and cheeses. Pregnant women who suffer from lactose intolerance can often tolerate smaller amounts of milk with meals, as well as aged cheeses, yogurt with active cultures or lactose-reduced milk. Other high-calcium food sources include fortified orange juice, cereals, breakfast bars and bread.

D. Vitamin and Mineral Supplements

The consumption of adequate calories to meet energy needs in addition to the increased absorption and efficiency of nutrient utilization that occurs in pregnancy is generally adequate to meet the nutritional needs for most nutrients. This is true if pregnant women select foods consistent with the Daily Food Guide Pyramid (Table 6.2).[42] However, vitamin and mineral supplementation may be appropriate for some nutrients and situations. Women most likely to benefit from vitamin and mineral supplements are those with inadequate dietary intake or food avoidances, who are thin or constantly trying to lose weight, or who abuse alcohol or other substances.[12] Guidance is necessary to prevent over-supplementation, particularly of vitamins A and D. Intake of vitamin A above 10,000 IU/d has been associated with birth defects,[43] while intake of vitamin D above 800 IU/d is associated with craniofacial anomalies in the offspring.[44]

TABLE 6.2
Daily Food Guide for Women

Food Group	Serving Size	Servings/day
Breads, cereal, rice, pasta (30 g)	1 slice of bread	6–11
	1/2 cup cooked rice, pasta, or cooked cereal (70 g)	
	1 oz (3/4 to 1 cup) dry cereal (30 g)	
	1/2 bun, bagel, or English muffin (30 g)	
	1 6-in. tortilla (30 g)	
	4 small plain crackers (15 g)	
Vegetables	1 cup raw leafy vegetables (55 g)	3–5
	1/2 cup other vegetables, raw or cooked (90 g)	
	3/4 cup vegetable juice (180 g)	
Fruits	1 medium apple, banana, or orange (180 g)	2–4
	1/2 cup chopped fruit (80 g)	
	3/4 cup fruit juice (185 g)	
Milk, yogurt, cheese (preferably fat-free or low-fat) (245 g)	1 cup milk or yogurt	3
	11/2 oz. natural cheese (42 g)	
	2 oz. processed cheese (56 g)	
Meat, poultry, fish, dry beans and peas, eggs and nuts (preferably lean or low-fat)	2–3 oz. lean meat, poultry, or fish (56–85 g)	2
	1/2 cup cooked dry beans or tofu (90 g)	
	1 egg (50 g), or 2 Tbsp peanut butter (32 g) = 1 oz. lean meat	
Fats, oils and sweets		use sparingly

Source: Modified from U.S. Department of Agriculture, Human Nutrition Information Service, The Food Guide Pyramid, Home and Garden Bulletin, No. 252 (HG-249), Hyattsville, MD, 1992.

1. Iron

The Centers for Disease Control recommends a routine low-dose iron supplement (30 mg/d) for all pregnant women, beginning with the first prenatal visit.[45] If anemia is positively diagnosed with hemoglobin and hematocrit screenings, 60–120 mg/d may be prescribed.[45] Routine iron supplementation during pregnancy remains a topic of debate, as there are many gaps in scientific knowledge regarding the adverse effects of maternal anemia and iron deficiency on maternal and fetal outcome. Substantial evidence suggests that iron deficiency during pregnancy is associated with adverse outcomes, while prenatal iron supplementation is not associated with significant risks.

2. Calcium

Calcium absorption is enhanced during pregnancy. Calcium requirements during pregnancy are equivalent to those in the nonpregnant state: 1000mg/d for women 19–50 years old and 1300 mg/d for adolescents aged 14–18.[41] This amount is achieved by consuming 3–4 servings of dairy products daily. However, calcium and vitamin D supplementation might be necessary for women who do not consume dairy products due to allergies or for other reasons. Research studies also suggest that adolescents and women at risk for pregnancy-induced hypertension might benefit from higher intakes of calcium.[45,46] In these instances, the Institute of Medicine (IOM) recommends a supplement providing 600 mg of elemental calcium daily.

3. Folate

The DRI for folate during pregnancy is 600 mcg/d.[37] Supplementation with folic acid during early gestation has been associated with decreased risk of recurrent neural tube defects.[5] Hence, supplementation of 4.0 mg/d is recommended for women with a history of NTD-affected pregnancy. The U.S. PHS recommends that all women of childbearing age consume 400 mcg of folic acid daily. Additional folic acid can be obtained by eating foods that are rich in folic acid (green leafy vegetables, citrus fruits and juices, whole wheat bread and legumes), taking a vitamin supplement, or both. Folic acid intake should be limited to 1000 mcg/d to avoid excess intake.

4. Zinc and Copper

Iron can interfere with the absorption of other minerals, particularly zinc and copper.[39] A 15 mg zinc and 2 mg copper supplement is recommended for women taking iron supplements of more than 30 mg daily. These amounts are commonly found in multivitamin supplements tailored for pregnant women.

5. Multivitamins

Routine use of multivitamin supplements has long been an accepted practice in obstetrical care. However, in low-risk women consuming a nutritionally adequate diet, this may be unnecessary. The Institute of Medicine (IOM) has recommended that health providers assess dietary practices and risk conditions and recommend a low-dose supplement when indicated.[47] Conditions warranting vitamin or mineral supplementation include failure to regularly consume a nutritionally adequate diet, multiple gestation, heavy cigarette smoking (20 or more per day), alcohol or drug abuse, complete vegetarianism or treatment of anemia with therapeutic doses of iron.[12]

6. Herbal Supplements

Many pregnant women regard herbal supplements as a safe alternative to taking over the counter drugs for relief from common pregnancy ailments such as morning sickness. The lay literature often provides misinformation regarding the use of herbal supplements during pregnancy.[48] In fact, few well-designed studies have examined the safety and efficacy of alternative therapies during pregnancy. One small clinical trial examined the effects of ginger on hyperemesis and reported improvement in symptoms.[49] However, the safety of ginger remains questionable as it affects thromboxane synthase, which could increase bleeding.[50] Pregnant women should be advised to avoid herbal treatments during pregnancy until their safety can be confirmed. Table 6.3 displays a list of medicinal herbs that may not be safe for use during pregnancy.

E. WEIGHT GAIN

Maternal weight gain during pregnancy is a strong predictor of fetal growth and health. Birthweight has long been recognized as an important determinant of infant morbidity and mortality. In addition, recent studies suggest that impaired intrauterine growth may predispose the fetus for cardiovascular, metabolic or endocrine disease later in life.[51] Recommendations for weight gain during pregnancy should be individualized according to pre-pregnancy BMI to improve pregnancy outcome, avoid excess maternal postpartum weight retention and reduce the risk of chronic disease in the offspring. Prenatal weight gain consistent with the IOM recommendations is associated with better pregnancy outcomes (see Table 6.4). Women who are underweight prior to pregnancy (BMI <19.8) are at greater risk for poor pregnancy outcome if weight gain is inadequate. However, even obese women (BMI >29) should gain at least 15 pounds, as those who fail to gain weight or lose weight are more likely to deliver low-birthweight infants.[52] Obese women should be cautioned to avoid excessive weight gain, as excess weight contributes to postpartum weight retention and also puts the infant at risk of being large for gestational age.[13] Being large for gestational age during infancy has been associated with excess body fat during childhood.[53] Previously, African-American women were recommended to gain weight at the upper end of the IOM range, as they are at high risk for delivering low-birthweight infants. However, recent evidence does not support this recommendation, as gaining weight in the upper end of the IOM ranges does not appear to provide consistent low-birthweight reduction for African-American women.[54] Also, a study examining recommendations for maternal weight gain for Chinese women concluded that recommended weight gain cutoff values for healthy pregnancy outcome differed from IOM recommendations due to differences in anthropometry

Table 6.3
Medicinal Herbs That May Not Be Safe for Use during Pregnancy and Lactation

Agnus castus, Aloes, Angelica, Apricot kernel, Asafoetida, Aristolchia, Avens

Blue Flag, Bogbean, Boldo, Boneset, Borage, Broom, Buchu, Buckthorn, Burdock

Calamus, Calendula, Cascara, German Chamomile, Roman Chamomile, Chaparral, Black
  Cohosh, Blue Cohosh, Cola, Coltsfoot, Comfrey, Cottonroot, Cornsilk, Crotalaria

Damiana, Devils Claw, Dong Quai, Dogbane

Ephedra, Eucalyptus, Eupatorium, Euphorbia

Fenugreek, Feverfew, Foxglove, Frangula, Fucus

Gentian, Germander, Ginseng, Golden Seal, Ground Ivy, Grounsel, Guarana

Hawthorne, Heliotropium, Hops, Horehound, Horsetail, Horseradish, Hydorcotyle

Jamaica Dogwood, Juniper

Liferoot, Licorice, Lobelia

Mandrake, Mate, Male Fern, Meadowsweet, Melliot, Mistletoe, Motherwort, Myrrh

Nettle

Osha

Passionflower, Pennyroyal, Petasites, Plantain, Pleurisy Root, Podophyllium, Pokeroot, Poplar,
  Prickly Ash, Pulsatilla

Queen's Delight

Rawort, Raspberry, Red Clover, Rhubarb, Rue

Sassafras, Scullcap, Senna, Shepherd's Purse, Skunk Cabbage, Stephania, Squill, St, John's Wort

Tansy, Tonka Bean

Uva-Ursi

Vervain

Wild Carrot, Willow, Wormwood

Yarrow, Yellow Dock, Yohimbe

Source: Foote, J. and Rengers, B., Medicinal herb use during pregnancy and lactation, *Perinatal Nutr. Report,* 5, 1, 1998.

Table 6.4
Recommended Weight Gain During Pregnancy

Prepregnant BMI	Weight Gain (total lb)	Trimester 1 (total lb)	Trimester 2,3 (lb/week)
Low (<10.9) (underweight)	28–40	5	1 or more
Normal (19.8–26.0)	25-35	3	1
High (26.1–29.0) (overweight)	15–25	2	0.66
Very High (>29) (obese)	at least 15	1.5	0.5

Source: Institute of Medicine, Nutrition During Pregnancy: Part I. Weight Gain, Part II. Nutrient Supplements, Committee on Nutrition Status During and Lactation, Food and Nutrition Board, National Academy Press, Washington, D.C., 1990.

across ethnic groups.[55] Excessive weight gain contributes more to postpartum weight retention and less to fetal growth in normal and overweight women.[56] This is especially problematic among teenagers who are still growing, particularly those who enter pregnancy with high BMI.[57]

In addition to total weight gain, the rate and pattern of weight gain has been shown to influence fetal growth and length of gestation. The appropriate rate of weight gain is largely dependent on the mother's pre-pregnancy weight. In general, pregnant women should gain 1.5–5 pounds during the first trimester and 0.5–1 pound per week during the second and third trimesters. Regardless of the mother's pre-pregnancy weight, inadequate weight gain during the second or third trimester increases the risk of intrauterine growth retardation.[58] Low weight gain during the third trimester is also associated with increased risk of preterm delivery.[59,60] The IOM recommended rates of weight gain during pregnancy (based on pre-pregnancy weight) are listed in Table 6.4.

G. EXERCISE

Moderate exercise is generally safe for healthy women with uncomplicated pregnancies.[61] Depending on its type, frequency, duration and intensity, exercise may confer health benefits to both mother and fetus.[62] Safe activities generally include walking, swimming, low-impact jogging or aerobics and riding on a stationary bike. Activities that may not be safe include ball games that increase the risk of abdominal trauma, weight-lifting, diving, martial arts, anaerobic exercises (sprinting), exercise above 2500 meters of altitude and any exercise with a high risk of falling or requiring balance, especially in late pregnancy. Exercise is contraindicated for women with pregnancy-induced hypertension, preeclampsia, preterm rupture of membranes, history of preterm labor, persistent second- or third-trimester bleeding, incompetent cervix or any sign of intrauterine growth retardation. Pregnant women who exercise must maintain an adequate intake of calories, nutrients and fluids.

H. SUBSTANCE USE

A range of effects, including spontaneous abortion, low birthweight and pre-term delivery, have been associated with prenatal use of illicit drugs including alcohol, tobacco, cocaine and marijuana.[8] In addition to direct adverse effects on the fetus, the nutrition-related consequences of tobacco, alcohol and drug use can further compromise pregnancy outcome. Potential effects of substance use on maternal nutritional status include decreased nutrient intake, reduced nutrient absorption, increased nutrient losses, or altered nutrient metabolism and utilization.

Cigarette smoking during pregnancy has been associated with low birthweight and may increase the risk of preterm delivery and perinatal mortality,[63] effects that cannot be corrected by simply increasing energy intake.[64] It is also associated with other adverse outcomes, including mental retardation.[65] In addition to direct exposure, passive exposure to cigarette smoke has also been associated with reduced fetal growth.[66]

Like cigarette smoke, marijuana smoking interferes with the supply of oxygen to the fetus and impairs fetal growth. Although findings are inconsistent, marijuana use during pregnancy has been associated with low birthweight, preterm delivery and neurobehavioral effects in the infant.[15] Cocaine exposure *in utero* has been linked to premature rupture of membranes, premature labor, intrauterine growth retardation and spontaneous abortion. In addition, infant effects of cocaine exposure include withdrawal, cerebral infarction and possible congenital defects.

An association of fetal alcohol exposure with fetal growth restriction and growth retardation is well established. Cranio-facial abnormalities have also been observed among infants exposed to alcohol during pregnancy. Other fetal alcohol effects include lifelong compromises in growth, health, behavior and cognitive ability.[67]

I. MORNING SICKNESS

Nausea and vomiting or "morning sickness" is one of the most common complaints of pregnancy, occuring in 50–70% of pregnant women.[68] The exact cause of morning sickness is unknown, but it is assumed to be related to hormonal changes that occur during pregnancy. Morning sickness is suggested to possibly provide benefit during early pregnancy by reducing maternal energy intake, thereby increasing placental weight. Morning sickness is associated with a decreased risk of miscarriage, preterm birth, low birthweight and perinatal death.[68] Milder cases of morning sickness can often be treated by consuming small frequent meals, avoiding offensive odors, drinking enough fluids and getting fresh air.[69] Consuming high carbohydrate foods, such as crackers, upon rising, and consuming liquids between meals also provides relief for some women. Severe nausea and vomiting, hyperemesis gravidum, often persisting beyond 14 weeks' gestation, is a more severe medical condition that could cause inadequate nutritional intake, weight loss, electrolyte or metabolic disturbances and dehydration, increasing risk to the mother and fetus.[70] This is a high-risk condition and usually requires hospitalization for anti-emetic therapy, rehydration and nutritional support.

J. CONSTIPATION

Constipation, characterized by infrequent or hard, dry stools may occur as a side effect of supplemental iron or as part of the normal digestive changes that occur during pregnancy.[12] Increasing intake of high-fiber foods such as fruits, vegetables and whole grains, increasing fluids and getting regular physical activity when possible should help to alleviate symptoms.

K. FOOD CRAVINGS, AVERSIONS AND PICA

Food cravings and aversions are very common during pregnancy.[71] Some commonly craved items include chocolate, citrus fruits, pickles, chips and ice cream. The most common aversions are to coffee, tea, fried or fatty foods, highly spiced foods, meat and eggs. Though results are inconclusive, research studies suggest that food cravings and aversions work to influence food consumption during pregnancy as necessary. Food cravings result in increased energy intake while food aversions cause decreased energy intake.

Pica refers to the compulsive consumption of nonfood substances over a sustained period of time.[72] Substances commonly consumed include ice or freezer frost, laundry starch, soap, ashes, chalk, paint or burnt matches. Abnormal consumption of food items such as cornstarch and baking soda also reflects pica. Pica has been associated with reduced serum ferritin and hemoglobin values in pregnant women and small head circumference in their offspring.[73] Pica is more common among African-American women and among women with a family or childhood history of the disorder.[73]

L. MEDICAL CONDITIONS

Offspring of women with pre-existing diabetes mellitus are at increased risk for congenital malformations, primarily due to poor preconceptional glucose control.[24] Thus, it is imperative for women with pre-existing diabetes to obtain good blood glucose control prior to conception. Gestational diabetes mellitus (GDM) appears in 2–3% of all pregnancies and increases the risk of macrosomia, difficult labor, infant shoulder dystocia (dislocation) and cesarean delivery.[74] Although symptoms of GDM commonly disappear after delivery, women with GDM during pregnancy are at increased risk of developing Type 2 diabetes later in life.[75] Also, maternal diabetes is associated with elevated blood pressure and overweight in childhood.[76,77] Gestational diabetes can often be controlled through diet and moderate exercise. However, for those pregnant women who do not obtain blood glucose control through lifestyle changes, insulin therapy might be indicated.

About 8–10% of pregnant women develop pregnancy-induced hypertension (PIH) during the course of pregnancy.[78] In severe cases, proteinuria, convulsions and coma may occur. However, even among women without severe preeclampsia, a steady increase in blood pressure throughout the course of pregnancy is associated with reduced birthweight, as PIH is thought to decrease blood flow and the supply of nutrients to the fetus.[79] Research studies have examined the impact of several nutrients on the course of PIH including calcium supplementation,[80] vitamins C and E,[81] sodium restriction and magnesium, zinc and fish oil supplementation.[82] To date, no specific therapy has proven to prevent or delay PIH or improve pregnancy outcomes.

Maternal nutrition status is of great concern with HIV-infected pregnant women. However, transmission of HIV from mother to child is equally as concerning. Transmission of HIV from mother to child ranges from 15–40% in the absence of antiretroviral treatment.[83] Medical advances, particularly the administration of antiretroviral drugs during pregnancy, labor and the postpartum period, in the United States and other developed countries have reduced the rates of transmission to 4–6%.[84] Maternal factors such as drug use, smoking, sexual practice, maternal immune status and poor nutrition all play a role in viral transmission. Women with HIV are likely to have multiple nutrition problems including protein-calorie, malnutrition, vitamin and mineral deficiencies and inadequate weight gain.[15] Consequently, intensive nutrition management is required for these women.

M. NUTRITION SERVICES

The IOM has recommended that all women receive nutrition assessment and individualized care during pregnancy, regardless of level of nutrition risk, socioeconomic status, health status, or type of care provider.[47] Nutrition services have proven effective in improving pregnancy outcome and cost. It has been observed that women who did not receive advice regarding vitamin use, proper diet, weight gain and avoidance of tobacco, alcohol and other drugs were 1.3 times more likely to deliver a low-birthweight infant.[85] Women at high risk for nutrition problems require intensive nutrition services and care (see Table 6.2).

Low-income women should be referred to the special supplemental nutrition program for Women, Infants and Children (WIC). Established in 1972, WIC targets low-income pregnant and postpartum women, and children up to age 5 at nutritional risk, and combines nutrition education with vouchers for certain nutritious foods. Evaluation of the effects of the WIC program on infant outcomes has provided varying results,[86] but the majority of studies have shown that women enrolled in WIC have fewer low-birthweight infants than women of similar socioeconomic status not enrolled in WIC.[87] Other benefits of WIC include increased use of prenatal care and increased Medicare savings.[88]

IV. LACTATION

A. BENEFITS

Breast milk is widely acknowledged to be the most complete form of nutrition for infants, with its wide range of benefits for infants' health, growth, immunity and development. Immunological benefit and reduction in severity of many acute and chronic diseases, including diarrhea, otitis media, asthma, lower respiratory tract infections and urinary tract infections have been associated with exclusive breast-feeding for at least 4 months.[89–91] There is also some suggestion that breastfeeding is protective against the development of overweight in young children.[89] A number of studies have suggested a positive association between breastfeeding and cognitive development in early and middle childhood.[92] A recent study found a significant association between duration of breastfeeding and intelligence in two independent samples of young adults.[93] Breastfeeding has also been shown to improve maternal health, with demonstrated effects that include reduction in postpartum bleeding, earlier return to prepregnancy weight, reduced risk of premenopausal breast cancer and reduced risk of osteoporosis.[8] Because of the benefits incurred, the American Academy of Pediatrics considers breastfeeding to be "the ideal method of feeding and nurturing infants" and recommends breastfeeding for at least 12 months.[90]

B. COMPOSITION

The composition of breast milk depends on maternal nutrition status, although an adequate volume of breast milk of appropriate nutrient composition, despite suboptimal dietary intakes, can be produced by drawing on maternal nutrient stores and reserves. Even in a mild energy deficit, while the volume of milk produced is reduced, the composition of the milk is rarely compromised. Consistently low dietary intakes of most vitamins, including B_6, A and D are reflected in decreased breast milk levels.[94] Long-term dietary inadequacies can cause depleted nutrient stores and altered breast milk composition. Severe malnutrition during lactation may interfere with breast milk production, secretion and possibly immunological properties.[94]

Nutrient needs during lactation are directly related to the volume of milk produced and the duration of lactation. In general, nutrient needs are highest during the first 6 months, when breast milk volume is approximately 20% higher than in the second 6 months.[31]

C. ENERGY

Until recently, safe methods for determining energy expenditure during lactation were unavailable. Hence, energy needs during lactation are estimated based on the factorial method. This method estimates the energy needs of lactation by adding the additional energy requirement of lactation to that of nonlactating women. Assuming that milk production is 80% efficient, 80 kcal are needed to produce 1 ml of breastmilk containing 70 kcal/ml. Thus, the energy needed to exclusively breastfeed a single infant during the first 6 months of lactation would be approximately 640 kcal/d and approximately 510 kcal/d during the second 6 months. The RDA of an additional 500 kcal/d also assumes that 250 kcal/d are mobilized from maternal fat stores.[31] This conservative estimate ensures adequate energy intake for lactating women and their infants. Younger adolescents and women who are underweight, gained inadequate weight during pregnancy and are highly physically active will require higher energy intakes during lactation.[94]

Studies of dietary intake of lactating women have rarely documented energy intakes that meet recommended levels.[95,96] Nevertheless, adequate lactational performance and infant growth have been documented with inadequate energy intake.[97] It is apparent that women use several mechanisms, including adjustments in energy intake and expenditure, to meet the energy needs of lactation. Goldberg et al.[98] determined that women increased food intake and decreased physical activity to meet the energy demands of lactation. Clearly, the components of energy expenditure vary greatly by individual. Hence, the adequacy of energy intake should be assessed based on the mother's overall nutritional status, weight status and the adequacy of the infant's growth.

D. PROTEIN

Based on the average protein content of breast milk (1.1 g/dl) and a 70% efficiency rate in converting dietary protein to breast milk protein, the RDA for lactation is 15 g additional protein per day.[31] U.S. women tend to have ample protein intakes and usually do not require additional amounts to meet this recommended level. Complete vegetarians or women with eating disorders may be at risk for insufficient protein intakes. Failure to consume the RDA for protein may result in significant mobilization of a woman's lean tissue stores. For instance, a 60-kg woman with 25% body fat could lose approximately 20% of tissue protein to support 6 months of breastfeeding.[94]

E. VITAMINS AND MINERALS

Inadequate dietary intakes of several vitamins and minerals have been reported for lactating women.[37,41,99,100] These include folate, thiamin, vitamin A, calcium, iron and zinc. If lactating women have dietary intakes that are adequate in energy and consistent with guidelines outlined by the Daily Food Guide Pyramid[42] (Table 6.1), it is likely that their nutritional requirements for vitamins and minerals will be met. The exceptions are for calcium and zinc, which have been found to be deficient in the diets of lactating women with adequate caloric intake (2700 kcal/day). Fortunately, low dietary intakes of calcium and zinc do not immediately affect their concentration in human milk, as they are maintained in maternal stores if dietary intake is inadequate. However, the long-term effects of low calcium intake during lactation on the mother's bone density are uncertain. Also, zinc plays a critical role in immune function and other pregnancy outcomes. Adequate intake of both nutrients should be encouraged. The DRI for calcium during lactation is 1000 mg/d for adults and 1300 mg/d for adolescents.[41] The RDA for zinc during lactation is 19 mg/d during the first 6 months and 16 mg/d during the second 6 months compared with 12 mg/d, which is recommended in the nonpregnant, nonlactating state.[31]

In contrast to calcium and zinc, low maternal thiamin intake can result in low thiamin levels in milk. Thiamin requirements are based on energy needs, which are increased during lactation. The DRI for thiamin includes a wide margin of safety to compensate for losses in milk. It is 1.5 mg/d during lactation, compared with 1.1 mg/d in the nonpregnant, nonlactating state.[37]

Inadequate maternal folate intake may cause depletion of maternal reserves to maintain folate levels in milk. In addition, body stores of folate are small and reserves could be depleted after only a few months of lactation. Low folate status is common among lactating women and adequate folate intake is necessary to protect the health of both mother and infant. The DRI for folate during lactation is 500 mcg/d, compared with 600 mcg/d during pregnancy and 400 microg/d in the nonpregnant, nonlactating state.[37] Lactating women should be encouraged to consume adequate amounts of folate-rich foods including leafy vegetables, fruit, liver, fortified cereals and legumes. For those lactating women with consistently low dietary intake of folate, nutritional counseling or supplementation might be warranted.

The iron demands of lactation are not significant, particularly if menstruation has not resumed.[94] However, depletion of maternal iron stores may occur if dietary intake is marginal. The RDA for iron is 15 mg/d and is not increased above requirements for nonpregnant women.[31]

F. VITAMIN AND MINERAL SUPPLEMENT

In general, well-nourished breastfeeding women do not need routine vitamin and mineral supplementation.[94] The nutrient demands of lactation can be met by the selection of foods in accordance with the Daily Food Guide Pyramid[42] (Table 6.1). Supplementation should target specific nutritional needs of individual women. Vitamin B_{12} supplementation may be indicated for complete vegetarians. Breastfed infants can suffer from B_{12} and vitamin D deficiencies even when the mother does not exhibit deficiency symptoms. Hence, vitamin D supplements might be warranted for mothers who receive inadequate exposure to sunlight or do not use vitamin D-fortified dairy products. Calcium supplementation might be necessary for women who are unable to consume at least 600 mg calcium/d due to food allergies or for other reasons. Women with restricted energy intake may also require supplementation, but should be cautioned against taking excessive supplemental amounts of vitamins A and D, as high levels of these vitamins are toxic and could be harmful to both mother and infant.

G. HERBAL SUPPLEMENTS

Scientific information about the use of herbal products during lactation is sparse. Little is known about the amount secreted in milk or the effects on term or preterm infants. Hence, herbs that are central nervous system stimulants, cathartic laxatives, hepatotoxic, carcinogenic, cytotoxic, mutagenic or that contain potentially toxic essential oils are not recommended during lactation. A list of herbs that should be avoided during pregnancy and lactation is provided in Table 6.3. Various herbal gels, ointments and creams are recommended for sore nipples. However, the nursing child could easily ingest any substance applied to the breast or nipples.[101] Hence, the use of herbal oil is not recommended. Regarding herbal teas, Lawrence[102] recommends using only those "that are prepared carefully, using only herbs for essence (e.g., Celestial Seasonings brand teas) and avoiding heavy doses of herbs with active principles."

H. WEIGHT STATUS

Breastfeeding has an average estimated energy cost of 750 kcal per day. In addition, mechanisms that favor the use of maternal fat stores and delivery of nutrients to the breast seem to occur during lactation.[103] Taken together, these mechanisms could enhance maternal weight loss. Earlier research suggested an average weight loss of 0.5 to 1.0 kg for 80% of lactating women during the first 4-6 months of lactation.[94] However, more recent studies indicate that despite mechanisms that favor weight loss during lactation, postpartum weight changes are rather small and inconsistent and do not differ between lactating and nonlactating women.[104] One explanation for this phenomenon is that changes in energy intake, energy expenditure and fat mobilization easily meet the increased energy demand. Nonetheless, overweight lactating women should be counseled to lose a maximum of 2 kg per month through a balanced diet low in fat and sugars and increased physical activity after lactation is well established. Milk production is not affected by gradual weight loss. Rigid dieting and weight loss products are contraindicated.[94] Postpartum weight loss is particularly important for women who had gestational diabetes during pregnancy, as they are at increased risk for developing type 2 diabetes, and for those who gained excess weight during the course of pregnancy.

I. EXERCISE

Increased postpartum physical activity may be effective in helping women to lose weight while improving their metabolic profile and increasing fat losses. In research studies, no adverse effects due to exercise have been observed on milk production, infant intake or infant growth.[105,106] Lactating women also appear to efficiently balance their energy intake to offset the excess energy expenditure due to exercise. One cross-sectional study examined the effects of exercise on weight and lactation and found that women who exercised vigorously increased their energy expenditure, but also increased their caloric intake.[106] The caloric deficit was the same in the exercising and nonexercising groups. Also, there was no significant difference in milk volume between the two groups. While exercise has many physiological benefits, lactating women with a goal of weight loss should be counseled to modestly restrict energy intake along with increased physical activity.

J. SUBSTANCE USE

Nicotine, alcohol, illicit drugs and caffeine are excreted in breast milk and have adverse effects on the infant. In addition, breast milk volume can be reduced by cigarette smoking, which inhibits prolactin levels, and by alcohol, which interferes with the milk ejection reflex. Breastfeeding women should be advised to avoid tobacco and illicit drugs and to avoid or limit alcohol intake and caffeine-containing beverages to one to two servings per day.[94]

K. NUTRITION SERVICES

All breastfeeding women should receive nutrition assessment, education and counseling. To achieve optimal infant growth and development and maternal health, those conditions indicating the need for intensive nutrition follow-up are listed in Table 6.2.

V. SUMMARY

Pregnancy and lactation are critical periods during which there is an increased need for nutrients. Nutrition plays a critical role in assuring the development of a healthy infant and in maintaining the health status of the mother. Preconceptional nutrition issues are important determinants of fetal outcome. Women who enter pregnancy undernourished have an increased risk of suboptimal fetal development and also of delivering a low-birthweight infant. Low birthweight during infancy is related to infant mortality and has been linked to coronary heart disease, type 2 diabetes, hypertension and hyperlipidemia in adult life. Maternal nutritional status during pregnancy is also related to infant birthweight and health and pregnancy outcomes. Finally, the postpartum period is a time when nutrient reserves should be restored and body weight modified if necessary. It is also an important time for women who choose to breastfeed, as optimal nutritional intake is needed for maternal health and the quality and quantity of milk production. Clearly, to maximize maternal and infant health, a focus on maternal nutrition is necessary before, during and after pregnancy.

REFERENCES

1. Rosenblat D.S., Inherited disorders of folate transport and metabolism, in *The Metabolic and Molecular Bases of Inherited Disease,* Scriver, C.R., Beaudet, A.L., Sly, W.S. and Valle, D., Eds., McGraw-Hill, New York, 1995: 3111.
2. Mudd S.H., Levy H.L. and Skovby F., Disorders of transsulfuration, in *The Metabolic and Molecular Bases of Inherited Disease*, Scriver, C.R., Beaudet, A.L., Sly, W.S. and Valle, D., Eds., McGraw-Hill, New York, 1995:1297.

3. Czeizel, A.E. and Dudas, I., Prevention of the first occurrence of neural tube defects by periconceptional vitamin supplementation, *New Engl. J. Med.*, 327, 1832, 1992.

4. Sulik, K.K. and Sadler, T.W., Postulated mechanisms underlying the development of neural tube defects, *Ann. N.Y. Acad. Sci.*, 678, 8, 1993.

5. MRC Vitamin Study Research Group, Prevention of neural tube defects: Results of the Medical Research Council vitamin study, *Lancet*, 338, 131, 1991.

6. Berry, R.J., Li, Z., Erickson, J.D. and Li, S., Prevention of neural tube defects with folic acid in China, *New Engl. J. Med*, 341, 1485, 1999.

7. Centers for Disease Control, Use of folic acid for the prevention of spina bifida and other neural tube defects, 1983–1991, *Morbid. Mortal. Wkly. Report*, 40, 513, 1991.

8. U.S. Department of Health and Human Services, *Healthy People 2010* (Conference Edition, in Two Volumes), Washington, D.C.: January 2000.

9. Abrams, B.F. and Laros, R.K., Prepregnancy weight, weight gain and birthweight, *Am. J. Obstet. Gynecol*, 154, 503, 1986.

10. Naeye, R.L., Maternal body weight and pregnancy outcome, *Am. J. Clin. Nutr.*, 52, 273, 1990.

11. Kirchengast, S. and Hartmann, B., Maternal prepregnancy weight status and pregnancy weight gain as major determinants for newborn weight and size, *Ann. Hum. Biolog.*, 25, 17, 1998.

12. Institute of Medicine, *Nutrition During Pregnancy: Part I. Weight Gain, Part II. Nutrient Supplements*. Committee on Nutrition Status During Pregnancy and Lactation, Food and Nutrition Board, National Academy Press, Washington, D.C., 1990.

13. Galtier-Dereure, F., Boegner, C. and Bringer, J., Obesity and pregnancy: Complications and cost, *Am. J. Clin. Nutr.*, 71, 1242S, 2000.

14. Norman, R.J. and Clark, A.M., Obesity and reproductive disorders: A review, *Repr. Fert.Dev.*, 10, 55, 1998.

15. Bendich, A., Lifestyle and environmental factors that can adversely affect maternal and nutritional status and pregnancy outcomes, *Ann. N.Y. Acad. Sci.*, 678, 255, 1993.

16. Shu, X.O., Hatch, M.C., Mills, J., Clemens, J. and Susser, M., Maternal smoking, alcohol drinking, caffeine consumption and fetal growth: Results from a prospective study, *Epidemiology*, 6, 115, 1995.

17. Scholl, T.O. and Reilly, T., Anemia, iron and pregnancy outcome, *J. Nutr.*, 130, 443S, 2000.

18. Allen, L.H., Anemia and iron deficiency: Effects on pregnancy outcome, *Am. J. Clin. Nutr.*, 719 (suppl), 1280S, 2000.

19. Scholl, T.O. and Hediger, M.L., Anemia and iron-deficiency anemia: Compilation of data on pregnancy outcome, *Am. J. Clin. Nutr.*, 59 (suppl), 492S, 1994.

20. Milman, N., Agger, A.O. and Nielsen, O.J., Iron supplementation during pregnancy: Effect on iron status markers, serum erythropoetin and human placental lactogen, *Dan. Med. Bull.*, 38, 471, 1991.

21. Institute of Medicine, *Iron Deficiency Anemia: Guidelines for Prevention, Detection and Management among U.S. Children and Women of Childbearing Age*, Food and Nutrition Board, National Academy Press, Washington, D.C., 1993.

22. Puolakka, J., Janne, O., Pakarinen, A. and Vihko, R., Serum ferritin as a measure of stores during and after normal pregnancy with and without iron supplements, *Acta. Obstet. Gynecol. Scand.*, 95 (suppl), 43, 1980.

23. Svanberg, B., Arvidsson B., Norrby, A., Rybo, G. and Solvell, L., Absorption of supplemental iron during pregnancy — A longitudinal study with repeated bone marrow studies and absorption measurements, *Acta. Obstet. Gynecol. Scand.*, 48 (suppl), 87, 1976.

24. American Diabetes Association, Preconception care of women with diabetes, *Diabetes Care*, 24 (suppl), 66S, 2001.

25. Holing, E.V., Beyer, C.S., Brown, C.A. and Connell, F.A., Why don't women with diabetes plan their pregnancies?, *Diabetes Care*, 21, 889, 1998.

26. Semba, R.D., Miotti, P.G. and Chipangwi, J.D., Infant mortality and vitamin A deficiency during human immunodeficiency virus infection, *Clin. Infect. Dis.*, 21, 966, 1995.

27. Position Paper of the American Dietetic Association: Promotion of breastfeeding, *J. Am. Diet. Assoc.*, 97, 662, 1997.

28. Howard, C., Howard, F., Lawrence, R. Andersen, E., DeBlieck, E. and Weitzman, M., Office prenatal formula advertising and its effect on breastfeeding patterns, *Ostet. Gynecol.*, 95, 296, 2000.

29. Chomitz, V.R., Cheung, L.W. and Lieberman, E, The role of lifestyle in preventing low birthweight, *Future Choices*, 5, 121, 1995.

30. Koop-Hoolihan, L.E., Van Loan, M.D., Wong, W.W. and King, J.C., Longitudinal assessment of energy balance in well-nourished pregnant women, *Am. J. Clin., Nutr.*, 69(4), 697, 1999.

31. National Research Council, *Recommended Dietary Allowances*, 10th ed., National Academy Press, Washington, D.C., 1989.

32. Gutierrez, Y., King, J.C., Nutrition during teenage pregnancy, *Ped. Ann.*, 22, 99, 1993.

33. Durnin, J.V., Energy requirements of pregnancy, *Diabetes*, 40 (suppl 2), 151 S, 1991.

34. U.S. Department of Health and Human Services, The Surgeon General's Report on Nutrition and Health, U.S. Public Health Service, Washington, D.C., 1998.

35. Tippett, K.S. and Cleveland, L.E., How current diets stack up: Comparison with the dietary guidelines, America's Eating Habits: Changes and Consequences, Agricultural Bulletin No. 750, U.S. Department of Agriculture, Washington, D.C., 2000.

36. Kirksey, A and Wasynczuk, A.Z., Norphologic, biochemical and functional consequences of vitamin B_6 deficits during central nervous system development, *Ann, N.Y. Acad. Sci.*, 678, 62, 1993.

37. Institute of Medicine, *Dietary Reference Intakes: Thiamin, Riboflavin, Niacin, Vitamin B_6, Folate, Vitamin B_{12}, Pantothenic Acid, Biotin and Choline*, National Academy Press, Washington, D.C., 1998.

38. Scholl, T.O. and Johnson, W.G., Folic acid: Influence on the outcome of pregnancy, *Am. J. Clin. Nutr.*, 71(5), 1295S, 2000.

39. Sheldon, W.L., Aspillaga, M.O., Smith, P.A. and Lind, T., The effect of oral iron supplementation on zinc and magnesium levels during pregnancy, *Br. J. Obstet. Gynaecol.*, 92, 892, 1985.

40. Jameson, S., Zinc status in pregnancy: The effect of zinc therapy on perinatal mortality, prematurity and placental ablation, *Ann. N.Y. Acad. Sci.*, 678, 178, 1993.

41. Institute of Medicine, *Dietary Reference Intakes: Calcium, Phosphorous, Magnesium, Vitamin D and Fluoride*, National Academy Press, Washington, D.C., 1999.

42. U.S. Department of Agriculture and U.S. Department of Health and Human Services, Nutrition and your health: Dietary guidelines for Americans, 2000.

43. Rothman, K.J., Moore, L.L., Singer, M.R., Nguyen, U.S., Manniino, S. and Milunsky, A., Teratogenicity of high vitamin A intake, *New Engl. J. Med.*, 333, 1369, 1995.

44. Schaeffer, D.M., Maternal nutritional factors and congenital anomalies: A guide for epidemiological investigation, *Ann. N.Y. Acad. Sci.*, 678, 205, 1993.

45. Centers for Disease Control, Recommendations to prevent and control iron deficiency in the United States, *Morbid. Mortal., Wkly. Report*, 47, 1, 1998.

46. Ritchie,L.D. and King, J.C., Dietary calcium and pregnancy-induced hypertension: Is there a relation?, *Am. J. Clin. Nutr.*, 71, 1371S, 2000.
47. Institute of Medicine, *Nutrition During Pregnancy and Lactation: An Implementation Guide*, National Academy Press, Washington, D.C., 1992.
48. Foote, J. and Rengers, B, Medicinal herb use during pregnancy and lactation, *Perinatal Nutr. Report*, 5, 1, 1998.
49. Fisher-Rasmussen, W., Kjaer, S.K., Dahl, C. and Asping, U., Ginger treatment of hyperemesis gravidarum, *Eur. J. Obstet. Gynecol. Reprod. Biolog.*, 38, 19, 1990.
50. Meltzer, D.I., Complementary therapies for nausea and vomiting during early pregnancy, *Fam. Pract.*, 17, 570, 2000.
51. Godfrey, K.M. and Barker, D.J., Fetal nutrition and adult disease, *Am. J. Clin. Nutr.*, 71, 1344S, 2000.
52. Edwards, L.E., Hellerstedt, W.L., Alton, I.R., Story M. and Himes, J.H., Pregnancy complications and birth outcomes in obese and normal-weight women: Effects of gestational weight change, *Obstet. Gynecol.*, 87, 389, 1996.
53. Hediger, M.L., Overpeck, M.D., McGlynn, A., Kucmarski, R.J., Maurer, K.R. and Davis, W.W., Growth and fatness at 3 to 6 years of age of children born small or large for gestational age, *Pediatrics*, 104, 33, 1999.
54. Scheive, L.A., Cogswell, M.E. and Scanlon, K.S., An empirical evaluation of the Institute of Medicine's pregnancy weight guidelines by race, *Obstet. Gynecol.*, 91, 878, 1998.
55. Wong, W., Tang, N.L.S., Lau, T.K. and Wong, T.W., A new recommendation for maternal weight gain in Chinese women, *J. Am. Diet. Assoc.*, 100, 791, 2000.
56. Luke, B., Hediger, M.L. and Scholl, T.O., Point of diminishing returns: When does gestational weight gain cease benefiting birthweight and begin adding to maternal obesity?, *J. Mat. Fetal Med.*, 5, 168, 1996.
57. Segel, J.S. and McAnarney, E.R., Adolescent pregnancy and subsequent obesity in African-American girls, *J. Adol. Hlth.*, 15, 491, 1994.
58. Strauss, R.S. and Dietz, W.H., Low maternal weight gain in the second or third trimester increases the risk for intrauterine growth retardation, *J. Nutr.*, 129,988, 1999.
59. Hickey, C.A., Cliver, S.P., McNeal, S.F., Hoffman, H.J. and Goldenberg, R.L., Prenatal weight gain patterns and spontaneous preterm birth among non-obese black and white women, *Obstet. Gynecol.*, 85, 909, 1995.
60. Carmichael, S.L. and Abrams, B., A critical review of the relationship between gestational weight gain and preterm delivery, *Obstet. Gynecol.*, 89, 865, 1997.
61. Hartmann, S. and Bung, P., Physical exercise during pregnancy — Physiological considerations and recommendations, *J. Perin. Med.*, 27, 204, 1999.
62. Clapp, J.F., Exercise during pregnancy: A clinical update, *Clin. Sports Med.*, 19, 273, 2000.
63. Groff, J.Y., Mullen, P.D., Mongoven, M. and Burau, K., Prenatal weight gain patterns and infant birthweight associated with maternal smoking, *Birth*, 24, 234, 1997.
64. Muscati, S.K., Koski, K.G. and Gray-Donald, K., Increased energy intake in pregnant smokers does not prevent human fetal growth retardation, *J. Nutr.*, 126, 2984, 1996.
65. Drews, C.D., Murphy, C.C., Yeargin-Allsopp, M. and Decoufle, P., The relationship between idiopathic mental retardation and maternal smoking during pregnancy, *Pediatrics*, 97, 547, 1996.
66. Roquer, J.M., Figueras, J., Botet, F. and Jimenez, Influence on fetal growth of exposure to tobacco smoke during pregnancy, *Acta. Paediatr.*, 84, 118, 1995.
67. Hannigan, J.H. and Armant, D.R., Alcohol and pregnancy and neonatal outcome, *Seminars in Neonatology*, 5, 243, 2000.

68. Huxley, R.R., Nausea and vomiting in early pregnancy: Its role in placental development, *Obstet. Gynecol.*, 95, 779, 2000.

69. Ward, E., Ed., Pregnancy nutrition: Good health for you and your baby, in *American Dietetic Association*, John Wiley & Sons, New York, 1998.

70. Broussard, C.N. and Richter, J.E., Nausea and vomiting of pregnancy, *Gastroent. Clin. N. Am.*, 27, 123, 1998.

71. Fairburn, C.G., Stein, A. and Jones, R., Eating habits and eating disorders during pregnancy, *Psychosom. Med.*, 54, 665, 1992.

72. Horner, R.D., Lackey, C.J., Kolaska, K. and Warren, K., Pica practices of pregnant women, *J Am. Diet. Assoc.*, 91, 34, 1991.

73. Edwards, C.H., Johnson, A.A., Knight, E.M., Oyemade, U.J., Cole, O.J., Westney, O.E., Jones, S., Laryea, H. and Westney, L.S., Pica in an urban environment, *J. Nutr.*, 124, 954S, 1994.

74. Casey, B.M., Lucas, M.J., McIntire D.D. and Leveno, K.J., Pregnancy outcomes in women with gestational diabetes compared with the general obstetric population, *Obstet. Gynecol.*, 90, 869, 1997.

75. American Diabetes Association, Gestational Diabetes Mellitus, *Diabetes Care*, 24, S77, 2001.

76. Cho, N.H., Silverman, B.L., Rizzo, T.A. and Metzger, B.E., Correlations between the intrauterine metabolic environment and blood pressure in adolescent offspring of diabetic mothers, *J. Pediatr.*, 136, 587, 2000.

77. Vohr, B.R., McGarvey, S.T. and Tucker, K. Effects of maternal gestational diabetes on offspring adiposity at 4–7 years of age, *Diabetes Care*, 22, 1284, 1999.

78. Wallenberg, H., Prevention of pre-eclampsia: Status and perspectives 2000, *Eur. J. Obstet. Gynecol. Reprod. Biol.*, 94, 13, 2001.

79. Churchill, D., Perry, I.J. and Beevers, B.G., Ambulatory blood pressure in pregnancy and fetal growth, *Lancet*, 349, 7, 1997.

80. Bucher, H.C., Cook, R.J., Guyatt, G.H., Lang, J.D., Cook, D.J., Hatala, R. and Hunt, D.L., Effects of dietary calcium supplementation on blood pressure: A meta-analysis of randomized controlled trials, *JAMA*, 275, 1016, 1996.

81. Chappell, L.C., Seed, P.T., Briley, A.L., Kelly, F.J., Lee, R., Hunt, B.J., Parmer, K., Bewley, S., Shennan, H., Steer, P.J. and Poston, L, Effect of antioxidants on the occurrence of pre-eclampsia in women at increased risk: A randomized trial, *Lancet*, 354, 810, 1999.

82. Dekker, G. and Sibai, B., Primary, secondary and tertiary prevention of pre-eclampsia, *Lancet*, 357, 209, 2001.

83. McIntyre, J., HIV in pregnancy: A review, World Health Organization, Joint United Nations Programme on HIV/AIDS, 1998.

84. Mofenson, L.M. and McIntyre, J.A., Advances and research directions in the prevention of mother-to-child HIV-1 transmission, *Lancet*, 355, 2237, 2000.

85. Kogan, M., Alexander, G., Kotelchuck, M. and Nagey, D., Relation of the content of prenatal care to the risk of low birthweight: Maternal reports of health behaviors, advice and initial prenatal care procedures *JAMA*, 271, 1340, 1994.

86. Besharov, D. and Germanic P., Is WIC as good as they say?, *Public Interest*, 134, 1, 1999.

87. Kowaleski-Jones and Duncan G., Effects of participation in the WIC program on birthweight: evidence from the National Longitudinal Survey of Youth, *Am. J. Pub. Health*, 92, 799, 2002.

88. Avruch, S. and Cakley, A., Savings achieved by giving WIC benefits to women prenatally, *Publ. Hlth. Reports*, 110, 27, 1995.

89. Hediger M.L., Overpeck, M.D., Kuczmarski, R.J. and Ruan, W.J., Association between infant breastfeeding and overweight in young children, *JAMA*, 285, 2453, 2001.

90. American Academy of Pediatrics National Research Council, *Nutrition During Lactation*, National Academy Press, Washington, D.C., 1991.

91. American Academy of Pediatrics, Work group on breastfeeding and the use of human milk, *Pediatrics*, 100, 1035, 1997.

92. Anderson, J.W., Johstone, B.M. and Remley, D.T., Breastfeeding and cognitive development: A meta-analysis, *Am. J. Clin. Nutr.*, 70, 525, 1999.

93. Mortenson, E.L., Michaelsen, K.F., Sanders, S.A. and Reinisch, J.M., The association between duration of breastfeeding and adult intelligence, *JAMA*, 287, 2365, 2001.

94. National Research Council, *Nutrition During Lactation*, National Academy Press, Washington, D.C., 1991.

95. Butte, N.F., Garza, C. and Stuff, J.E., Effect of maternal diet and body composition on lactational performance, *Am. J. Clin. Nutr.*, 39, 296, 1984.

96. Brewer, M.M., Bates, M.R. and Vannot, L.P., Postpartum changes in maternal weight and body fat deposits in lactating vs. nonlactating women, *Am. J. Clin. Nutr*, 49, 259, 1989.

97. Butte N.F., Garza, C. and Smith, E.O., Human milk intake and growth in exclusively breastfed infants, *J. Pediatr.*, 104, 187, 1984.

98. Goldberg, G.R., Prentice, A.M. and Coward, W.A., Longitudinal assessment of energy expenditure during pregnancy by the doubly labeled water method, *Am. J. Clin. Nutr.*, 57, 494, 1993.

99. Institute of Medicine, *Dietary Reference Intakes for Vitamin C, Vitamin E, Selenium and Carotenoids*, National Academy Press, Washington, D.C., 2000.

100. Institute of Medicine, *Dietary Reference Intakes for Vitamin A, Vitamin K, Arsenic, Boron, Chromium, Copper, Iodine, Iron, Manganese, Molybdenum, Nickel, Silicon, Vanadium and Zinc*, National Academy Press, Washington, D.C., 2001.

101. Humphrey, S., Sage advice on herbs and breastfeeding, *LEAVEN*, 34, 43, 1998.

102. Lawrence, R.A. and Lawrence, R.M. *Breastfeeding: A Guide for the Medical Professional*, Mosby, St. Louis, 1999.

103. Macnamara, J.P., Role and regulation of metabolism in adipose tissue during lactation, *J. Nutr. Biochem.*, 6, 120, 1995.

104. Butte, N.F. and Hopkinson, J.M., Body composition changes during lactation are highly variable among women, *J. Nutr.*, 128, 381S, 1998.

105. Lovelady, C.A., Lonnerdal, B. and Dewey, K.G., Lactation performance of exercising women, *Am. J. Clin. Nutr.*, 52, 103, 1990.

106. Dewey, K.G. and McCrory, M.A., Effects of dieting and physical activity on pregnancy and lactation, *Am. J. Clin. Nutr.*, 59, 446S, 1994.

7 Hormonal Oral Contraception and Nutrition: Vitamins and Minerals

Priscille G. Massé and Carole C. Tranchant

CONTENTS

0-8493-1337-6/03/$0.00+$1.50
© 2004 by CRC Press LLC

I. INTRODUCTION

Introduction of the birth-control pill (oral contraceptives (OCs)) into our modern society almost 40 years ago stands out as an epochal event in human history.[1] The use of OCs has never ceased to grow since then. It impacted various aspects of social life, including women's careers and role in the family, the size of families and gender relationships. Modern women became sexually active earlier, delaying the birth of their first child and limiting their total number of children. Today, approximately 14 million women in the U.S. and 150 million worldwide, averaging 85% of reproductive-age women, choose OCs for birth control because of their convenience and efficiency. These statistics reflect changes in economics with the increase in family income and the need to reduce the costs associated with childbearing and childrearing.[2] The decrease in unintended pregnancies over the past years has been attributed to the more widespread use of contraception and increased use of more effective methods such as OCs.[3]

II. COMPOSITION AND TRENDS

OCs are among the most thoroughly studied drugs. The new generation of OCs includes both the low-dose combined estrogen-progestogen (progestin) pill, which contains less than 50 µg estrogen and less than 1.5 mg progestogen, and the progestogen-only pill. All of the combined steroid preparations contain an estrogen component (e.g., ethinyl estradiol or mestranol) and a progestogen (progestin) (e.g., norethindrone acetate, norethynodrel or norgestrel). The progestins may differ, although those derived from 19-nortestosterone are essentially the same. This progestative steroid exhibits a progesterone-like activity and is used because progesterone itself is inactive when taken orally. Due to extensive metabolism, the fate of progestogens in the body is more complex than the fate of synthetic estrogens. More than 30 metabolites have been identified for the various progestogens.

More than two dozen preparations are currently marketed. The majority are modifications of the "first generation" higher-dose combined estrogen-progestogen. The estrogen dose found in today's OCs has been reduced to <20% of the dose employed in the earliest preparations. Over the last 15 years, the dose of estrogen has been reduced to the minimum required to suppress follicular development (equivalent to 20 µg ethinylestradiol). In the most recent formulations, daily doses of ethinyl estradiol, the most widely used estrogen, are in the 20–40 µg range.[4] A low dose of estrogen is considered 35 µg or less. Dose reduction has also been applied to the progestin component, with modern formulations now containing <10% of the original doses. The newer low-dose OCs are efficacious, reliable and have good cycle control and minimal metabolic impact. New "third-"generation gestogens, such as desogestrel, gestodene and norgestimate, have been introduced to reduce the incidence of side effects associated with the androgenic effect of 19-nor derived gestogens, such as the alterations of lipid and carbohydrate metabolism.[4–7] A newly approved progestin, drospirenone, differs from other progestins in that it has both anti-mineralocorticoid and anti-androgenic activities. Symptoms such as bloating and breast tenderness are lessened by its diuretic effect.

During the past decade, the major development in hormone contraceptive technology has been the introduction of triphasic preparations, e.g., Triphasil® (Wyeth-Ayerst Laboratories), which has been studied recently for both metabolic and related psychological side effects (see Section IVA.1.a). These new combinations of low-dose hormones are specifically tailored to minimize estrogen- and progestogen-related side effects, to mimic the woman's physiologic hormonal cycle and to provide effective contraception. This contraceptive regimen consists of three phases, each with a different progestin dose. In some formulations, the estrogen dose is increased in the second phase as well. All triphasic and most modern monophasic OCs include ethinyl estradiol as the estrogenic constituent. All five progestins used in triphasic OCs are 19-nortestosterone derivatives. The three newer progestins (desogestrel, gestodene and norgestimate) can be considered derivatives of norgestrel, with structural changes that result in reduced androgenic side effects without the loss of menstrual cycle control. Overall, cycle control appears to be somewhat better for the triphasics containing the newer progestins than for the formulations containing norethindrone or norgestrel.[4]

Further refinements of hormonal contraception, which have taken place over the last 10 years and which will be developed further, are new delivery systems of the steroids by non-oral routes, e.g., percutaneously or vaginally. Examples include: the combination transdermal patch, the monthly combination injectable marketed as Lunelle® (Pharmacia), the vaginal ring marketed as NuvaRing® (Organon) and the single-rod implant. These new contraceptive methods bypass the first pass through the liver and, hence, have an impact on metabolism.[8] With such delivery systems, the dose of hormone can be reduced considerably in comparison with the dose required using the oral route. The efficacy, compliance, safety and cycle control of these new contraceptive methods have been well studied. However, to our knowledge, relevant metabolic and nutritional studies are still lacking. This is why only oral contraception will be discussed in the present chapter. The emphasis has been placed on OC-induced metabolic and related psychological side effects, with a particular emphasis on vitamins and minerals.

III. ESTABLISHMENT OF METABOLIC CHANGES

The assessment of any drug-induced metabolic effects implies the evaluation of the nutritional status, which requires laboratory tests on easily available body fluids such as blood and urine. The tests should be specific, simple and inexpensive and should reveal tissue depletion at an early stage. The choice of the blood component is guided by the concentration of the vitamin in it and by its sensitivity to deficiency states. Vitamin B_{12} measurements are generally made using the serum or plasma, whereas, for most other water-soluble vitamins, plasma as well as blood cells are used. For fat-soluble vitamins, only plasma is used because the concentrations of these vitamins or their metabolites in blood cells are very low.[9] Under some circumstances, the distribution of vitamins between tissues is known to be altered. One such example is OC use.

In the case of vitamins, nutritional status can be evaluated basically by two types of biochemical tests:

1. Tests based on the measurement of either the vitamin or its metabolites in blood or urine:
   - In metabolic tests, a rise in the concentration of a metabolite in blood or urine as a result of a vitamin deficiency-mediated enzymatic lesion is measured, preferably after administering a load of an appropriate precursor. Examples of such tests are the tryptophan load test inherent to the evaluation of pyridoxine status (e.g., urinary level of xanthurenic acid), the histidine and valine load tests to assess folate and vitamin B_{12} status by the formiminoglutamic acid (abbreviated as FIGLU) and methylmalonic acid excretions in urine, respectively.
2. Tests based on the measurement of one or more of the enzymatic and metabolic functions of the vitamin (functional tests):
   - In the case of the B complex vitamins, it has been possible to develop functional tests, since most of their biochemical functions are well established. In the interpretation of test results, it is advisable to take into account the basal enzyme activity as well as its activation with coenzyme, known as the *in vitro* stimulation test, which is expressed as "activation coefficient" (AC). Examples of functional enzymatic tests are transketolase for thiamin, glutathione reductase for riboflavin, and alanine (ALT) and aspartate (AST) aminotransferases for pyridoxine (vitamin B_6), commonly known as GPT and GOT transaminases, respectively.

Sauberlich[10] has described tentative guidelines for the interpretation of laboratory tests currently available for assessing vitamin nutrition status. Table 7.1 indicates some tests pertinent to our discussion. This table will be referred to throughout this chapter.

A. Overview of OC-Induced Metabolic Changes

The enthusiastic acceptance and widespread use of OCs have withdrawn attention from their potential side effects. This subject has been documented previously on several occasions. Either estrogens or progestogens, or their combination, modulate a number of physiological processes that are metabolic and nutritional in nature. In general, their ingestion has been shown to significantly or nonsignificantly affect a number of metabolic processes in either a disadvantageous or a beneficial manner. Examples will be given to highlight some cases pertaining to vitamins and minerals.

The significance of the alterations in nutrient metabolism becomes a matter of concern when OCs are used on a long-term basis. Table 7.2 summarizes the recognized metabolic modifications that may occur in women upon exposure to "the pill." In brief, serum concentrations tend to rise for iron, copper and vitamin A (retinol), while reductions are reported in circulating levels of selected B vitamins, ascorbic acid (vitamin C) and zinc.[11-15] The most significant decreases are found in water-soluble vitamins, namely, thiamin (vitamin B_1), riboflavin (vitamin B_2), pyridoxine (vitamin B_6), cobalamin (vitamin B_{12}) and folate. Clinical effects of severe vitamin

TABLE 7.1
Normal Values for Pertinent Blood Vitamin Levels, their Inherent Enzyme Tests and Urinary Excretion or their Metabolites in Adults

	Acceptable (low risk)
Erythrocyte aspartate aminotransferase (AC)*	< 1.80
Erythrocyte alanine aminotransferase (AC)	< 1.25
Plasma vitamin B_6 (PLP)** (nmol/L)	≤ 30
Serum folate (nmol/L)	≤ 13.4
Erythrocyte folate (nmol/L)	≤ 356
Serum vitamin B_{12} (pmol/L)	≤ 147
Urinary metabolites	
Total vitamin B_6 (μmol/day)	> 0.5
Pyridoxic acid (nmol/nmol creatinine)	128-680
Xanthurenic acid (μmol/day)	< 65
Methylmalonic acid (μg/mg creatinine)	< 5

* AC: Activation coefficient.
** PLP: Pyridoxal phosphate.

Adapted from Sauberlich, H.E., *Laboratory Tests for the Assessment of Nutritional Status. Second Edition*, CRC Press, Boca Raton, FL, 1999.

deficiencies are rare (Table 7.3). However, a marginal (or subclinical) vitamin deficiency can occur. Marginal deficiency describes a condition in which vitamin status is poor (depleted reserves) but no overt symptoms of a deficiency are present. The increases in vitamin A, iron and copper are not large enough to cause clinical effects and may even be beneficial in some instances. The changes in vitamin A and copper can be explained by an increase in serum-binding proteins, retinal-binding protein (RBP) and ceruloplasmin, respectively.[16] The elevation of serum iron will be discussed more thoroughly in Section V.

IV. EFFECTS OF OCs ON VITAMIN NUTRITION

Several studies have been conducted on the effects of OCs on several vitamins, namely, vitamin A, thiamin, riboflavin, pyridoxine, folate, cobalamin, vitamin C, α-tocopherol (vitamin E) and vitamin K.[12,17,18] However, some studies have been criticized for methodological reasons. For instance, an early study on vitamin E that revealed that OC-users had significantly lower values than nonuser controls, was

TABLE 7.2
Oral Contraceptives and Nutritional Status

Nutrient	Observed Modifications in Nutritional Status
Vitamins	↑ circulating levels of vitamin A. ↓ circulating levels of carotene, vitamin E, thiamine, riboflavin, folate, vitamin B_{12}, vitamin B_6, vitamin C. ↑ *in vitro* stimulation of erythrocyte B_1-dependent transketolase, B_2-dependent glutathione reductase and B_6-dependent aminotransferases with thiamine, riboflavin and pyridoxine (vitamin B_6), respectively. Biochemical signs of vitamin B_6 deficiency in some women (low urinary pyridoxic acid, plasma pyridoxal phosphate (PLP) and erythrocyte aminotransferases); occasionally accompanied by depression.
Minerals	↓ circulating levels of calcium, phosphorus, magnesium and zinc. ↑ circulating levels of iron and copper.

based on a nonspecific spectrophotometric technique and the use of high-dose OCs only.[19] This chapter will focus on vitamins B_6, B_{12} and folate due to:

1. The greater number of studies available
2. The significance of their metabolic alterations in terms of psychological side effects
3. The role of these vitamins in homocysteine metabolism in the contemporary context of homocysteine as a risk factor for cardiovascular disease

TABLE 7.3
Some Vitamin Deficiency Diseases and their Symptoms

Vitamin	Deficiency disease/major symptoms
A (retinol)	Xerophthalmia, night blindness, blindness
B_1 (thiamin)	Beriberi, numbness, muscle weakness, cardiac disturbance Wernicke's encephalopathy, polyneuropathy
B_2 (riboflavin)	Glossitis, dermatitis, cheilosis
Niacin	Pellagra, dermatitis, diarrhea, mental disturbance
B_6 (pyridoxine)	Sideroblastic (microcytic) anemia, dermatitis, depression, convulsions
B_{12} (cobalamin)	Pernicious (macrocytic) anemia, peripheral neuritis, spinal cord degeneration
C (ascorbic acid)	Scurvy, sore gums, capillary bleeding
Folate	Anemia, megaloblastic (macrocytic) anemia

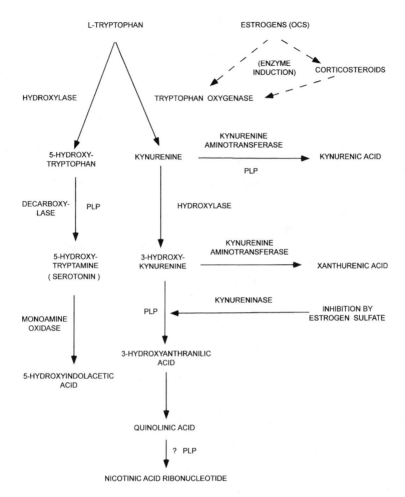

FIGURE 7.1 Tryptophan metabolism in liver and in brain. (From Bamji, M.S., in *Vitamins in Human Biology and Medicine*, Briggs, M.H., Ed., CRC Press, Boca Raton, FL, 1981. With permission). PLP: Pyridoxal phosphate (vitamin B_6).

A. Impairment of Vitamin B_6 Status

1. Indirect Evidence: Abnormalities in Tryptophan Metabolism

As mentioned in Section III, one indirect biochemical method to evaluate vitamin B_6 status consists of measuring the amount of xanthurenic acid (XA) excreted in urine after administration of a tryptophan load test. One of the main roles of vitamin B_6 after it is converted to the coenzyme (active) form pyridoxal phosphate (PLP), is to act as a catalyst in the formation of niacin from tryptophan, an essential amino acid. This metabolic pathway in the liver is illustrated in Figure 7.1. The first enzyme of this pathway, tryptophan pyrrolase (TPase), also named tryptophan oxygenase, appears to be particularly susceptible to the direct effect of OCs or to their secondary stimulating action on glucocorticoid secretion by adrenal glands. In effect, plasma cortisol was found to be significantly elevated in pill users.[20,21] Whatever the mechanism, this induction of hepatic TPase directs more tryptophan than usual into the niacin pathway, which results in a higher metabolic demand for vitamin B_6, since a number of the steps of this pathway are B_6 dependent. The results are the accumulation of tryptophan intermediates and a consequent relative deficiency of vitamin B_6.

The suspicion that OCs might affect vitamin B_6 status arose in part from the analogy drawn with the state of pregnancy (50-fold increased secretion of endogenous estrogen). In fact, the same abnormality in the tryptophan pathway has been demonstrated in women taking a variety of combined estrogen-progestogen contraceptive preparations.[22] This disturbance has been demonstrated after a tryptophan load and also without loading.[17] Several investigators have consistently shown that urinary excretion of XA in women taking OCs is higher than in nonusers.[23–25] For years, this increase in the excretion of XA was interpreted as evidence for pyridoxine deficiency, although, at that time, the mode of action by which estrogen modifies tryptophan metabolism was not clear. Various investigators have proposed that the activation of liver tryptophan catabolism by estrogen was the result of increased TPase activity.[26–29] Consequently, an oral load of tryptophan will cause a relative shortage of PLP coenzyme due to a higher activity of aminotransferases (refer to Figure 7.1) required to transaminate the extra amount of kynurenine and hydroxykynurenine deriving from the accelerated degradation of tryptophan.

The validity of the tryptophan load test as an index of vitamin B_6 deficiency has often been questioned. One study showed that the urinary excretion of XA was poorly correlated with plasma PLP.[30] Leklem[31] reported a significant difference between users of OCs and nonusers in the tryptophan load test, but no significant difference in other indices of B_6 status, such as urinary cystathionine (Figure 7.2), urinary pyridoxic acid, plasma PLP and erythrocyte aminotransferase (ALT and AST) activities. The use of the tryptophan load as an index of B_6 status was also criticized on the grounds that inhibition of kynureninase by estrogens or their metabolites would give results indistinguishable from a true vitamin B_6 deficiency. In effect, as kynureninase is a PLP-dependent enzyme, its activity is also impaired in this deficiency, leading to increased excretion of kynurenic and XA acids.

A relative vitamin B_6 deficiency at the level of B_6-dependent kynureninase might well be responsible for the accumulation of tryptophan metabolites (Figure 7.1). In 1982, Bender et al.[32] extrapolated from their study on rats that abnormalities of tryptophan metabolism in women taking estrogens can be accounted for by the inhibition of this enzyme by estrogen metabolites, and not by a stimulation of TPase activity as was initially thought. In a further experiment, Bender even concluded that there is also inhibition rather than stimulation of TPase.[33] It is noteworthy that the inhibition of both enzymes noted in the aforementioned studies has been demonstrated in rats when given estradiol at a high dose (500 μg/kg body weight, which is much more than the dose used clinically). Thus, there seems to be some disagreement at the present time over the fact that consumption of OCs can contribute to vitamin B_6 deficiency as a result of the perturbation in tryptophan metabolism. However, it is generally agreed that the tryptophan load test is not a reliable indicator of vitamin B_6 nutritional status. This test exhibits a number of problems that have been reviewed by Bender.[34]

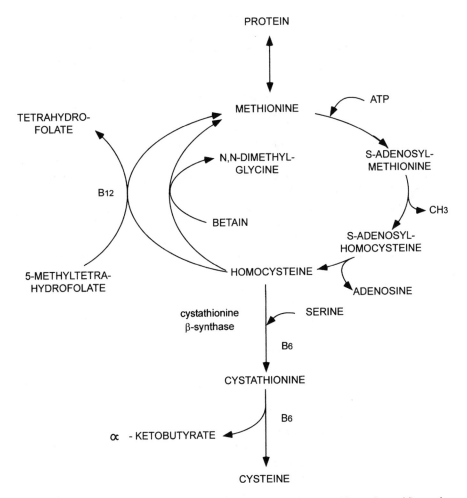

FIGURE 7.2 Role of vitamins B_6, B_{12} and folate in homocysteine (sulfur amino acid) metabolism. (From Smolin, L.A. and Benevenga, N.J., *J. Nutr.*, 114, 103, 1984. With permission).

a. OC-Induced Psychological Side effects

The clinical significance of the tryptophan metabolic abnormality is that the increased TPase activity, as shown by several investigators, may be the cause of the depression observed among women taking OCs.[35] The synthetic estrogens and high amount of endogenous estrogen secreted during pregnancy, by stimulating TPase contribute to the diversion of tryptophan metabolism from its minor brain serotonin (5-hydroxytryptamine or 5-HT) pathway to its major kynurenine-niacin pathway in the liver.[36] This shift of tryptophan metabolism toward the kynurenine-niacin pathway, which is evidenced by increased urinary xanthurenic acid excretion, is at the expense of serotonin synthesis in the brain (Figure 7.1). The reduced 24-h urinary output of 5-hydroxyindolacetic acid (5-HIAA), the end product of 5-HT, has been demonstrated by Shaarawy et al.[20] The exact biochemical mechanism by which OCs lower serotonin in the central nervous system and subsequently induce depression in some OC users is not completely understood. Direct links are also possible. First, a direct inhibition of cerebral uptake of tryptophan by the synthetic OC steroids may reduce the amount of tryptophan available for 5-HT synthesis.[37] Second, 5-hydroxytryptophan decarboxylase (a B_6-dependent enzyme, also named aromatic amino acid decarboxylase), which is involved in serotonin synthesis, may be susceptible to competition for PLP by estrogen conjugates.

It is generally accepted nowadays that the biochemical basis of depressive illness is due to impaired synthesis of one or more neurotransmitter amines.[34] Serotonin (5-HT) is one and dopamine is another whose precursor amino acid is tyrosine. Both need to be decarboxylated by the same B_6-dependent enzyme (aromatic amino acid decarboxylase). It is logical, therefore, that the activity of this enzyme is reduced in vitamin B_6 deficiency, thereby reducing the synthesis of the brain amines (neurotransmitters). But according to Bender,[34] the rate-limiting step in these syntheses is not the decarboxylation step for which vitamin B_6 is coenzyme, but the initial hydroxylation reaction of the parent amino acids (tryptophan and tyrosine, respectively) which requires vitamin C. A variety of other mechanisms may be involved too. A number of metabolites affecting brain functions originate from tryptophan metabolism.[38] It is possible that OC-induced psychological side effects are the result of the buildup of circulating neuroactive compounds from this metabolism, such as kynurenine, hydroxykynurenine and quinolinic acid (Figure 7.1).[39] These metabolites compete with tryptophan, the precursor of serotonin, for uptake into the brain.[40] Vitamins other than pyridoxine and vitamin C can also affect the functioning of the central nervous system. For instance, borderline low or deficient serum or red blood cell folate levels have been detected in 15–38% of adults diagnosed with depressive disorders.[41]

Depression has been recognized as a complication of estrogen-progestogen contraceptives, although only a small number of women develop this syndrome. Its incidence is still disputed, but it probably occurs in about 5 to 9% of women on OCs,[37,42–44] whereas the global estimate of women more or less affected by depression increases from 10 to 20%.[45] Recent literature suggests that depression associated with OCs may differ significantly from nonorganic major depressive episodes.[46] There may be a genetic predisposition involved.[47] Psychological studies have focused on the depressive syndrome, although other various emotional states (e.g., nervousness, anxiety, irritability) do occur. In fact, psychological side effects related to OC use are multidimensional in nature.[48] However, the role of OCs as distinct from reactions to life events has not yet been adequately defined in the scientific literature. Although data support a relationship between OCs and psychological well-being, even with the advent of low dose OCs the incidence of psychological side effects seems to decrease and interest in the effect of OCs on the central nervous system has begun to dwindle.

In agreement with Kutner and Brown's study,[49] Massé and Roberge,[50] also using the MMPI (Minnesota Multiphasic Personality Inventory) test, have been unable to confirm the existence of psychological disturbances during the use of oral contraception. In this study, none of the OC users suffered depression, but they were found to have a lower performance on the social introversion (Si) scale.[50] This finding was confirmed by a lower T-score on the correction (K) scale. A moderate elevation of this score can be observed in social, dynamic and enthusiastic persons.[51] In another study on younger women (21.8 ± 2.6 years of age) who were prescribed OCs (Triphasil®) for the first time, the same investigators did not detect psychological changes at an early stage of utilization, e.g., at the sixth menstrual cycle.[52]

The strength of the aforementioned psychological studies lies in the use of the same objective and comprehensive rating instrument (the MMPI). The likelihood of OC-induced psychological side effects has been explored further in our laboratories using more sensitive biochemical means.[21] Plasma ratio of tryptophan to the sum of specific large neutral amino acid competitors, used as an indicator for brain tryptophan availability for serotonin synthesis, was unchanged, whereas its tyrosine counterpart, used as an indicator for brain tyrosine availability for dopamine synthesis, was significantly reduced.[21] This latter finding is in agreement with Møller,[53] who also showed a significant reduction in plasma tryptophan confirming a catabolic enhancement of the tryptophan-kynurenine pathway. In view of the interest in low levels of neurotransmitters in the etiology of depression, several groups have also looked at plasma tryptophan levels and the plasma ratio of tryptophan to large neutral amino acids in depressed patients. Values were found to be low in depression.[54] However, according to Sidransky,[55] the magnitude of the decline is too small to cause an appreciable decline in brain serotonin.

2.   Direct Evidence: Abnormalities in Vitamin B_6 Metabolism

Some controversy also exists where the B_6-dependent ALT and AST enzyme activities are used to assess vitamin B_6 status. When a significant change in basal or activated enzymatic activity is reported, both enzymes are generally affected. The scientific literature pertaining to the activity of these enzymes in serum is exhaustive but shows disparate results. This biochemical parameter that reflects liver functions is known to be a poor indicator of B_6 nutritional status. As judged by the basal activity of specific ALT aminotransferase in erythrocytes (red blood cells), the B_6 status of OC users is either similar to nonusers[56,57] or different enough to be considered significant.[23,58] The basal activity of specific AST aminotransferase in erythrocytes indicated a deficiency in OC users consuming a nonsupplemented diet.[24,59,60] Van der Vange et al.[61] reported no significant change in the activation coefficient (AC) (a more complete and reliable parameter than the basal activity) of this enzyme in erythrocytes after 6 months of low-dose oral contraception. Subjects were taking seven different varieties of monophasic, biphasic and triphasic OC preparations. The follow-up study of Massé et al.[62] confirmed the negative finding of van der Vange et al.[61] However, one case of vitamin B_6 deficiency was reported as judged by erythrocyte AST-AC and plasma PLP. The strengths of the latter study were that only one OC preparation (Triphasil®) was used and that subjects had never used OCs in the past.

Alternative approaches to the assessment of vitamin B_6 status are direct measurements of the vitamin and its metabolites. Attempts to define the nutritional status of vitamin B_6 during oral contraception by biochemical analysis, particularly in blood, but also in urine, have also led to a range of conclusions. Both enzymatic and microbiological assays have been used. The latter method often lacks specificity, which may account for some conflicting results. Chemical HPLC methods have proven most reliable and reproducible.

In several human studies, the concentration of the active form of vitamin B_6 (PLP) in plasma, which is often used as a biochemical indicator of B_6 status, was found to be significantly lower in OC users than in nonusers.[30,60,63-65] It is noteworthy that most of these women returned to their normal PLP values by the sixth month of OC utilization. A similar observation was also made, more recently, by van der Vange et al.[61] According to their more recent OC study, no real difference exists between OC users and nonusers in regard to plasma PLP level.[61] Massé et al.'s[62] specific study on Triphasil®, which was based on biochemical parameters such as plasma and erythrocyte PLP levels as an adjunct to the *in vitro* stimulated activity of AST aminotransferase in erythrocytes, also showed no significant changes after six consecutive menstrual cycles. Only one subject out of 14 exhibited a decline in erythrocyte PLP level at the first menstrual cycle. There was no return to normal values at the sixth month of OC use. This finding was consistent with a continuous elevation of AST-AC (activation coefficient) throughout the study. In addition to using other B_6-specific biochemical criteria, several investigators also studied the urinary excretion of 4-pyridoxic acid. Generally, OCs do not change the level of this metabolite, despite the excretion of abnormal amounts of tryptophan metabolites.[48,63,66,67] Although a high percentage (evaluated to be approximately 80% by Luhby et al.[68]) of women who take OCs exhibit abnormal tryptophan metabolism, only a minority show biochemical evidence of vitamin B_6 deficiency, the exact number depending on the criterion used. It seems that the biochemical alterations of vitamin B_6 metabolism in OC users are diverse.

There is also a possibility that OCs interfere with and impair folate and vitamin B_{12} metabolism, as will be described in the next two sections. These sections will show that several investigators have reported contradictory findings. These discrepancies, independent of the biochemical indicators used, have created some confusion and controversy.

B. IMPAIRMENT OF FOLATE STATUS

Clinical and biochemical indicators frequently examined to assess the folate nutritional status have been the following:

1. The incidence of megaloblastic anemia and cervical dysplasia
2. Serum and erythrocyte folate concentrations
3. The urinary excretion of formiminoglutamic acid (FIGLU)
4. The intestinal absorption of polyglutamates, which are the major dietary sources of folate.

Numerous cases of megaloblastic anemia attributed to OCs have been reported.[69] In some of these cases, other contributory factors, such as a mild malabsorption syndrome or dietary folate deficiency existed and it is not clear whether megaloblastic anemia would have occurred in the absence of these factors. The literature pertinent to the association between OC use and folate status is divergent. Some reports which have demonstrated that women using OCs have a lower serum level of folate than nonusers[70,71] have been contradicted by other reports showing no statistical difference.[72–74] The study of Massé et al.[52] on Triphasil® showed a 18% trend toward a reduction in serum folate, but the difference did not reach statistical significance due to small sample size. The subject is also considered controversial when the erythrocyte (red blood cell) level (a better biochemical marker than serum level and more representative of tissue metabolism) is used to assess nutritional status. A number of investigators have reported that the mean red cell level of folate in groups of women taking OCs, as assessed by microbiological techniques, was significantly lower than that of control groups.[71,75–77] Other studies have failed to show any statistical differences.[65,78]

Although conflicting data still exist as to the effects of OCs on folate status, the majority of reports tend to support the observation that the lowering of folate concentration is accompanied by an increase in urinary FIGLU excretion. FIGLU is an intermediary product of the metabolism of histidine that requires folate to be further metabolized. Shojania[75] found that women using OCs excreted significantly more FIGLU in their urine after a histidine load than controls and that the levels excreted decreased to normal within 2 to 4 months after OC use was stopped. It is not clear whether this increase is due to folate deficiency induced by OCs or to a physiologic effect that mimics early pregnancy. A higher level of FIGLU is also excreted during pregnancy.[79]

Polyglutamates, the major dietary source of folate, must be enzymatically degraded in the small intestine before absorption takes place. Initially, the inhibition of the activity of folate conjugase by OCs and the consequent malabsorption of folate polyglutamates seemed to have provided a satisfying explanation for the impairment of folate metabolism. An early study has described cases of women on OCs showing a defect in utilization or absorption between polyglutamates and monoglutamate.[80] Moreover, the difference in the intestinal absorption between the usual dietary folate and folic acid in therapeutic vitamin preparations, in OC users, has been underlined in several medical reports.[65,75–79] However, subsequent reports failed to show (1) any malabsorption of folate polyglutamates in OC users, (2) neither any change in the conversion of formyl to methyltetrahydrofolate, a vital step for final intestinal absorption, nor (3) any inhibitory effect of OCs and derivative compounds on folate conjugase.[81,82] The mechanism of the impairment of folate metabolism by OCs, both in experimental animals and in humans, remains unclear. The hormonal alterations found during pregnancy do not selectively change polyglutamate absorption, suggesting that oral synthetic estrogens and progestogens may act in a different manner from the naturally occurring hormones, at least as far as intestinal absorption of folate is concerned. Another mechanism has been proposed for the impairment of OC-induced folate metabolism. The increased excretion of folates in the urine, which is also reported in pregnant women, may in part explain the lower levels of folate in serum and erythrocytes of some OC users.[83]

C. Impairment of Vitamin B_{12} Status

OC users have also been reported to exhibit significantly reduced levels of vitamin B_{12} whether the level is determined by microbiological[76,78,84] or radioisotope[84–86] assays. It is difficult to explain the mechanism behind this phenomenon. Serum levels of vitamin B_{12} may be lowered — to subnormal values in some cases — but this finding is not necessarily associated with evidence of tissue depletion (sign of a true deficiency). However, the clinician may suggest that the patient temporarily stop taking "the pill" to see if the serum level of vitamin B_{12} remains decreased. The Schilling test (a radioactive absorption assay) is usually performed to exclude the possibility that the problem is caused by vitamin B_{12} malabsorption. In their recent study on Triphasil®, Massé et al.[52] found that serum vitamin B_{12} level was reduced by 26% but the difference was not significant (due to high variance of data) despite the fact that the blood sample was withdrawn at the same period of menstrual cycle for all subjects.

Besides malabsorption problems, proposed explanations for vitamin B_{12} reduction have included an increased renal excretion and an impaired production of vitamin binders. Hjelt et al.[87] measured vitamin B_{12} absorption and excretion by means of a sensitive whole-body counting technique. Since none of the OC users suffered from dietary insufficiency, the findings of normal absorption and excretion indicated that the vitamin B_{12} stores were adequate. This is in accordance with other studies that have found a normal Schilling test and no changes in erythrocyte levels and in urinary excretion of methylmalonic acid (another biochemical marker for vitamin B_{12} status).[84,85,87]

The low serum vitamin B_{12} level is most likely associated with defective serum vitamin B_{12} binders. In fact, OCs can inhibit the production of transcobalamin I (TC-I), a glycoprotein synthesized by leukocytes. This binder, which is 70 to 100% saturated, is not essential for vitamin B_{12} transport to the tissues and is more concerned with its transport in plasma. Total serum level of TC-I has been found to be reduced[84] or not significantly changed[85,86] in OC users. Since about 90% of vitamin B_{12} is bound to TC-I, a low level of the binder may contribute to the low serum level of vitamin B_{12}. Transcobalamin II is a beta globulin and is 90 to 95% unsaturated, but it plays the major role in vitamin B_{12} transport to the tissues. Larsson-Cohn[88] suggested that OC treatment increases the tissue avidity for vitamin B_{12}, resulting in a redistribution of the vitamin within the different tissue compartments. This is unlikely to occur, according to Shojania and Wylie,[84] because TC-II is unaffected by OCs.

D. Interrelationships between Vitamins B_6, B_{12} and Folate

These three vitamins are involved as coenzymes in homocysteine metabolism (Figure 7.2). Vitamin B_{12} and folate are mutually essential to convert their metabolically inactive form to active form, methylcobalamin and tetrahydrofolate, respectively (Figure 7.2). Kornberg et al.[89] reported the case of a 34-year-old woman who had developed megaloblastic anemia and peripheral polyneuropathy following the use of OCs for 4 years. Both levels of folate and vitamin B_{12} were low in this patient. The poor response to vitamin B_{12} alone and the development of anemia and polyneuropathy 4 months after cessation of vitamin B_{12} therapy suggested that folate deficiency was the primary problem. However, according to Wertalik et al.,[85] oral administration of folic acid has no effect on serum vitamin B_{12} values, suggesting that low serum vitamin B_{12} associated with OC is not secondary to folate deficiency.

Although OCs are widely used, symptoms of folate deficiency rarely develop. It is possible that a minor effect of the drug may unmask a preexistent subclinical vitamin deficiency caused by nutritional factors, hidden malabsorption or increased metabolism. There may also be some relation between the low serum levels of vitamin B_{12} and impaired pyridoxine (tryptophan) metabolism. Boots et al.[90] demonstrated that baboons treated with OCs had lower serum vitamin B_{12} levels than controls, but that the lowering of serum vitamin B_{12} levels could be prevented with pyridoxine.

1. Homocysteine (and Copper): Risks of Cardiovascular Disease

It has been reported that deficiencies in folate and vitamin B_{12} can lead to pathological homocysteinemia with levels comparable to those found in heterozygotic homocystinuric patients.[91–96] Based on these observations, one can hypothesize that the occurrence of vascular events reported during the use of OCs may be induced, at least partially, by pathological homocysteinemia caused by depressed levels of one of the three vitamins playing an important role in the metabolism of homocysteine (Figure 7.2). Steegers-Theunissen et al.[65] showed that the homocysteine levels in fasting serum of long-term users of a monophasic sub-50 OC (Marvelon®), on the third day of the menstrual cycle, were significantly higher in comparison with control women not taking OCs. However, this difference was not significant in the high hormonal phase (50 μg), i.e., on the 21st day. Serum and red blood cell folate and vitamin B_{12} levels were not reduced. However, on both days, the fasting whole-blood PLP concentrations were slightly but significantly lower in OC users. A possible explanation of the difference observed in serum homocysteine levels between the two groups is this decrease in the PLP concentration of OC users. This active form of vitamin B_6 acts as a coenzyme in the conversion of homocysteine to cystathionine[97] (Figure 7.2). The Third National Health and Nutrition Examination Survey (NHANES III) revealed recently that higher estrogen status was associated with a lower serum homocysteine concentration, independent of nutritional status.[98]

As for homocysteine, intriguingly, the increase in serum copper is more pronounced in women using low-estrogen-dose OCs (≤45 μg ethinyl estradiol) than in women using OCs containing 50 μg ethinyl estradiol.[15] This differential increase is more likely explained by the androgenic activity of the combined progestin used. While elevated serum copper concentration was found in users of all types of OCs, the increase appears to be relatively high among women taking OCs containing the third-generation progestin desogestrel, which has a partially anti-androgenic capacity. Whether elevated serum copper concentration during OC use leads to an increased cardiovascular risk is a question that cannot be answered with the data currently at hand. Nevertheless, given the mounting evidence about the cardiovascular risk associated with high-serum copper, the serum copper concentration in women who use OCs, especially anti-androgen effective type, should not be neglected.[99] Taken together, the available data suggest that the possible risk of vascular complications in women receiving triphasic OCs is likely to be comparable to that observed for women using monophasic counterparts containing similar doses of ethinyl estradiol.[4]

V. EFFECTS OF OCs ON MINERAL NUTRITION

Although the metabolic side effects of OCs have been studied for a number of years, reports are scarce with regard to minerals as opposed to vitamins. For instance, as shown in Table 7.2, which mentions a few, OCs can depress the level of zinc and elevate those of copper and iron, which have been the most studied minerals by far. This new section will underline some advantageous sides of OCs other than its contraceptive action.

A. BODY IRON STORES

First, the notable effect of OCs with regard to iron is the reduction in menstrual blood loss that occurs in about 60 to 80% of the women who use them. This is the origin of the statement that the use of oral hormonal contraceptives has a protective effect against iron deficiency.[100] The mode of action of this reduction is known to be due to several different factors. Atrophy of the endometrium is considered the main reason for the reduction in menstrual blood loss during oral contraception. The contraceptive steroids are also known to influence coagulation and fibrinolysis as well as prostaglandin synthesis, which may also contribute to the observed changes in the menstrual blood loss.[101,102]

OC users may lose one third to one half the menstrual blood iron of non-OC users.[103,104] Most studies on this subject were performed several years ago in women using combined OCs containing quantities of estrogen and progestogen well in excess of those found in modern OCs currently in use. However, a recent study has shown comparable results with a modern low-dose combined OC containing 30 μg estradiol and 0.15 mg desogestrel.[105] In this study, the menstrual blood loss was reduced by approximately 44%. If there is such a marked reduction in menstrual blood loss and consequently in iron excretion, the iron status of women of child-bearing age would be significantly improved. This will be particularly beneficial in the prevention of anemia during pregnancy and for teenagers using OCs. In fact, iron requirements of this latter target group are not adequately met due to notoriously bad food habits.

Although the use of steroid contraceptives has been often associated with an improved iron status, there are conflicting data in the literature regarding the effect of OCs on hemoglobin content and blood and tissue iron levels.[106,107] Walters and Lim[108] performed a longitudinal study that showed that hemoglobin level was reduced significantly during OC use because of a 10% increase in plasma volume. This 10% increase in plasma volume was accompanied by a decrease in hemoglobin of 0.3 mg/dL and a decrease in hematocrit of 1.2%, which is less than a 10% difference. It is possible that the change in plasma volume could be responsible for masking any benefits that OC use might entail regarding iron status.

Both serum iron and total iron-binding capacity (TIBC) are elevated in OC users.[16] However, it has been observed that, although changes in TIBC or transferrin occur very rapidly after the onset of treatment with contraceptive drugs, this increase is not followed immediately by an increase in serum iron. Thus, the possibility remains that there may be separate mechanisms affecting serum iron levels and iron-binding capacities.[109] The mechanism by which serum transferrin and TIBC levels are raised may be a function of the stimulatory effect of estrogen on the liver biosynthesis of protein.[110] Moreover, little is known about the mechanism(s) controlling fluctuations in serum iron levels, but fever, time of day and day of the menstrual cycle, as well as iron deficiency, are well-known factors associated with variations in serum iron levels.[111–113]

Serum ferritin is the most reliable single parameter for determination of iron status. Pilon et al.[114] found that, for a given individual, serum ferritin varied less from day to day than did serum iron and percent iron saturation. In the study by Frassinelli-Gunderson et al.,[115] a comparison of serum ferritin and of other parameters of iron status was made between a group of 46 women taking OCs continuously for 2 years or more and 71 women who never took OCs. The mean serum ferritin level of the OC users was significantly higher than that of the control group. Their serum transferrin and serum iron values were also significantly greater than those of the control nonusers, as demonstrated by other investigators.[116] Hemoglobin was identical in both groups. The major differences between the study groups were: (1) the lesser quantity and shorter duration of menstrual blood loss for OC users, (2) the longer menstrual cycle for the controls and (3) the higher heme iron content of the OC users' diet. The heme iron content of the diet was about 0.5 mg/day higher for the OC users, but this alone could not account for the magnitude of the difference in serum ferritin levels. In effect, since the total iron content of the diet was not significantly different, the net amount of absorbed iron would be about 0.05 mg higher for the OC users based on the assumption that the absorption of heme iron is about 20% and about 10% for non-heme iron. The additional 0.05 mg of iron per day over 3 years would then result in a storage of about 55 mg of iron, which is still well below the estimated 113 mg of additional iron stored by the OC users.

In a cross-sectional study on the effects of long-term (4 years on average) use of OCs, Massé and Roberge[116] found that serum ferritin level of OC users was comparable to that of non-OC users. However, their mean serum iron concentration was significantly higher. The discrepancy between these two sets of biochemical data may reflect a shift of minerals from one body pool to another, as postulated by Lei et al.[117] Body iron reserves, as assessed by serum ferritin levels, were considered to be low in both groups of women, although their dietary intakes were adequate.[118] This finding may reflect a lack of readily available iron (heme iron) in their diet. Most of the iron in plant sources is in the less bioavailable non-heme form. To provide a more accurate means of estimating the adequacy of diets with respect to iron metabolism, it has been proposed to discriminate the chemical nature of iron ingested (heme and non-heme) and to take into consideration the dietary vitamin C intake, because this vitamin can enhance the intestinal absorption of non-heme iron.[119,120]

Massé and Roberge's study[50] on the short-term use of Triphasil® also revealed a 1.5-fold increase (although not significant) in the serum ferritin concentration that occurred early after the sixth month of administration. Serum ferritin levels fluctuated very much (as judged by high variance of data) despite the blood sample's being withdrawn during the same period of the menstrual cycle for all subjects. This study confirmed the previous finding that iron body reserves in women, as assessed by serum ferritin, are borderline, irrespective of the choice of the contraception method, even when OC users exhibit an elevation of their serum ferritin. The mechanisms behind this increase observed in OC users have not yet been elucidated. More evidence is required, first of all, to substantiate the physiological impact of this metabolic difference between OC users and nonusers. A correlation analysis showed a relationship (although not significant) between psychometric data (T-score) on MMPI clinical scales and iron status, that is, a lower performance on some clinical scales (particularly those used to detect symptoms such as irritability, aggressiveness and anxiety) in women having lower serum iron and ferritin concentrations.[50] More studies are also needed to understand why the ferritin concentration in the OC users decreases to levels that are similar to those of nonusers during iron supplementation (ferrous fumarate equivalent to 16 mg of iron).[121] To conclude that the higher serum ferritin level actually represents a greater amount of stored iron for OC users, further studies are needed to determine whether induction of apoferritin synthesis can be produced by sex steroids independent from iron.

B. BONE HEALTH STATUS

Enhanced bone mineralization among OC users is biologically plausible because estrogen has a direct positive inhibitory effect on bone resorption. In a study by Pasco et al.,[122] women (age range: 20–69 years) exposed to OCs had a 3.3% greater bone mineral density (BMD) at the lumbar spine. The bone density was higher with increased duration of exposure (5 years).[123] To better understand the effect of OCs on bone health, Zitterman[124] studied calcium renal excretion and biochemical markers of bone formation and resorption. He observed a reduction in urinary calcium loss and a slow bone turnover (less resorption) in young OC users (25.5 years ± 0.8). The risk of postmenopausal bone loss could be reduced for past long-term users (6 years or more) according to Kritz-Silverstein and Barrett-Connor.[125] They examined bone mineral density of 239 postmenopausal women, 35.1% of whom reported prior oral contraceptive use. Women who had used OCs for 6 or more years had significantly higher bone densities of the lumbar spine and femoral neck than women who never were on OCs. A population-based study among Swedish postmenopausal women showed that women who had ever used a high-dose OC had a 44% lower risk for hip fractures than never-users.[126] Data from another study on a cohort of 46,000 women do not support the hypothesis that pill use protects women against the occurrence of osteoporotic fractures in later life.[127] Whether premenopausal estrogen exposure in the form of OCs reduces the risk of osteoporotic fractures remains uncertain.

Cross-sectional studies of bone density among pill users have yielded discrepant results, depending on the dose used, the age of subjects and their physical activity. The bone-mass improvement in past OC users seems to be associated with OCs containing mestranol in dosage of 100 μg daily, not with OCs containing lower doses of mestranol or ethinyl estradiol. In a 2-year study of 200–300 healthy young women aged 20–39 years, no effect of OCs on BMD was seen.[128] Polatti et al.[129] demonstrated a significant increase in bone mass content in young (between 19 and 23 years of age) non-OC users, as expected for this age, but no significant bone change in the OC group occurred after 5 years of a monophasic (20 μg ethinyl estradiol + 0.15 mg desogestrel) treatment. In other words, the use of OCs prevented the occurrence of the physiologic peak of bone mass in these young women. A similar striking finding in another study was that in women (20–35 years old) doing long-term exercise while taking low-dose OCs over a long period of time, no beneficial effect of physical activity on BMD development could be observed by Hartard et al.[130] This unexpected negative impact of exercise in combination with OC use on spinal and femoral neck BMD, also observed by other investigators in women of similar age group, suggests that exercising young women who take OCs compromise the attainment of their bone mass peak.[131,132]

The effect of OCs on bone health is still inconclusive. Few recent studies[130–132] have suggested that exercising young women who take OCs compromise attainment of their bone-mass peak. The question arises as to whether sexually active women taking low-dose OC at an earlier age will develop adequate bones.

C. BREAST-MILK NUTRITIVE COMPOSITION

There are numerous studies of the effects of OCs on the nutritive composition of breast milk . As mentioned above, the use of OCs seems to affect mineral metabolism, with a particularly marked effect on iron. Recently, Baheiraei et al.[133] showed a significantly reduced concentration of magnesium in 26th-week breast milk of Iranian women taking progestogen-only contraceptives. No explanation was proposed and no statistical correlation analysis was performed to relate this change with the noncoincidental elevation of triglyceride concentrations that was found. Biochemically, magnesium and triglycerides are interrelated because magnesium is directly involved in lipid (triglyceride) synthesis. Moreover, the investigators did not take into consideration the maternal variables that might affect lactation and milk components. So many other factors — undernutrition, stage of lactation and hormones involved (e.g., prolactin), adolescent motherhood, gestation length and parity as maternal constitutional variables, in addition to environmental variables such as dietary intakes, smoking, vegetarianism, to name a few — influence milk composition. To add to this complexity, the reported concentrations of minerals in breast milk, for instance iron and copper, show a wide natural variation. Altogether, these factors made clear-cut conclusions impossible.

One would suspect the progestogen component with androgenic activity to be a more likely culprit for the mineral elevation than estrogen. However, progestogens are less likely to interfere with lactation[134] and their effects on mineral metabolism are not as marked as those of estrogens.[16] Recent studies showed no effect on iron, copper and magnesium concentrations in breast milk during the first 6 months of lactation in women taking either a combination pill (30 µg ethinyl estradiol and 0.15 mg levonorgestrel) or a mini-pill (0.35 mg norethindrone).[135,136] In a recent review of the literature, Dórea concluded that prolonged use of OCs before and during lactation does not consistently affect the concentrations of either iron or copper in breast milk.[137]

VI. IMPACT OF OCs ON NUTRITIONAL REQUIREMENTS

Although the effects of OCs on several metabolic routes have been well documented, little information exists about their impact on nutritional requirements. Since the reduction of serum vitamin B_{12} has been observed within a few months of the administration of OCs and since the possibility does exist that related folate deficiency-induced megaloblastic anemia might result from long-term use, it has been proposed that the requirement for vitamin B_{12} of women on OCs be considered to be the same as those of pregnant women.[138] As previously mentioned, the first factor thought to be the cause of higher serum iron level in women taking OCs is that progestogens cause atrophy of the endometrium and induce a scanty withdrawal bleeding that is less than in a normal cycle. This is why the nutritional iron requirement of women — in other words, their dietary need for iron — might be lowered while taking OCs.[12,138] This contention is supported by the observation that steroid contraceptives not only decrease the menstrual blood loss, but also increase iron absorption from the gut.[107]

A wealth of research articles have dealt with the effects of OC use on pyridoxine (vitamin B_6) status. This considerable interest was triggered by reports in the 1960s that women using oral contraception exhibited abnormal tryptophan metabolism, which was corrected by a vitamin B_6 supplement.[139] If XA excretion is used as the sole criterion, one might indeed conclude that a significant proportion of OC users require additional vitamin B_6 beyond what they normally consume. However, nutritionists universally agree with the conclusion that XA (a tryptophan metabolite) is not a good indicator of vitamin B_6 status. The use of a more direct and accurate biochemical indicator, namely plasma PLP level, provided the evidence that a significant number of OC users do not require additional dietary pyridoxine.[30] Moreover, the results of depletion and repletion studies based on a diversity of parameters are not in favor of an increased requirement during oral contraception.[25,66,140,141] Donald and Bossé[141] concluded that the requirement for this vitamin, in the majority of cases, was close to that for women not using oral contraception. According to the American National Academy of Sciences, there is no evidence to support a greater dietary allowance for OC users based on the fact that their plasma PLP levels are not deficient and therefore their vitamin B_6 status does not appear to be compromised.[142]

However, there are several observations justifying the concern for an adequate nutritional requirement for vitamin B_6 during oral contraception. One is that lower plasma PLP levels (although not statistically significant) have consistently been observed in some OC users (about 10 to 20%). Second, the level of PLP in whole blood was found to be lowered significantly[65,143] and erythrocyte PLP concentration as well, albeit slightly.[140] The latter biochemical parameter is a very good indicator of tissue metabolism, but unfortunately, for lack of well-established normal reference values, is not usually used for assessing vitamin B_6 status. Third, a B_6-dependent enzyme such as ALT, considered to have a relatively constant activity as opposed to AST, which can be influenced directly by sex steroids, can be *in vitro* stimulated with PLP. This is an excellent method to confirm a metabolic lack of vitamin B_6, as already discussed in a previous section. Finally, the effect of long-term use of OCs on the vitamin B_6 status of future pregnant and lactating women is a real concern to nutritionists. According to a report by Roepke and Kirksey,[144] these women may be at risk of developing vitamin B_6 deficiency after a long-term use of OCs. These investigators suggested that long-term use of OCs before conception reduces the reserves of vitamin B_6, thereby compounding the effects of hormonal changes that affect vitamin B_6 in normal pregnancy. According to Miller,[145] vitamin B_6 status should be monitored and evaluated in women using OCs, especially those who are postponing pregnancy and intending to breast-feed their infants. Reynolds et al.[146] revealed that the dietary vitamin B_6 intakes of upper-income-class pregnant and lactating women were only half of the current recommended dietary allowances.

A. PERTINENCE OF ORAL SUPPLEMENTATION

The elevation of iron body stores upon OC use entails health considerations. Women taking OCs should have their iron levels monitored and should talk to their physician before using iron-containing supplements. Supplementation with iron might impose a risk of iron overload for some OC users, except for those who have borderline or deficient iron stores. General nutritional iron supplementation or fortification is not justified, as this would imply unnecessary treatment in those 50–60% of women who have replete iron stores.[100] Any proposal for further enrichment of food with iron needs to be reassessed in light of the recent study showing a 3.5 times greater risk of myocardial infarction for past OC users (depending on the duration of its use).[147] Vitamin A levels can also be increased during oral contraception.[12,14,78] According to Amatayakul et al.,[148] serum vitamin A can be elevated as high as 40% above those of control subjects. Caution is needed regarding daily supplementation of this vitamin, especially periconceptionally, to avoid toxic or teratogenic levels. Routine supplementation of 1,000 IU of vitamin A does not approach these levels.

Folate deficiency may not necessarily be the cause of megaloblastic anemia if it is present in OC users. Certain underlying disorders in absorption and metabolism may be the principal factors involved. Other factors, such as insufficient diet, alcoholism and disease, can also be related to megaloblastic anemia. Folic acid supplementation is advisable for high-risk groups, such as women who become pregnant within 6 months after the interruption of OC utilization and women with increased folate needs caused by repeated pregnancies, malnutrition, iron deficiency, malnutrition, or anticonvulsant drug use. It is well known that pregnancy increases the metabolic demand for this vitamin.[9] Folate deficiency during pregnancy is a real public health concern because of the risk of neural tube defect (*spina bifida*) in the newborn.[149] Women living in marginal economic conditions and teenagers having poor dietary habits and taking the pill need a folic acid supplement. Martinez and Roe[150] suggest a daily dose varying between 50 µg and 1 mg.

A high dose (10 mg folic acid tablet) has been tested to reduce the progression of cervical dysplasia and to help reduce the risk of cervical cancer in women taking OCs. At present, there is epidemiologic evidence that OC use is associated with this form of cancer. Moreover, histological biopsy previously revealed that megaloblastic features are "deceptively similar" to those observed in early cervical cancer. OCs are known to increase the rate of cell division of cervical cells, hence escalating the need for adequate folate intake. In their study, Butterworth et al.[151] found that low red blood cell folate level enhances the effect of other risk factors, such as the number of sexual partners, smoking and parity. Folate deficiency appears to play a crucial role early in cervical carcinogenesis by facilitating the incorporation of HPV (human papillomavirus) genomes at a fragile chromosomal site.[152] In a previous study, Butterworth et al.[153] measured red blood cell folate concentration and assigned biopsy scores to 47 cervical dysplasia patients and controls. Initially, folate concentrations were lower in OC users than nonusers and lowest in users with dysplasia. After a double-blind 3-month placebo-controlled trial using 10 mg folic acid, treated subjects had significantly better biopsy scores than controls. According to a more recent study, the same investigators concluded that folate deficiency may be involved as a co-carcinogen during the initiation of cervical dysplasia, but folic acid supplements do not alter the course of the established disease.[154] A summary of early reports concluded that approximately one fifth of OC users had megaloblastic changes in the cervicovaginal epithelium that were completely reversed by folic acid supplementation.[155] A striking finding is that these changes were found even in women with normal serum folate levels. This finding suggests that other factors such as homocysteine and copper are involved, as revealed in a recent study.[156]

Lower cobalamin (vitamin B_{12}) concentrations in OC users are seen both in populations with adequate and inadequate nutritional conditions. According to Hjelt et al.,[87] absorption and excretion of this vitamin in OC users are not different from other women. No sign of pernicious anemia has ever been associated with OCs. According to Mooij et al.,[78] multivitamin supplementation did not change the vitamin B_{12} concentration, suggesting that the lower vitamin B_{12} in OC users does not reflect a situation of higher vitamin B_{12} demand.

Significant improvements in vitamin B_6 status occur when pyridoxine hydrochloride is administered, usually at dose levels of 10 to 40 mg daily. Several years ago, Rose and Adams[139] showed that the administration of only 10 mg vitamin B_6 supplement could restore tryptophan metabolism to normal when a relatively high dose of estrogen (50 µg ethinyl estradiol or more) was used. Improvement in the metabolic response of subjects to OCs containing a relatively low dose (30 µg ethinyl estradiol) has also been reported.[13] Daily administration of 40 mg not only restores normal tryptophan biochemical values but also relieves the clinical symptoms (including glucose intolerance) in those vitamin B_6-deficient women taking OCs.[44] A 150 mg daily dose of vitamin B_6 was administered for 30 days to 124 women including low-dose OC users (30 µg ethinyl estradiol) in a randomized triple-blinded placebo-controlled trial of 124 women. A nonsignificant decrease in the severity of all symptoms (nausea, dizziness, depression, irritability) was found in both groups suggesting more a placebo effect than a pharmacological effect.[157]

Winston[158] made the first attempt to treat OC-induced depression with a vitamin B_6 supplement. In 1969, he reported beneficial effect with a 50 mg dose administered daily. Subsequently, Baumblatt and Winston[159] observed that the administration of vitamin B_6 supplement to 58 women taking OCs who complained of premenstrual depression relieved the symptoms in 18 and resulted in an improvement in a further 26. According to these studies, vitamin B_6 therapy seemed to be successful in alleviating the symptoms of depression, although they have been criticized for not being well controlled. In Massé and Roberge's nutritional intervention study,[160] OC users and nonusers were given a 100 mg vitamin B_6 supplement during a complete menstrual cycle. Significant positive changes were observed at the end of the nutritional intervention for half of the 10 clinical MMPI scales in both groups and plasma

PLP levels were increased threefold. No case of deficient or marginal values was reported. Although the mean T-score on the depression (D) scale was not modified by the B_6 supplement, it improved significantly in subjects having a baseline T-score equal or superior to 60 — whatever the groups. In the group of depressed women studied by Adams et al.[161] only those having absolute vitamin B_6 deficiency responded to the administration of pyridoxine supplement.

A positive psychological response to supplemental dose of pyridoxine may be attributed to the stimulating dopaminergic activity of this vitamin in the central nervous system, as has been demonstrated by pharmacological studies on humans and animals.[162–164] In effect, this vitamin is a coenzyme in the decarboxylation reaction that converts dopa to dopamine. Massé and Roberge's study[160] suggests a role for the vitamin B_6 supplement as a psychostimulant agent.

VII. CONCLUSIONS

The nutritional status of a woman reflects her dietary habits, which are influenced by several factors and life styles, including consumption of "the pill." Numerous biochemical studies have clearly demonstrated that the use of OCs is associated with decreased or increased plasma levels of some vitamins and minerals. OC users represent a selected group at risk of poor vitamin status in the U.S. population.[165] For example, the percentage of population having an inadequate vitamin B_6 and folate status is estimated to be 10.4. In view of the role of these vitamins in the growth and functioning of the central nervous system and in homocysteine metabolism, adequate nutritional status of all pregnant and lactating women in general, and those who use OCs before conception in particular, should be of concern.

OCs are not harmful to infants but, because estrogen diminishes the maternal milk supply, these products should be avoided by breastfeeding mothers whenever possible, especially during the first 2 months of breastfeeding.[166] The opinion is divergent on this matter. According to Shenfield and Griffin,[167] concentrations of OC-steroid hormones secreted in breast milk are small and mothers taking them can breastfeed safely.

While the absence of obvious malnutrition is considered to represent good nutrition, the importance of preventing functional metabolic disturbances that can evolve into overt clinical symptoms has been recognized.[168] This is why women should be encouraged to adopt good dietary habits during oral contraception. Table 7.4 summarizes the best dietary sources of nutrients that are susceptible to the influence of OCs. New Dietary Reference Intakes (DRI) (formerly known as Recommended Dietary Allowances or RDA) of the American National Academy of Sciences (1999)[169] are also indicated (see also Appendix to this volume). Consumption of the foods proposed is encouraged or discouraged during oral contraception to minimize the risks of nutritional deficiencies or excess (e.g., vitamin A and iron). There is little or no need for nutritive supplements for OC users who have an adequate diet. Vitamin and mineral supplementation are indicated only if deficiency symptoms become apparent and cannot be corrected through dietary adjustments. At present, supplements are advised only for high-risk groups where other factors such as diet, previous pregnancies and disease could increase the chances for a deficiency to

TABLE 7.4
Major Dietary Sources of Vitamins and Minerals at Risk of Deficiency or Excess During Oral Contraception and Respective Nutritional Recommendations for Adult Women and Teenagers*

	DRI**	
Vitamin A and carotenes	800 µg RE	Milk, butter, fortified margarine, liver, eggs, leafy green and yellow vegetables (e.g., carrots)
Vitamin E	8 mg TE	Vegetable oils, margarine, leafy green vegetables, wheat germ, whole-grain products, liver, egg yolk, nuts
Thiamin	1.1 (1.0) mg	Enriched bread and cereals, liver, peas and lima beans, leafy green vegetables
Riboflavin	1.1 (1.0) mg	Eggs, liver, lean meats, enriched bread and cereals, leafy green vegetables, milk
Vitamin B_6	1.3 (1.2) mg	Liver, meats, fish, eggs, whole grain cereals, green leafy and yellow vegetables, bananas, grapes, pears
Vitamin B_{12}	2.4 µg	Liver, other meats, clams, sardines, salmon, oysters, herring, other fish, cheese, milk, eggs
Ascorbic acid (Vitamin C)***	60 mg	Lemons, oranges, grapefruit, tangerines strawberries, cantaloupe, citrus fruit juices, canned fruit beverages fortified with vitamin C, sweet peppers, broccoli, Brussels sprouts, cabbage, turnip greens, collards, collard greens, cauliflower, spinach, kale, tomatoes
Folate***	400 µg	Liver (beef, calf, lamb, pork, chicken), asparagus, spinach, lettuce, onions, Brussels sprouts, cauliflower, broccoli, cabbage, peas, beans, nuts, orange juice, berries
Iron	10.9 (11.4) mg	Red meats, fish, poultry, shellfish, eggs, legumes
Zinc	12 mg	Liver, other animal protein foods
Calcium	1000 (1300) mg	Milk, buttermilk, ice cream and ice milk, cheese, cottage cheese
Magnesium	320 (360) mg	Dried beans and peas, soybeans, nuts

*Dietary reference intakes (DRI) for teenagers 14–18 years of age are in parentheses.

**Dietary Reference Intakes (DRI), National Academy of Sciences, National Academy Press, Washington, D.C., 1999.

***Major losses occur due to storage or cooking.

RE = Retinol equivalents.

TE = Tocopherol equivalents.

develop. If a woman becomes pregnant within 6 months of discontinuing OCs, she should be considered at risk for nutritional depletion, especially if she has been using them for several years.[170]

Since OC-induced metabolic changes can occur within the first few months, screening for side effects may be done routinely after 6 months of use. Nutritional status should be reassessed after 5 years of use or more often.

REFERENCES

1. Tyrer, L., Introduction of the pill and its impact, *Contraception*, 59, 11S, 1999.
2. Archer, D.F., New contraceptive options, *Clin. Obstet. Gynecol.*, 44, 122, 2001.
3. Parker Jones, K., Oral contraception: Current use and attitudes, *Contraception*, 59, 17S, 1999.
4. Cedars, M.I., Triphasic oral contraceptives: Review and comparison of various regimens, *Fertil. Steril.*, 77, 2002.
5. van Rooijen, M., von Schoultz, B., Silveira, A., Hamsten, A. and Bremme, K., Different effects of oral contraceptives containing levonorgestrel or desogestrel on plasma lipoproteins and coagulation factor VII, *Am. J. Obstet. Gynecol.*, 186, 44, 2002.
6. Troisi, R.J., Cowie, C.C. and Harris, M.I., Oral contraceptive use and glucose metabolism in a national sample of women in the United States, *Am. J. Obstet. Gynecol.*, 183, 389, 2000.
7. Gupta, S. and Harding, K, Contraception and cardiovascular disorders, *Br. J. Fam. Plann.*, 25, 13, 1999.
8. Baird, D.T., Overview of advances in contraception, *Br. Med. Bull.*, 56, 704, 2000.
9. Bamji, M.S., Laboratory tests for the assessment of vitamin nutritional status, in *Vitamins in Human Biology and Medicine*, Briggs, M.H., Ed., CRC Press, Boca Raton, FL, 1981.
10. Sauberlich, H.E., *Laboratory Tests for the Assessment of Nutritional Status. Second Edition*, CRC Press, Boca Raton, FL, 1999.
11. Worthington, B.S., Nutrition during pregnancy, lactation and oral contraception, *Nurs. Clin. North Am.*, 14, 269, 1979.
12. Webb, J.L., Nutritional effects of oral contraceptive use. A review, *J. Reprod. Med.*, 25, 150, 1980.
13. Prema, K., Ramalakshmi, B.A. and Babu, S., Serum copper and zinc in hormonal contraceptive users, *Fertil. Steril.*, 33, 267, 1980.
14. Thorp, V.J., Effect of oral contraceptive agents on vitamin and mineral requirements, *J. Am. Diet. Assoc.*, 76, 581, 1980.
15. Berg, G., Kohlmeier, L. and Brenner, H., Effect of oral contraceptive progestins on serum copper concentration, *Eur. J. Clin. Nutr.*, 52, 711, 1998.
16. Amatayakul, K., Metabolism: Vitamins and trace elements, in *Pharmacology of Contraceptive Steroids*, Goldzieher, J.W., Ed., Raven Press, New York, 1994, 363.
17. Tonkin, S.Y., Oral contraceptives and vitamin status, in *Vitamins in Human Biology and Medicine*, Briggs, M.H., Ed., CRC Press, Boca Raton, FL, 1981, 29.
18. Tyrer, L.B., Nutrition and the pill, *J. Reprod. Med.*, 29, 547, 1984.
19. Tangney, C.C. and Driskell, J.A., Vitamin E status of young women on combined-type oral contraceptives, *Contraception*, 17, 499, 1978.
20. Shaarawy, M., Fayard, M., Nagui, A.R. and Azim, S.A., Serotonin metabolism and depression in oral contraceptive users, *Contraception*, 26, 193, 1982.
21. Massé, P.G., Livingstone, M.M., Duguay, C. and Beaulieu, G., Testing the tyrosine/catecholamine hypothesis of oral contraceptive-induced psychological side effects: A controlled study on Triphasil®, *Ann. Nutr. Metab.*, 45, 102, 2001.
22. Rose, D.P., Excretion of xanthurenic acid in the urine of women taking progestogen-oestrogen preparations, *Nature*, 210, 196, 1966.
23. Faisy, A. and Mahtab, B.S., Vitamin supplements to women using oral contraceptives, *Contraception*, 14, 309, 1976.

24. Faisy, A., Bamji, M.S. and Iyengar, L., Effect of oral contraceptive agents on vitamin nutrition status, *Am. J. Clin. Nutr.*, 28, 606, 1975.

25. Leklem, J.E., Brown, R.R., Rose, D.P., Linkswiler, H.M. and Arend, R.A., Metabolism of tryptophan and niacin in oral contraceptive users receiving controlled intakes of vitamin B$_6$, *Am. J. Clin. Nutr.*, 28, 146, 1975.

26. Rose, D.P., The influence of oestrogens on tryptophan metabolism in man, *Clin. Sci.*, 31, 265, 1966.

27. Leonard, B.E. and Hamburger, A.D., Sex hormones, tryptophan oxygenase activity and cerebral monoamine metabolism in the rat, *Biochem. Soc. Trans.*, 2, 1351, 1974.

28. Manning, B.D. and Mason, M., Kynurenine metabolism in rats: Some hormonal factors affecting enzyme activities, *Life Sci.*, 17, 225, 1975.

29. Kanke, Y., Suzuki, K., Hirakawa, S. and Goto, S., Oral contraceptive steroids: Effects on iron and zinc levels and on tryptophan pyrrolase and alkaline phosphatase activities in tissues of iron-deficient anemic rats, *Am. J. Clin. Nutr.*, 33, 1244, 1980.

30. Lumeng, L., Cleary, R.E. and Li, T.K., Effect of oral contraceptives on the plasma concentration of pyridoxal phosphate, *Am. J. Clin. Nutr.*, 27, 326, 1974.

31. Leklem, J.E., Vitamin B$_6$ requirement and oral contraceptive use — a concern? *J. Nutr.*, 116, 475, 1986.

32. Bender, D.A., Tagoe, C.E. and Vale, J.A., Effects of oestrogen administration on vitamin B$_6$ and tryptophan metabolism in the rat, *Br. J. Nutr.*, 47, 609, 1982.

33. Bender, D.A., Inhibition of kynureninase by oestrogen conjugates: Evidence that oestrogens do not cause vitamin B$_6$ deficiency, *Prog. Clin. Biol. Res.*, 144A, 351, 1984.

34. Bender, D.A., Oestrogens and vitamin B$_6$ — Actions and interactions, *World Rev. Nutr. Diet*, 51, 140, 1987.

35. Herzberg, B.N., Johnson, A.L. and Brown, S., Depressive symptoms and oral contraceptives, *Br. J. Med.*, 4, 142, 1970.

36. Rose, D.P. and Braidman, I.P., Excretion of tryptophan metabolites as affected by pregnancy, contraceptive steroids and steroids, *Am. J. Clin. Nutr.*, 24, 673, 1971.

37. Malek-Ahmadi, P. and Behrmann, P.J., Depressive syndrome induced by oral contraceptives, *Dis. Nerv. Sys.*, 37, 406, 1976.

38. Moroni, F., Tryptophan metabolism and brain function: Focus on kynurenine and other indole metabolites, *Eur. J. Pharmacol.*, 375, 87, 1999.

39. van de Kamp, J.L. and Smolen, A., Response of kynurenine pathway enzymes to pregnancy and dietary level of vitamin B$_6$, *Pharmacol. Biochem. Behav.*, 51, 753, 1995.

40. Holman, P., Pyridoxine – Vitamin B$_6$, *J. Austral. Coll. Nutr. Environ. Med.*, 14, 5, 1995.

41. Alpert, J.E. and Fava, M., Nutrition and depression: The role of folate, *Nutr. Rev.*, 55, 145, 1997.

42. De Lia, J.E. and Emery, M.G., Clinical pharmacology and common minor side effects of oral contraceptives, in *Clinical Obstetrics and Gynecology — Update on Oral Contraception*, Beck, W.W., Ed., Harper & Row, Scranton, PA, 1981, 879.

43. Herzberg, B. and Copper, A., Changes in psychological symptoms in women taking oral contraceptives, *Br. J. Psychiat.*, 116, 161, 1970.

44. Bermond, P., Therapy of side effects of oral contraceptive agents with vitamin B$_6$, *Acta Vitaminol. Enzymol.*, 4, 45, 1982.

45. Weissman, M.M., Leaf, P.J., Holzer, C.E., Myers, J.K. and Tischler, G.L., The epidemiology of depression. An update on sex differences in rates, *J. Affect. Disord.*, 7, 179, 1984.

46. Patten, S.B. and Lamarre, C.J., Can drug-induced depression be identified by their clinical features? *Can. J. Psychiat.*, 37, 213, 1992.
47. Kendler, K.S., Martin, N.G., Heath, A.C., Handelsman, D. and Eaves, L.J., A twin study of the psychiatric side effects of oral contraceptives, *J. Nerv. Ment. Dis.*, 176, 15, 1988.
48. Chang, A.M.Z., Chick, P. and Milburn, S., Mood changes as reported by women taking the oral contraceptive pill, *Aust. N.Z. Obstet. Gynaecol.*, 22, 78, 1982.
49. Kutner, S.J. and Brown, W.L., Types of oral contraceptives, depression and premenstrual symptoms, *J. Nerv. Ment. Dis.*, 155, 153, 1972.
50. Massé, P.G. and Roberge, A.G., Relationship between oral contraceptives, iron status and psychoaffective behavior, *J. Nutr. Med.*, 2, 273, 1991.
51. Gilberstadt, H. and Duker, J., *Handbook for Clinical and Actuarial MMPI Interpretation*, W.B. Saunders, New York, 1982.
52. Massé, P.G., van den Berg, H., Livingstone, M.M., Duguay, C. and Beaulieu, G., Nutritional and psychological status of young women after a short-term use of a triphasic contraceptive steroid preparation, *Int. J. Vitam. Nutr. Res.*, 68, 203, 1998.
53. Møller, S.E., Effect of oral contraceptives on tryptophan and tyrosine availability: Evidence for a possible contribution to mental depression, *Neuropsychobiology*, 7, 192, 1981.
54. Lucca, A., Lucini, V., Piatti, E., Ronchi, P. and Smeraldi, E., Plasma tryptophan levels and plasma tryptophan/neutral amino acids ratio in patients with mood disorder, patients with obsessive-compulsive disorder and normal subjects, *J. Psychiatr. Res.*, 44, 85, 1992.
55. Sidransky, H., *Tryptophan: Biochemical and Health Implications*, CRC Press, Boca Raton, FL, 2002.
56. Joshi, U.M., Lahiri, A., Kora, S., Dikshit, S.S. and Virkar, K., Short-term effect of Ovral and Norgestrel on the vitamin B_6 and B_1 status of women, *Contraception*, 12, 425, 1975.
57. Miller, L.T., Dow, M.J. and Kokkeler, S.C., Methionine metabolism and vitamin B_6 status in women using oral contraceptives, *Am. J. Clin. Nutr.*, 31, 619, 1978.
58. Driskell, J.A., Geders, J.M. and Urban, M.C., Vitamin B_6 status of young men, women and women using oral contraceptives, *J. Lab. Clin. Med.*, 87, 813, 1976.
59. Kishi, H., Kishi, T., Williams, R.H., Watanabe, T., Folkers, K. and Stahl, M.L., Deficiency of vitamin B_6 in women taking contraceptive formulations, *Res. Commun. Chem. Pathol. Pharmacol.*, 17, 283, 1977.
60. Prasad, A.S., Lei, K.Y., Oberleas, D., Moghissi, K.S. and Stryker, J.C., Effect of oral contraceptive agents on nutrients. II. Vitamins, *Am. J. Clin. Nutr.*, 28, 385, 1975.
61. van der Vange, N., van den Berg, H., Kloosterboer, H.J. and Haspels, A.A., Effects of seven low-dose combined contraceptives on vitamin B_6 status, *Contraception*, 40, 377, 1989.
62. Massé, P.G., van den Berg, H., Duguay, C., Beaulieu, G. and Simard, J.M., Early effect of a low dose (30 micrograms) ethinyl estradiol-containing Triphasil® on vitamin B_6 status. A follow-up study on six menstrual cycles, *Int. J. Vitam. Nutr. Res.*, 66, 46, 1996.
63. Miller, L.T., Benson, E.M., Edwards, M.A. and Young, J., Vitamin B_6 metabolism in women using oral contraceptives, *Am. J. Clin. Nutr.*, 27, 797, 1974.
64. Shane, B. and Contractor, S.F., Assessment of vitamin B_6 status. Studies on pregnant women and oral contraceptive users, *Am. J. Clin. Nutr.*, 28, 739, 1975.

65. Steegers-Theunissen, R.P.M., Boers, G.H.J., Steegers, E.A.P., Trijbels, F.J.M., Thomas, C.M.G. and Eskes, T.K., Effects of sub-50 oral contraceptives on homocysteine metabolism: A preliminary study, *Contraception*, 45, 129, 1992.

66. Brown, R.R., Rose, D.P., Leklem, J.E., Linkswiler, H. and Anand, R., Urinary 4-pyridoxic acid and plasma pyridoxal phosphate and erythrocyte aminotransferase levels in oral contraceptive users receiving controlled intakes of vitamin B_6, *Am. J. Clin. Nutr.*, 28, 385, 1975.

67. Leklem, J.E., Brown, R.R., Rose, D.P. and Linkswiler, H.M., Vitamin B_6 requirements of women using oral contraceptives, *Am. J. Clin. Nutr.*, 28, 535, 1975.

68. Luhby, A.L., Brin, M., Gordon, M., Davis, P., Murphy, M. and Spiegel, H., Vitamin B_6 metabolism in users of oral contraceptive agents. I. Abnormal urinary xanthurenic acid excretion and its correction by pyridoxine, *Am. J. Clin. Nutr.*, 24, 684, 1971.

69. Shojania, A.M., Oral contraceptives: effects on folate and vitamin B_{12} metabolism, *Can. Med. Assoc. J.*, 126, 244, 1982.

70. Prasad, A.S., Lei, K.Y., Moghissi, K.S., Stryker, J.C. and Oberleas, D., Effect of oral contraceptives on nutrient. III. Vitamins B_6, B_{12} and folic acid, *Am. J. Obstet. Gynecol.*, 125, 1063, 1976.

71. Pietarinen, G.J., Leichter, J. and Pratt, R.F., Dietary folate intake and concentration of folate in serum and erythrocytes in women using oral contraceptives, *Am. J. Clin. Nutr.*, 30, 375, 1977.

72. Paine, C.J., Crafton, W.D., Dickson, V.L. and Eichner, E.R., Oral contraceptives, serum folate and hematological status, *JAMA*, 231, 731, 1975.

73. Ross, C.E., Stone, M.K., Reagan, J.W., Wentz, W.B. and Kellermeyer, R.W., Lack of influence of oral contraceptives on serum folate, hematologic values and cervical cytology, *Semin. Hematol.*, 13, 233, 1976.

74. Rhode, B.M., Cooper, B.A. and Farmer, F.A., Effect of orange juice, folic acid and oral contraceptives on serum folate in women taking a folate-restricted diet, *J. Am. Coll. Nutr.*, 2, 221, 1983.

75. Shojania, A.M., The effect of oral contraceptives on folate metabolism, *Am. J. Obstet. Gynecol.*, 111, 782, 1971.

76. Areekul, S., Panatampon, P., Doungbarn, J., Yamarat, P. and Vongyuthithum, M., Serum vitamin B_{12}, serum and red cell folic acid binding proteins in women taking oral contraceptives, *S.E. Asian J. Trop. Med. Pub. Hlth.*, 8, 480, 1977.

77. Ahmed, F., Bamji, M.S. and Iyengar, L., Effect of oral contraceptive agents on vitamin nutrition status, *Am. J. Clin. Nutr.*, 28, 606, 1975.

78. Mooij, P.N.M., Thomas, C.M.G., Doesburg, W.H. and Eskes, T.K., Multivitamin supplementation in oral contraceptive users, *Contraception*, 44, 277, 1991.

79. Courtney, M.G., McPartlin, J.M., McNulty, H.M., Scott, J.M. and Weir, D.G., The cause of folate deficiency in pregnancy is increased catabolism of the vitamin, *Gastroenterology*, 92, 1355, 1987.

80. Streiff, R.R., Folate deficiency and oral contraceptives, *JAMA*, 214, 105, 1970.

81. Stephens, M.E.M., Craft, I., Peters, T.J. and Hoffbrand, A.V., Oral contraceptives and folate metabolism, *Clin. Sci.*, 42, 405, 1972.

82. Butterworth, C.E. Jr., Krumdieck, C.L., Stinson, H.N. and Cornwell, P.E., A study of the effect of oral contraceptive agents on the absorption, metabolic conversion and urinary excretion of a naturally occurring folate (citrovorum factor), *Ala. J. Med. Sci.*, 12, 330, 1975.

83. Fleming, A.F., Urinary excretion of folate in pregnancy, *J. Obstet. Gynecol. Br. Com.*, 79, 916, 1972.

84. Shojania, A.M. and Wylie, B., The effect of oral contraceptives on vitamin B_{12} metabolism, *Am. J. Obstet. Gynecol.*, 135, 129, 1979.
85. Wertalik, L.F., Metz, E.N., LoBuglio, A.F. and Balcerzak, S.P., Decreased serum B_{12} levels with oral contraceptive use, *JAMA*, 221, 1371, 1972.
86. Costanzi, J.J., Young, B.K. and Carmel, R., Serum vitamin B_{12} and B_{12}-binding protein levels associated with oral contraceptives, *Texas Rep. Biol. Med.*, 36, 69, 1978.
87. Hjelt, K., Brynskov, J., Hippe, E., Lundström, P. and Munck, O., Oral contraceptives and the cobalamin (vitamin B_{12}) metabolism, *Acta Obstet. Gynecol. Scand.*, 64, 59, 1985.
88. Larsson-Cohn, U., Oral contraceptives and vitamins: A review, *Am. J. Obstet. Gynecol.*, 121, 84, 1975.
89. Kornberg, A., Segal, R., Theitler, J., Yona, R. and Kaufman, S., Folic acid deficiency, megaloblastic anemia and peripheral polyneuropathy due to oral contraceptives, *Israel J. Med. Sci.*, 25, 142, 1989.
90. Boots, L., Cornwell, P.E. and Beck, L.R., Effect of ethynodiol diacetate and mestranol on serum folic acid and vitamin B_{12} levels and tryptophan metabolism in baboons, *Am. J. Clin. Nutr.*, 28, 354, 1975.
91. Stabler, S.P., Marcell, P.D., Podell, E.R., Allen, R.H., Savage, D.G. and Lindenbaum, J., Elevation of total homocysteine in the serum of patients with cobalamin or folate deficiency detected by a capillary gas chromotography mass spectrometry, *J. Clin. Invest.*, 81, 466, 1988.
92. Brattström, L.E., Israelsson, B., Lindgärde, F. and Hultberg, B., Higher total plasma homocysteine in vitamin B_{12} deficiency than in heterozygosity for homocystinuria due to cystathionine β-synthase deficiency, *Metabolism*, 37, 175, 1988.
93. Böttiger, L.E., Boman, G., Eklund, G. and Westerholm, B., Oral contraceptives and thromboembolic disease: Effects of lowering estrogen content, *Lancet*, 1, 1097, 1980.
94. Maguire, M.G., Tonascia, J., Sartwell, P.E., Stolley, P.D. and Tockman, M.S., Increased risk of thrombosis due to oral contraceptives: A further report, *Am. J. Epidemiol.*, 110, 188, 1979.
95. Mishell, D.R., Contraception, *N. Engl. J. Med.*, 320, 777, 1989.
96. Vessey, M.P., Oral contraceptives and cardiovascular disease: Some questions and answers, *Br. Med. J.*, 284, 615, 1982.
97. Smolin, L.A. and Benevenga, N.J., Factors affecting the accumulation of homocysteine in rats deficient in vitamin B_6, *J. Nutr.*, 114, 103, 1984.
98. Morris, M.S., Jacques, P.F., Selhub, J. and Rosenberg, I.H., Total homocysteine and estrogen status indicators in the Third National Health and Nutrition Examination Survey, *Am. J. Epidemiol.*, 152, 140, 2000.
99. Reunanen, A., Knekt, P., Marniemi, J., Mäki, J., Maatela, J. and Aromaa, A., Serum calcium, magnesium, copper and zinc and the risk of cardiovascular death, *Eur. J. Clin. Nutr.*, 50, 431, 1996.
100. Milman, N., Clausen, J. and Byg, K.-E., Iron status in 268 Danish women aged 18–30 years: Influence of menstruation, contraceptive method and iron supplementation, *Ann. Hematol.*, 77, 13, 1998.
101. Siegban, A. and Ruusuvaara, L., Age dependence of blood fibrinolytic components and the effects of low-dose contraceptives on coagulation and fibrinolysis in teenagers, *Thromb. Haemostas.*, 60, 361, 1988.
102. Lundström, V. and Gréen, K., Endogenous levels of prostaglandin F_2 and its metabolites in plasma and endometrium of normal and dysmenorrheic women, *Am. J. Obstet. Gynecol.*, 130, 640, 1978.

103. Thein, M., Beaton, G.H., Milne, H. and Veen, M.J., Oral contraceptive drugs: Some observations on their effect on menstrual loss and hematological indices, *Can. Med. Assoc. J.*, 101, 73, 1969.

104. Newton, J., Barnard, G. and Collins, W., A rapid method for measuring menstrual blood loss using automatic extraction, *Contraception*, 16, 269, 1977.

105. Larsson, G., Milsom, I., Lindstedt, G. and Rybo, G., The influence of a low-dose combined oral contraceptive on menstrual blood loss and iron status, *Contraception*, 46, 327, 1992.

106. Briggs, M. and Staniford, M., Oral contraceptives and blood-iron, *Lancet*, 2, 742, 1969.

107. Margen, S. and King, J.C., Effect of oral contraceptive agents on the metabolism of some trace minerals, *Am. J. Clin. Nutr.*, 28, 392, 1975.

108. Walters, W.A.W. and Lim, Y.L., Haemodynamic changes in women taking oral contraceptives, *J. Obstet. Gynaecol. Br. Com.*, 77, 1007, 1970.

109. Zilva, J.F., Oral contraceptives and serum proteins, *Br. Med. J.*, 3, 521, 1970.

110. McKnight, G.S., Lee, D.C. and Palmiter, R.D., Transferrin gene expression. Regulation of mRNA transcription in chick liver by steroid hormones and iron deficiency, *J. Biol. Chem.*, 255, 148, 1980.

111. Elin, R.J., Wolff, S.M. and Finch, C.A., Effect of induced fever on serum iron and ferritin concentrations in man, *Blood*, 49, 147, 1977.

112. Mardell, M. and Zilva, J.F., Effect of oral contraceptives on the variations in serum-iron during the menstrual cycle, *Lancet*, 2, 1325, 1967.

113. Cook, J.D., Finch, C.A. and Smith, N.J., Evaluation of the iron status of a population, *Blood*, 48, 449, 1976.

114. Pilon, V.A., Howanitz, P.J., Howanitz, J.H. and Domres, N., Day-to-day variation in serum ferritin concentration in healthy subjects, *Clin. Chem.*, 27, 78, 1981.

115. Frassinelli-Gunderson, E.P., Margen, S. and Brown, J.R., Iron stores in users of oral contraceptive agents, *Am. J. Clin. Nutr.*, 41, 703, 1985.

116. Massé, P.G. and Roberge, A.G., Long-term effect of low-dose combined steroid contraceptives on body iron status, *Contraception*, 46, 243, 1992.

117. Lei, K.J., Prasad, A.S., Bowersox, E. and Oberleas, D., Oral contraceptives, norethindrone and mestranol: Effects on tissue levels of minerals, *Am. J. Physiol.*, 231, 98, 1976.

118. Massé, P.G., Nutrient intakes of women who use oral contraceptives, *J. Am. Diet. Assoc.*, 91, 1118, 1991.

119. Monsen, E.R., Halberg, L., Larysse, M., Hegsted, D.M., Cook, J.D., Mertz, W. and Finch, C.A., Estimation of available dietary iron, *Am. J. Clin. Nutr.*, 31, 134, 1978.

120. Henderson-Sabry, J. and Grief, H., Calculated available iron, heme iron and non-heme iron in diets of a group of men, *J. Can. Diet. Assoc.*, 43, 132, 1982.

121. Mooij, P.N.M., Thomas, C.M.G., Doesburg, W.H. and Eskes, T.K.A.B., The effects of oral contraceptives and multivitamin supplementation on serum ferritin and hematological parameters, *Int. J. Clin. Pharmacol. Ther. Toxicol.*, 30, 57, 1992.

122. Pasco, J.A., Kotowicz, M.A., Henry, M.J., Panahi, S., Seeman, E. and Nicholson, G.C., Oral contraceptives and bone mineral density: A population-based study, *Am. J. Obstet. Gynecol.*, 182, 265, 2000.

123. Burkman, R.T., Oral contraceptives: Current status, *Clin. Obstet. Gynecol.*, 44, 62, 2001.

124. Zittermann, A., Decreased urinary calcium loss and low bone turnover in young oral contraceptive users, *Metabolism*, 49, 1078, 2000.

125. Kritz-Silverstein, D. and Barrett-Connor, E., Bone mineral density in postmenopausal women as determined by prior oral contraceptive use, *Am. J. Pub. Hlth.*, 83, 100, 1993.

126. Michaëlsson, K., Baron, J.A., Farahmand, B.Y., Persson, I. and Ljunghall, S., Oral-contraceptive use and risk of hip fracture: A case-control study, *Lancet*, 353, 1481, 1999.

127. Cooper, C., Hannaford, P., Croft, P. and Kay, C.R., Oral contraceptive pill use and fractures in women: A prospective study, *Bone*, 14, 41, 1993.

128. Mazess, R. and Barden, H.S., Bone density in premenopausal women: Effects of age, dietary intake, physical activity, smoking and birth-control pills, *Am. J. Clin. Nutr.*, 53, 132, 1991.

129. Polatti, F., Perotti, F., Filippa, N., Gallina, D. and Nappi, R.E., Bone mass and long-term monophasic oral contraceptive treatment in young women, *Contraception*, 51, 221, 1995.

130. Hartard, M., Bottermann, P., Bartenstein, P., Jeschke, D. and Schwaiger, M., Effects on bone mineral density of low-dosed oral contraceptives compared to and combined with physical activity, *Contraception*, 55, 87, 1997.

131. Weaver, C.M., Teegarden, D., Lyle, R., McCabe, G., McCabe, L.D., Proulx, W., Kern, M., Sedlock, D. anderson, D.D., Hillberry, B.M., Peacock, M. and Johnston, C.C., Impact of exercise on bone health and contraindication of oral contraceptive use in young women, *Med. Sci. Sports Exerc.*, 33, 873, 2001.

132. Burr, D.B., Yoshikawa, T., Teegarden, D., Lyle, R., McCabe, G., McCabe, L.D. and Weaver, C.M., Exercise and oral contraceptive use suppress the normal age-related increase in bone mass and strength of the femoral neck in women 18–31 years of age, *Bone*, 27, 855, 2000.

133. Baheiraei, A., Ardsetani, N. and Ghazizadeh, Sh., Effects of progestogen-only contraceptives on breastfeeding and infant growth, *Int. J. Gynecol. Obstet.*, 74, 203, 2001.

134. Hull, V.J., Research on the effects of hormonal contraceptives on lactation: Current findings, methodological considerations and future priorities, *World Health Stat. Q.*, 36, 168, 1983.

135. Dórea, J.G. and Miazaki, E.S., The effects of oral contraceptive use on iron and copper concentrations in breast milk, *Fertil. Steril.*, 72, 297, 1999.

136. Dórea, J.G., Oral contraceptives do not affect magnesium in breast milk, *Int. J. Gynecol. Obstet.*, 71, 25, 2000.

137. Dórea, J.G., Iron and copper in human milk, *Nutrition*, 16, 209, 2000.

138. Theur, R.C., Effect of oral contraceptive agents on vitamin and mineral needs: A review, *J. Reprod. Med.*, 8, 13, 1972.

139. Rose, D.P. and Adams, P.W., Oral contraceptives and tryptophan metabolism: Effect of estrogen with a low progestogen and a low progestogen (megesterol acetate) given alone, *J. Clin. Pathol.*, 25, 252, 1972.

140. Bossé, T.R. and Donald, E.A., The vitamin B_6 requirement in oral contraceptive users. I. Assessment by pyridoxal level and transferase activity in erythrocytes, *Am. J. Clin. Nutr.*, 32, 1015, 1979.

141. Donald, E.A. and Bossé, T.R., The vitamin B_6 requirement in oral contraceptive users, *Am. J. Clin. Nutr.*, 32, 1023, 1979.

142. Food and Nutrition Board, *Dietary Reference Intakes for Thiamin, Riboflavin, Niacin, Vitamin B_6, Folate, Vitamin B_{12}, Pantothenic Acid, Biotin and Choline*, National Academy Press, Washington, D.C., 2000.

143. Amatayakul, K., Uttaravichai, L., Singkamani, R. and Ruckphapunt, S., Vitamin metabolism and the effects of multivitamin supplementation in oral contraceptive users, *Contraception*, 30, 179, 1984.

144. Roepke, J.L.B. and Kirksey, A., Vitamin B_6 nutriture during pregnancy and lactation. II. The effect of long-term use of oral contraceptives, *Am. J. Clin. Nutr.*, 32, 2257, 1979.

145. Miller, L.T., Do oral contraceptive agents affect nutrient requirements — Vitamin B_6? *J. Nutr.*, 116, 1344, 1986.

146. Reynolds, R.D., Polansky, M. and Moser, P.B., Analyzed vitamin B_6 intakes of pregnant and postpartum lactating and nonlactating women, *J. Am. Diet. Assoc.*, 84, 1339, 1984.

147. Slone, D., Shapiro, S. and Miettinen, O.S., Risk of myocardial infarction in relation to current and discontinued use of oral contraceptives, *New Engl. J. Med.*, 305, 1531, 1981.

148. Amatayakul, K., Underwood, B.A., Ruckphaopunt, S., Singkamani, R., Linpisarn, S., Leelapat, P. and Thanangkul, O., Oral contraceptives: Effect of long-term use on liver vitamin A storage assessed by the relative dose response test, *Am. J. Clin. Nutr.*, 49, 845, 1989.

149. Butterworth, C.E. Jr. and Bendich A., Folic acid and the prevention of birth defects, *Ann. Rev. Nutr.*, 16, 73, 1996.

150. Martinez, O. and Roe, D.A., Effect of oral contraceptives on blood folate levels in pregnancy, *Am. J. Obstet. Gynecol.*, 128, 255, 1977.

151. Butterworth, C.E. Jr., Hatch, K.D., Macaluso, M., Cole, P., Sauberlich, H.E., Soong, S.J., Borst, M. and Baker, V.V., Folate deficiency and cervical dysplasia, *JAMA,* 267, 528, 1992.

152. Butterworth, C.E. Jr., Effect of folate on cervical cancer, *Ann. N. Y. Acad. Sci.*, 669, 293, 1992.

153. Butterworth, C.E. Jr., Hatch, K.D., Gore, H., Mueller, H. and Krumdieck, C.L., Improvement in cervical dysplasia associated with folic acid therapy in users of oral contraceptives, *Am. J. Clin. Nutr.*, 35, 73, 1982.

154. Butterworth, C.E. Jr., Hatch, K.D., Soong, S.-J., Cole, P., Tamura, T., Sauberlich, H.E., Borst, M., Macaluso, M. and Baker, V.V., Oral folic acid supplementation for cervical dysplasia: A clinical intervention trial, *Am. J. Obstet. Gynecol.*, 166, 803, 1992.

155. Lindenbaum, J., Whitehead, N. and Reyner, F., Oral contraceptive hormones, folate metabolism and the cervical epithelium, *Am. J. Clin. Nutr.*, 28, 346, 1975.

156. Thomson, S.W., Heimburger, D.C., Cornwell, P.E., Turner, M.E., Sauberlich, H.E., Fox, L.M. and Butterworth, C.E. Jr., Correlates of total plasma homocysteine: Folic acid, copper and cervical dysplasia, *Nutrition*, 16, 411, 2000.

157. Villegas-Salas, E., Ponce de León R., Juárez-Perez, M.A. and Grubb, G.S., Effect of vitamin B_6 on the side effects of low-dose combined oral contraceptive, *Contraception*, 55, 245, 1997.

158. Winston, F., Oral contraceptives, pyridoxine and depression, *Am. J. Psychiat.*, 130, 1217, 1973.

159. Baumblatt, M.J. and Winston, F., Pyridoxine and the pill, *Lancet*, 2, 832, 1970.

160. Massé, P.G. and Roberge, A.G., The psychoaffective profile of women taking oral contraceptives in relation to vitamin B_6 status, in *Current Topics in Nutrition and Disease: Clinical and Physiological Applications of Vitamin B_6 — Vol. 19, Proc. Third Int. Conf. on Vitamin B_6*, Reynolds, R.D. and Leklem, J.E., Eds., Alan R. Liss, New York, 1988, 381.

161. Adams, P.W., Rose, D.P., Folkard, J., Wynn, V., Seed, M. and Strong, R., Effect of pyridoxine hydrochloride (vitamin B_6) upon depression associated with oral contraception, *Lancet*, 28, 897, 1973.

162. LeChat, P.G., Streichenberger, G., Boismare, F. and Letteron, N., Modification par la pyridoxine des propriétés pharmacologiques antiparkinsoniennes de la L-Dopa, *J. Pharmacol.*, 28, 479, 1977.

163. Roberge, A.G., Differentiation in brain and liver DOPA/5-HTP decarboxylase activity after L-DOPA administration with or without pyridoxine in cats, *J. Neurochem.*, 28, 479, 1977.

164. Cassachia, M., Boni, B. and Meco, G., Pyridoxine and depression: Neuroendocrine aspects, *Acta Vitaminol. Enzymol.*, 4, 55, 1982.

165. Gaby, S.K., Bendich, A., Singh, V.N. and Machlin, L.J., *Vitamin Intake and Health: A Scientific Review*, Marcel Dekker, New York, 1991, 7.

166. Spencer, J.P., Gonzales, L.S. and Barnhart, D.J., Medications in the breastfeeding mother, *Am. Fam. Physician*, 64, 119, 2001.

167. Shenfield, G.M. and Griffin, J.M., Clinical pharmacokinetics of contraceptive steroids. An update, *Pharmacokinetics*, 20, 15, 1991.

168. Pietrzik, K., Concept of borderline vitamin deficiencies, *Int. J. Vitam. Nutr. Res. Suppl.*, 27, 61, 1985.

169. Food and Nutrition Board, *Dietary Reference Intakes (DRI)*, National Academy of Sciences, National Academy Press, Washington, D.C., 1999.

170. Massey, L.K. and Davison, M.A., Effects of oral contraceptives on nutritional status, *Am. Fam. Physician*, 19, 119, 1979.

8 Menopause and Nutrition

Jennifer C. Lovejoy and Michael Hamilton

CONTENTS

I. INTRODUCTION

With improvements in medical care and hygiene, women in most developed countries will live for many years beyond menopause. As a result, nutrition plays an increasingly important role in maintaining the health of women during their postmenopausal years. Many of the diseases commonly found in postmenopausal women, including osteoporosis, cancer, noninsulin-dependent diabetes mellitus (Type 2 diabetes) and cardiovascular disease, have a nutritional basis or component. Nutritional or lifestyle modifications during the postmenopausal years can often help prevent or delay the onset of chronic diseases associated with aging.

II. NUTRITION AND HEALTH RISKS IN THE POSTMENOPAUSAL WOMAN

A. OBESITY

Obesity is a risk factor for a number of chronic diseases common among older women, including cardiovascular disease, Type 2 diabetes and cancer.[1] Most studies have shown that menopause is associated with a modest increase in body weight (~1–2 kg); however, for some women, the weight gain is more substantial.[2] For example, in a longitudinal study of ~500 perimenopausal women, the average weight gain in the group was 2.25 kg; however, 20% of the population gained 4.5 kg or more.[3]

Hormonal changes at menopause may influence cravings for high-sugar or high-fat foods that impact weight gain. In female rats, high levels of estradiol during the follicular phase of the estrous cycle are associated with increased preference for sweet flavors and decreased appetite for fat, while during the luteal phase, fat preference and intake increase.[4,5] In women, some studies have also reported increased sweet preference in the follicular or periovulatory phases.[6] Ovariectomy increases food consumption in female rodents and monkeys, while a single injection of estradiol in ovariectomized female monkeys produces a significant decrease in food intake.[4] Thus, it is possible that the reduction of estrogen levels after menopause may alter food intake and macronutrient preference, making it difficult for some women to maintain appropriate caloric intake.

Changes in lean body mass at menopause may also impact weight gain. There appear to be specific decreases in lean body mass in postmenopausal women.[7] Since decreases in lean mass are strongly associated with lower basal metabolic rate, such changes will lead to positive energy balance if not offset by decreases in food intake. Physical activity, especially that targeted at maintaining muscle mass, is important to offset menopause-associated decreases in lean body mass.

B. CARDIOVASCULAR DISEASE

Postmenopausal women are at greater risk for cardiovascular disease than younger women.[8] Although much of this increased risk is due to the loss of the protective effect of estrogen, nutritional factors also play a role in cardiovascular health.

The role of low-fat diets in preventing cardiovascular disease is controversial. While low-fat diets lower total and LDL-cholesterol, they have also been shown in some clinical studies to reduce HDL-cholesterol and increase triglycerides.[9] However, the majority of studies that have shown adverse effects of low-fat diets on serum lipids have kept body weight stable during the study. When body weight is allowed to fluctuate naturally, it tends to decrease slightly on low-fat diets.[10] Under these circumstances, we have recently shown that a low-fat diet fed for 9 months accompanied by weight loss does not result in decreased HDL-cholesterol or increased triglycerides.[11] Similar findings were observed in the Dietary Approaches to Stop Hypertension (DASH) trial.[12] The DASH diet is a low-fat diet enriched in fruits, vegetables and calcium (mainly from low-fat dairy products). The DASH study demonstrated that low-fat, low-sodium, high-calcium diets improve both blood pressure and serum lipids.[12,13]

Increased body weight per se has been shown to be an independent risk factor for dyslipidemia in the longitudinal Healthy Women Study.[14] In this study, women who gained weight during the perimenopause had a significant increase in serum cholesterol, while those who maintained or lost body weight did not. Given the potential of low-fat diets to reduce calorie intake and assist in maintenance of a healthy body weight,[10] their use by postmenopausal women should be encouraged.

Soy protein, a natural source of phytoestrogens (plant-derived estrogen-like compounds), has also been shown to have cardiovascular benefits. In a meta-analysis of controlled clinical trials, consumption of soy protein (from 31–47 g/day) was shown to reduce total cholesterol by 23.3 mg/dl (9.3%), LDL-cholesterol by 21.7 mg/dl (12.9%) and triglycerides by 13.3 mg/dl (10.5%) relative to consumption of animal protein (casein).[15] While the benefits of soy were greater in individuals with higher serum cholesterol, there were no differences in the effects by age or amount of soy protein consumed. A more recent study also demonstrated that consumption of soy protein produced beneficial effects on serum lipid profile that were not significantly different from the changes seen in women treated with hormone replacement therapy.[16] Epidemiological data also confirm that higher dietary phytoestrogen intakes are associated with lower cardiovascular risk scores in postmenopausal women in the Framingham Study.[17]

In addition to benefits on serum lipids and lipoproteins, phytoestrogens also may have beneficial effects on vascular reactivity. Impaired vascular reactivity has been associated with menopause and can lead to hypertension and cardiovascular disease in older women. Nestel et al. studied the vascular effects of soy isoflavones in perimenopausal and menopausal women not taking hormones.[18] They observed that arterial compliance measured by ultrasound increased by 26% following 5–10 weeks of phytoestrogen supplementation. Animal studies suggest that dietary soy protein may be as effective as hormone replacement therapy in improving vascular reactivity. Clarkson et al.[19] studied coronary artery reactivity in ovariectomized female rhesus monkeys given conjugated equine estrogen (CEE), CEE plus medroxyprogesterone acetate or soy protein. Monkeys fed soy protein had a 12% increase in coronary artery dilation from control, compared with a 10% increase in monkeys receiving CEE and a 4% increase in monkeys receiving CEE plus progesterone. Thus, overall, consumption of soy protein appears to have substantial benefits for cardiovascular health and should be strongly encouraged in postmenopausal women.

Finally, moderate alcohol consumption has been shown to increase HDL-cholesterol and lower LDL-cholesterol in women[20] and is associated with reduced risk of coronary heart disease.[21] However, because alcohol intake also contributes to excess calories and has been related to increased breast cancer risk (see below), no strong conclusion regarding alcohol intake in postmenopausal women can be drawn at this time. Nonetheless, women who currently consume alcoholic beverages in moderation may reap some cardiovascular benefits.

C. TYPE 2 DIABETES

The prevalence of Type 2 diabetes increases with age in both men and women,[22] however, several studies have suggested that menopause per se results in increased insulin resistance,[23] a strong risk factor for Type 2 diabetes. Menopause may therefore increase risk for Type 2 diabetes in women independent of the aging process.

Both insulin resistance and Type 2 diabetes are strongly influenced by nutrition. Obesity is a major nutrition-related risk factor for Type 2 diabetes and most patients with diabetes are (or have been) obese.[24] Obesity commonly results in insulin resistance, which may explain the close association between obesity and Type 2 diabetes. Thus, avoiding excess weight gain during the postmenopausal years is key to reducing diabetes risk.

Dietary fat intake also plays a role in the development of insulin resistance and Type 2 diabetes[25]. Most studies,[26,27] although not all, support a positive association between total fat intake and degree of insulin resistance in non-diabetic individuals. Additionally, several epidemiological studies have suggested that higher intakes of dietary fat predict the development of Type 2 diabetes[28,29] and two recent epidemiological studies have shown positive associations between total fat intake and glycated hemoglobin levels in healthy men and women.[30,31] The type of fat consumed is also important, with saturated and monounsaturated fats conveying a greater risk for insulin resistance and/or diabetes than polyunsaturated and omega-3 fatty acids.[25] Thus, a low fat diet (particularly one low in saturated fats) is prudent for the postmenopausal women in terms of preventing diabetes, in addition to the considerations of heart disease and obesity mentioned above. Low-fat diets high in complex carbohydrates and fiber may further reduce diabetes risk since low-fiber (high glycemic index) diets have been associated with increased diabetes risk.[32]

Limited data suggest that soy protein may protect against the development of insulin resistance at menopause. Soy protein consumption results in a lowering of the insulin/glucagon ratio, primarily due to a decrease in fasting insulin.[33] Improved peripheral insulin sensitivity and improved glucose tolerance have also been observed in rodents fed high soy protein diets compared to high casein diets.[34] In ovariectomized female monkeys, consumption of soy protein resulted in substantial increases in whole-body insulin sensitivity relative to casein consumption.[35] The effect of soy protein on insulin sensitivity and Type 2 diabetes risk has not been studied in humans to our knowledge.

Moderate alcohol consumption has been shown in epidemiological studies of both men [36] and women [37] to be associated with reduced risk of diabetes. Recently, a randomized, controlled clinical study of 51 postmenopausal women demonstrated that consumption of 30 g/d of alcohol (equivalent to approximately 2 alcoholic drinks per day) reduced fasting insulin concentration by 19% and increased insulin sensitivity by 7%.[38] This amount of alcohol also significantly lowered serum triglyceride concentrations by 10%. Thus, as with cardiovascular disease, for women who choose to consume alcohol, there may be some metabolic benefits to modest alcohol intake.

D. OSTEOPOROSIS

Postmenopausal osteoporosis and related hip and spine fracture are significant health risks in older women. In addition to the bone loss that occurs at menopause due to declining estrogen levels, nutritional factors earlier in life are thought to play a major role in the likelihood of developing osteoporosis and fractures. Dietary calcium intake is a major factor in both the development of peak bone mass early in life and also in protecting against bone loss after menopause.[39] Women with low calcium intakes have lower bone density than those with high calcium intakes, however, postmenopausal bone loss occurs despite normal-high calcium intakes.[40,41] Supplementation with calcium and vitamin D has been shown to preserve and perhaps even increase bone mass in elderly women [42] while vitamin D alone has been shown to reduce hip fracture incidence in women living in northern climates where winter sun exposure is low.[43]

Phosphorus, which is high in meat products and many carbonated soft drinks, causes calcium loss. A low calcium-phosphate ratio, typically the result of excess consumption of high phosphorus foods, increases parathyroid hormone concentration causing calcium depletion from bone.[44] High-phosphorus, low-calcium diets are inversely associated with bone density in perimenopausal women, while calcium and phosphorus intakes independently do not predict bone density.[45] Thus, in addition to increasing calcium intake, postmenopausal women should limit consumption of phosphoric-acid containing soft drinks.

High intakes of protein, particularly animal protein, increase urinary calcium losses [46] and cause bone loss in older women.[47] Furthermore, women with higher ratios of animal to vegetable protein intake have 3.7 times greater risk of hip fracture.[47] In contrast, a recent study suggested that animal protein intake was positively correlated and vegetable protein negatively correlated, with bone mineral density in the spine and hip after adjusting for confounding variables.[48] Furthermore, higher protein intakes, when combined with increased calcium intake, may have a beneficial effect on bone in elderly women.[49]

Recently, there has been some indication that soy protein may be protective against bone loss.[50] Potter et. al.[51] demonstrated that supplementing with soy isoflavones resulted in an increase in vertebral bone density relative to casein supplement over 24 weeks in postmenopausal women. Alekel et al. similarly showed that consumption of a soy protein isolate for 24 weeks attenuated bone loss in the lumbar spine of perimenopausal women.[52] Interestingly, a Japanese study reported that dietary soy intake had a stronger positive impact on bone mineral density and bone resorption in postmenopausal women than energy, protein or calcium intakes.[53]

Adequate protein intakes are clearly essential for bone health and proper functioning of many physiologic systems in older women. However, excess protein intake (>50 g/day for women over 51 years), which is not uncommon in the U.S. and Europe, should be avoided and, when possible, preference should be given to consuming vegetable rather than animal protein.

E. CANCER

Rates of cancer in women increase with increasing age, although the role of menopause per se in this increase may vary depending on the type of cancer. Many cancers are recognized as having a nutritional component, therefore, healthy nutrition during the postmenopausal years may help offset cancer risk.

Obesity is a risk factor for development of both breast and endometrial cancer.[54] Additionally, breast cancer mortality is higher in obese postmenopausal women than in those of normal body weight.[55] Obesity also increases risk for colorectal cancer, which, although not specifically a "women's cancer," is the second most common cancer in women after breast cancer.[56]

The role of dietary fat intake in the development of breast cancer is controversial. Early epidemiological studies suggested a relationship between total fat intake[57] or intake of fried foods[58] and breast cancer. Although some more recent studies have not found an association between fat intake and breast cancer,[59] others have confirmed the relationship between total fat intake[60,61] or saturated fat intake[62] and breast cancer. Associations between increased fat intake (particularly animal fat intake) and ovarian cancer[63] and endometrial cancer[64] have also been reported although, as with breast cancer, these associations are not consistent across all studies.

Diets high in fruits and vegetables may be protective against breast and other cancers.[65] This effect is likely to be due to the high concentrations of antioxidant vitamins and minerals (such as vitamin C, E, carotenoids and selenium) in fruits and vegetables; however, other phytonutrients as well as the high fiber content of vegetables and fruits may also be important for cancer prevention. Additionally, since diets high in meat are associated with breast cancer,[66] vegetables and fruits may reduce cancer risk by replacing meat or other fat sources in the diet.

Soy protein consumption has been associated with reduced risk for certain cancers.[67] The incidence of breast cancer is significantly lower in populations that consume more soy products.[68] In the U.S., however, where soy consumption is generally low, there does not appear to be an association between phytoestrogen intake and breast cancer,[69] thus it may be that higher intakes of soy are necessary to achieve a protective effect. Animal studies largely confirm the beneficial effects of soy phytoestrogens on cancer risk. Genistein, an isoflavone in soy, decreases tumor volume and tumor blood vessel density in female nude mice injected with breast cancer cells, and increases breast tumor cell death in tissue culture in a dose-dependent manner.[70] Genistein has also been found to suppress estrogen-dependent tumor proliferation *in vivo*,[71] although some studies have reported that certain doses of genistein stimulate tumor growth *in vivo*.[72] Because, besides isoflavones, there are numerous other compounds in soy that have anticancer effects (e.g., Bowman-Birk inhibitor, inositol hexaphosphate and β-sitosterol),[73] it may be that the adverse effects seen in some *in vivo* studies with high-dose pure isoflavones would not occur if intact soy protein were used. More research is needed to determine the exact effects of isoflavones in breast cancer.

Alcohol intake in women has been associated with an increased risk of breast cancer.[74] This increased risk is seen even in women who consume as little as 8 g of alcohol per day, a group that had a 50% increased risk of breast cancer in one study.[75] On the other hand, alcohol intake does not appear to increase risk for endometrial cancer[76] and even high levels of alcohol consumption are only modestly associated with the incidence of ovarian cancer.[77] Thus, despite the apparent benefits of moderate alcohol consumption on cardiovascular disease and diabetes risk, encouraging alcohol intake in postmenopausal women should be viewed with caution because of the possible increase in breast cancer risk.

III. NUTRITION AND MENOPAUSAL SYMPTOMS
AND COMPLAINTS

The symptoms of menopause include vasomotor flushes, vaginal dryness, skin changes and cognitive and mood changes. Accepted remedies for these symptoms include hormone replacement therapy in addition to a wide variety of largely untested complementary methods such as herbal remedies, vitamins and other dietary supplements. The use of soy products has been studied with regard to reducing symptoms of hot flushes and improving cognition. The data on soy and hot flushes are largely equivocal, with most studies showing similar or only slightly greater symptom improvement with soy compared with control.[78,79] However, several randomized placebo-controlled clinical trials have found statistically significant improvements in hot flush frequency or severity during soy or isoflavone supplementation.[80,81]

Several herbal preparations, including black cohosh (*Cimicifuga racemosa*) and red clover (*Trifolium pratense*) are also high in isoflavones and may have benefits on menopausal symptoms. In a study of 60 surgically menopausal women under age 40, black cohosh produced improvements in self-reported menopausal symptoms similar to that reported with hormone replacement therapy.[82] Similarly, in 50 postmenopausal women with menopausal complaints, 3 months of treatment with black cohosh significantly improved symptom scores on a variety of clinical and psychological measures.[83]

Few studies address the effect of phytoestrogens on cognitive performance. A recent study in rodents indicated that both estradiol and soy protein improve performance during a radial arm maze test that assesses working memory.[84] These researchers have also shown favorable changes in brain markers associated with Alzheimer's disease in rats fed soy protein.[85] Clinical research addressing the effects of soy on human memory and cognition is lacking and is clearly an important area for future study.

IV. GENERAL PRINCIPLES FOR MAINTAINING
HEALTH AFTER MENOPAUSE

A. WEIGHT CONTROL

As discussed above, weight gain during the transition to menopause is modest in most women, although some will experience more significant weight gains during this period. However, because weight gain and obesity are associated with greater health risks, postmenopausal women should be aware of their weight and lifestyle factors that affect weight. Unfortunately, the majority of women do not enter menopause at a healthy weight. A 10-year longitudinal study of women ages 30–55 years revealed an average weight gain of 4.4 lb. (2 kg.), but an incidence of major weight gain (i.e., greater than 10 kg or 22 lbs.) of 12% in white women and 17% in African-American women.[86] Time trends show that the prevalence of obesity (Body Mass Index or BMI > 30 kg/m^2) in middle-aged women has increased significantly from 1960 to 1994.[87] The prevalence of BMI>30 kg/m^2 was 27% in 40–49-year-old women and 36% in 50–59 year olds in 1994, roughly a 60% increase from 1960 survey data in both age groups. Prevalence rates of overweight and obesity are significantly higher in low-income women and those belonging to minority groups, specifically African-American and Mexican-American women.[87] Therefore, in spite of evidence that the healthiest BMI for older women is 19–24 kg/m^2,[88,89] significant numbers of women are entering menopause at body weights that increase health risk, making treatment of excess body weight a major public health goal in this age group.

The intensity of any therapeutic intervention will depend on a woman's personal and family history of risk factors, body fat distribution (upper- vs. lower-body fat) and lifestyle factors such as smoking and physical activity. For example, there should be more concern about a woman who has a BMI of 26 kg/m^2, a waist circumference >88 cm (indicating a significant amount of visceral abdominal fat), who smokes, is sedentary and whose parents have diabetes and coronary heart disease, than a nonsmoking, physically active woman with a BMI of 32 kg/ m^2 whose parents lived into their 80s and 90s and who has a lower-body distribution of fat.[90,91] It is also important to assess osteoporosis risk before initiating a weight loss program since weight loss may decrease bone mineral density (BMD), although this loss appears to be attenuated by physical activity.[92] It is worth noting that significant visceral obesity may make measurement of lumbar spine density by imaging techniques slightly more difficult.[93]

Finally, because industrialized nations have attracted large numbers of immigrants from many parts of the world, western nations are becoming multiethnic societies with demonstrated differences in health risk among women based on ethnicity.[94-96] Even in healthy African-Americans, Asians and Caucasians within given BMI ranges and age groups, there are differences in percent body fat and health risks.[97] Not surprisingly then, it has been suggested that uniform standards for defining overweight, obesity and health risk may not be appropriate in all populations.[98]

Having briefly described the complexity and number of variables associated with weight and health risk, it is important to return to a few basic principles that make intuitive sense. Women who enter menopause at a normal body weight should strive to maintain that weight, while those who are overweight or obese should first of all gain no more weight and preferably lose weight, with a goal of losing and maintaining a 10–15% loss from initial weight. This amount of weight loss, while less than most women hope for,[99] has been shown to result in significant health benefits and, just as importantly, is a loss that is realistic and achievable.[100,101] The strategies by which these goals can be achieved are conceptually simple: controlling caloric intake and the adoption of a physically active lifestyle. However, for those who are unsuccessful in adopting healthier nutrition and physical activity habits, medications are available that can help patients to more effectively decrease caloric intake. Currently available obesity drugs include sibutramine, a centrally acting appetite suppressant, and orlistat, a lipase inhibitor that reduces the absorption of dietary fat. Medications are indicated only in those with a BMI greater than 30 kg/m^2, but may be prescribed in those with a BMI as low as 27 kg/m^2 if obesity comorbidities that affect cardiovascular health or quality of life are present. Obesity surgery (gastric restriction or gastric bypass) is indicated in patients with a BMI of greater than 40 kg/m^2 or as low as 35 kg/m^2 in the presence of obesity comorbidities. Surgery is the most effective treatment for patients with these levels of obesity and should be discussed as a possible option in appropriately selected patients.

B. DIET

The elements of a healthy diet in postmenopausal women are essentially the same as for women of all ages, except that the previously discussed health problems and their prevention take on greater immediacy because of the impact of advancing age. Therefore, the prevention and control of the metabolic syndrome, coronary heart disease and osteoporosis assume greater importance in postmenopausal women, especially those with a family history of these problems.

The rationale for adopting a diet that is low in saturated fat and simple sugars, high in complex carbohydrates and includes generous amounts of vegetables and fruits has been presented in an earlier section of this chapter. Essentially, the food pyramid describes the healthiest diet, but with these modifications: (1) the base of the pyramid should strongly emphasize that unrefined complex carbohydrates are preferred and (2) vegetable sources of protein, particularly soy protein, offer an advantage over animal sources of protein. Calcium from natural sources should be a major component of the diet in women of all ages but particularly so for post-menopausal women. A calcium supplement may be needed to achieve the Recommended Daily Allowance of at least 1200–1500 mg daily. Some authorities recommend a multivitamin daily, even for those whose diet is varied and well balanced.[102]

Because so many women are concerned about gaining weight during menopause and because almost half of all women who enter menopause are either overweight or obese, it may be useful to briefly mention a few basics concerning diet and weight control:

To maintain weight, one must consume no more calories than are expended throughout the day. To lose weight, one must consume fewer calories than are expended during the day. Estimating caloric requirements (i.e., total daily caloric expenditure) is therefore important. Although daily energy requirements are difficult to estimate without sophisticated testing procedures, one can obtain a rough estimate by multiplying body weight in pounds by 10 kcal/lb (or body weight in kilograms by about 22 kcal/lb), although this estimate will be inappropriately low for someone who is normal weight or relatively muscular and lean. Alternatively, one can estimate metabolic rate from the revised WHO equations. For women aged 31–60 years, basal metabolic rate (BMR) can be calculated as:

$$BMR = (0.0342 \times \text{actual weight in kg} + 3.5377) \times 240 \text{ kcal/d}$$

Total energy requirements are then obtained by multiplying BMR by an activity factor of 1.3 (sedentary), 1.5 (moderate activity) or 1.7 (very heavy work or leisure activity). To maintain weight, one must eat approximately the same number of calories as the estimated daily requirement. To lose weight, one must consume less.

Caloric restriction should generally not exceed 500 below estimated daily requirements. Obviously, a well-balanced and varied diet will be the healthiest. On a reduced-calorie diet, it is prudent to take a multivitamin as well as a calcium supplement since some nutritional requirements may not be met when food intake is decreased, even with the most careful dietary plans. As mentioned, weight loss can lead to a decrease in BMD. Although obesity decreases the risk of osteoporosis, potential loss of BMD must be weighed against the benefits of weight loss. Physical activity attenuates the loss of BMD with weight loss.[92]

Meal replacements can be effective for both acute weight loss and weight maintenance. One study showed that replacing two meals and two snacks daily with a commercially available liquid meal and snack bar for an initial 3 months, followed by a 24-month maintenance phase using replacements for just one meal and one snack daily resulted in the maintenance of a 11.3% loss from initial weight, compared with a 5.9% loss in the control group assigned to conventional meals.[103]

Although high-fat, low-carbohydrate diets have enjoyed renewed favor in the last several years, there is no consistent evidence that the proportion of macronutrients in the diet makes any difference with respect to weight maintenance or loss.[104] However, many patients who do go on low-carbohydrate, higher-fat and -protein diets report dramatic weight losses, at least initially. Such losses can probably be attributed to a substantial decrease in caloric intake resulting from the elimination of carbohydrates, which normally compose 50% of caloric intake, as well as the satiating effect of animal protein, which is generally allowed in liberal amounts on these diets.[105] The long-term health effects of low-carbohydrate, higher-fat diets are of concern with respect to cardiovascular risk; however, as mentioned, this issue is still controversial since low-fat, high-carbohydrate diets increase triglycerides and reduce HDL levels,[106] particularly in patients who are insulin resistant and neither gaining nor losing weight.[107] A reasonable course to suggest is that a low-fat diet rich in complex carbohydrates is perfectly appropriate during weight loss,[11] but that, during weight maintenance, it may be preferable to follow the generally recommended 30%-fat diet, low in saturated fats with a relative increase in monounsaturated fats, along with a liberal intake of unrefined complex carbohydrates and fiber in the form of whole grains, vegetables and fruits.

Lifestyles have changed for many working families, who increasingly depend on foods prepared outside the home. Statistics from the U.S. Department of Labor Bureau of Labor Statistics show that women's food budget spent on eating out increased from 27% to 38% between 1974 and 1994.[108] In this study, compared with those who ate out fewer than five times per week, women who ate out 6–13 times per week ate more calories (2057 kcal vs. 1769 kcal), more fat (80 g vs. 61 g) but only slightly more carbohydrate and protein. From a practical standpoint, how often people eat out may not change, but education concerning healthier selections, both in the choice of restaurants and menu items, may help people limit the damage from the large portions and energy dense selections that restaurants offer.

C. Physical Activity

The health benefits of physical activity are well known in terms of cardiovascular risk[109–111] and diabetes.[37] In women, physical activity assumes even greater importance with increasing age because of the increased risk of cardiovascular disease and osteoporosis associated with menopause.

While diet is a critical component of any weight-loss effort or of weight maintenance, the increasing prevalence of overweight and obesity in the United States and other industrialized nations over the last 50–100 years cannot be attributed to a major increase in food intake in the average person since caloric intake from 1965 to 1995 has, on average, changed very little.[112]

Many experts believe that the increasing prevalence of overweight and obesity is instead due to a decrease in physical activity over the past decades. The magnitude of the decline in physical activity is difficult to document, but W.P. James has estimated that, in Britain since 1970, daily energy expenditure from physical activity has fallen by 800 kcal.[113] Anyone over the age of 30 can probably recall several activities of daily life that require less effort to accomplish today than in childhood days. For example, 50 years ago, when women were generally responsible for maintaining the home, laundry was done by hand with a washing board, clothes were twisted until nearly dry and finally carried to the clothesline to be hung. These are all fairly strenuous tasks estimated to require an energy expenditure of 1500 kcal for a week's worth of household clothes.[114] Today, washing the same amount with a washer and dryer probably requires an energy expenditure of no more than 270 kcal. Considering that spontaneous physical activity, also called "nonexercise activity thermogenesis" or NEAT ("fidgeting" in lay terms), can burn as much as 241–453 kcal in a day,[115] it is not surprising that the adoption of labor-saving devices has had an impact on energy expenditure and weight over the last several decades.

Therefore, the adoption of a program of physical activity that involves not just formal exercise but also an effort to increase the amount of energy expended in the activities of daily life (such as walking, climbing stairs, carrying one's bags and, in general, refusing the physical assistance of others to do things one can do for oneself), can do much to recapture the opportunities for physical activity that were taken from us by the invention and widespread use of labor-saving devices.

Physical activity increases caloric expenditure and minimizes the loss of lean tissue that normally occurs with weight loss (the tissue composition of weight loss or gain resulting from changes in food intake is about 75% fat and 25% lean tissue). While physical activity alone has only a modest impact in producing initial weight loss, it appears to be essential in maintaining weight loss.[116] Even repeated small amounts of physical activity have an effect on energy expenditure; studies have shown that the benefits of exercise can be attained in shorter segments i.e., exercising three times per day in 10-min sessions instead of exercising 30-min once per day.[117] Therefore, the exercise prescription can be adapted to the patient's lifestyle and level of conditioning.[118]

Aerobic activities will have the greatest impact on cardiovascular health, but in terms of weight loss, the total calories expended determine the effect on weight. Physical activities carried out with less intensity over a longer period of time will burn approximately the same number of calories as the same activity at a higher intensity over a shorter period of time. Walking 1 mile (1.6 km), for example, will burn approximately the same number of calories as jogging 1 mile (about 100 kcals depending on body weight).

Resistance exercises build lean tissue and can help attenuate the normal loss of lean tissue that occurs with menopause.[7] Resistance training has special benefits in terms of quality of life to people over 60 years who are generally less interested in running a marathon than continuing to enjoy the activities of daily life, i.e., having the strength and flexibility to climb stairs, shop, step out of a shower without falling and to travel to visit friends and family, whether far or near. Resistance exercises also reduce the risk of osteoporosis, as do impact exercises.

Since prevention of weight gain is possibly the most important goal for postmenopausal women, whether normal weight or overweight, it is instructive to review the experience of persons in the National Weight Control Registry who have lost weight and maintained their loss for a significant period of time.[116] In a study of 3000 subjects who have maintained an average weight loss of 66 lbs (30 kg) for more than 5 years, the major ingredients of success were (1) following a diet low in fat (24% of total calories from fat), (2) self-monitoring of body weight (daily) and food intake and (3) consistent physical activity. Of interest, the level of physical activity reported was considerably higher than the 30 minutes a day recommended to the general public. Women reported expending 2545 kcal per week in physical activity (equivalent to walking about 25 miles or 40 km) and men, 3293 kcal per week. Walking was an important physical activity in over 75% of subjects. Twenty-four percent of men and 20% of women reported weight lifting. Subjects reported that considerable effort was required to maintain weight loss but that, after 2 years of maintenance, these efforts seemed easier to sustain. Of interest, almost half reported being overweight children and 46% reported having one obese parent and 26% having two obese parents.

Finally, physical activity as reflected by fitness level may be related to better adherence to a healthy diet.[119] In one study, fitness in women was associated with reduced intake of saturated fat and increased consumption of dietary fiber, minerals and vitamins.

D. STRESS MANAGEMENT

Stress is part of the human condition and can affect behavior in many ways, including altering food intake and physical activity. For many individuals, the best-intentioned nutrition and physical activity plans often fail in the face of a stressful event. It is intuitively apparent that the effect of stress on food intake is due to emotional arousal and the relief afforded by eating, especially in those who overeat in response to stress. Studies indicate, however, that physiological and hormonal mechanisms also play an important role. Glucocorticoids have been associated with increased food intake[120] and steroid therapy is known to have appetite-stimulating effects. In a recent study of women aged 30–45 years, caloric intake was greatest in women who had the greatest increase in cortisol secretion (determined by salivary cortisol) in response to a standard mental stress compared with women who were low-cortisol reactors in response to the same stressor.[121] On control days (days without an administered stress stimulus) high- and low-cortisol reactors ate approximately the same number of calories. However, high-cortisol reactors ate more sweet foods on both stress days and control days. In another study of the effect of a mental stress on food intake, those whose response to stress was greatest (as determined by blood pressure, heart rate and mood) ate more sweet and high-fat foods.[122] One study of workplace stress showed that periods of high stress, as defined by longer working hours, was associated with a higher intake of saturated fat and sugar. Furthermore, restrained eaters (those who habitually try to limit their food intake) were more likely to overeat in response to work stress.[123]

The effect of stress on physical activity habits is also intuitively apparent. While some respond to stress by increasing their level of physical activity, it is probably more common that most will become less physically active during periods of stress, in spite of the fact that physical activity has been shown to reduce stress and the risk of cardiovascular disease, diabetes and osteoporosis. Thus, stress can have a significant effect on behavior with respect to nutrition and physical activity.

Managing stress is a more difficult issue and has become a huge industry in the United States, with self-help books, seminars and workshops abounding. For some, these avenues are readily available, but for many women, these resources are not accessible because of economic, social or cultural barriers. Nevertheless, providing referral to appropriate community resources when available, along with practical advice about nutrition and physical activity, sends a message: Nutrition, physical activity and how one manages one's life are important to health and quality of life.

V. SUMMARY AND CONCLUSIONS

Maintaining healthy nutrition throughout the menopause transition and postmenopausal years can have many beneficial effects on both chronic disease risk and quality of life in women. The effects of different dietary factors on health risks common in postmenopausal women are summarized in Table 8.1. Dietary recommendations for postmenopausal women largely parallel recommendations for all adults, i.e., eating a

TABLE 8.1
Relationship Between Specific Nutrients or Dietary Components and Disease Risk

	Obesity	Cardiovascular disease	Diabetes	Osteoporosis	Cancer
Dietary fat	↑	↑	↑	No effect	↑
Dietary protein	??*	No effect	No effect	↑	No effect
Calcium	??**	↓	No effect	↓	No effect
Fruits/ Vegetables	↓	↓	↓	No effect	↓
Soy protein	??***				↑
Omega-3 fatty acids	↓	↓	??****	??****	↓
Alcohol	↑	↓	↓	No effect	↑

*Dietary protein may help reduce obesity by reducing hunger and increasing thermogenesis.[124]
**Recent studies have suggested that calcium intake is associated with lower Body Mass Index in some populations, however it is not clear if this is generally true or what the mechanism would be.[125]
***Soy protein has been associated with lower body fat in animals and may increase thermogenesis in humans.[124,126]
****Animal studies and a few clinical trials have suggested that long-chain omega-3 fatty acids (particularly docosahexaenoic acid, DHA) may have beneficial effects on insulin sensitivity[25] and bone.[127]

relatively low-fat diet high in vegetables, fruits, complex carbohydrates and omega-3 fatty acid sources such as fish. However, postmenopausal women need to pay greater attention to increasing calcium intake and avoiding excess protein in order to maintain bone in the absence of estrogen. Additionally, there are many benefits to increasing phytoestrogen consumption in the postmenopausal years, including reducing risk for heart disease and possibly diabetes, increasing bone density and managing menopausal symptoms. Finally, because menopause appears to confer an increased risk for weight gain and decreased estrogen causes unfavorable shifts in fat distribution to the abdominal area, weight management during menopause should be a paramount consideration for women and the health professionals who care for them.

REFERENCES

1. National Institutes of Health. Clinical guidelines on the identification, evaluation and treatment of overweight and obesity in adults — the evidence report. *Obes. Res.* 6 Suppl 2: 51S-209S, 1998.
2. Tchernof A. and Poehlman E.T. Effects of the menopause transition on body fatness and body fat distribution. *Obes. Res.* 6: 246–254, 1998.
3. Wing R.R., Matthews K.A., Kuller L.H., Meilahn E.N. and Plantinga P.L. Weight gain at the time of menopause. *Arch. Intern. Med.* 151: 97-102, 1991.
4. Wade G. Sex hormones, regulatory behaviors and body weight. *Adv. Study Behav.* 6: 201-279, 1976.
5. Geiselman P.J., Martin J.R., Vanderweele D.A. and Novin D. Dietary self-selection in cycling and neonatally ovariectomized rats. *Appetite* 2: 87-101, 1981.
6. Wright P. and Crow R. Menstrual cycle: Effect on sweetness preferences in women. *Horm Behav.* 4: 387, 1973.
7. Douchi T., Yamamoto S., Nakamura S., Ijuin T., Oki T., Maruta K. and Nagata Y. The effect of menopause on regional and total body lean mass. *Maturitas.* 29: 247–252, 1998.
8. Sullivan J.M. and Fowlkes L.P. The clinical aspects of estrogen and the cardiovascular system. *Obstet Gynecol.* 87: 36S–43S, 1996.
9. Clarke R., Frost C., Collins R., Appleby P. and Peto R. Dietary lipids and blood cholesterol: Quantitative meta-analysis of metabolic ward studies. *Brit. Med. J.* 314: 112–117, 1997.
10. Bray G.A. and Popkin B.M. Dietary fat intake does affect obesity! *Am J Clin Nutr.* 68: 1157–1173, 1998.
11. Lovejoy J.C., Lefevre M., Bray G.A., Most-Windhauser M., Denkins Y.M., Rood J.C. and Peters J. Beneficial effect of a low-fat diet on health risk factors is mediated by weight loss in middle age men. *Obes Res.* 8: 56S, 2000.
12. Appel L.J., Moore T.J., Obarzanek E., Vollmer W.M., Svetkey L.P., Sacks F.M., Bray G.A., Vogt T.M., Cutler J.A., Windhauser M.M., Lin P.H. and Karanja N. A clinical trial of the effects of dietary patterns on blood pressure. DASH Collaborative Research Group. *New Engl J Med.* 336: 1117–1124, 1997.
13. Obarzanek E., Sacks F.M., Vollmer W.M., Bray G.A., Miller E.R., III, Lin P.H., Karanja N.M., Most-Windhauser M.M., Moore T.J., Swain J.F., Bales C.W., Proschan M.A.; DASH Research Group: Effects on blood lipids of a blood pressure-lowering diet: The Dietary Approaches to Stop Hypertension (DASH) Trial. *Amer. J. Clin. Nutr.* 74: 80–89, 2001.

14. Kuller L.H., Simkin-Silverman L.R., Wing R.R., Meilahn E.N. and Ives D.G. Women's Healthy Lifestyle Project: A randomized clinical trial: Results at 54 months. *Circulation* 103: 32–37, 2001.

15. Anderson J.W., Johnstone B.M. and Cook-Newell M.E. Meta-analysis of the effects of soy protein intake on serum lipids. *New Engl. J. Med.* 333: 276–282, 1995.

16. Chiechi L.M., Secreto G., Vimercati A., Greco P., Venturelli E., Pansini F., Fanelli M., Loizzi P., Selvaggi L. The effects of a soy rich diet on serum lipids: the Menfis randomized trial. *Maturitas* 41: 97–104, 2002.

17. deKleijn M.J.J., van der Schouw Y.T., Wilson P.W.F., Grobbee D.E., Jacques P.F., Dietary intake of phytoestrogens is associated with a favorable metabolic cardiovascular risk profile in postmenopausal U.S. women: The Framingham Study. *J. Nutr.* 132: 276–282, 2002.

18. Nestel P.J., Yamashita T., Sasahara T., Pomeroy S., Dart A., Komesaroff P., Owen A. and Abbey M. Soy isoflavones improve systemic arterial compliance but not plasma lipids in menopausal and perimenopausal women. *Arterioscler. Thromb. Vasc Biol.* 17: 3392–3398, 1997.

19. Clarkson T.B., Anthony M.S., Williams J.K., Honore E.K. and Cline J.M. The potential of soybean phytoestrogens for postmenopausal hormone replacement therapy. *Proc. Soc. Exp. Biol. Med.* 217: 365–368, 1998.

20. van der Gaag M.S., Sierksma A., Schaafsma G., van Tol A., Geelhoed-Mieras T., Bakker M. and Hendriks H.F. Moderate alcohol consumption and changes in postprandial lipoproteins of premenopausal and postmenopausal women: a diet-controlled, randomized intervention study. *J. Womens Health Gend. Based Med.* 9: 607–616, 2000.

21. Fuchs C.S., Stampfer M.J., Colditz G.A., Giovannucci E.L., Manson J.E., Kawachi I., Hunter D..J, Hankinson S.E., Hennekens C.H. and Rosner B. Alcohol consumption and mortality among women. *New Engl. J. Med.* 332: 1245–1250, 1995.

22. Diabetes in America. National Diabetes Data Group. National Institutes of Health: 87–88, 1995.

23. DeNino W.F., Tchernof A., Dionne I.J., Toth M.J., Ades P.A., Sites C.K. and Poehlman E.T. Contribution of abdominal adiposity to age-related differences in insulin sensitivity and plasma lipids in healthy nonobese women. *Diabetes Care.* 24: 925–932, 2001.

24. Pi-Sunyer F.X. Health implications of obesity. *Amer. J. Clin. Nutr.* 53: 1595S–1603S, 1991.

25. Lovejoy J.C. Dietary fatty acids and insulin resistance. *Curr. Atheroscler.* Rep. 1: 215–220, 1999.

26. Fukagawa N.K. Anderson J.W., Hageman G., Young V.R. and Minaker K.L. High-carbohydrate, high-fiber diets increase peripheral insulin sensitivity in healthy young and old adults. *Am. J. Clin. Nutr.* 52: 524–528, 1990.

27. Lovejoy J.C., Windhauser M.M., Rood J.C. and de la Bretonne J.A. Effect of a controlled high-fat versus low-fat diet on insulin sensitivity and leptin levels in African-American and Caucasian women. *Metabolism.* 47: 1520–1524, 1998.

28. Feskens E.J., Virtanen S.M., Rasanen L., Tuomilehto J., Stengard J., Pekkanen J., Nissinen A. and Kromhout D. Dietary factors determining diabetes and impaired glucose tolerance. A 20-year follow-up of the Finnish and Dutch cohorts of the Seven Countries Study. *Diabetes Care.* 18: 1104–1112, 1995.

29. Mayer-Davis E.J., Monaco J.H., Hoen H.M., Carmichael S., Vitolins M.Z., Rewers M.J., Haffner S.M., Ayad M.F., Bergman R.N. and Karter A.J. Dietary fat and insulin sensitivity in a triethnic population: The role of obesity. The Insulin Resistance Atherosclerosis Study (IRAS). *Am. J. Clin. Nutr.* 65: 79–87, 1997.

30. Harding A.H., Sargeant L.A., Welch A., Oakes S., Luben R.N., Bingham S., Day N.E., Khaw K.T. and Wareham N.J. Fat consumption and HbA(1c) levels: The EPIC-Norfolk study. *Diabetes Care.* 24: 1911–1916, 2001.

31. Gulliford M.C., Ukoumunne O.C., Determinants of glycated haemoglobin in the general population: Associations with diet, alcohol and cigarette smoking. *Eur. J. Clin. Nutr.* 55: 615–623, 2001.

32. Salmeron J., Manson J.E., Stampfer M.J., Colditz G.A., Wing A.L. and Willett W.C. Dietary fiber, glycemic load and risk of non-insulin-dependent diabetes mellitus in women. *J. Am. Med. Assoc.* 277: 472–477, 1997.

33. Sanchez A. and Hubbard R.W. Plasma amino acids and the insulin/glucagon ratio as an explanation for the dietary protein modulation of atherosclerosis. *Med. Hypotheses.* 36: 27–32, 1991.

34. Lavigne C., Marette A., Jacques H., Cod and soy proteins compared with casein improved gluocse tolerance and insulin sensitivity in rats. *Am. J. Physiol.* 278: E491–E500, 2000.

35. Wagner J.D., Cefalu W.T., Anthony M.S., Litwak K.N., Zhang L. and Clarkson T.B. Dietary soy protein and estrogen replacement therapy improve cardiovascular risk factors and decrease aortic cholesteryl ester content in ovariectomized cynomolgus monkeys. *Metabolism* 46: 698–705, 1997.

36. Wei M., Gibbons L.W., Mitchell T.L., Kampert J.B. and Blair S.N. Alcohol intake and incidence of Type 2 diabetes in men. *Diabetes Care* 23: 18–22, 2000.

37. Hu F.B., Manson J.E., Stampfer M..J, Colditz G., Liu S., Solomon C.G. and Willett W.C. Diet, lifestyle and the risk of Type 2 diabetes mellitus in women. *New Engl. J. Med.* 345: 790–797, 2001.

38. Davies M.J., Baer D.J., Judd J.T., Brown E.D., Campbell W.S., Taylor P.R., Effects of moderate alcohol intake on fasting insulin and glucose concentrations and insulin sensitivity in postmenopausal women. *J. Am. Med. Assoc.* 287: 2559–2562, 2002

39. Lloyd T. andon M.B., Rollings N. et al. Calcium supplementation and bone mineral density in adolescent girls. *J. Am. Med. Assoc.* 270: 841–844, 1993.

40. Reed J.A. Anderson J.J., Tylavsky F.A. and Gallagher P.N., Jr. Comparative changes in radial-bone density of elderly female lacto-ovovegetarians and omnivores. *Am. J. Clin. Nutr.* 59: 1197S–1202S, 1994.

41. Riggs B.L., O'Fallon W.M., Muhs J., O'Connor M.K., Kumar R. and Melton L.J., III. Long-term effects of calcium supplementation on serum parathyroid hormone level, bone turnover and bone loss in elderly women. *J. Bone Miner. Res.* 13: 168–174, 1998.

42. Chapuy M.C., Arlot M.E., Duboeuf F., Brun J., Crouzet B., Arnaud S., Delmas P.D. and Meunier P.J. Vitamin D3 and calcium to prevent hip fractures in the elderly woman. *New Engl. J. Med.* 327: 1637–1642, 1992.

43. Heikinheimo R.J., Inkovaara J.A., Harju E.J., Haavisto M.V., Kaarela R.H., Kataja J.M., Kokko A.M., Kolho L.A. and Rajala S.A. Annual injection of vitamin D and fractures of aged bones. *Calc. Tissue Int.* 51: 105–110, 1992.

44. Calvo M.S., Kumar R. and Heath H. Persistently elevated parathyroid hormone secretion and action in young women after four weeks of ingesting high phosphorus, low calcium diets. *J. Clin. Endocrinol. Metab.* 70: 1334–1340, 1990.

45. Brot C., Jorgensen N., Madsen O.R., Jensen L.B. and Sorensen O.H. Relationships between bone mineral density, serum vitamin D metabolites and calcium:phosphorus intake in healthy perimenopausal women. *J. Intern. Med.* 245: 509–516, 1999.

46. Kerstetter J.E. and Allen L.H. Dietary protein increases urinary calcium. *J. Nutr.* 120: 134–136, 1990.

47. Sellmeyer D.E., Stone K.L., Sebastian A. and Cummings S.R. A high ratio of dietary animal to vegetable protein increases the rate of bone loss and the risk of fracture in postmenopausal women. Study of Osteoporotic Fractures Research Group. *Am. J. Clin. Nutr.* 73: 118–122, 2001.

48. Promislow J.H., Goodman-Gruen D., Slymen D.J., Barrett-Connor E., Protein consumption and bone mineral density in the elderly: The Rancho Bernardo study. *Am. J. Epidemiol.* 155: 636–644, 2002.

49. Dawson-Hughes B., Harris S.S., Calcium intake influences the association of protein intake with rates of bone loss in elderly men and women. *Am. J. Clin. Nutr.* 75: 773–779, 2002.

50. Scheiber M.D. and Rebar R.W. Isoflavones and postmenopausal bone health: A viable alternative to estrogen therapy? *Menopause.* 6: 233–241, 1999.

51. Potter S.M., Baum J.A., Teng H., Stillman R.J., Shay N.F. and Erdman J.W., Jr. Soy protein and isoflavones: Their effects on blood lipids and bone density in postmenopausal women. *Am. J. Clin. Nutr.* 68: 1375S–1379S, 1998.

52. Alekel D.L., Germain A.S., Peterson C.T., Hanson K.B., Stewart J.W. and Toda T. Isoflavone-rich soy protein isolate attenuates bone loss in the lumbar spine of perimenopausal women. *Am. J. Clin. Nutr.* 72: 844–852, 2000.

53. Horiuchi T., Onouchi T., Takahashi M., Ito H. and Orimo H. Effect of soy protein on bone metabolism in postmenopausal Japanese women. *Osteoporos Int.* 11: 721–724, 2000.

54. Schindler A.E. Obesity and cancer risk in women. *Arch. Gynecol. Obstet.* 261: 21–24, 1997.

55. Zhang S., Folsom A.R., Sellers T.A., Kushi L.H. and Potter J.D. Better breast cancer survival for postmenopausal women who are less overweight and eat less fat. The Iowa Women's Health Study. *Cancer.* 76: 275–283, 1995.

56. Slattery M.L., Potter J., Caan B., Edwards S., Coates A., Ma K.N. and Berry T.D. Energy balance and colon cancer — beyond physical activity. *Cancer Res.* 57: 75–80, 1997.

57. Phillips R.L. Role of life-style and dietary habits in risk of cancer among Seventh-Day Adventists. *Cancer Res.* 35: 3513–3522, 1975.

58. Miller A.B., Kelly A., Choi N.W., Matthews V., Morgan R.W., Munan L., Burch J.D., Feather J., Howe G.R. and Jain M. A study of diet and breast cancer. *Am. J. Epidemiol.* 107: 499–509, 1978.

59. Lee M.M. and Lin S.S. Dietary fat and breast cancer. *Ann. Rev. Nutr.* 20: 221–248, 2000.

60. Kushi L.H., Sellers T.A., Potter J.D., Nelson C.L., Munger R.G., Kaye S.A. and Folsom A.R. Dietary fat and postmenopausal breast cancer. *J. Natl. Cancer Inst.* 84: 1092–1099, 1992.

61. Barrett-Connor E. and Friedlander N.J. Dietary fat, calories and the risk of breast cancer in postmenopausal women: A prospective population-based study. *J. Am. Coll. Nutr.* 12: 390–399, 1993.

62. Smith-Warner S.A., Spiegelman D., Adami H.O., Beeson W.L., van den Brandt P.A., Folsom A.R., Fraser G.E., Freudenheim J.L., Goldbohm R.A., Graham S., Kushi L.H., Miller A.B., Rohan T.E., Speizer F.E., Toniolo P., Willett W.C., Wolk A., Zeleniuch-Jacquotte A., Hunter D.J. Types of dietary fat and breast cancer: A pooled analysis of cohort studies. *Int. J. Cancer.* 92: 767–774, 2001.

63. Cramer D.W., Welch W.R., Hutchison G.B., Willett W. and Scully R.E. Dietary animal fat in relation to ovarian cancer risk. *Obstet. Gynecol.* 63: 833–838, 1984.

64. Potischman N., Swanson C.A., Brinton L.A., McAdams M., Barrett R.J., Berman M.L., Mortel R., Twiggs L.B., Wilbanks G.D. and Hoover R.N. Dietary associations in a case-control study of endometrial cancer. *Cancer Causes Control.* 4: 239–250, 1993.

65. Gandini S., Merzenich H., Robertson C. and Boyle P. Meta-analysis of studies on breast cancer risk and diet: The role of fruit and vegetable consumption and the intake of associated micronutrients. *Eur. J. Cancer.* 36: 636–646, 2000.

66. Bingham S.A. High-meat diets and cancer risk. *Proc. Nutr. Soc.* 58: 243–248, 1999.

67. Messina M.J., Persky V., Setchell K.D. and Barnes S. Soy intake and cancer risk: A review of the *in vitro* and *in vivo* data. *Nutr. Cancer.* 21: 113–131, 1994.

68. Wu A.H., Ziegler R.G., Horn-Ross P.L., Nomura A.M., West D.W., Kolonel L.N., Rosenthal J.F, Hoover RN and Pike MC: Tofu and risk of breast cancer in Asian-Americans. *Cancer Epidemiol. Biomarkers Prev.* 5: 901–6, 1996.

69. Horn-Ross P.L., John E.M., Lee M., Stewart S.L., Koo J, Sakoda L.C., Shiau A.C., Goldstein J., Davis P. and Perez-Stable E.J. Phytoestrogen consumption and breast cancer risk in a multiethnic population: The Bay Area Breast Cancer Study. *Am. J. Epidemiol.* 154: 434–441, 2001.

70. Shao Z.M., Wu J., Shen Z.Z. and Barsky S.H. Genistein exerts multiple suppressive effects on human breast carcinoma cells. *Cancer Res.* 58: 4851–4857, 1998.

71. Constantinou A.I., Krygier A.E. and Mehta R.R. Genistein induces maturation of cultured human breast cancer cells and prevents tumor growth in nude mice. *Am. J. Clin. Nutr.* 68: 1426S–1430S, 1998.

72. Allred C.D., Allred K.F., Ju Y.H., Virant S.M. and Helferich W.G. Soy diets containing varying amounts of genistein stimulate growth of estrogen-dependent (MCF-7) tumors in a dose-dependent manner. *Cancer Res.* 61: 5045–5050, 2001.

73. Kennedy A.R. The evidence for soybean products as cancer preventive agents. *J. Nutr.* 125: 733S–743S, 1995.

74. Longnecker M.P. Alcoholic beverage consumption in relation to risk of breast cancer: Meta-analysis and review. *Cancer Causes Cont.* 5: 73–82, 1994.

75. Martin-Moreno J.M., Boyle P., Gorgojo L., Willett W.C., Gonzalez., Villar F. and Maisonneuve P. Alcoholic beverage consumption and risk of breast cancer in Spain. *Cancer Causes Cont.* 4: 345–353, 1993.

76. Gapstur S.M., Potter J.D., Sellers T.A., Kushi L.H. and Folsom A.R. Alcohol consumption and postmenopausal endometrial cancer: Results from the Iowa Women's Health Study. *Cancer Causes Cont.* 4: 323–329, 1993.

77. La Vecchia C., Negri E., Franceschi S., Parazzini F., Gentile A. and Fasoli M. Alcohol and epithelial ovarian cancer. *J. Clin. Epidemiol.* 45: 1025–1030, 1992.

78. Quella S.K., Loprinzi C.L., Barton D.L., Knost J.A., Sloan J.A., LaVasseur B.I., Swan D., Krupp K.R., Miller K.D. and Novotny P.J. Evaluation of soy phytoestrogens for the treatment of hot flashes in breast cancer survivors: A North Central Cancer Treatment Group Trial. *J. Clin. Oncol.* 18: 1068–1074, 2000.

79. St. Germain A., Peterson C.T., Robinson J.G. and Alekel D.L. Isoflavone-rich or isoflavone-poor soy protein does not reduce menopausal symptoms during 24 weeks of treatment. *Menopause.* 8: 17–26, 2001.

80. Washburn S., Burke G.L., Morgan T. and Anthony M. Effect of soy protein supplementation on serum lipoproteins, blood pressure and menopausal symptoms in perimenopausal women. *Menopause.* 6: 7–13, 1999.

81. Upmalis D.H., Lobo R., Bradley L., Warren M., Cone F.L.and Lamia C.A. Vasomotor symptom relief by soy isoflavone extract tablets in postmenopausal women: A multicenter, double-blind, randomized, placebo-controlled study. *Menopause* 7: 236–242, 2000.
82. Lehmann-Willenbrock E., Riedel H.H., Clinical and endocrinologic studies of the treatment of ovarian insufficiency manifestations following hysterectomy with intact adnexa. *Zentralbl Gynakol* 1988; 100: 611–618.
83. Vorberg G. Treatment of menopausal symptoms. *ZFA* 1984; 60: 626–629.
84. Pan Y., Anthony M., Watson S. and Clarkson T.B. Soy phytoestrogens improve radial arm maze performance in ovariectomized retired breeder rats and do not attenuate benefits of 17-beta-estradiol treatment. *Menopause.* 7: 230–235, 2000.
85. Pan Y., Anthony M. and Clarkson T.B. Evidence for up-regulation of brain-derived neurotrophic factor mRNA by soy phytoestrogens in the frontal cortex of retired breeder female rats. *Neurosci. Lett.* 261: 17–20, 1999.
86. Williamson D.F., Kahn H.S. and Byers T. The 10-yr incidence of obesity and major weight gain in black and white U.S. women aged 30–55 y. *Am. J. Clin. Nutr.* 53: 1515S–1518S, 1991.
87. Flegal K.M., Carroll M.D., Kuczmarski R.J. and Johnson C.L. Overweight and obesity in the United States: Prevalence and trends, 1960–1994. *Int. J. Obes. Relat. Metab. Disord.* 22: 39–47, 1998.
88. Brown W.J., Dobson A.J. and Mishra G. What is a healthy weight for middle aged women? *Int. J. Obes. Relat. Metab. Disord.* 22: 520–8, 1998.
89. Stevens J. Impact of age on associations between weight and mortality. *Nutr Rev.* 58: 129–37, 2000.
90. Lissner L., Bjorkelund C., Heitmann B.L., Seidell J.C. and Bengtsson C. Larger hip circumference independently predicts health and longevity in a Swedish female cohort. *Obes Res.* 9: 644–6, 2001.
91. Seidell J.C., Perusse L., Despres J.P. and Bouchard C. Waist and hip circumferences have independent and opposite effects on cardiovascular disease risk factors: the Quebec Family Study. *Am. J. Clin. Nutr.* 74: 315–21, 2001.
92. Salamone L.M., Cauley J.A., Black D.M., Simkin-Silverman.L, Lang W., Gregg E., Palermo L., Epstein R.S., Kuller L.H. and Wing R. Effect of a lifestyle intervention on bone mineral density in premenopausal women: A randomized trial. *Am. J. Clin. Nutr.* 70: 97–103, 1999.
93. Brooks E.R., Heltz D., Wozniak P., Partington C., Lovejoy J.C., Lateral spine densitometry in obese women. *Calc. Tiss. Intl.* 63: 173–176, 1998.
94. Stevens J,. Plankey MW., Williamson D.F., Thun M.J., Rust P.F., Palesch Y. and O'Neil P.M. The body mass index–mortality relationship in white and African American women. *Obes Res.* 6: 268–277, 1998.
95. Park Y.W., Allison D.B., Heymsfield S.B.and Gallagher D. Larger amounts of visceral adipose tissue in Asian Americans. *Obes. Res.* 9: 381–387, 2001.
96. Kamath S.K., Hussain E.A., Amin D., Mortillaro E., West B., Peterson C.T., Aryee F., Murillo G. and Alekel D.L. Cardiovascular disease risk factors in 2 distinct ethnic groups: Indian and Pakistani compared with American premenopausal women. *Am. J. Clin. Nutr.* 69: 621–631, 1999.
97. Gallagher D., Heymsfield S.B., Heo M., Jebb S.A., Murgatroyd P.R. and Sakamoto Y. Healthy percentage body fat ranges: an approach for developing guidelines based on body mass index. *Am. J. Clin. Nutr.* 72: 694–701, 2000.
98. Deurenberg P. Universal cut-off BMI points for obesity are not appropriate. *Brit. J. Nutr.* 85: 135–136, 2001.

99. Foster G.D., Wadden T.A., Vogt R.A. and Brewer G. What is a reasonable weight loss? Patients' expectations and evaluations of obesity treatment outcomes. *J. Consult. Clin. Psychol.* 65: 79–85, 1997.

100. Blackburn G. Effect of degree of weight loss on health benefits. *Obes. Res.* 3 Suppl 2: 211S–216S, 1995.

101. Institute of Medicine. *Weighing the Options.* Washington, D.C., National Academy Press, 1995.

102. Willett W.C. and Stampfer M.J. Clinical practice. What vitamins should I be taking, doctor? *New Engl. J. Med.* 345: 1819–1824, 2001.

103. Ditschuneit H.H., Flechtner-Mors M., Johnson T.D. and Adler G. Metabolic and weight-loss effects of a long-term dietary intervention in obese patients. *Am. J. Clin. Nutr.* 69: 198–204, 1999.

104. Leibel R.L., Hirsch J., Appel B.E. and Checani G.C. Energy intake required to maintain body weight is not affected by wide variation in diet composition. *Am. J. Clin. Nutr.* 55: 350–355, 1992.

105. Freedman M.R., King J. and Kennedy E. Popular diets: A scientific review. *Obes. Res.* 9 Suppl 1: 1S–40S., 2001.

106. Parks E.J. and Hellerstein M.K. Carbohydrate-induced hypertriacylglycerolemia: Historical perspective and review of biological mechanisms. *Am. J. Clin. Nutr.* 71: 412–433, 2000.

107. Baum C.L.and Brown M. Low-fat, high-carbohydrate diets and atherogenic risk. *Nutr. Rev.* 58: 148–151, 2000.

108. Clemens L.H., Slawson D.L. and Klesges R.C. The effect of eating out on quality of diet in premenopausal women. *J. Am. Diet. Assoc.* 99: 442–444, 1999.

109. Glassberg H. and Balady G.J. Exercise and heart disease in women: Why, how and how much? *Cardiol. Rev.* 7: 301–308, 1999.

110. Kohl H.W., 3rd. Physical activity and cardiovascular disease: evidence for a dose response. *Med. Sci. Sports Exerc.* 33: S472–83; discussion S493–494, 2001.

111. Will J.C., Massoudi B., Mokdad A., Ford E.S., Rosamond W., Stoddard A.M., Palombo S.R., Holliday J., Byers T., Ammerman A., Troped P., Sorensen G. Reducing risk for cardiovascular disease in uninsured women: Combined results from two WISEWOMAN projects. *J. Am. Med. Womens Assoc.* 56: 161–165, 2001.

112. Lichtenstein A.H., Kennedy.E, Barrier P., Danford D., Ernst N.D., Grundy S.M., Leveille G.A., Van Horn L., Williams C.L. and Booth S.. Dietary fat consumption and health. *Nutr. Rev.* 56: S3–19, 1998.

113. James W.P. A public health approach to the problem of obesity. *Int. J. Obes.* 19 Suppl 3: S37–45, 1995.

114. Martinez J.A. Body-weight regulation: Causes of obesity. *Proc. Nutr. Soc.* 59: 337–345., 2000.

115. Zurlo F., Ferraro R.T., Fontvielle A.M., Rising R., Bogardus C. and Ravussin E. Spontaneous physical activity and obesity: cross-sectional and longitudinal studies in Pima Indians. *Am. J. Physiol.* 263: E296–300, 1992.

116. Wing R.R. and Hill J.O. Successful weight loss maintenance. *Ann Rev Nutr.* 21: 323–341, 2001.

117. Schmidt W.D., Biwer C.J. and Kalscheuer L.K. Effects of long versus short bout exercise on fitness and weight loss in overweight females. *J. Am. Coll. Nutr.* 20: 494–501, 2001.

118. NIH Consensus Development Panel on Physical Activity and Cardiovascular Health. Physical activity and cardiovascular health. *J. Am. Med. Assoc.* 276: 241–246, 1996.

119. Brodney S., McPherson R.S., Carpenter R.S., Welten D. and Blair S.N. Nutrient intake of physically fit and unfit men and women. *Med. Sci. Sports Exerc.* 33: 459–467, 2001.
120. Cavagnini F., Croci M., Putignano P., Petroni M.L. and Invitti C. Glucocorticoids and neuroendocrine function. *Int. J. Obes.* 24 Suppl 2: S77–79, 2000.
121. Epel E., Lapidus R., McEwen B. and Brownell K. Stress may add bite to appetite in women: A laboratory study of stress-induced cortisol and eating behavior. *Psychoneuroendocrinology.* 26: 37–49, 2001.
122. Oliver G., Wardle J. and Gibson E.L. Stress and food choice: A laboratory study. *Psychosom. Med.* 62: 853–65, 2000.
123. Wardle J., Steptoe A., Oliver G. and Lipsey Z. Stress, dietary restraint and food intake. *J. Psychosom. Res.* 48: 195–202, 2000.
124. Mikkelsen P.B., Toubro S. and Astrup A., Protein Effect of fat-reduced diets on 24-h energy expenditure: comparisons between animal protein, vegetable protein and carbohydrate. *Am. J. Clin. Nutr.* 72: 1135–41, 2000.
125. Zemel M.B., Shi H., Greer B., Dirienzo D. and Zemel P.C. Regulation of adiposity by dietary calcium. *FASEB J.* 14: 1132–1138, 2000.
126. Aoyama T., Fukui K., Takamatsu K., Hashimoto Y., Yamamoto T., Soy protein isolate and its hydrolysate reduce body fat of dietary obese rats and genetically obese mice (yellow KK). *Nutrition* 16: 349–354, 2000.
127. Watkins B.A., Yong L., Lippman H.E., Seifert M.F., Omega-3 polyunsaturated fatty acids and skeletal health. *Exp. Biol. Med.* 226: 485–497, 2001.

9 Nutritional Considerations of Older Women

Helen Smiciklas-Wright, Jenny H. Ledikwe,
Gordon L. Jensen and Janet M. Friedmann

CONTENTS

I. INTRODUCTION

The first goal of Healthy People 2010 is to increase the quality as well as the years of healthy life. Here the emphasis is on health status and nature of life, not just longevity.

— Healthy People 2010 Objectives, 2000.[1]

Quality of life can be affected by many factors in the lives of older women. Rowe and Kahn defined successful aging to include avoidance of disease and disability, maintenance of physical and mental functions and active engagement with others and with productive activities.[2] Nutrition can play an important role in maintaining quality of life.[3–5] We have learned a great deal in recent years about how nutrition affects the health of older women, knowledge that has been used to revise and improve recommendations of intakes of foods, nutrients and other food components. We have also learned that many older women recognize nutrition as important to their health and are willing to make dietary changes to improve their own health and that of other family members.[6,7] This chapter summarizes dietary recommendations for older women, reviews rationale and tools for identification of older persons at risk for poor nutritional status and considers recommendations for nutritional care. We begin with a brief review of the demographic and health characteristics that may impact life quality of older women.

II. SELECTED CHARACTERISTICS

The American Association for World Health describes aging as a women's issue.[8] This is based on the reality that women live longer than men. Differences in life expectancy exist with regard to race as well as gender. White women and men in the United States have a life expectancy of about 80 and 74 years respectively, while black women and men have a life expectancy of about 74 and 65 years, respectively.[9] Currently, women compose 58% of those age 65 or older and 70% of those age 85 and older.[10]

Aging is often accompanied by a change in marital status, especially for older women. At ages 65 to 74 years, 32% of women are widowed as compared with only 9% of men.[9] In this same age group, 55% of women and 79% of men are married but, for those 85 years and older, this drops to 13% for women and 50% for men. Many factors associated with marital status may put women at nutritional risk. Older women are more likely to live alone than older men and are more likely to be poor. In turn, women living alone and those who are poor are at high risk of food insecurity and poor diets.[11,12]

Many older women remain quite healthy with few serious disabilities. At 70 years of age, women have an average expected life of 14 more years, 11 years of which are likely to be active.[13] Women are more likely than men to report that they need assistance or special equipment to perform routine activities like walking, climbing stairs and stooping.[10] About 12% of older white women and 16% of black women report some limitation of activity due to chronic health conditions.[14] In addition to physical problems, about 20% of women 65 years and older report severe depressive symptoms.[10] The ability to function well both physically and mentally is most likely to be affected by chronic diseases. The major chronic conditions that afflict women are arthritis, high blood pressure, heart disease, diabetes, cancer, stroke, Alzheimer's disease and visual impairments.[7,10,14] Chronic conditions are associated with expensive health care and poor quality of life for older women. The remainder of this discussion will review the role of nutrition in reducing disease risk and improving heath status.

III. NUTRITION AND QUALITY OF LIFE

Diet can improve quality of life by reducing the risks for major disabling diseases such as heart disease, diabetes and cancers. The landmark 1989 publication *Diet and Health: Implications of Reducing Chronic Disease Risk*[15] provided a number of dietary recommendations that have been promoted more recently in publications such as the *Dietary Guidelines for Americans*.[16] These recommendations include:

- Balancing food intake and physical activity to maintain an appropriate body weight
- Increasing intake of complex carbohydrates such as whole grain cereals
- Increasing intake of fruits and vegetables
- Reducing fat intake, especially the saturated fats, more recent guidelines recommend reductions in trans fatty acids
- Maintaining adequate calcium intake

Some of the most recent research confirms the importance of these recommendations for reducing disease risks such as high blood pressure and diabetes and reducing disabilities through better disease management. Both hypertensive heart disease and diabetes are leading causes of functional incapacity and death in older women.[17] The Dietary Approaches to Stop Hypertension (DASH) study was conducted to compare the impact of three different dietary patterns on blood pressure.[18] The three diets included: (1) a control diet that was low in fruits, vegetables and dairy products, with a fat content typical for Americans; (2) a diet rich in fruits and vegetables and (3) a combination diet that was high in fruits, vegetables and low-fat dairy products. A diet high in fruits, vegetables and low-fat dairy products was shown to reduce blood pressure in people with hypertension and also those with normal blood pressure levels. Another clinical trial, The Diabetes Prevention Program (DPP), also showed that diet is extremely important in preventing diabetes.[19] While these clinical trials were not designed specifically for older adults, there is no reason to believe that these general dietary recommendations would not benefit older women.

The evidence that good nutritional status can reduce chronic disease risk is strong. Nutrition can improve overall health and well-being of older women in many ways. It can reduce the decline in immune function that is often seen in older persons. Krause and colleagues compared immune functions of younger women (20–40 years) and older women (62–88 years) who were healthy and well nourished.[20] There were almost no differences in immune function measures between the younger and the well-nourished older women. The researchers concluded that a decline in immune status is not inevitable with age, but is more likely to be evident in persons with poor health and nutritional status.

Nutrition may help to reduce visual problems that can be so disabling with age. Cataract damage to the lens and age-related macular degeneration of the retina are leading causes of vision loss in older adults. The health of the eye may be prolonged by reducing oxidative damage. Dietary antioxidants such as carotenoids, vitamin C and vitamin E may protect the eye during aging.[21,22]

High cognitive function is essential for healthy aging. Nutritionists have long known that severe nutrient deficiencies can affect mental abilities such as memory, reasoning, verbal fluency and spatial associations. Mental disabilities can have profound effects on independence such as remembering to take medications, recognizing directions and depression. Nutrition is one of many factors that determine how well the mind functions. Various nutrients such as vitamins B_{12}, B_6 and folate can protect mental functions in older age.[23,24] Low levels of these three nutrients can increase serum levels of plasma homocysteine, which appears to be a strong risk factor for dementia and Alzheimer's disease.[25] Recent evidence indicates that antioxidant nutrients such as vitamin C and vitamin E may lower the risk of Alzheimer disease; however, antioxidants from foods, as opposed to supplements, may be more efficacious.[26,27]

IV. NUTRITIONAL REQUIREMENTS

A. NUTRIENT RECOMMENDATIONS

Since 1941, the Food and Nutrition Board of the National Academy of Sciences' Institute of Medicine has published periodic reports entitled Recommended Dietary Allowances to provide recommendations regarding dietary intake. The 10th edition was published in 1989.[28] In an effort to update and expand dietary recommendations, a new set of reports entitled Dietary Reference Intakes (DRIs) is being developed and released.[29,34]

The new reference values are being released in a series of DRI reports, each focusing on a specific group of nutrients or dietary components. Each DRI report is prepared by a separate committee of leading scientists and contains a comprehensive literature review, the data on which each reference value is based and areas in which future research is needed. Thus far, DRI reports have been released establishing updated recommendations for vitamins and most elements as well as for enerby and micronutrients (See Table 9.1).[30-34] Additionally, DRI reports are expected to be released revising recommendations for energy and macronutrient intake and establishing recommendations for electrolytes and water as well as other food components such as phytochemicals and alcohol.[29]

TABLE 9.1
Dietary Reference Intake Reports Released by Spring 2002

Year	Nutrients Covered
1997	Calcium, phosphorus, magnesium, vitamin D and fluoride
1998	Thiamin, riboflavin, niacin, vitamin B_6, folate, vitamin B_{12}, pantothenic acid, biotin and choline
2000	Vitamin C, vitamin E, selenium and carotenoids
2001	Vitamin A, vitamin K, arsenic, boron, chromium, copper, iodine, iron, manganese, molybdenum, nickel, silicon, vanadium and zinc.
2002	Energy, carbohydrates, fiber, fat, protein and amino acids

B. Energy and Macronutrients

Caloric requirements decrease with age due to an age-related reduction of lean muscle mass as well as a tendency to decrease physical activity. The recommended energy intake is set at 2403 kcal for women 19 years old, with a reduction of 7 kcal for each year above 19.[30] Recommendations may change when the energy DRIs are released. Setting a recommendation for energy intake is quite challenging, as energy needs are affected by many factors, including an individual's health status and activity level, which can vary greatly for older women. Both over- and under-consumption of energy can be problematic for older women. Over-consumption can contribute to obesity, a serious medical condition and major risk factor for mortality and morbidity.[36] Under-consumption of energy can lead to weight loss, frailty, fatigue and low micronutrient intake.

Dietary carbohydrates are important sources of energy. The recommended carbohydrate intake for women 51 years and older is 130 grams per day. Is it is generally recommended that 55% to 60% of total calories come from carbohydrates. There is increasing evidence that fiber has an important role in health through reducing blood cholesterol and improving glycemic control.[37] The American Dietetic Association and the National Cancer Institute recommend consumption of 20–35 grams of fiber per day for healthy adults.[37] The DRI for fiber for older women is 21 grams per day. Average fiber consumption is 14 grams for older females.[38]

Dietary fat provides energy and essential fatty acids and also aids in the absorption of fat-soluble vitamins. No RDA has been set for fat intake. The 2000 Dietary Guidelines for Americans recommends choosing a diet that provides no more than 30% of total calories from fat, with less that 10% of calories coming from saturated fat and less than 300 mg/day from cholesterol.[16] Intake of fat, particularly saturated fat and trans fat, has been associated with several disease states including cardiovascular disease, obesity and hypertension.[39] Nationally representative data indicate that total fat accounts for about 32% of the total calories consumed by older women, with slightly more than 10% of total calories coming from saturated fat.[38] Mean intake of cholesterol for older women is approximately 200 mg per day.[38]

Protein requirements for older adults are based on minimizing age-related loss of skeletal muscle. The RDA for protein in older adults is 0.8 grams per kilogram of body weight, which is about 54 grams for a 150-lb (68-kg) woman.[30] Average protein intake is 52.6 grams for older females.[38] Defining protein requirements for older adults has been challenging and controversial.[40] A recent reevaluation of studies of older adults concluded that daily protein requirements should be increased to 1.0–1.25 g/kg, which would be approximately 77 grams for a 150-lb woman.[41] However, other studies with older adults indicate that 0.8 g/kg is adequate.[40] It is important to remember that the recommended intakes are set for healthy individuals. Illness and other stress, such as surgery, can increase or decrease protein requirements.

C. Micronutrients

DRI values have been released for vitamins and most minerals (Table 9.2).[31–34] The DRIs compose a set of reference values used for planning and assessing the diets

TABLE 9.2
Recommendations for Selected Nutrients, Females aged 51–70 and > 70 years

Nutrient	RDA[a]	AI[b]	UL[c]
Vitamin A (μg/d)	700	-	3,000[d]
Vitamin C (mg/d)	75	-	2,000
Vitamin D[e] (μg/d)	-	10/15	50
Vitamin E (mg/d)	15	-	1,000[f]
Vitamin K (μg/d)	-	90	-
Thiamin (mg/d)	1.1	-	-
Riboflavin (mg/d)	1.1	-	-
Niacin (mg/d)	14	-	35
Vitamin B$_6$ (mg/d)	1.5	-	100[g]
Folate (μg/d)	400	-	1,000[h]
Vitamin B$_{12}$ (μg/d)	2.4	-	-
Calcium (mg/d)	-	1,200	2,500
Iron (mg/d)	8	-	45
Magnesium (mg/d)	320	-	350[i]
Zinc (mg/d)	8	-	40

[a] Recommended Dietary Allowance
[b] Adequate Intake
[c] Upper Limit
[d] As preformed vitamin A
[e] For those aged 51–70 yrs. and > 70 yrs. the recommendation is 10 μg/d and 15 μg/d, respectively.
[f] From any form of supplementary α-tocopherol
[g] As pyridoxine
[h] From fortified foods or supplements
[i] From supplemental magnesium

of healthy individuals and groups of individuals. The DRI values included not only the traditional Recommended Daily Allowance (RDA), but also three new reference values: Estimated Average Requirement (EAR), Adequate Intake (AI), Tolerable Upper Limit (UL):

- The EAR is an average daily intake level estimated to meet nutrient requirements for half of all healthy individuals and is used for assessing the adequacy of individual and group intakes.
- The RDA is determined by adding a specific value to the EAR to derive the average daily dietary intake level estimated to meet nutrient requirements of nearly all healthy individuals. As with previous recommendations, the RDA is an intake value healthy individuals should strive to achieve.
- The AI is used if data are insufficient to establish an EAR/RDA; an AI value is established based on estimates of nutrient intake by healthy

individuals. The AI is also a recommended intake value for healthy individuals.

- The UL is the highest level of daily intake likely to pose no risk of adverse health effects for most individuals. UL values do not represent a desired intake level and are becoming more important as the use of dietary supplements and the number of fortified foods increases. Sufficient data are not available for the development of UL values for all nutrients and the lack of a UL value does not mean there is no potential for adverse effects resulting from high intake.

Reference values for older adults have been set for two age categories: 51–70 years and over 70 years. The Institute of Medicine has recently released a report entitled *Dietary Reference Intakes Applications in Dietary Assessment,* which provides guidance for using the new DRI reference values for assessing and planning of individual and group intakes.[42]

While caloric needs decrease with age, micronutrient needs generally do not. For many, nutrients recommendations are the same for older and younger adults, but older adults do have higher intake recommendations for several nutrients, including calcium, vitamin D and vitamin B_6. Separate recommendations are made for adults aged 51–70 years and for those over the age of 70 years. However, at the present time, values are virtually identical, with the exception of vitamin D, which is higher for those over the age of 70 years. Meeting DRI micronutrient levels with limited caloric intake is difficult. Recommendations and current intake values for several key micronutrients are discussed below.

Calcium plays important roles in bone health, muscle and nerve function and blood pressure. The AI for calcium is set at 1200 mg/day for women ages 51 and older, which is 200 mg/day higher than for younger women and represents a substantial increase from the 1989 RDA of 800 mg/day.[28,34] The new recommendation is based mainly on data from controlled trials indicating that intakes greater than 1000 mg/day reduce bone loss, and takes into account the decrease in calcium absorption thought to occur with age.[34] It is difficult for older women to achieve appropriate levels of calcium intake from food sources. At least four calcium-rich dairy servings are needed to supply 1200 mg of calcium. Nationally representative data indicate that older women consume about 600 mg of calcium from foods each day, which is substantially less than the current recommendation.[38] Lactose intolerance, which increases with age, may further reduce consumption of dairy products.[43] The use of reduced-lactose dairy products, supplemental lactase, calcium-fortified foods or calcium supplements may help older women achieve desired intake levels. Excess calcium intake should be avoided, as it increases risk of kidney stone formation. The UL for calcium is 2500mg/day.[34]

Vitamin D is important in calcium absorption and bone health. The AI for vitamin D is 10 µg (400 IU)/day for women ages 51 through 70 and 15 µg (600 IU)/day for women ages 71 and older.[34] These values, which are a substantial increase from the 1989 RDA recommendation of 5 µg (200 IU) daily, are based mainly on plasma vitamin D concentrations and bone loss.[28,34] The AI value increases with age, accounting for the decrease in sun exposure that generally occurs with aging, as well as physiological changes such as decreased capacity for vitamin D synthesis and conversion to the active metabolite. Vitamin D is found naturally in very few foods; primary sources are fortified dairy and cereal products. Intakes of vitamin D appear to be quite low, less than 5 µg a day for older women.[34,44] While there is little risk of excessive intakes from natural food sources, individuals using multiple supplements may be at risk for hypercalcemia (high plasma calcium levels), metastatic calcification and other problems. The UL is 50 µg/day.[34]

A deficiency in vitamin B_6 increases homocysteine levels, an independent risk factor for cardiovascular disease, and may also have a role in maintaining cognitive function. The RDA for women ages 51 and older is 1.5 mg/day, which is based on plasma nutrient levels.[33] This value is higher than the RDA for younger women and is slightly lower than the 1998 RDA of 1.6 mg/day.[28,33] While nationally representative data indicate that average intake for older women is approximately 1.5 mg/day, a portion of older women do have intakes below recommended levels.[33,38,45] While there been no adverse effects associated with high intakes of vitamin B_6 from food sources, large supplemental doses have been associated with nerve damage and skin lesions. The UL for vitamin B_6 is 100 mg/day.[33]

Low folate status can lead to megaloblastic anemia and higher homocysteine levels. The RDA for women ages 51 years and older is 400 µg/day of dietary folate equivalents.[33] Dietary folate equivalents are a new measure of dietary folate, which adjusts for the lower bioavailability of folate naturally occurring in foods as compared with the form of folate added to fortified foods and found in dietary supplements. The amount of folate recommended is the same for older and younger adults, as folate absorption and utilization are not thought to be reduced with aging. The new recommendation, which is substantially higher than the 180 µg of folate recommended in 1989, is based on metabolic studies as well as epidemiological data.[28,33] Nationally representative data indicate that intake for older women is slightly over 200 µg/day, however, this underestimates current folate intake as data were collected before the mandatory fortification of cereal grains.[38] In a sample of older adults, it was estimated that folate fortification will increase folate intake by 28%.[46] Excessive folate intake can possibly mask vitamin B_{12} deficiency. Unrecognized B_{12} deficiency can culminate in irreversible neurological injury. The UL for folate from fortified foods and supplements is 1000 µg/day, exclusive of food intake.[33]

Low vitamin B_{12} can cause pernicious anemia, lead to neurological problems and may also increase homocysteine levels. The RDA for older adults is 2.4 µg/day, which is based on maintaining adequate hematological concentrations.[33] The recommendation is the same for younger and older adults, but the DRI committee recommends that fortified foods or supplements be used to meet much of the requirement for older individuals. An estimated 10–30% of older people have atrophic gastritis, which decreases absorption of naturally occurring vitamin B_{12} but not the form found in fortified products and dietary supplements. Nationally representative data indicate that mean intake from food was over 4 µg of vitamin B_{12} a day, but data are not available for the amount provided by fortified foods. As no adverse effects have been associated with excess intakes from food or supplements in healthy individuals, a UL was not set.[33]

Vitamin E is an antioxidant. The RDA is 15 mg of α-tocopherol a day for all adults, as intake and utilization is not thought to change with age.[32] While there is a growing body of data suggesting that elevated intakes of vitamin E may lower risk of chronic disease, such as heart disease, the DRI committee judged the scientific evidence to be too nonspecific to be used as the basis for setting recommended levels of intake at this time.[32] Nationally representative data indicate that mean intake for older women is around or less than 7 mg α-tocopherol equivalents a day, which overestimates α-tocopherol intake as it also includes other naturally occurring forms of vitamin E such as β-, γ- and δ- tocopherol.[38] There is no evidence of adverse reactions from consumption of vitamin E naturally occurring in foods; a UL is set at 1000 mg/day of any form of supplemental α-tocopherol.[32]

D. Food Patterns

Dietary patterns consider the entire diet rather than just one food or nutrient and provide a more comprehensive method for planning and assessing dietary intakes. Dietary patterns that emphasize the intake of nutrient-dense foods are important in helping older adults meet vitamin and mineral requirements. The importance of dietary patterns has been highlighted by several recent studies. The DASH Trial has shown that diets high in fruits, vegetables and low-fat dairy products can reduce blood pressure in both normotensive and hypertensive individuals.[18] Likewise, a study by Kant et al. demonstrated that high intakes of fruit, vegetables, low-fat dairy and lean meats reduce mortality risk.[47]

The heterogeneous nature of the older adult population makes it impossible to advocate one dietary plan for all women over the age of 65, but there are several nutritional guides that can be useful for older adults. These include the Dietary Guidelines for Americans[16] and the Food Guide Pyramid.[48] The USDA Human Nutrition Research Center on Aging at Tufts University has released a modified food pyramid for adults 70 years and over.[35] The modified pyramid, shown in Figure 9.1, is similar to the USDA Food Guide Pyramid,[48] but also includes a row of water glasses along the bottom of the pyramid to emphasize the need for eight 8-oz (227-ml) glasses of fluid each day, a fiber symbol signifying food groups with high-fiber options and a flag on top of the pyramid indicating the need for supplemental calcium, vitamin D and vitamin B_{12}.[35] For specific guidance on individual dietary plans, older adults should consult a registered dietitian to meet their particular and unique needs.

A variety of dietary quality scores have been used as indicators of dietary patterns. Nutrient adequacy ratios (NAR), the amount of a particular nutrient in the diet divided by a dietary standard and mean adequacy ratios, the mean NAR for several nutrients, are methods of comparing an individual's intake with a dietary standard such as an RDA.[49] Another way to examine the quality of an individual's diet is to calculate the number of servings from each food group and compare this with food grouping standards such as the USDA Food Guide Pyramid.[48] Sophisti-cated diet quality scores have been developed that take into account not just nutrients or food group servings alone but also an aggregation of these two assessments into one score. For example, the Healthy Eating Index score, created by the USDA, takes

TUFTS

Food Guide Pyramid for Older Adults

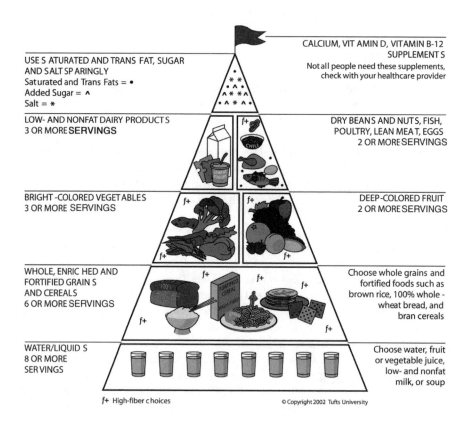

f+ High-fiber choices   © Copyright 2002 Tufts University

For additional copies visit us on the web at http://nutrition. tufts.edu

FIGURE 9.1 Tufts Modified Food Pyramid for Mature (70+) Adults. (The Gerald J. and Dorothy R. Friedman School of Nutrition Science and Policy at Tufts University. With permission.)

into account servings from the major food groups of the Food Guide Pyramid as well as a dietary variety and health-risk-related nutrient intakes.[50] This more comprehensive line of attack, as well as others that have been developed,[51] is becoming an increasingly popular approach to the interpretation of the dietary patterns of individuals and groups of individuals.

V. DIETARY SUPPLEMENTS

Dietary supplements are widely consumed by older Americans. These include single nutrient supplements such as calcium; multinutrient supplements such as a multivitamin-mineral combinations and herbal supplements, as well as supplements that contain both nutrient and herbal constituents.

A. NUTRIENTS

Obtaining vitamins and minerals from a wide variety of foods is generally the best way to meet micronutrient requirements.[52] However, it may be difficult for some older women to obtain adequate amounts of vitamins and minerals from their diet alone. The use of a daily multivitamin-mineral supplement may be a fairly economical and efficient method to achieve desired levels of micronutrient intake.

Many older women are using supplements. Older adults and women have repeatedly been shown to be among the highest users of nutritional supplements.[53–57] Nationally representative data indicate that about 50% of older women use supplements;[58] however, use varies among older adults between 20% and 70%, depending on the population sampled.[53–55,57,59,60] A study of rural older adults in North Carolina, suggest that women are almost three times as likely to take vitamin-mineral supplements as older men.[55] The most commonly consumed supplements are multivitamin-mineral supplements.[53–55,59,61,62] followed by single nutrient supplements.

Several demographic and lifestyle characteristics have been associated with supplement use. Married individuals as well as those with higher levels of education or income are likely to report using dietary supplements.[54,55,57] Other characteristics associated with supplement use include being nonHispanic white, living in the west, having a low BMI, being physically active and not smoking.[58,63] Individuals who rate their health status as very good or excellent are more likely to take supplements than those with a lower self-rated health status.[58]

Reasons for taking a dietary supplement are complex. While physicians and nurses are primary sources of information on general health, family and friends are a common source of information when beginning to use a supplement.[61] Many supplement users cite "feeling better" as a major reason for taking a supplement[61] and believe that supplements are good for their health and well-being and may prevent chronic diseases.[57] Several studies indicate that supplement users have strong health beliefs about these products,[57,61,64] with the majority of users believing manufacturers' claims in advertisements.[57] Women with the strongest belief in the effectiveness of supplements have been shown to use a wider array of supplements.[64] Furthermore, many supplement users have reported feeling so strongly about the use of supplements that they would continue use even if shown to be ineffective in scientifically conducted clinical studies.[57]

Interestingly, there is not a direct association between using a nutritional supplement and having a nutrient-poor diet.[54,55,62] Among a sample of rural older adults, supplement users were more likely to have adequate diets than those not taking supplements.[55] Data from a U.S. national survey also indicate that supplement users have healthier diets with lower fat intake, higher fiber intake and higher vitamin intake from food than nonusers.[54]

The potential benefits of supplement use have been the subject of much ongoing research. Over the past 10 years, evidence has been accumulating that supplement use may have beneficial effects.[65–72] Studies have investigated the effect of supplements on various outcome measures including plasma biomarkers, immune function, cognitive status, morbidity and mortality.

Several studies have shown that vitamin and mineral supplementation can improve plasma nutrient concentrations. An observational study of 100 older adults participating in the New Mexico Aging Process Study found that those individuals using supplements containing B vitamins had higher serum vitamin B_{12} and folate concentrations than nonusers.[65] Results from a long-term controlled trial with hospitalized older adults indicated that supplementation with select trace elements (zinc and selenium) and antioxidant vitamins (β-carotene, vitamins C and E) increase the serum concentrations of these nutrients as compared with the placebo group.[66] Similarly, healthy older adults in a controlled trial receiving a multivitamin-mineral supplement formulated at about 100% of the RDA had higher plasma markers of vitamins D, B_6, B_{12} and C and folate as well as a lower prevalence of suboptimal plasma levels of vitamins E, B_{12} and C than those in the placebo group.[67] Additionally, several studies have also provided evidence that supplement use in older adults can reduce plasma homocysteine levels, an independent risk factor for vascular disease.[65,67,68]

Effects on immune function have varied. A study by McKay et al. found short-term use of multivitamin-mineral supplement formulated at about 100% of the RDA did not affect measures of antioxidant status or immune function in free-living older adults.[73] However, in a long-term trial with free-living older adults using a multivitamin/mineral supplement formulated at about 100% of the RDA for most nutrients and higher amounts of vitamin E and beta carotene, subjects in the supplement group were less likely than those in the placebo group to experience infection and had improvements in several measures of antioxidant status.[69] Girodon et al. reported a long-term multicenter trial with institutionalized older adults using a supplement with select trace elements (zinc and selenium) and/or antioxidant vitamins (β-carotene, vitamins C and E) and found no effect of supplementation on delayed-type hypersensitivity skin response, but antibody concentrations following a flu vaccination were higher in those receiving a supplement than in those receiving a placebo.[70] In a group of hospitalized older adults, Girodon et al. found that a similar vitamin-mineral formulation improved measures of antioxidant status.[66]

Studies investigating the effect of vitamin and mineral supplementation on cognitive status have also yielded mixed results. A study by Baker et al. reported that supplementation with a high-dose multivitamin-mineral supplement for 1 year yielded no improvement in cognitive function in a group of 20 older adults.[74] Conversely, a year-long study by Chandra et al. did find that older adults receiving a multivitamin-mineral supplement showed a significant improvement on multiple cognitive tests.[71] Clearly, more research is needed to draw a definitive conclusion regarding the beneficial effects of dietary supplements on cognitive function.

While few studies have examined the beneficial effects of dietary supplements on morbidity and mortality, some compelling evidence has been provided by Mark et al. in a randomized trial in rural China with more than 3000 men and women taking a supplement formulated at two to three times the RDA. In this population with a micronutrient-poor diet, the presence of elevated systolic and diastolic blood pressure was less common in the supplement group than in the placebo group. The supplemented group also experienced a slight reduction in overall mortality, especially for cerebrovascular disease deaths. This study provides some evidence that supplement use may reduce mortality from cerebrovascular disease and the prevalence of hypertension in individuals with micronutrient-poor diet.[72]

Studies on the effects of supplement use are difficult to interpret due to conflicting results. Factors that vary across studies are likely to contribute to the differences in research findings, including vitamin formulations, length of study, subject health[20] and outcome measure. While it does appear that supplement use is beneficial in helping prevent nutritional deficiencies, more research is needed to make definitive conclusions regarding disease prevention.

B. HERBAL SUPPLEMENTS

The use of alternative therapies such as herbs and botanicals is increasing.[56] Relatively little is known about the herbal supplement practices of older adults as there is very little data available on use of herbals and other nonvitamin, nonmineral supplements. However, there is evidence that many older women are using herbal supplements.[56,75] In a nationally representative survey in which participants were asked about their use of dietary supplements, people over the age of 45 were more likely to report use of herbal supplements than younger individuals.[76] Even though these products are becoming increasingly popular, the efficacy and safety of these products must be questioned.

For most, there is simply a lack of strong, consistent evidence that various herbal products are effective. For example, despite the widespread commercial marketing of garlic to lower cholesterol levels, studies have shown conflicting results.[77-83] Similarly, there have been inconsistent results for the effectiveness of Ginkgo biloba,[84-87] St. John's Wort,[88-91] and Echinacea[92-95] on various health-related outcomes. Manufacturers are allowed to place certain health claims as well as structure and function claims on supplement labels. While the FDA can object to any claims made on supplement labels, claims that appear in other places such as advertisements are not regulated.

Safety is an important issue regarding the use of herbal supplements by older adults. While many consumers assume that herbal preparations are tested for safety, these products are not subject to the same rigorous evaluation as prescription or over-the-counter medications. Manufacturers are expected to provide evidence to the Food and Drug Administration (FDA) that their products are reasonably expected to be safe; however, the burden of proof is on the FDA to show that a product is unsafe. The risk of herb–drug interactions is higher for older than younger individuals due to a higher use of other medications. Furthermore, many individuals fail to inform physicians about their use of herbal supplements, creating a particularly hazardous situation.[56]

C. Summary

Older women comprise a very heterogeneous population, including healthy, active individuals, frail institutionalized individuals and the wide spectrum in between. The American Dietetic Association's position statement on dietary supplements states that vitamins and minerals from supplements can help some people meet their nutritional needs.[52] The decision to use a dietary supplement should be made on an individual's needs based on advice from a healthcare provider who is knowledgeable about supplements. It is important for older people to report the type and amount of supplements they are using to their health care provider,[96] as there is a potential for drug–supplement interactions and physiological changes may lead to the accumulation of nutrients at potentially toxic levels. Additionally, as the supplement market continues to expand, it is becoming easier for people to get confused, especially as more supplements are available and as herbal supplements are being combined with vitamin-mineral supplements. Unfortunately, many people do not inform their physician of their use of supplements.[56,57] Based on extrapolations from a nationwide survey, it is estimated that nearly 3 million older adults are at risk for potentially adverse interactions involving prescription medications and herbs or high-dose vitamin supplements.[56] Continuing research to determine the efficacy and safety of both nutrient and herbal supplements will be valuable in helping consumers and health care providers make informed decisions.

VI. NUTRITION RISK FACTORS AND SCREENING

Malnutrition is often undetected in older women.[97,98] Inadequate dietary intake unquestionably impacts the health of our nation's older adults. It is estimated that 85% of noninstitutionalized older adults have one or more chronic health conditions that could improve with proper nutrition.[99] Davies and Knutson[100] define a nutritional risk factor as a "major, identifiable biological or environmental circumstance or event that increases the risk of malnutrition and therefore suggests the need for special care and attention." Many of the factors that have been associated with nutrition risk are listed in Figure 9.2.

A. Risk Factors

Various physiological changes that affect nutrient intake and status occur with aging. Sensory impairments, including declines in taste and olfaction acuity, can decrease enjoyment of food, reduce appetite and lead to changes in intake patterns.[101] Oral health problems, such as tooth loss, ill-fitting dentures and difficulty swallowing, can make chewing uncomfortable and limit food selection.[102,103] Aging-related digestive changes are thought to be minimal, but include a reduction in absorptive surface area of the small intestine, which can decrease nutrient absorption, and reductions in pancreatic enzyme production, which can reduce digestion and lessen the amount of micronutrients available for absorption.[104] Changes that can cause constipation and diverticular disease, which may decrease food intake, also occur in the large intestine. Additionally, estimated to occur in

- Physiological Changes
  - Sensory changes
  - Oral-health problems
  - Digestive changes
- Health Status
  - Polypharmacy
  - Functional limitations
  - Cognitive impairment
- Psychosocial Factors
  - Social isolation
  - Inadequate nutrition knowledge
  - Limited financial resources/food insecurity
  - Depression
- Poor Diet Quality
- Weight status
  - Underweight
  - Overweight
  - Weight change

FIGURE 9.2 Factors associated with nutritionally at-risk older adults.

10–30% of older adults,[35] atrophic gastritis, a condition associated with infection of the stomach with *Helicobactor pylori,* can cause (1) abdominal discomfort and nausea, diminishing appetite; (2) diarrhea, increasing nutrient losses; (3) increased gastric pH, decreasing absorption of some vitamins (protein-bound vitamin B_{12}) and minerals and (4) bacterial overgrowth, reducing the concentration of micronutrients available for the body to absorb. Also, lactose intolerance increases with age, which may limit intake of dairy products.[43]

Several health-related factors are likely to increase nutrition risk. Older adults are particularly susceptible to illness, which can lead to a decreased desire to eat and may alter nutrient needs. Poor health can also increase the number and types of prescription medications an individual takes, leading to polypharmacy, or taking many medications. Side effects of different medications include xerostomia (dry mouth), nausea, abdominal pain, bloating, depression and alteration of taste sensation; all of which can reduce nutrient intake. Functional limitations that decrease ability to carry out instrumental activities of daily living (IADLs) such as food shopping and meal preparation, or activities of daily living (ADLs) such as self-feeding or walking, may cause difficulty in acquiring nutritious foods from grocery stores and may make the older person less able to prepare nutritious meals. Also, severe cognitive impairment, as may be observed with advanced Alzheimer's disease, can inhibit one's ability to meet nutrient needs.

Psychosocial factors that can adversely affect dietary intake include social isolation, limited nutrition knowledge, depression and food insecurity. Social isolation can decrease motivation to prepare meals and make dining a less gratifying occasion, thus decreasing appetite. Some older adults may not have the appropriate knowledge and skills to prepare nutritious meals, particularly widowed individuals who have relied on others for meal preparation. Bereavement, illness and medication use can cause depression, which may manifest in decreased appetite. After people retire, a decrease in income is common, which may force older adults to make difficult decisions regarding the purchase of nutritious foods.

Poor diet quality increases the risk of not meeting vitamin and mineral needs. As mentioned previously, muscle mass declines with aging, which contributes to decreased energy requirements for older individuals. While caloric needs decrease, vitamin and mineral needs generally do not. Older individuals who consume low-nutrient-dense foods decrease their ability to meet micronutrient needs.

Underweight, overweight and weight change have been associated with adverse health outcomes.[105–120] Older adulthood is often inaccurately associated with frailty, as some individuals are quite robust and physically active at advanced ages. Low body weight represents an unquestionable health risk,[116,118–122] but high body weights are a more common public health problem in this age cohort.[123] Data from the third National Health and Nutrition Examination Survey indicate that over 60% of older Americans are overweight or obese.[124] Furthermore, the prevalence of obesity in this population is increasing.[125] This trend has numerous adverse consequences and is a considerable public health concern, given that elevated weight status increases risk of co-morbidities,[114] functional decline, [126–128] impaired quality of life,[129] increased use of healthcare resources[130] and mortality.[106]

B. SCREENING TOOLS

Older persons at nutrition risk often go undetected. The early identification of older adults particularly susceptible to adverse health outcomes provides the foundation for the implementation of appropriate interventions to mitigate adverse health outcomes associated with poor nutrient intake.[131,132] Nutrition screening, the process of identifying characteristics known to be associated with dietary or nutritional problems, is important in distinguishing those older adults who are at highest risk of developing nutrition-related health problems. In addition to traditionally used anthropometric measures, dietary assessment and biochemical indicators, multi-item screening tools that combine these and other potential risk indicators are being used to identify older adults at nutritional risk.

The Nutrition Screening Initiative (NSI) was formed in 1990 as a collaborative effort involving the American Academy of Family Physicians, the American Dietetic Association and the National Council on the Aging to identify, intervene and treat nutritional problems in older adults before health and quality of life are seriously impaired.[133] The NSI developed and distributed a three-tier set of screening instruments: the DETERMINE checklist, the Level I screen and the Level II screen.[131,132] The DETERMINE checklist is a public awareness tool to help identify potential risks; it does not provide a detailed risk assessment. The Level I and Level II screens are intended to be used as nutritional risk assessment tools. The Level I was developed for use by health care professionals, whereas the Level II was intended for use by medical and nutrition professionals. The Level II, the most comprehensive of the three tools, includes assessment of body composition, laboratory data, drug use, oral health, eating habits, living environment, functional and cognitive status. While the

NSI instruments are being widely used,[131,132] they have been criticized for having a low positive predictive value.[134,135] However, several studies indicate that specific LII items, including using multiple medications, high BMI, elevated cholesterol and eating alone, are associated with functional limitations,[136] healthcare charges[136] and hospitalization.[137] This indicates that, while the instruments are not ideal screening tools, several of the items have important utility. Other screening instruments such as the Mini-Nutrition Assessment are available,[138] however, their effectiveness can also be questioned.[139] Further research exploring the clinical relevance of nutrition-related factors is needed to help explain and confirm the extent of health endangerment that accompanies nutritional risk among older adults.[140]

VII. CONTINUUM OF CARE

Aging has been described as a continuum extending from independence to intervention to interdependence.[141] A "continuum of care" has been proposed by the American Dietetic Association to promote an improved quality and dignity of life across the aging continuum through a well-coordinated care system that includes medical services, social support services and food and nutrition services.[141] Food and nutrition services spanning the continuum of care should include nutrition education, food assistance programs and medical nutrition therapy.

Federal programs such as the Food Guide Pyramid[48] and nutrition labels on foods[142] can provide general information about better food choices. However, many older women need additional guidance to interpret concepts such as appropriate serving sizes or percent daily values.[143] Various educational programs that incorporate group sessions[144,145] or newsletters[6] can lead to better knowledge about food selection and can motivate older women to make dietary changes. Well-designed medical nutrition therapies can lead to improved medical outcome measures such as fasting blood glucose and serum lipid levels.[146] Additionally, several managed care models have demonstrated the effectiveness of integrating nutrition screening for older persons with medical nutrition therapy and other clinical and social services.[147]

Food assistance programs have been implemented from federal to local levels to reduce food insecurity and malnutrition in elderly persons. Food insecurity is defined as the lack of availability of nutritionally adequate and safe food and limited ability to acquire acceptable foods in socially acceptable ways.[148] Some degree of food insecurity is reported for about 5–10% of older adults with much higher prevalence in minority and poor elderly.[149] Wolfe and colleagues described a progression of severity for food-insecure older persons from compromised diet quality to food anxiety, socially unacceptable meals, use of emergency food services and finally, actual hunger.[150]

The Elderly Nutrition Program (ENP), which celebrated its 30th anniversary in 2002,[151] and the Food Stamp Program are the major federal programs designed to reduce hunger and malnutrition. Lee and Frongillo assessed the impact of food assistance programs on nutritional and health status of older Americans.[152] Those authors found that many older adults who were identified as food insecure did not use food assistance programs. Furthermore, the impact of these programs was not greater for food-insecure than food-secure persons. The authors proposed that one interpretation could be that these programs may protect food-insecure persons from further nutritional problems but also recognized the need for more research to improve program effectiveness.

This review has touched on only a few of the food and nutrition services available to elderly persons. In its position paper on nutrition and aging, the American Dietetic Assciation noted that many services are provided through separate systems and stressed the need for a coordinated delivery of nutritional, medical and supportive services to achieve a true continuum of care.[141]

VIII. SUMMARY

Older women of the 21st century are a diverse group, differing socioeconomically and genetically as well as in their medical and nutritional histories and health habits. This chapter reviews factors that place older women at nutritional risk and presents recommendations and guidance for nutritional well-being. Sociodemographic characteristics such as living alone and reduced income, especially among the very old, may affect nutritional well-being by limiting access to food, decreasing motivation to prepare food and increasing food insecurity. Chronic disease states and medication use, which are common in older women, may impair physical and mental activities and alter appetite and food preferences. However, the management and homeostatic control of many of the diseases common among older women can be improved through prudent dietary choices.

Recommended intakes for most nutrients have been revised recently and published in a series of Dietary Reference Intake (DRI) reports. Recommendations are provided for two older age groups: 51–70 years and over 70 years. The recommendations reflect the importance of maintaining immunocompetence, vision, skeletal integrity and cardiovascular and cognitive function across the age spectrum. Consequently, with the exception of iron and chromium, recommended micronutrient intakes do not decrease for older women. In fact, higher levels of calcium, vitamin D and vitamin B_6 are recommended for older than younger women. Guidelines for achieving dietary adequacy, such as the Modified Food Pyramid for Mature (70+) Adults (Figure 9.1) can assist older adults and caregivers in selecting nutritionally dense foods. This chapter also includes a review of supplement use by older adults. Supplementation of nutrients such as calcium, vitamin D and vitamin B_{12} may be advisable to help some older women achieve dietary adequacy.

In the final section of the chapter, a case is made for integration of food, nutritional, medical and social services that can assist older adults in achieving the Healthy People 2010 goal of increasing quality as well as years of life.

REFERENCES

1. U.S. Department of Health and Human Services, *Healthy people 2010: understanding and improving health,* 2nd ed. Washington, D.C., 2000.
2. Rowe, J.W. and Kahn, R.L., Successful aging, *Gerontologist,* 37, 433, 1997.

3. Amarantos, E., Martinez, A. and Dwyer, J., Nutrition and quality of life in older adults, *J. Gerontol. A Biol. Sci. Med. Sci.*, 56, 54, 2001.

4. Drewnowski, A. and Evans, W.J., Nutrition, physical activity and quality of life in older adults: Summary, *J. Gerontol. A Biol. Sci. Med. Sci.*, 56, 89, 2001.

5. Thomas, D.R., The critical link between health-related quality of life and age-related changes in physical activity and nutrition, *J. Gerontol. A Biol. Sci. Med. Sci.*, 56, M599, 2001.

6. Taylor-Davis, S., Smiciklas-Wright, H., Warland, R., Achterberg, C., Jensen, G.L., Sayer, A. and Shannon, B., Responses of older adults to theory-based nutrition newsletters, *J. Am. Diet. Assoc.*, 100, 656, 2000.

7. Abusabha, R., Hsieh, K.H. and Achterberg, C., Dietary fat reduction strategies used by a group of adults aged 50 years and older, *J. Am. Diet. Assoc.*, 101, 1024, 2001.

8. American Association for World Health, Healthy aging, healthy living — start now, Washington, D.C., 1999.

9. Wagener, D.K., Molla, M.T., Crimmins, E.M., Pamuk, E. and Madans, J.H., Summary measures of population health: Addressing the first goal of healthy people 2010, improving health expectancy, National Center for Health Statistics, Hyattsville, MD, 2001.

10. Federal Interagency Forum on Aging Related Statistics, *Older Americans 2000: Key Indicators of Well-Being*, U.S. Government Printing Office, Washington, D.C., 2000.

11. Davis, M.A., Murphy, S.P., Neuhaus, J.M., Gee, L. and Quiroga, S.S., Living arrangements affect dietary quality for U.S. adults aged 50 years and older: NHANES III 1988–1994, *J. Nutr.*, 130, 2256, 2000.

12. Lee, J.S. and Frongillo, E.A., Jr., Nutritional and health consequences are associated with food insecurity among U.S. elderly persons, *J. Nutr.*, 131, 1503, 2001.

13. Crimmins, E.M., Hayward, M.D. and Saito, Y., Differentials in active life expectancy in the older population of the United States, *J. Gerontol. B. Psychol. Sci. Soc. Sci.*, 51, S111, 1996.

14. Johnson, R.J. and Wolinsky, F.D., Gender, race and health: The structure of health status among older adults, *Gerontologist*, 34, 24, 1994.

15. National Research Council, *Diet and Health: Implications for Reducing Chronic Disease Risk*, National Academy Press, Washington, D.C., 1989.

16. U.S. Department of Agriculture and U.S. Department of Health and Human Services, *Nutrition and Your Health: Dietary Guidelines for Americans*, U.S. Government Printing Office, Washington, D.C., 2000.

17. Hoyert, D.L., Arias, E., Smith, B.L., Murphy, S.L. and Kochanek, K.D., Deaths: Final data for 1999. National Vital Statistics Reports National Center for Health Statistics, Hyattsville, MD, 2001.

18. Harsha, D.W., Lin, P.H., Obarzanek, E., Karanja, N.M., Moore, T.J. and Caballero, B., Dietary approaches to stop hypertension: A summary of study results. DASH Collaborative Research Group, *J. Am. Diet. Assoc.*, 99, S35, 1999.

19. Knowler, W.C., Barrett-Connor, E., Fowler, S.E., Hamman, R.F., Lachin, J.M., Walker, E.A. and Nathan, D.M., Reduction in the incidence of type 2 diabetes with lifestyle intervention or metformin, *New Engl. J. Med.*, 346, 393, 2002.

20. Krause, D., Mastro, A.M., Handte, G., Smiciklas-Wright, H., Miles, M.P. and Ahluwalia, N., Immune function did not decline with aging in apparently healthy, well-nourished women, *Mech. Aging Dev.*, 112, 43, 1999.

21. Taylor, A., Jacques, P.F., Chylack, L.T., Jr., Hankinson, S.E., Khu, P.M., Rogers, G., Friend, J., Tung, W., Wolfe, J.K., Padhye, N. and Willett, W.C., Long-term intake of vitamins and carotenoids and odds of early age-related cortical and posterior subcapsular lens opacities, *Am. J. Clin. Nutr.*, 75, 540, 2002.

22. Valero, M.P., Fletcher, A.E., De Stavola, B.L., Vioque, J. and Alepuz, V.C., Vitamin C is associated with reduced risk of cataract in a Mediterranean population, *J. Nutr.*, 132, 1299, 2002.

23. Duthie, S.J., Whalley, L.J., Collins, A.R., Leaper, S., Berger, K. and Deary, I.J., Homocysteine, B vitamin status and cognitive function in the elderly, *Am. J. Clin. Nutr.*, 75, 908, 2002.

24. Bryan, J., Calvaresi, E. and Hughes, D., Short-term folate, vitamin B-12 or vitamin B-6 supplementation slightly affects memory performance but not mood in women of various ages, *J. Nutr.*, 132, 1345, 2002.

25. Seshadri, S., Beiser, A., Selhub, J., Jacques, P.F., Rosenberg, I.H., D'Agostino, R.B., Wilson, P.W. and Wolf, P.A., Plasma homocysteine as a risk factor for dementia and Alzheimer's disease, *New Engl. J. Med.*, 346, 476, 2002.

26. Morris, M.C., Evans, D.A., Bienias, J.L., Tangney, C.C., Bennett, D.A., Aggarwal, N., Wilson, R.S. and Scherr, P.A., Dietary intake of antioxidant nutrients and the risk of incident Alzheimer's disease in a biracial community study, *JAMA*, 287, 3230, 2002.

27. Engelhart, M.J., Geerlings, M.I., Ruitenberg, A., van Swieten, J.C., Hofman, A., Witteman, J.C. and Breteler, M.M., Dietary intake of antioxidants and risk of Alzheimer's disease, *JAMA*, 287, 3223, 2002.

28. Food and Nutrition Board, *Recommended Dietary Allowances*, 10th ed. National Academy Press, Washington, D.C., 1989.

29. Monsen, E.R., New Dietary Reference Intakes proposed to replace the Recommended Dietary Allowances, *J. Am. Diet. Assoc.*, 96, 754, 1996.

30. Food and Nutrition Board, *Dietary Reference Intakes for Energy, Carbohydrates, Fiber, Fat, Protein and Amino Acids*. National Academy Press, Washington, D.C. 2002.

31. Food and Nutrition Board, *Dietary Reference Intakes for Vitamin A, Vitamin K, Arsenic, Boron, Chromium, Copper, Iodine, Iron, Molybdenum, Nickel, Silicon, Vanadium and Zinc*, National Academy Press, Washington, D.C., 2001.

32. Food and Nutrition Board, *Dietary Reference Intakes for Vitamin C, Vitamin E, Selenium and Carotenoids*, National Academy Press, Washington, D.C., 2000.

33. Food and Nutrition Board, *Dietary Reference Intakes for Thiamin, Riboflavin, Niacin, Vitamin B_6, Folate, Vitamin B_{12}, Pantothenic Acid, Biotin and Choline*, National Academy Press, Washington, D.C., 1998.

34. Food and Nutrition Board, *Dietary Reference Intakes for Calcium, Phosphorus, Magnesium, Vitamin D and Fluoride*, National Academy Press, Washington, D.C., 1997.

35. Russell, R.M. and Rasmussen, H., The impact of nutritional needs of older adults on recommended food intakes, *Nutr. Clin. Care.*, 2, 164, 1999.

36. National Institutes of Health, *Clinical Guidelines on the Identification, Evaluation and Treatment of Overweight and Obesity in Adults: the Evidence Report*, National Heart Lung and Blood Institute, Rockville, MD, 1998.

37. Marlett, J.A., McBurney, M.I. and Slavin, J.L., Position of the American dietetic association: Health implications of dietary fiber, *J. Am. Diet. Assoc.*, 102, 993, 2002.

38. U.S. Department of Agriculture, A.R.S., *Food and Nutrient Intakes by Individuals in the United States, by Sex and Age, 1994–96*, U.S. Department of Agriculture, Washington, D.C., 1998.

39. Willett, W.C., Stampfer, M.J., Manson, J.E., Colditz, G.A., Speizer, F.E., Rosner, B.A., Sampson, L.A. and Hennekens, C.H., Intake of trans fatty acids and risk of coronary heart disease among women, *Lancet*, 341, 581, 1993.

40. Millward, D.J., Fereday, A., Gibson, N. and Pacy, P.J., Aging, protein requirements and protein turnover, *Am. J. Clin. Nutr.,* 66, 774, 1997.

41. Campbell, W.W., Crim, M.C., Dallal, G.E., Young, V.R. and Evans, W.J., Increased protein requirements in elderly people: New data and retrospective reassessments, *Am. J. Clin. Nutr.,* 60, 501, 1994.

42. Food and Nutrition Board, *Dietary Reference Intakes Applications in Dietary Assessment,* National Academy Press, Washington, D.C., 2000.

43. Elbon, S.M., Johnson, M.A. and Fischer, J.G., Milk consumption in older Americans, *Am. J. Public Health,* 88, 1221, 1998.

44. Bates, C., Prentice, A. and Finch, S., Gender differences in food and nutrient intakes and status indices from the National Diet and Nutrition Survey of people aged 65 years and over, *Eur. J. Clin. Nutr.,* 53, 694, 1999.

45. Ryan, A.S., Craig, L.D. and Finn, S.C., Nutrient intakes and dietary patterns of older Americans: A national study, *J. Gerontol.,* 47, M145, 1992.

46. Koehler, K.M., Pareo-Tubbeh, S.L., Romero, L.J., Baumgartner, R.N. and Garry, P.J., Folate nutrition and older adults: Challenges and opportunities, *J. Am. Diet. Assoc.,* 97, 167, 1997.

47. Kant, A.K., Schatzkin, A., Graubard, B.I. and Schairer, C., A prospective study of diet quality and mortality in women, *JAMA,* 283, 2109, 2000.

48. U.S. Department of Agriculture, *The Food Guide Pyramid: A Guide to Daily Food Choices,* Nutrition Information Service, 1992.

49. Smiciklas-Wright, H., Mitchell, D. and Ledikwe, J.H. Dietary intake assessment: Methods for adults, in *CRC Handbook of Nutrition and Food,* Berdanier, C.D., Ed., CRC Press, Boca Raton, Fl, 2001, 477.

50. Bowman, S.A., Lino, M., Gerrior, S.A. and Basiotis, P.P., *The Healthy Eating Index: 1994–96, CNPP-5,* US Department of Agriculture, Center for Nutrition Policy and Promotion, 1998.

51. Haines, P.S., Siega-Riz, A.M. and Popkin, B.M., The Diet Quality Index revised: A measurement instrument for populations, *J. Am. Diet. Assoc.,* 99, 697, 1999.

52. Position of the American Dietetic Association: Food fortification and dietary supplements, *J. Am. Diet. Assoc.,* 101, 115, 2001.

53. Patterson, R.E., Neuhouser, M.L., White, E., Kristal, A.R. and Potter, J.D., Measurement error from assessing use of vitamin supplements at one point in time, *Epidemiology,* 9, 567, 1998.

54. Slesinski, M.J., Subar, A.F. and Kahle, L.L., Dietary intake of fat, fiber and other nutrients is related to the use of vitamin and mineral supplements in the United States: the 1992 National Health Interview Survey, *J. Nutr.,* 126, 3001, 1996.

55. Vitolins, M.Z., Quandt, S.A., Case, L.D., Bell, R.A., Arcury, T.A. and McDonald, J., Vitamin and mineral supplement use by older rural adults, *J. Gerontol.,* 55A, M613, 2000.

56. Eisenberg, D.M., Davis, R.B., Ettner, S.L., Appel, S., Wilkey, S., Van Rompay, M. and Kessler, R.C., Trends in alternative medicine use in the United States, 1990–1997: results of a follow-up national survey, *JAMA,* 280, 1569, 1998.

57. Blendon, R.J., DesRoches, C.M., Benson, J.M., Brodie, M. and Altman, D.E., Americans' views on the use and regulation of dietary supplements, *Arch. Intern. Med.,* 161, 805, 2001.

58. Ervin, R.B., Wright, J.D. and Kennedy-Stephenson, J., *Use of dietary supplements in the United States, 1988–94,* Department of Health and Human Services, National Center for Health Statistics, Hyattsville, MD, 1999.

59. Slesinski, M.J., Subar, A.F. and Kahle, L.L., Trends in use of vitamin and mineral supplements in the United State: The 1987 and 1992 National Health Interview Surveys, *J. Am. Diet. Assoc.*, 95, 921, 1995.

60. Oakland, M.J. and Thomsen, P.A., Beliefs about and usage of vitamin/mineral supplements by elderly participants of rural congregate meal programs in central Iowa, *J. Am. Diet. Assoc.*, 90, 715, 1990.

61. Neuhouser, M.L., Patterson, R.E. and Levy, L., Motivations for using vitamin and mineral supplements, *J. Am. Diet. Assoc.*, 99, 851, 1999.

62. White-O'Connor, B., Sobal, J. and Muncie, H.L., Dietary habits, weight history and vitamin supplement use in elderly osteoarthritis patients, *J. Am. Diet. Assoc.*, 89, 378, 1989.

63. Lyle, B.J., Mares-Perlman, J.A., Klein, B.E., Klein, R. and Greger, J.L., Supplement users differ from nonusers in demographic, lifestyle, dietary and health characteristics, *J. Nutr.*, 128, 2355, 1998.

64. Raab, C.A., Vitamin and mineral supplement usage patterns and health beliefs of women, *J. Am. Diet. Assoc.*, 87, 775, 1987.

65. Koehler, K.M., Romero, L.J., Stauber, P.M., Pareo-Tubbeh, S.L., Liang, H.C., Baumgartner, R.N., Garry, P.J., Allen, R.H. and Stabler, S.P., Vitamin supplementation and other variables affecting serum homocysteine and methylmalonic acid concentrations in elderly men and women, *J. Am. Coll. Nutr.*, 15, 364, 1996.

66. Girodon, F., Blache, D., Monget, A.L., Lombart, M., Brunet-Lecompte, P., Arnaud, J., Richard, M.J. and Galan, P., Effect of a two-year supplementation with low doses of antioxidant vitamins and/or minerals in elderly subjects on levels of nutrients and antioxidant defense parameters, *J. Am. Coll. Nutr.*, 16, 357, 1997.

67. McKay, D.L., Perrone, G., Rasmussen, H., Dallal, G. and Blumberg, J.B., Multivitamin/mineral supplementation improves plasma B-vitamin status and homocysteine concentration in healthy older adults consuming a folate-fortified diet, *J. Nutr.*, 130, 3090, 2000.

68. Naurath, H.J., Joosten, E., Riezler, R., Stabler, S.P., Allen, R.H. and Lindenbaum, J., Effects of vitamin B_{12}, folate and vitamin B_6 supplements in elderly people with normal serum vitamin concentrations, *Lancet,* 346, 85, 1995.

69. Chandra, R.K., Effect of vitamin and trace-element supplementation on immune responses and infection in elderly subjects, *Lancet,* 340, 1124, 1992.

70. Girodon, F., Galan, P., Monget, A.L., Boutron-Ruault, M.C., Brunet-Lecomte, P., Preziosi, P., Arnaud, J., Manuguerra, J.C. and Herchberg, S., Impact of trace elements and vitamin supplementation on immunity and infections in institutionalized elderly patients: a randomized controlled trial. MIN. VIT. AOX. geriatric network, *Arch. Intern. Med.*, 159, 748, 1999.

71. Chandra, R.K., Effect of vitamin and trace-element supplementation on cognitive function in elderly subjects, *Nutrition,* 17, 709, 2001.

72. Mark, S.D., Wang, W., Fraumeni, J.F., Jr., Li, J.Y., Taylor, P.R., Wang, G.Q., Guo, W., Dawsey, S.M., Li, B. and Blot, W.J., Lowered risks of hypertension and cerebrovascular disease after vitamin/mineral supplementation: The Linxian Nutrition Intervention Trial, *Am. J. Epidemiol.*, 143, 658, 1996.

73. McKay, D.L., Perrone, G., Rasmussen, H., Dallal, G., Hartman, W., Cao, G., Prior, R.L., Roubenoff, R. and Blumberg, J.B., The effects of a multivitamin/mineral supplement on micronutrient status, antioxidant capacity and cytokine production in healthy older adults consuming a fortified diet, *J. Am. Coll. Nutr.*, 19, 613, 2000.

74. Baker, H., De Angelis, B., Baker, E.R., Frank, O. and Jaslowdagger, S.P., Lack of effect of 1 year intake of a high-dose vitamin and mineral supplement on cognitive function of elderly women, *Gerontology,* 45, 195, 1999.

75. Radimer, K.L., Subar, A.F. and Thompson, F.E., Nonvitamin, nonmineral dietary supplements: issues and findings from NHANES III, *J. Am. Diet. Assoc.,* 100, 447, 2000.

76. Radimer, K.L., Nonvitamin, nonmineral dietary supplements: Issues and findings from NHANES III, *J. Am. Diet. Assoc.,* 100, 447, 2000.

77. Berthold, H.K., Sudhop, T. and von Bergmann, K., Effect of a garlic oil preparation on serum lipoproteins and cholesterol metabolism: A randomized controlled trial, *JAMA,* 279, 1900, 1998.

78. Gardner, C.D., Chatterjee, L.M. and Carlson, J.J., The effect of a garlic preparation on plasma lipid levels in moderately hypercholesterolemic adults, *Atherosclerosis,* 154, 213, 2001.

79. Isaacsohn, J.L., Moser, M., Stein, E.A., Dudley, K., Davey, J.A., Liskov, E. and Black, H.R., Garlic powder and plasma lipids and lipoproteins: A multicenter, randomized, placebo-controlled trial, *Arch. Intern. Med.,* 158, 1189, 1998.

80. Simons, L.A., Balasubramaniam, S., von Konigsmark, M., Parfitt, A., Simons, J. and Peters, W., On the effect of garlic on plasma lipids and lipoproteins in mild hypercholesterolaemia, *Atherosclerosis,* 113, 219, 1995.

81. Adesh, K., Can garlic reduce levels of serum lipids? A controlled clinical study, *Am. J. Med.,* 94, 632, 1993.

82. Adler, A.J. and Holub, B.J., Effect of garlic and fish-oil supplementation on serum lipid and lipoprotein concentrations in hypercholesterolemic men, *Am. J. Clin. Nutr.,* 65, 445, 1997.

83. Steiner, M., Khan, A.H., Holbert, D. and Lin, R.I., A double-blind crossover study in moderately hypercholesterolemic men that compared the effect of aged garlic extract and placebo administration on blood lipids, *Am. J. Clin. Nutr.,* 64, 866, 1996.

84. Le Bars, P.L., Katz, M.M., Berman, N., Itil, T.M., Freedman, A.M. and Schatzberg, A.F., A placebo-controlled, double-blind, randomized trial of an extract of Ginkgo biloba for dementia. North American EGb Study Group, *JAMA,* 278, 1327, 1997.

85. Maurer, K., Clinical efficacy of ginkgo biloba special extract Egb 761 in dementia of the Alzheimer type., *J. Psychiatr. Res.,* 31, 645, 1997.

86. Kanowski, S., Herrmann, W.M., Stephan, K., Wierich, W. and Horr, R., Proof of efficacy of the ginkgo biloba special extract EGb 761 in outpatients suffering from mild to moderate primary degenerative dementia of the Alzheimer type or multi-infarct dementia, *Pharmacopsychiatry,* 29, 47, 1996.

87. van Dongen, M.C., van Rossum, E., Kessels, A.G., Sielhorse, H.J. and Knipschild, P.G., The efficacy of ginkgo for elderly people with dementia and age-associated memory impairment: New results of a randomized clinical trial, *J. Am. Geriatr. Soc.,* 48, 1183, 2000.

88. Linde, K., Ramirez, G., Mulrow, C.D., Pauls, A., Weidenhammer, W. and Melchart, D., St John's wort for depression — an overview and meta-analysis of randomised clinical trials, *Brit. Med. J.,* 313, 253, 1996.

89. Philipp, M., Kohnen, R. and Hiller, K.O., Hypericum extract versus imipramine or placebo in patients with moderate depression: randomised multicentre study of treatment for eight weeks, *Brit. Med. J.,* 319, 1534, 1999.

90. Woelk, H., Comparison of St John's wort and imipramine for treating depression: randomised controlled trial, *Brit. Med. J.,* 321, 536, 2000.

91. Shelton, R.C., Keller, M.B., Gelenberg, A., Dunner, D.L., Hirschfeld, R., Thase, M.E., Russell, J., Lydiard, R.B., Crits-Cristoph, P., Gallop, R., Todd, L., Hellerstein, D., Goodnick, P., Keitner, G., Stahl, S.M. and Halbreich, U., Effectiveness of St. John's wort in major depression: A randomized controlled trial, *JAMA,* 285, 1978, 2001.

92. Melchart, D., Walther, E., Linde, K., Brandmaier, R. and Lersch, C., Echinacea root extracts for the prevention of upper respiratory tract infections: A double-blind, placebo-controlled randomized trial, *Arch. Fam. Med.,* 7, 541, 1998.

93. Brinkeborn, R.M., Shah, D.V. and Degenring, F.H., Echinaforce and other Echinacea fresh plant preparations in the treatment of the common cold. A randomized, placebo controlled, double-blind clinical trial, *Phytomedicine,* 6, 1, 1999.

94. Dorn, M., Placebo-controlled, double-blind study of Echinaceae pallidae radix in upper respiratory tract infections, *Complement. Ther. Med.,* 5, 40, 1997.

95. Lindenmuth, G.F. and Lindenmuth, E.B., The efficacy of echinacea compound herbal tea preparation on the severity and duration of upper respiratory and flu symptoms: A randomized, double-blind placebo-controlled study, *J. Altern. Complement. Med.,* 6, 327, 2000.

96. Tripp, F., The use of dietary supplements in the elderly: Current issues and recommendations, *J. Am. Diet. Assoc.,*97, S181, 1997.

97. Burns, J.T. and Jensen, G.L., Malnutrition among geriatric patients admitted to medical and surgical services in a tertiary care hospital: Frequency, recognition and associated disposition and reimbursement outcomes, *Nutrition,* 11, 245, 1995.

98. Mowe, M. and Bohmer, T., The prevalence of undiagnosed protein-calorie undernutrition in a population of hospitalized elderly patients, *J. Am. Geriatr. Soc.,* 39, 1089, 1991.

99. Food and Nutrition Board, *The Role of Nutrition in Maintaining Health in the Nation's Elderly: Evaluating Coverage of Nutrition Services for the Medicare Population,* National Academy Press, Washington, D.C., 2000.

100. Davies, L. and Knutson, K.C., Warning signals for malnutrition in the elderly, *J. Am. Diet. Assoc.,* 91, 1413, 1991.

101. Rolls, B.J., Do chemosensory changes influence food intake in the elderly?, *Physiol. Behav.,* 66, 193, 1999.

102. Frongillo, E.A., Jr., Rauschenbach, B S., Roe, D.A. and Williamson, D.F., Characteristics related to elderly persons' not eating for 1 or more days: Implications for meal programs, *Am. J. Public Health,* 82, 600, 1992.

103. Posner, B.M., Jette, A., Smigelski, C., Miller, D. and Mitchell, P., Nutritional risk in New England elders, *J. Gerontol.,* 49, M123, 1994.

104. Jensen, G.L., McGee, M. and Binkley, J., Nutrition in the elderly, *Gastroenterol. Clin. North Am.,* 30, 313, 2001.

105. Allison, D.B., Fontaine, K.R., Manson, J.E., Stevens, J. and VanItallie, T.B., Annual deaths attributable to obesity in the United States, *JAMA,* 282, 1530, 1999.

106. Calle, E.E., Thun, M.J., Petrelli, J.M., Rodriguez, C. and Heath, C.W., Jr., Body-mass index and mortality in a prospective cohort of U.S. adults, *New Engl. J. Med.,* 341, 1097, 1999.

107. Franklin, C.A. and Karkeck, J., Weight loss and senile dementia in an institutionalized elderly population, *J. Am. Diet. Assoc.,* 89, 790, 1989.

108. Aronoff, N.J., Geliebter, A. and Zammit, G., Gender and body mass index as related to the night-eating syndrome in obese outpatients, *J. Am. Diet. Assoc.,* 101, 102, 2001.

109. Gryglewska, B., Grodzicki, T. and Kocemba, J., Obesity and blood pressure in the elderly free-living population, *J. Hum. Hypertens.,* 12, 645, 1998.

110. Jensen, G.L. and Rogers, J., Obesity in older persons, *J. Am. Diet. Assoc.*, 98, 1308, 1998.

111. Kohrt, W.M., Abdominal obesity and associated cardiovascular comorbidities in the elderly, *Coron. Artery Dis.*, 9, 489, 1998.

112. Kolotkin, R.L., Head, S., Hamilton, M. and Tse, C.K., Assessing impact of weight on quality of life, *Obes. Res.*, 3, 49, 1995.

113. Kubena, K.S., McIntosh, W.A., Georghiades, M.B. and Landmann, W.A., Anthropometry and health in the elderly, *J. Am. Diet. Assoc.*, 91, 1402, 1991.

114. Must, A., Spadano, J., Coakley, E.H., Field, A.E., Colditz, G. and Dietz, W.H., The disease burden associated with overweight and obesity, *JAMA*, 282, 1523, 1999.

115. Nguyen, T.V., Sambrook, P.N. and Eisman, J.A., Bone loss, physical activity and weight change in elderly women: The Dubbo Osteoporosis Epidemiology Study, *J. Bone Miner. Res.*, 13, 1458, 1998.

116. Payette, H., Coulombe, C., Boutier, V. and Gray-Donald, K., Weight loss and mortality among free-living frail elders: A prospective study, *J. Gerontol. A Biol. Sci. Med. Sci.*, 54, M440, 1999.

117. Tayback, M., Kumanyika, S. and Chee, E., Body weight as a risk factor in the elderly, *Arch. Intern. Med.*, 150, 1065, 1990.

118. Wallace, J.I. and Schwartz, R.S. Involuntary weight loss in the elderly, in *Handbook of Nutrition in the Aged*, 2nd ed., Watson, R.R., Ed., CRC Press, Boca Raton, FL, 99, 1994.

119. Wallace, J.I. and Schwartz, R.S., Involuntary weight loss in elderly outpatients: Recognition, etiologies and treatment, *Clin. Geriatr. Med.*, 13, 717, 1997.

120. Yaari, S. and Goldbourt, U., Voluntary and involuntary weight loss: associations with long term mortality in 9,228 middle-aged and elderly men, *Am. J. Epidemiol.*, 148, 546, 1998.

121. Marton, K.I., Sox, H.C., Jr. and Krupp, J.R., Involuntary weight loss: diagnostic and prognostic significance, *Ann. Intern. Med.*, 95, 568, 1981.

122. Taylor, P.R., Albanes, D. and Tangrea, J.A., To supplement or not to supplement, that is the question, *Cancer Causes Control*, 8, 685, 1997.

123. Ledikwe, J.H., Smiciklas-Wright, H., Mitchell, D., Friedmann, J. M. and Still, C. D., Body mass index more associated with nutrition risk in rural older women than men, *FASEB J.*, 16, 2002.

124. Kuczmarski, R.J., Carroll, M.D., Flegal, K.M. and Troiano, R.P., Varying body mass index cutoff points to describe overweight prevalence among U.S. adults: NHANES III (1988 to 1994), *Obes. Res.*, 5, 542, 1997.

125. Flegal, K.M., Carroll, M.D., Kuczmarski, R.J. and Johnson, C.L., Overweight and obesity in the United States: Prevalence and trends, 1960–1994, *Int. J. Obes. Relat. Metab. Disord.*, 22, 39, 1998.

126. Jensen, G.L. and Friedmann, J.M., Obesity is associated with functional decline among community dwelling rural older persons, *J. Am. Geriatr. Soc.*, 50, 918, 2002.

127. Friedmann, J.M., Elasy, T. and Jensen, G.L., The relationship between body mass index and self-reported functional limitation among older adults: A gender difference, *J. Am. Geriatr. Soc.*, 49, 398, 2001.

128. Launer, L.J., Harris, T., Rumpel, C. and Madans, J., Body mass index, weight change and risk of mobility disability in middle-aged and older women. The epidemiologic follow-up study of NHANES I, *JAMA*, 271, 1093, 1994.

129. Ford, E.S., Moriarty, D.G., Zack, M.M., Mokdad, A.H. and Chapman, D.P., Self-reported body mass index and health-related quality of life: findings from the behavioral risk factor surveillance system, *Obes. Res.*, 9, 21, 2001.

130. Wolf, A.M. and Colditz, G.A., Current estimates of the economic cost of obesity in the United States, *Obes. Res.,* 6, 97, 1998.

131. Wellman, N.S., The Nutrition Screening Initiative, *Nutr. Rev.,* 52, S44, 1994.

132. White, J.V., Dwyer, J.T., Posner, B.M., Ham, R., Lipschitz, D.A. and Wellman, N.S., Nutrition Screening Initiative: Development and implementation of the public awareness checklist and screening tools, *J. Am. Diet. Assoc.,* 92, 163, 1992.

133. The Nutrition Screening Initiative, *Incorporating Nutrition Screening and Interventions into Medical Practice,* The Nutrition Screening Initiative, Washington, D.C., 1994.

134. Rush, D., Evaluating the Nutrition Screening Initiative, *Am. J. Public Health,* 83, 944, 1993.

135. Mitchell, D.C., Smiciklas-Wright, H., Friedmann, J.M. and Jensen, G.L., Dietary intake assessed by the Nutrition Screening Initiative Level II Screen is a sensitive but not a specific indicator of nutrition risk in older adults, *J. Am. Diet. Assoc.,* 102, 842, 2002.

136. Jensen, G.L., Kita, K., Fish, J., Heydt, D. and Frey, C., Nutrition risk screening characteristics of rural older persons: Relation to functional limitations and health care charges, *Am. J. Clin. Nutr.,* 66, 819, 1997.

137. Jensen, G.L., Friedmann, J.M., Coleman, C.D. and Smiciklas-Wright, H., Screening for hospitalization and nutritional risks among community-dwelling older persons, *Am. J. Clin. Nutr.,* 74, 201, 2001.

138. Guigoz, Y., Vellas, B. and Garry, P.J., Assessing the nutritional status of the elderly: The Mini Nutritional Assessment as part of the geriatric evaluation, *Nutr. Rev.,* 54, S59, 1996.

139. Reuben, D.B., Greendale, G.A. and Harrison, G.G., Nutrition screening in older persons, *J. Am. Geriatr. Soc.,* 43, 415, 1995.

140. Bales, C.W., What does it mean to be "at nutritional risk?" Seeking clarity on behalf of the elderly, *Am. J. Clin. Nutr.,* 74, 155, 2001.

141. Position of the American Dietetic Association: Nutrition, aging and the continuum of care, *J. Am. Diet. Assoc.,* 100, 580, 2000.

142. Nutrition labeling and education act of 1990, Pub. no. 1001-535, 104 stat 2353, 1990.

143. Levy, L., Patterson, R.E., Kristal, A.R. and Li, S.S., How well do consumers understand percentage daily value on food labels?, *Am. J. Health Promot.,* 14, 157, 2000.

144. Miller, C.K., Jensen, G.L. and Achterberg, C.L., Evaluation of a food label nutrition intervention for women with type 2 diabetes mellitus, *J. Am. Diet. Assoc.,* 99, 323, 1999.

145. Mitic, W., Nutrition education for older adults: Implementation of a nutrition instruction program, *Health Educ.,* 16, 7, 1985.

146. Franz, M.J., Monk, A., Barry, B., McClain, K., Weaver, T., Cooper, N., Upham, P., Bergenstal, R. and Mazze, R.S., Effectiveness of medical nutrition therapy provided by dietitians in the management of non-insulin-dependent diabetes mellitus: A randomized, controlled clinical trial, *J. Am. Diet. Assoc.,* 95, 1009, 1995.

147. Klein, G.L., Kita, K., Fish, J., Sinkus, B. and Jensen, G.L., Nutrition and health for older persons in rural America: A managed care model, *J. Am. Diet. Assoc.,* 97, 885, 1997.

148. Wolfe, W., Olson, C.M., Kendall, A. and Frongillo, E.A., Jr., Understanding food insecurity in the elderly: A conceptual framework, *J. Nutr. Ed.,* 28, 92, 1996.

149. Cohen, B.E. and Schulte, M.E., *Hunger and Food Insecurity among the Elderly,* The Urban Institute, Washington, D.C., 1993.

150. Wolfe, W.S., Olson, C.M., Kendall, A. and Frongillo, E.A., Jr., Hunger and food insecurity in the elderly: Its nature and measurement, *J. Aging Health,* 10, 327, 1998.

151. Millen, B.E., Ohls, J.C., Ponza, M. and McCool, A.C., The elderly nutrition program: An effective national framework for preventive nutrition interventions, *J. Am. Diet. Assoc.,* 102, 234, 2002.

152. Lee, J.S. and Frongillo, E.A., Jr., Understanding needs is important for assessing the impact of food assistance program participation on nutritional and health status in U.S. elderly persons, *J. Nutr.,* 131, 765, 2001.

10 Eating Disorders: Metabolic Complications and Therapy

Kelly K. Hill, Daniell B. Hill, Lisa Gaetke, Marion P. McClain and Craig J. McClain

CONTENTS

I. INTRODUCTION

Eating disorders are increasingly problematic in the United States. Magazines, television, movies, certain athletes, etc., all promote an unrealistic image of very thin people. Eating disorders, which primarily affect women, carry a high morbidity and the highest rate of mortality of any psychiatric illness. It has been estimated that more than 3% of young women have these disorders and probably twice that number have a clinically important variant.[1] Males have these conditions as well, but in much smaller numbers. This chapter will focus on anorexia nervosa (AN) and bulimia nervosa (BN), as virtually all research on eating disorders (ED) has focused on one or both of these conditions. Other known ED conditions — not-otherwise-specified and binge-eating disorder — will not be reviewed because of the limited research in these areas.

Because there is no consensus regarding the pathogenesis of EDs, the development of an ED is probably a combination of psychological, biological, genetic, environmental and social factors.[2-8] These factors include: affective disorders, anxiety disorders, obsessive-compulsive disorder and personality disorders; genetics; athletic endeavors; ballet or gymnastics and substance abuse. Neurotransmitters may play a role in the pathogenesis of eating disorders — norepinephrine and serotonin have both been implicated.[9-11] Some studies have examined brain changes in patients with anorexia nervosa but the meaning of the findings is unclear.[12,13] This chapter will review the definitions and differential diagnosis of eating disorders, complicatons of EDs and potential treatments for these problems.

II. DEFINITIONS

The Diagnostic and Statistical Manual-IV (DSM-IV) defines four diagnostic criteria for anorexia nervosa (AN):

1. Refusal to maintain weight within a normal range for height and age (more than 15% below ideal body weight (IBW))
2. Fear of weight gain
3. Severe body image disturbance in which body image is the predominant measure of self-worth, and denial of the seriousness of the illness
4. Absence of the menstrual cycle (amenorrhea) greater than three cycles for females

The two subtypes of anorexia nervosa are restricting and binge eating or purging. Patients with the restricting type of AN use only diet restriction to reduce their weight, while those with the binge/purge subtype may either binge or use purging (e.g., vomiting, laxatives, diuretics) to control weight. Thus, a patient who binges and purges but is at least 15% below IBW and meets the other psychological criteria can still be considered to be anorexic.

By definition, the AN patient is malnourished, weighing below a minimally normal level for age and height. These patients usually accomplish weight loss by drastically reducing their daily intake, restricting their diet to only a few very low-calorie foods. For example, a typical daily intake for such an individual might include: breakfast consisting of 8 ounces (250 ml) of coffee (black), followed by 8 ounces of diet coke, lunch would be skipped, afternoon refreshment two glasses (500 ml) of water, dinner consisting of chicken broth and tossed salad without dressing.

The fear of fatness seen in this population is irrational. These individuals fear being fat even though they are in an emaciated state. They are not reassured by weight loss and the fear often intensifies with continued weight loss. Frequently, the patient with anorexia nervosa is focused on a particular body part such as hips, thighs, or stomach. The rigorous exercise schedules commonly practiced by this population often are an attempt to "fix" the unacceptable areas. The self-worth of these individuals is very dependent on their body weight and shape. Weight loss is experienced as an achievement and demonstrates superior self-discipline, whereas weight gain is perceived as an unacceptable failure.

The DSM-IV criteria for bulimia nervosa (BN) are the following:

- Episodes of binge eating with a sense of loss of control
- Binge eating followed by a compensatory behavior of purging (self-induced vomiting, laxative or diuretic abuse) or nonpurging (excessive exercise, fasting or strict diets)
- Binges and the resulting compensatory behavior must occur a minimum of two times per week for 3 months
- Dissatisfaction with body shape and weight

A binge is eating a large amount of food in a short, discrete amount of time. A detailed history of a typical binge or of the last binge episode is essential. A typical binge might be a whole bag of cookies, a gallon of ice cream (3.7 L) and six candy bars consumed in 2 hours. At the start of the binge, patients feel a loss of control over their eating. Usually the patients say that after the first bite they cannot stop the binging. Some individual patients identify "trigger foods" (typically sweet or salty) and indicate that eating any sweet food, such as a piece of candy, triggers a binge.

The bulimic patient is terrified of the fattening effects of the binge and will engage in several behaviors to negate these. Initially, patients survive on a small amount of food between binges. They may consume only 800 kcals in a typical day and engage in excessive exercise. Vomiting is frequently used. The vomiting may occur either after binges, after normal meals, or after any eating. Severe bulimics will engage in a series of purging behaviors. They may vomit, use laxatives or a diuretic. Bulimics talk about seeking an "empty" feeling after a binge and these purging behaviors bring a tremendous release of tension. These individuals feel they can "have their cake and eat it too."

Bulimia nervosa is more common than AN. Generally, BN is found in approximately 3% of young females. As with AN, BN is less common in males. Certain groups are particularly at risk, such as cheerleaders, gymnasts, models and dancers. Any activity that places an emphasis on body weight presents a risk.

III. DIFFERENTIAL DIAGNOSIS

The most common medical illnesses confused with AN are other psychiatric disorders, diabetes mellitus, hyperthyroidism, certain cancers including brain tumors, and various GI disorders. Other psychiatric syndromes such as depression also may cause loss of appetite with subsequent weight loss. Yet, with depression alone, the other ED criteria are seldom present. Some schizophrenic patients present with abnormal eating habits, but these tend to be very bizarre and the other criteria for a diagnosis of AN or BN are seldom present.

TABLE 10.1
Gastrointestinal Diseases Simulating Eating Disorders

1.	Inflammatory bowel disease (e.g., Crohn's disease, ulcerative colitis)
2.	Irritable bowel syndrome
3.	Intestinal motility disorders (e.g., achalasia, gastroparesis)
4.	Acid peptic disease (e.g., esophagitis, ulcers, etc.)
5.	Malabsorptive status (sprue)
6.	Pancreatic disease (e.g., pancreatitis presenting with increased amylase, nausea and vomiting)
7.	Hepatitis (e.g., viral hepatitis presenting with nausea, vomiting and anorexia)
8.	Gallbladder disease (e.g., cholecystitis)

A host of GI diseases are in the differential diagnosis of eating disorders (Table 10.1). Probably one of the most difficult diseases to distinguish from an eating disorder is inflammatory bowel disease, especially Crohn's disease.[14,15] Crohn's disease can present with weight loss, anorexia, nausea, vomiting and diarrhea. Inflammatory bowel disease classically presents between 15 and 35 years of age. Thus, the age of onset for inflammatory bowel disease and eating disorders is very similar. Both groups of patients tend to be compulsive and high achievers. Irritable bowel syndrome (also known as functional bowel) may be confused with eating disorders. Indeed, many ED patients also have irritable bowel symptoms.[16] This is especially true for BN (relative risk ratio ~ 3.5). Patients with irritable bowel syndrome often have vague complaints of abdominal cramping and discomfort, diarrhea alternating with constipation, gas, bloating, etc. Irritable bowel syndrome is a very common problem seen in a wide variety of clinical settings and by a variety of health care providers. Thus, patients need a careful medical evaluation before the diagnosis of an eating disorder is determined. Acid peptic disease is another group of problems that can be confused with eating disorders. Esophagitis, gastritis, gastric ulcers and duodenal ulcers can present with abdominal pain, nausea, vomiting and weight loss and thus simulate symptoms of eating disorders. Intestinal motility disorders such as achalasia, gastroparesis and pseudoobstruction are often confused with eating disorders. Moreover, gastroparesis can occur in patients with eating disorders. Malabsorptive states such as sprue (presenting with diarrhea and weight loss) must be included in the differential diagnosis. Pancreatitis, cholecystitis and hepatitis all can be associated with nausea, vomiting, anorexia and abdominal pain (see Table 10.1).

IV. MEDICAL COMPLICATIONS

Eating disorders are unique among psychiatric illnesses because of the severe medical complications that result from the abnormal eating behavior and weight-reduction methods utilized by this population. Anorexia nervosa is one of the deadliest of psychiatric disorders.[17] The majority of the physical sequelae of AN are related to the effects of starvation and can be reversed by restoration of a balanced, healthy diet and weight. However, there are important differences between AN and starvation. In anorexia nervosa, protein intake is usually adequate, but there is limited consumption of carbohydrates, fats and, thus, calories.[18] In starvation, the diet is lacking in protein, vitamins and calories. Therefore, some immunological and hematological abnormalities are specific to AN, while others are also seen in starvation and malnutrition.[18]

There is a great deal of overlap between the medical complications seen in BN with those seen in anorexia nervosa. BN patients are at risk to suffer from the complications described for the AN patient because they, too, have an abnormal nutritional intake and engage in destructive methods for weight control. Important physical signs that suggest the diagnosis of BN include dental erosions, hypertrophy of the parotid glands and skin changes over the dorsum of the hand caused by self-induced vomiting.[19] Major grouping of medical complications are discussed below.

A. Gastrointestinal Complications

The gastrointestinal problems associated with eating disorders are many and varied.[16,20] Chami et al. found that the most important determinant of gastrointestinal symptoms appears to be depression.[21] Winstead and Willard[22] surveyed 14 ED patients for their histories of seeking treatment for physical problems. They found that 62% had sought out a gastroenterologist or primary care physician with a GI complaint and that 46% had sought treatment of their GI complaint before seeking treatment for their eating disorder. This section will review GI complications observed in eating disorders based on an anatomic distribution (see Table 10.2).

Dental and oral problems associated with frequent vomiting are a problem both in patients with BN and those anorexics with self-induced vomiting. This relates mainly to the effects of gastric acid on the teeth with subsequent enamel injury.[23,24] Bulimics also may ingest large amounts of carbohydrates and thus may be more predisposed to dental caries.[23,24] Mendell and Logemann[25] studied the relationship between bulimia and abnormalities in swallowing function. They identified abnormalities in the oral cavity and oropharynx, changes in taste, tissue changes and potential motility disorders that could impact swallowing function. Parotid enlargement is a potential complication of AN and BN.[26] In our experience, parotid enlargement in most ED patients relates to bulimia, and the parotid enlargement improves

TABLE 10.2
Relative GI Disturbances in Eating Disorders

	AN (restrictors)	AN (purgers)	BN
Dental	−	+	+
Parotid	−	+	+
Esophagitis	−	+	+
Altered gastric emptying	+	+	+
Delayed gastric transit	+	+	+
Elevated amylase, pancreatic diseases	+/−	+	+

clinically with hospitalization and careful monitoring to prevent purging. Many patients with eating disorders and parotid enlargement have hyperamylasemia[27,28] that is salivary in origin. However, because these patients have associated complaints of nausea and vomiting, they may be mistakenly diagnosed as having pancreatitis unless a serum lipase or salivary isoamylase test is performed.[27–29] We measured amylase, lipase and isoamylase activity in 17 consecutive patients admitted to our ED unit.[27] Six patients had elevated total serum amylase activity and five of these six had isolated increases in their salivary isoamylase activity. Another six patients had normal serum total amylase activity, but modest elevations in the salivary isoamylase fraction. Thus, distinguishing the origin of the amylase is quite important in evaluating an ED patient with hyperamylasemia.

Data regarding esophageal abnormalities in eating disorders are conflicting. Some investigators have reported a high frequency of esophagitis and ulcers in patients with BN, but other investigators have been unable to identify important esophageal abnormalities on upper GI endoscopy.[30–32] It has been our clinical observation that esophagitis and esophageal ulceration are not frequent complications in patients with eating disorders. Of major concern relating to the esophagus are reports by some investigators regarding esophageal dysmotility in patients with AN and BN. One group reported that approximately one-third of bulimic patients had major esophageal dysmotility including achalasia.[33] Other groups have reported similar findings in AN.[34]

Abnormal gastric emptying of solid food is frequently observed in AN, affecting up to 80% of patients with this condition.[33–38] Most patients have delayed gastric emptying, although a few appear to actually have increased gastric emptying.[33–38] Alterations in antral motility are thought to be responsible for gastric emptying problems and delayed emptying can be treated with prokinetic agents such as metoclopramide. Similar gastric emptying disturbances also have been reported in patients with BN. Hutson and Wald[39] performed a dual radioisotope technique to assess gastric emptying in ED patients and found that gastric emptying in bulimics was similar to controls, but AN patients had markedly delayed gastric emptying. Kamal et al.[40] also showed delayed transit times in ED patients compared with controls, but the levels did not reach statistical significance. Koch et al.[41] reported that hospitalized BN patients had exaggerated perceptions of stomach fullness and satiety in response to water, abnormal gastric myoelectrical activity and accelerated lag phase of gastric emptying. Occasionally, disastrous consequences occur with marked dilatation of the stomach and gastric rupture in AN.[42] This necessitates care in refeeding very malnourished AN patients. We frequently place post-pyloric feeding tubes if we are using enteral feeding solutions in order to bypass the problem of impaired gastric emptying.

Endoscopic findings of gastritis, gastric ulcer, or duodenal ulcer are infrequent and usually are not a cause of the common GI symptoms reported by these patients. Helicobacter pylori is a gram-negative bacteria that resides beneath the mucus layer of the stomach. The presence of this bacteria in the stomach can be associated with symptoms of bloating, anorexia and nausea, and *H. pylori* is highly associated with the development of peptic ulcer disease. Studies from our laboratory show that the incidence of *H. pylori* infection is no higher in ED patients than in age- and sex-matched controls.[43]

Only a limited number of studies evaluating small intestine function and motility in ED patients have been performed. Haller et al. [44] reported that AN patients generally had normal or slightly delayed small intestine transit as determined by barium meal. Hirakawa et al.[45] evaluated small bowel transit time as assessed by breath hydrogen measurements in 10 patients with AN. Gastrocecal transit time was significantly delayed in AN patients compared with normal volunteers. Abnormalities in hypothalamic-pituitary function or thyroid function due to starvation, impaired sensitivity of cholinergic receptors, or impaired autonomic function have been suggested as possible mechanisms for the delayed intestinal transit in these subjects.

Laxative abuse is quite common in ED patients.[30] This abuse may lead to electrolyte abnormalities, especially hypokalemia in some ED patients. The colon may be dilated, atonic and lack haustrations. Rarely, rectal impaction can occur in AN patients with very poor oral intake.

Abnormalities of the pancreas as assessed biochemically, by ultrasound and by computerized tomography (CT) scan have been reported in patients with eating disorders.[27–29,46] In AN patients studied by Cox et al.,[46] seven of ten had ultrasonic or biochemical abnormalities in the pancreas. Seven patients had elevated amylase:creatinine clearance ratios and three had elevated serum amylase concentrations. Three also had reduced echogenicity of the pancreas. These abnormalities resolved after refeeding. We reported ultrasound and CT abnormalities of the pancreas in two patients who underwent exploratory laparotomy, with no significant pancreatic pathology being noted.[29] Both patients were inappropriately diagnosed as having pancreatic disorders because of biochemical and radiologic abnormalities when, in fact, both had eating disorders. Thus, true pancreatic abnormalities may complicate eating disorders. However, most frequently, ED patients are erroneously diagnosed as having pancreatic disease because of an elevated serum amylase that is actually salivary and not pancreatic in origin, as discussed previously.

Finally, in AN patients, there have been case reports of rare GI complications such as small bowel obstruction,[47] severe liver dysfunction,[48] gastrectasia with tight pyloric stenosis[49] and pancreatic damage caused by laxative abuse.[50] Gwirtsman et al.[51] reported a patient with both anorexia nervosa and Wilson's disease.

B. RENAL ABNORMALITIES

Several reports have detailed urologic or renal complications in patients with EDs. The lower urinary tract is estrogen sensitive and female patients with AN are hypoestrogenemic. Thus, they may tend to suffer an increased incidence of lower urinary tract symptoms. Indeed, Hextall et al.[52] studied 29 women with AN and found that the majority had significant irritative urinary symptoms, the most frequent of which were frequency, urgency and nocturia.

Some of the important recently reported renal complications include: nephrolithiasis,[53] hypopotassemia and distal renal tubular acidosis,[54] secondary gout and pseudo syndrome,[55] acute renal failure,[56] acute renal failure resulting from rhabdomyolysis,[57,58] nephropathy associated with electrolyte disorders,[59] ammonium urate urinary stones[60] and potentially life-threatening hypophosphatemia associated with proximal tubular dysfunction.[61]

Electrolyte abnormalities occur more frequently in ED patients who abuse laxatives or diuretics and who engage in self-induced vomiting. Indeed, hypokalemia in an outpatient with an eating disorder suggests persistent purging. With the subsequent volume depletion, there is a disproportionate increase in blood urea nitrogen compared with creatinine.[62]

When there is long-standing abuse of laxatives and diuretics, hypokalemic nephropathy can occur and can lead to chronic renal failure with polyuria, polydipsia and elevated serum creatinine.[63] Ishikawa et al. [64] reported a patient with a history of AN who developed licorice-induced hypokalemic myopathy. Even with potassium replacement, the patient remained hypokalemic and had impaired renal function with inability to concentrate and acidify the urine. Renal biopsy revealed intense degeneration and vacuolation of the tubules (normal glomerus) that was consistent with hypokalemic nephropathy.

Two types of peripheral edema may occur, often when the patient is being refed.[65] A benign form, with normal plasma protein and albumin levels, is of unclear etiology and usually presents no adverse clinical sequelae. A more ominous form can follow chronic laxative abuse and vigorous purging. This may lead to hypoproteinemia with subsequent hypovolemia with fluid shifts. Occasionally, these patients may develop shock, renal failure and cardiovascular collapse.[63]

C. SKELETAL COMPLICATIONS

Osteoporosis is traditionally considered a disease of aging, but it has been long recognized that young patients with anorexia nervosa often suffer from osteoporosis. In 1992, Kiriike et al.[66] determined that the severe weight loss, low physical activity, longer duration of amenorrhea and deficiency of estrogen contributed to bone loss in AN. These young patients may not achieve peak bone mass, may suffer premature bone fractures and may not even achieve full potential height.

In 1995, Carmichael and Carmichael[67] examined bone mineral density in patients with anorexia nervosa, bulimia and anorexia/bulimia. Patients with AN had the lowest bone density, while overt osteopenia was uncommon in anorexia/bulimia and in bulimia. Hypercortisolism was found to be the best laboratory indicator for assessing the risk of osteopenia in the AN patients. A 1997 study found that, while bone density was reduced in AN patients, physical activity had a significant positive effect on bone density.[68] In 1997, Ward, Brown and Treasure[69] found that osteopenia persisted in female anorexics even after recovery, and they suggested the use of oral contraceptives (for estrogen) in these patients.

Castro et al.[70] examined predictors of bone mineral density in adolescents with AN and found that several predictors were correlated with reduced bone density: more than 12 months since the onset of AN; more than 6 months of amenorrhea, body mass index (BMI) <15, calcium intake of <600 mg/day, and less than 3 hr/week of physical activity. Several recent studies have examined bone changes in anorexia and concluded that early in AN there is not a significant bone loss, but the longer the condition continues, the more likely there will be significant bone density loss.[71–79] Male anorexics are also at risk for osteopenia and osteoporosis.[72,79]

Osteomalacia has also been reported in a patient with AN.[80] Fractures may occur after 7–15 years duration of the AN[81] and, crucial for an increase in bone density, is restoration of weight and resumption of menstruation.[81] A further long-term follow-up study of a cohort of AN patients found that the cumulative incidence of any bone fracture at 40 years post diagnosis of AN was 57%.[82] Thus, these patients are clearly at an increased risk even in the face of weight restoration. A report in 2000 examined bone density of recovered AN patients[83] and found that femur bone mineral density was still significantly less among recovered AN patients, even without post-illness fractures. Other studies have found a normalizing of bone mass after recovery.[71]

A study[76] of bone mineral density over time in patients with bulimia found that osteopenia was uncommon in these patients. In normal weight bulimics, osteopenia is not common.[84–86] Bulimics who have a history of anorexia do evidence osteopenia and osteoporosis.[76,84–86] Weight- bearing exercise can prevent or attenuate bone loss at specific skeletal sites in bulimic patients.[85]

Several studies have examined the effects of hormone replacement therapy on bone density.[87–89] These studies indicate that hormone replacement therapy can attenuate, but not necessarily reverse the effects of bone loss in young women with anorexia. Reduced bone size and reduced volumetric bone mineral density contribute significantly to loss of bone density,[87] and other factors, such as length of amenorrhea, years of estrogen exposure after weight gain, low levels of IGF-1, lowest BMI and body weight as a percentage of ideal body weight independently affect bone recovery.[88,89]

Weight gain and dietary intervention have also been studied for their effects on bone turnover/density.[90–94] Caillot-Augusseau et al.[90] found that weight gain, due to refeeding only, reversed the AN-induced uncoupling of bone remodeling and restored circadian variation of a bone resorption marker. There is conflicting evidence regarding the ability to regain bone mass once weight has been restored and menses have returned, but the potential for recovery of bone mass may exist for some period of time after refeeding.[91–94]

D. CARDIAC/LIPID ABNORMALITIES

Cardiac abnormalities represent one of the most serious and life-threatening complications of eating disorders. Cardiac abnormalities include bradycardia, tachycardia, hypotension, ventricular arrhythmias, mitral valve prolapse and cardiac failure.[18,9 5] Moodie[96] in 1987 outlined the association between AN and the heart and found that patients with AN have a small heart on chest x-ray, with a reduction in myocardial mass. Numerous electrocardiographic abnormalities occur including low voltage bradycardia, T-wave inversions and ST segment depression. The most lethal findings are arrhythmias, ranging from supraventricular premature contractions to ventricular tachycardia.18,97 Prolonged QT intervals are not common, but are thought to be one etiology of sudden death. The most common cardiac finding is bradycardia of less than 60 beats per minute, found in up to 87% of patients.

Hypotension (blood pressure less than 90/60 mmHg) is seen in up to 85% of patients. One probable cause is related to chronic volume depletion, which can cause dizziness/syncope.[18]

Biadi et al.[98] reported that patients with AN showed a lower heart rate and systolic blood pressure at peak exercise, lower work load and other measures of cardiac function. They concluded that the data indicated an abnormal working capacity and cardiovascular response to exercise in AN patients.

These patients are at risk for electrolyte abnormalities that may result in arrhythmias. If patients engage in purging behavior, they may develop elevated serum bicarbonate and metabolic alkalosis.[20] Other abnormalities include hypochloremia and hypokalemia, which may be further exacerbated by laxative abuse. Less frequently found are low serum bicarbonate, hypomagnesemia and hyponatremia. Severe hypophosphatemia can occur and must be carefully monitored during the refeeding process.[99] Severe electrolyte and acid-base imbalances are the most frequent cause of death.[100]

Schocken et al. [101] examined both AN and protein-calorie malnutrition and noted rhythm disturbances, mitral valve prolapse, systolic and diastolic ventricular dysfunction, with diminished exercise capacity in both states. They also noted that congestive heart failure may occur, especially during refeeding. This is analogous to that seen in prisoners of war and concentration camp survivors following World War II. Ipecac abuse to induce vomiting also can cause irreversible myocardial damage.[19]

The few reports in the literature regarding serum lipid levels and EDs consistently demonstrate normal to high levels of cholesterol and triglycerides.[102–104] In BN patients, the higher cholesterol levels are thought to relate to the nutrient intake during bingeing.[103] Since AN patients take in restricted amounts of dietary fats, the finding of normal to high serum lipids is not clearly understood.[104] AN patients with initial high cholesterol levels have the worst nutritional status and high cholesterol levels are not related to a *de novo* synthesis. This profile returns to normal with refeeding.[104]

E. HEMATOLOGICAL COMPLICATIONS

Research from as far back as the mid 1970s indicated that patients with AN exhibit abnormalities of the hematologic system.[105] The major abnormalities include mild anemia[105,106] and low total leukocyte count.[106] Some patients develop bone marrow hypoplasia.[106–108] Hemolytic anemia has occurred in association with hypophosphatemia with refeeding.[109] Bone marrow hypoplasia seems to be reversible with intensive nutritional intervention[107] or recombinant human erythropoietin.[108] Phosphate supplementation should be considered in the refeeding of severely malnourished patients[109] and careful monitoring of minerals and electrolytes is vital in these patients (discussed in Treatment section).

Some patients with BN also demonstrate low hemoglobin and low vitamin B_{12} levels.[110] In the study by Gendall et al.,[110] low prealbumin levels were associated with more episodes of binge eating and vomiting, but only 4.3% of patients had low prealbumin levels. Low albumin was associated with increased vomiting.[110]

F. Immune Dysfunction

Nutrients play key roles in the development and function of the human immune system. Eating disorder patients have altered and often diminished nutrient intake. In spite of the undernourished state of AN and BN patients, they often appear to retain immunocompetence.[111] Various subsets of T cells have been studied regarding their relative ratios in ED patients.[112–115] Marcos et al.[116] evaluated the immunocompetence of patients with BN and found that lymphocyte subsets CD2 and CD4 were lower than in controls and CD8 was unchanged. Thus, the CD4:CD8 ratio was also lower. The B lymphocyte subset was increased and innate immunity was impaired. Nova and co-workers[111] studied both AN and BN patients and found that duration of the eating disorder and the time when appropriate treatment is achieved are likely contributors to the alterations seen in the CD4:CD8 ratio. A significant inverse correlation between spontaneous NK cell activity and baseline serum cortisol also has been reported.[117] Abnormal cytokine metabolism has been implicated as one mechanism for anorexia and wasting in ED, but the observed abnormalities have been modest. One study examined the possible relationship between the hypothalamic-pituitary-adrenal axis and the immune response by studying serum cortisol concentractions, plasma ACTH and TNF-α and IL-1β production by *ex-vivo* unstimulated and LPS-stimulated peripheral mononuclear cells.[118] They found a positive correlation between IL-1β release in unstimulated supernatants of mononuclear cell cultures and serum cortisol levels in AN patients, while there was a trend toward a negative correlation in normal subjects.[118] They also found a slight, but not statistically significant, positive correlation between IL-1β and plasma ACTH, as well as between TNF-α and serum cortisol. They concluded that the normal relationship between pro-inflammatory cytokine release and cortisol secretion is deranged in AN. Other studies have also found cytokine dysregulation.[119–121]

G. Endocrine Complications

The individual with AN has numerous endocrine changes that are probably related to malnutrition, low body fat and psychological factors. Multiple recent studies detail abnormalities in the hypothalmic pituitary-ovarian axis in AN and BN.[1–5,7] By definition, AN patients are amenorrheic due to low body weight. With major loss of fat stores, conversion of androgens to estrogens is decreased because this function normally occurs in adipose tissue. Some studies have reported that 90% of AN patients will begin menstruating when their body fat increases to about 22% of total body weight.

In approximately 16% of AN patients, amenorrhea develops before any weight loss. Amenorrhea may continue after weight restoration in some patients, supporting the hypothesis that the disturbance of hypothalamic function is secondary to psychological stress.[18] Therefore, some patients must have restoration of weight as well as improvement in psychological functioning to regain normal menses.

The AN patient can also suffer from hypothalamic hypogonadism, with low basal levels of plasma luteinizing hormone (LH) and follicle stimulating hormone (FSH). The episodic release of these hormones can also be altered. The pattern of

LH release is similar to that seen in puberty. These changes usually normalize with weight restoration.[18]

Fertility is abnormal and pregnancy is rare, since, by definition, AN patients are amenorrheic. The ovaries and uterus may be small and again normalize with weight gain (ovarian growth being related to gonadotropin functioning and uterine size to estrogen levels).[18] Breast mass may be reduced and there may be an associated decreased libido and atrophy of the vaginal mucosa. In the male AN patient, serum testosterone levels are decreased.[18] Plasma testosterone levels were decreased in AN, but not in BN women.[122]

Abnormalities of the hypothalmic-pituitary-adrenal axis are also well documented, with elevated cerebrospinal fluid levels of corticotropin releasing hormone (CRF) and elevated plasma cortisol levels following dexamethasone suppression.[118,123–126] Patients do not demonstrate cushingoid features on physical exam in spite of the modestly elevated plasma cortisols, but some of the observed metabolic abnormalities such as bone loss may be worsened due to excess cortisol. Katz[127] described a patient with AN and Cushing's disease and suggested that increased hypothalamic-pituitary corticotropin stimulation in association with the AN may have activated an occult inactive pituitary basophil adenoma in this patient that subsequently was evidenced by the overproduction of ACTH by the tumor.

Anorexia nervosa patients have altered glucose metabolism. In a study published in 2001, Gniuli and coauthors[128] reported blunted glucose metabolism and low glucose-induced thermogenesis. Cuntz et al.[129] found that pancreatic size correlates highly with BMI and with the actual amount of digested food. They suggest that pancreatic size might be useful in assessing normalization of the eating patterns. Nozaki et al.[130] suggest that in AN, the low insulin response to oral glucose seen in the flat type group may be due to a disturbance of GI factors (such as motility) and that the delayed type group has a beta-cell failure corrected by weight gain and has insulin resistance requiring a longer recovery time. They suggest that these abnormalities are related to the duration of AN.

Growth hormone (GH) is frequently oversecreted and insulin-like growth factor-1 (IGF-1) is very low as a result of undernutrition and acquired peripheral GH resistance. IGF-1 synthesis and release both appear to be markedly impaired.[131] Importantly, IGF-1 mediates many of the anabolic aspects of GH. Gianotti et al. [132] examined IGF-1 and GH in other catabolic conditions, such as trauma, sepsis, major burns, postsurgery patients, liver cirrhosis and severe GH deficiency. IGF-1 levels were depressed in AN patients, similar to these other catabolic states. This depressed IGF-1 may play a role in many of the metabolic complications of AN, ranging from poor weight gain with refeeding to bone disease. Hotta et al. [133] found that IGF-1 and IGFBP-3 (binding protein) levels were lower in AN patients with a BMI < 16.5, but IGF-1 and its binding proteins were normal in AN patients whose BMI was greater than 16.5.

There may be disturbed thyroid function in eating disorders. Thyroxine levels (T4) may be mildly depressed (but this generally is not clinically important). Free tri-iodothyronine (T3) levels may be 50% of those found in non-anorexic populations, secondary to diminished peripheral conversion of T4 to T3. Thyroxine stimulating hormone (TSH) levels are usually in the normal range. However, there may be abnormal responses to stimulation tests.[18]

Leptin is a hormone secreted by adipocytes. Circulating leptin levels are thought to control appetite (leptin decreases food intake) and have a usual circadian rhythm in normal subjects. In patients with eating disorders, this pattern seems to be altered. Several studies have examined leptin levels in ED patients.[134–138] Early on, leptin was shown to be associated with BMI, but not specific eating pathology in ED patients.[139] Other investigators showed that the log of the serum leptin level correlated with triiodothyronine (T3) levels and that body fat mass and eating behavior score were significant determinants of leptin levels.[140] Eckert et al.[141] studied serum leptin and insulin-like growth factor I (IGF-1) before and after weight gain in AN patients. In untreated AN patients, leptin levels were significantly lower than those in normal body weight controls (p<.001). They found that at very low BMIs, there seems to be a threshold beneath which leptin does not decrease. Thus, the correlation between leptin and BMI does not continue at these low BMIs. Leptin levels increased significantly with refeeding and showed a significant correlation with BMI after refeeding. Serum leptin and IGF-1 were highly correlated, even controlling for body weight during starvation, but not after refeeding or in normal weight controls. Leptin appears to be related to menstrual status in that a threshold level may be necessary for normal menstruation and, if that level is present, even in the face of low body weight, menstruation will occur.[142]

H. Dermatologic Complications

Because of inadequate nutrition, ED patients are at increased risk for many possible dermatologic consequences. Cutaneous signs often seen include xerosis of the skin, white dermographism, diffuse hypertrichosis, acrocyanosis, scars, diffuse effluvium, artifacts, brittle nails, anychophagia, carotenoderma, generalized pruritus, hyperpigmentation, striae distensae, factitial dermatitis, seborrheic dermatitis and poor wound healing.[143–149] Schulze et al.[143] found a significant correlation between hypertrichosis and amenorrhea or a BMI < 16. Hediger[145] also noted the importance of a BMI < 16 for the more frequent appearance of skin problems. Many of the skin manifestations can resolve with weight gain in AN or with cessation of purging in BN.

I. Selected Nutritional Abnormalities

Obviously, ED patients have disturbed dietary practices. In an effort to quantify eating patterns in subjects who showed psychological evidence of anorexia, Evers[150] studied the dietary intake in female university dancers and found that 70% consumed less than two thirds the RDA for at least one nutrient and 24% consumed less than two thirds RDA for three or more nutrients. van der Ster Wallin[151] and associates studied the food selection in AN and BN patients and controls and found that bulimics had lower relative and absolute intake of carbohydrates from bread and cereals. They found only minor differences among the three groups with respect to nutrient density, and energy percentages of protein, fat and carbohydrates were similar among the groups. Gendall et al.[152] studied BN patients and found that nonbinge eating had low energy intake and low intake of iron, calcium and zinc. Binge eating was characterized by high sucrose and saturated fatty acid content and overcompensated for the low energy intakes of the nonbinge eating.

Energy requirements are also disturbed in these patients. Dempsey et al.[153] measured resting energy expenditure (REE) in four AN patients before initiation of nutritional therapy and weekly thereafter. Before therapy, REE was 70% of the predicted level and rose to 102% of the predicted value after initiation of nutritional therapy. The caloric requirements for weight gain in these patients can be quite high. Walker et al.[154] found that a mean excess of 5026 Kcals was required per kg of weight gain during the first 15 days of standard refeeding protocol and this figure increased to 7428 Kcals/kg during the following 19 days. Normal-weight bulimic patients have been found to have reduced caloric needs to maintain weight.[155]

The implications of these derangements in energy expenditure in AN and BN patients are significant. The enormous caloric requirement for weight gain in AN patients may serve to undermine their efforts at weight gain. The decreased metabolic rate observed in some bulimic patients and the resulting difficulties in maintaining desired weight may perpetuate the purging behavior that the medical staff is attempting to discourage. Careful consideration of these abnormalities in energy expenditure is important in designing the optimal nutritional therapy for ED patients.

Micronutrient status may also be disturbed in these patients (Table 10.3 summarizes the current knowledge).

TABLE 10.3
Selected Nutrients That Are Altered in ED Patients

Minerals	Alterations in ED patients
Zinc[152,177,178,185–188,192–195]	marginal status, increased needs with refeeding, deficiency can cause anorexia and inhibit weight gain
Copper [178,185,192]	marginal status, deficiency can cause anemia, neutropenia, increased cholesterol
Calcium[94,150,152,185]	marginal status, deficiency may accelerate bone disease
Phosphorous [109,160]	marginal status, deficiency frequently may occur with aggressive refeeding

Water-soluble vitamins	Alterations in ED patients
Folate [152,177]	marginal status, may cause anemia
Niacin [150]	rare cases of pellagra
Thiamine [150,177,196]	rare cases of Wernicke's encephalopathy
B_{12} [185,197]	rare case of neurologic problems
B_6, Riboflavin [177,178]	intake depressed, complications rare

Fat-soluble vitamins	Alterations in ED patients
Vitamin A [150,152]	increased serum carotene, may develop yellowish skin color, intake may be subnormal
Vitamin D, E, K [177,181,198]	usually normal serum levels, dietary intake may be reduced

V. TREATMENT

Eating disorders are multifactorial conditions encompassing psychiatric, medical and nutritional facets. A team approach is the most comprehensive and thus the most likely to be a successful avenue to treatment. The team generally comprises a mental health professional familiar with eating disorders, a medical physician with expertise concerning the many medical complications of ED and a nutritionist with experience in ED.[156] The nutritional management of the underweight patient with AN is critical for recovery and long-term prognosis. Both AN and BN patients may be hospitalized because of comorbid psychiatric problems such as suicide, ideation and depression.

Without treatment, up to 20% of people with serious eating disorders die. With treatment, that number falls to 2–3%. With treatment, about 60% of people with eating disorders recover. They maintain healthy weight. They eat a varied diet of normal foods and do not choose exclusively low-calorie and nonfat items. They participate in friendships and romantic relationships. They create families and careers. Many say they feel they are stronger people and more insightful about life in general and themselves in particular than they would have been without the disorder.[157]

In spite of treatment, about 20% of people with eating disorders make only partial recoveries. They remain too much focused on food and weight. They participate only peripherally in friendships and romantic relationships. They may hold jobs but seldom have meaningful careers. Much of each paycheck goes to diet books, laxatives, jazzercise classes and binge food.[157]

The remaining 20% do not improve, even with treatment. They are seen repeatedly in emergency rooms, ED programs and mental health clinics. Their quietly desperate lives revolve around food and weight concerns, spiraling down into depression, loneliness and feelings of helplessness and hopelessness.[157]

Poor outcome in AN is associated with later age of onset, longer duration, lower minimal body weight and psychiatric comorbidity. The 10-year mortality may be as high as 6.6% in AN. Women with AN may have up to a 10-fold increase in mortality compared with other women of their same age group. In BN, up to 30% continue to engage in recurrent binge eating and purging behaviors after 10 years of follow-up. Substance abuse and long duration of the disorder are predictors of poor outcome.

The American Psychiatric Association has developed practice guidelines for ED[158] that call for a multifactorial approach. These guidelines are summarized below.

All patients should have a psychiatric management plan. Important components include the establishment and maintenance of a therapeutic alliance; coordination of care with others on the team; assessment and monitoring of eating disorder symptoms and behaviors; assessment and monitoring of the patient's general medical condition; assessment and monitoring of the patient's psychiatric status and safety and provision of family assessment and treatment.[158] This requires careful and consistent interaction with the patient and family.

For anorexia nervosa the goals of treatment should be:

- Restore patients to a healthy weight with a return of menses and normal ovulation (females) or normal sex drive (males) and a return to normal physical and sexual growth and development in children and adolescents.
- Treatment of medical/physical complications of the eating disorder.
- Enhancement of the patient's motivation to cooperate in the restoration of healthy eating patterns and to participate in treatment.
- Provision of education/nutrition counseling.
- Correction of core maladaptive thoughts, attitudes and feelings.
- Treatment of associated psychiatric conditions (e.g., defects in mood regulation, self-esteem and behavior).
- Enlisting family support and providing family counseling.
- Prevention of relapse.[158]

A program of nutritional rehabilitation and management should be established for all patients. AN patients usually have some alterations in their nutritional status that may already have led to medical complications (or have the potential to do so). Thus, nutrition management must be an integral part of the treatment program. Medications should not be used as the sole or primary treatment for AN.[159] The role for antidepressants is best assessed following weight gain. Inpatient ED therapy is often more effective than outpatient, but, because of insurance concerns, this option is often not available to patients. However, for AN patients with severe or life-threatening medical complications, hospitalization must be initiated. Patients should be hospitalized if they are 25% or more under ideal body weight (emaciated); having hypoglycemia, syncope or grayouts; if there are severe fluid and electrolyte abnormalities (e.g., dehydration); if there is a cardiac arrhythmia, hypotension, hypothermia or vasomotor instability; or if there is refractory vomiting.

For bulimia nervosa, the goals of treatment should be:

- Reduction in or elimination of binge-eating and purging behaviors
- Improvement in attitudes related to the eating disorder
- Minimization of food restriction
- Increasing the variety of foods eaten
- Encouragement of healthy, but not excessive, exercise
- Treatment of medical complications
- Addressing of underlying behaviors, developmental issues, identity formation, etc.[158]

Many BN patients are near normal weight, but have disturbed eating patterns and thus nutritional concerns. These must be addressed through nutrition counseling and medical treatment of any physical complications of the bulimia. Medications, primarily antidepressants, are used to reduce the frequency of disturbed eating behaviors. Additionally, medications may be employed to alleviate symptoms that may be coexistent with the eating disorder, such as depression, anxiety, obsession, or impulsivity.[15]

Bulimia nervosa patients rarely encounter significant medical complications during nutritional therapy in the absence of laxative, alcohol or drug abuse, psychosis, suicidality or major personality disturbance. The initial period of refeeding an AN patient, however, can be among the most risky phases of their illness. Minerals and electrolytes such as phosphorous and potassium should be carefully followed.[160] These patients must be monitored for signs of congestive heart failure and excessive peripheral edema.

Patients often complain of nausea, vomiting and bloating, which can interfere with nutrition support; gastric motility problems are common. Some studies suggest pro-motility agents can be helpful in treating this dysmotility associated with eating disorders. Superior mesenteric artery (SMA) syndrome has been reported in AN patients.[161] If these problems interfere with oral intake, nasoenteric tubes are often helpful for nutrition support.[162] We often endoscopically place small-bore feeding tubes deep into the small intestine, thus bypassing an atonic stomach or SMA obstruction. Initial daily caloric intake goals should be 30–40 kcal/kg body weight. The goal weight gain should be 2–3 pounds per week (1–1.5 kg).[163] Measured energy expenditure (MEE) initially is often low, even when corrected for lean body mass. However, in clinical experience, these patients often require inordinate amounts of calories to gain weight. MEE may increase, indicating that some patients become hypermetabolic during refeeding and recovery phases. Patients are encouraged to take regular food. However, if they are not eating within 24 hours, a nasoenteric feeding tube is placed and a standard isocaloric/isoosmolar formula is started. Studies have shown that the closer the AN patient is to achieving ideal body weight at the time of discharge, the better the chances for long-term recovery.[164–166] This is especially true with a first-time treatment.[167] For BN patients, intensive nutrition and psychiatric therapy is useful.

Energy requirements for ED patients are important aspects of their treatment regimens. To refeed either AN or BN patients adequately and to help them begin to eat in a normal fashion, it is important to assess their pretreatment energy expenditure as well as concurrently with treatment. Several groups have examined this problem from various aspects. Schebendach et al.[168] examined both AN and BN patients and used both indirect calorimetry and the Harris-Benedict equation to calculate energy requirements for the patients. They found that actual measured energy expenditure was less than that predicted by the Harris-Benedict equation for AN, but similar in BN. Others have found that REE is lower in normal-weight bulimics than controls and that the equations used to predict REE are not accurate.[169–174]

A detailed study of changes in body composition and resting energy expenditure in anorexic patients after a weight gain of at least 15%[175] showed that REE increased with weight gain and that most of the weight regained was in fat mass and most of the body water was in extra cellular water, which may help explain the hyperhydra-tion and clinical problems associated with the refeeding syndrome. Interestingly, bone density was not significantly different after weight gain. Rigaud et al.[176] studied REE in malnourished near-death patients who were refed and compared it with REE of anorexia patients. They found that near-death patients (BMI 9.77 ± 0.1) had high REE and high protein catabolism, whereas the AN patients were low. During refeed-ing, REE decreased in the dying patients and increased in the AN patients.

A. NUTRITIONAL THERAPY

Suboptimal vitamin intake or status is common in ED patients.[177–185] Nutrition intervention has been tried as a therapy for ED. We reported on the zinc status of

AN and BN patients before and after treatment that included zinc supplementation.[186] We found that zinc supplementation increased the serum zinc and urine zinc levels in supplemented patients. Birmingham and co-workers[187] also tried a controlled trial of zinc in AN and found the rate of increase in BMI of the zinc-supplemented group was twice that of the placebo group. Su and Birmingham[188] concluded that zinc supplementation should be included in the treatment regimens of AN patients. Zinc therapy during refeeding makes teliological sense because of the important role of zinc in multiple enzyme systems and protein metabolism. We have also given growth hormone (GH) therapy to inpatients with AN and observed more rapid weight gain and cardiac stabilization in a pilot study.[189]

Various studies have examined the utility of combined cognitive and nutritional therapy in AN and BN with mixed results.[156,186–188,190,191] Thus, there is still much investigative work to be accomplished to decide whether nutritional therapy will help in treating these patients.

Psychiatric treatment is very important during inpatient hospitalizations, especially if patients have been admitted because of suicide ideation or severe exacerbations of comorbid psychiatric issues. For patients with AN, intensive, individual and family psychotherapy should be initiated as soon as practical after the patient is medically stable.

B. Psychiatric Intervention

The mental health provider must be one who is experienced with ED. Individual and family cognitive behavior therapy are the mainstays of treatment of ED. These have been found to be especially helpful in the treatment of BN. Family involvement is crucial for successful psychotherapy. The mental health provider should also guide the team regarding comorbid psychiatric issues, the severity of the ED and underlying psychiatric conditions. Cognitive behavioral therapy helps patients manage anxiety relating to eating and poor body image by developing more adaptive thoughts and coping strategies. Cognitive behavioral therapy has been found to be more effective than simple behavioral therapy or interpersonal psychotherapy for patients with BN. However, local experience may vary and there is no clear evidence that any specific form of psychotherapy is superior for all patients. Pharmacologic intervention may be necessary in some ED patients. The American Psychiatric Association guidelines reviews accepted therapy.[158]

VI. CONCLUSION

Eating disorders, particularly anorexia nervosa and bulimia nervosa, are complex, multifactorial conditions with multiple complications and comorbidities. Some medical complications have long-term consequences for the ED patient. For example, osteopenia and osteoporosis are serious long-term complications. Some medical complications can be life-threatening (e.g., cardiac arrhythmias, refeeding syndrome). Additionally, comorbid psychiatric conditions may persist and require long-term follow-up. A team of psychiatric, medical and nutritional professionals is key to achieving the best treatment outcome for patients.

A great deal of research is ongoing into the etiology, complications and treatment modalities of these disorders. Some progress has been made, but these illnesses remain difficult to diagnose and treat successfully. Individual differences among patients make a single "cure" unlikely. Thus, the team of providers (psychiatric, medical and nutritional providers) familiar with eating disorders is the most promising approach to treating these patients.

REFERENCES

1. Becker, A.E., Grinspoon, S.K., Klibanski, A. and Herzog, D.B., Eating disorders, *N Engl J Med* 340, 1092–8, 1999.
2. Patton, G.C., Selzer, R., Coffey, C., Carlin, J.B. and Wolfe, R., Onset of adolescent eating disorders: Population based cohort study over 3 years, *Br Med J* 318, 765–8, 1999.
3. Nattiv, A., Agostini, R., Drinkwater, B. and Yeager, K.K., The female athlete triad. The interrelatedness of disordered eating, amenorrhea and osteoporosis, *Clin Sports Med* 13, 405–18, 1994.
4. Woodside, D.B., A review of anorexia nervosa and bulimia nervosa, *Curr Probl Pediatr* 25, 67–89, 1995.
5. Strober, M., Family-genetic studies of eating disorders, *J Clin Psychiat* 52, 9–12, 1991.
6. Kendler, K.S., MacLean, C., Neale, M., Kessler, R., Heath, A. and Eaves, L., The genetic epidemiology of bulimia nervosa, *Am J Psychiat* 148, 1627–37, 1991.
7. Herzog, D.B., Nussbaum, K.M. and Marmor, A.K., Comorbidity and outcome in eating disorders, *Psychiat Clin N Am* 19, 843–59, 1996.
8. Halmi, K.A., Eckert, E., Marchi, P., Sampugnaro, V., Apple, R. and Cohen, J., Comorbidity of psychiatric diagnoses in anorexia nervosa, *Arch Gen Psychiat* 48, 712–8, 1991.
9. Pirke, K.M., Central and peripheral noradrenalin regulation in eating disorders, *Psychiat Res* 62, 43–9, 1996.
10. Kaye, W.H., Persistent alterations in behavior and serotonin activity after recovery from anorexia and bulimia nervosa, *Ann N Y Acad Sci* 817, 162–78, 1997.
11. Kaye, W.H., Gwirtsman, H.E., George, D.T. and Ebert, M.H., Altered serotonin activity in anorexia nervosa after long-term weight restoration. Does elevated cerebrospinal fluid 5-hydroxyindoleacetic acid level correlate with rigid and obsessive behavior? *Arch Gen Psychiat* 48, 556–62, 1991.
12. Katzman, D.K., Lambe, E.K., Mikulis, D.J., Ridgley, J.N., Goldbloom, D.S. and Zipursky, R.B., Cerebral gray matter and white matter volume deficits in adolescent girls with anorexia nervosa, *J Pediatr* 129, 794–803, 1996.
13. Lambe, E.K., Katzman, D.K., Mikulis, D.J., Kennedy, S.H. and Zipursky, R.B., Cerebral gray matter volume deficits after weight recovery from anorexia nervosa, *Arch Gen Psychiat* 54, 537–42, 1997.
14. Jenkins, A.P., Treasure, J. and Thompson, R.P., Crohn's disease presenting as anorexia nervosa, *Br Med J (Clin Res Ed)* 296, 699–700, 1988.
15. Hershman, M.J. and Hershman, M., Anorexia nervosa and Crohn's disease, *Br J Clin Pract* 39, 157, 159, 1985.
16. Chial, H.J., McAlpine, D.E. and Camilleri, M., Anorexia nervosa: Manifestations and management for the gastroenterologist, *Am J Gastroent* 97, 255–69, 2002.

17. Theander, S., Outcome and prognosis in anorexia nervosa and bulimia: Some results of previous investigations compared with those of a Swedish long-term study, *J Psychiat Res* 19, 493–508, 1985.

18. Sharp, C.W. and Freeman, C.P., The medical complications of anorexia nervosa, *Br J Psychiat* 162, 452–62, 1993.

19. Herzog, D., Bradburn, I., *The Nature of Anorexia Nervosa and Bulimia Nervosa in Adolescents in Feeding Problems and Eating Disorders in Children and Adolescents* Harwood Academic Publishers, Switzerland, 1992.

20. McClain, C.J., Humphries, L.L., Hill, K.K. and Nickl, N.J., Gastrointestinal and nutritional aspects of eating disorders, *J Am Coll Nutr* 12, 466–74, 1993.

21. Chami, T.N., Andersen, A.E., Crowell, M.D., Schuster, M.M. and Whitehead, W.E., Gastrointestinal symptoms in bulimia nervosa: effects of treatment, *Am J Gastroent* 90, 88–92, 1995.

22. Winstead, N.S. and Willard, S.G., Frequency of physician visits for GI complaints by anorexic and bulimic patients, *Am J Gastroent* 96, 1667–8, 2001.

23. Hellstrom, I., Oral complications in anorexia nervosa, *Scand J Dent Res* 85, 71–86, 1977.

24. House, R.C., Grisius, R., Bliziotes, M.M. and Licht, J.H., Perimolysis: unveiling the surreptitious vomiter, *Oral Surg Oral Med Oral Pathol* 51, 152–5, 1981.

25. Mendell, D.A. and Logemann, J.A., Bulimia and swallowing: Cause for concern, *Int J Eat Disord* 30, 252–8, 2001.

26. Levin, P.A., Falko, J.M., Dixon, K., Gallup, E.M. and Saunders, W., Benign parotid enlargement in bulimia, *Ann Intern Med* 93, 827–9, 1980.

27. Humphries, L.L., Adams, L.J., Eckfeldt, J.H., Levitt, M.D. and McClain, C.J., Hyperamylasemia in patients with eating disorders, *Ann Intern Med* 106, 50–2, 1987.

28. Levine, J.M., Walton, B.E., Franko, D.L., Jimerson, D.C., Serum amylase in bulimia nervosa: clinical status and pathophysiology, *Int J Eat Disord* 12, 431–439, 1992.

29. Gilinsky, N.H., Humphries, L.L., Fried, A.M., McClain, C.J., Computed tomographic abnormalities of the pancreas in eating disorders: a report of two cases with normal laparotomy, *Int J Eat Disord* 7, 567–572, 1988.

30. Cuellar, R.E. and Van Thiel, D.H., Gastrointestinal consequences of the eating disorders: anorexia nervosa and bulimia, *Am J Gastroent* 81, 1113–24, 1986.

31. Cuellar, R.E., Kaye, W.H., Hsu, L.K. and Van Thiel, D.H., Upper gastrointestinal tract dysfunction in bulimia, *Dig Dis Sci* 33, 1549–53, 1988.

32. Kiss, A., Wiesnagrotzki, S., Abatzi, T.A., Meryn, S., Haubenstock, A. and Base, W., Upper gastrointestinal endoscopy findings in patients with long-standing bulimia nervosa, *Gastrointest Endosc* 35, 516–8, 1989.

33. Kiss, A., Bergmann, H., Abatzi, T.A., Schneider, C., Wiesnagrotzki, S., Hobart, J., Steiner-Mittelbach, G., Gaupmann, G., Kugi, A., Stacher-Janotta, G. and et al. Oesophageal and gastric motor activity in patients with bulimia nervosa, *Gut* 31, 259–65, 1990.

34. Stacher, G., Kiss, A., Wiesnagrotzki, S., Bergmann, H., Hobart, J. and Schneider, C., Oesophageal and gastric motility disorders in patients categorised as having primary anorexia nervosa, *Gut* 27, 1120–6, 1986.

35. McCallum, R.W., Grill, B.B., Lange, R., Planky, M., Glass, E.E. and Greenfeld, D.G., Definition of a gastric emptying abnormality in patients with anorexia nervosa, *Dig Dis Sci* 30, 713–22, 1985.

36. Domstad, P.A., Shih, W.J., Humphries, L., DeLand, F.H. and Digenis, G.A., Radionuclide gastric emptying studies in patients with anorexia nervosa, *J Nucl Med* 28, 816–9, 1987.

37. Shih, W.J., Humphries, L., Digenis, G.A., Castellanos, F.X., Domstad, P.A. and DeLand, F.H., Tc-99m labeled triethelene tetraamine polysterene resin gastric emptying studies in bulimia patients, *Eur J Nucl Med* 13, 192–6, 1987.
38. Stacher, G., Bergmann, H., Wiesnagrotzki, S., Steiner-Mittelbach, G., Kiss, A., Abatzi, T-A., Primary anorexia nervosa: gastric emptying and antral motor activity in 53 patients, *Int J Eat Disord* 11, 163–172, 1992.
39. Hutson, W.R. and Wald, A., Gastric emptying in patients with bulimia nervosa and anorexia nervosa, *Am J Gastroent* 85, 41–6, 1990.
40. Kamal, N., Chami, T., and ersen, A., Rosell, F.A., Schuster, M.M. and Whitehead, W.E., Delayed gastrointestinal transit times in anorexia nervosa and bulimia nervosa, *Gastroenterology* 101, 1320–4, 1991.
41. Koch, K.L., Bingaman, S., Tan, L. and Stern, R.M., Visceral perceptions and gastric myoelectrical activity in healthy women and in patients with bulimia nervosa, *Neurogastroenterol Motil* 10, 3–10, 1998.
42. Russell, G.F., Acute dilatation of the stomach in a patient with anorexia nervosa, *Br J Psychiat* 112, 203–7, 1966.
43. Hill, K.K., Hill, D.B., Humphries, L.L., Maloney, M.J. and McClain, C.J., A role for Helicobacter pylori in the gastrointestinal complaints of ED patients?, *Int J Eat Disord* 25, 109–12, 1999.
44. Haller, J.O., Slovis, T.L., Baker, D.H., Berdon, W.E. and Silverman, J.A., Anorexia nervosa — the paucity of radiologic findings in more than fifty patients, *Pediatr Radiol* 5, 145–7, 1977.
45. Hirakawa, M., Okada, T., Iida, M., Tamai, H., Kobayashi, N., Nakagawa, T. and Fujishima, M., Small bowel transit time measured by hydrogen breath test in patients with anorexia nervosa, *Dig Dis Sci* 35, 733–6, 1990.
46. Cox, K.L., Cannon, R.A., Ament, M.E., Phillips, H.E. and Schaffer, C.B., Biochemical and ultrasonic abnormalities of the pancreas in anorexia nervosa, *Dig Dis Sci* 28, 225–9, 1983.
47. Stheneur, C., Rey, C., Pariente, D. and Alvin, P., Acute gastric dilatation with superior mesenteric artery syndrome in a young girl with anorexia nervosa, *Arch Pediatr* 2, 973–6, 1995.
48. Furuta, S., Ozawa, Y., Maejima, K., Tashiro, H., Kitahora, T., Hasegawa, K., Kuroda, S. and Ikuta, N., Anorexia nervosa with severe liver dysfunction and subsequent critical complications, *Intern Med* 38, 575–9, 1999.
49. De Caprio, C., Pasanisi, F. and Contaldo, F., Gastrointestinal complications in a patient with eating disorders, *Eat Weight Disord* 5, 228–30, 2000.
50. Brown, N.W., Treasure, J.L. and Campbell, I.C., Evidence for long-term pancreatic damage caused by laxative abuse in subjects recovered from anorexia nervosa, *Int J Eat Disord* 29, 236–8, 2001.
51. Gwirtsman, H.E., Prager, J. and Henkin, R., Case report of anorexia nervosa associated with Wilson's disease, *Int J Eat Disord* 13, 241–4, 1993.
52. Boos, K., Hextall, A., Cardozo, L., Toozs-Hobson, P., and Anders, K. and Treasure, J., Lower urinary tract symptoms and their impact on women with anorexia nervosa, *Br J Obstet Gynaecol* 106, 501–4, 1999.
53. Silber, T.J. and Kass, E.J., Anorexia nervosa and nephrolithiasis, *J Adolesc Health Care* 5, 50–2, 1984.
54. Pines, A., Kaplinsky, N., Olchovsky, D., Frankl, O., Goldfarb, D. and Iaina, A., Anorexia nervosa, laxative abuse, hypopotassemia and distal renal tubular acidosis, *Isr J Med Sci* 21, 50–2, 1985.

55. Adam, O. and Goebel, F.D., Secondary gout and pseudo-Bartter syndrome in females with laxative abuse, *Klin Wochenschr* 65, 833–9, 1987.
56. Copeland, P.M., Renal failure associated with laxative abuse, *Psychother Psychosom* 62, 200–2, 1994.
57. Abe, K., Mezaki, T., Hirono, N., Udaka, F. and Kameyama, M., A case of anorexia nervosa with acute renal failure resulting from rhabdomyolysis, *Acta Neurol Scand* 81, 82–3, 1990.
58. Wada, S., Nagase, T., Koike, Y., Kugai, N. and Nagata, N., A case of anorexia nervosa with acute renal failure induced by rhabdomyolysis: Possible involvement of hypophosphatemia or phosphate depletion, *Intern Med* 31, 478–82, 1992.
59. Tsuchiya, K., Nakauchi, M., Hondo, I. and Nihei, H., [Nephropathy associated with electrolyte disorders], *Nippon Rinsho* 53, 1995–2000, 1995.
60. Komori, K., Arai, H., Gotoh, T., Imazu, T., Honda, M. and Fujioka, H., [A case of ammonium urate urinary stones with anorexia nervosa], *Hinyokika Kiyo* 46, 627–9, 2000.
61. Alexandridis, G., Liamis, G. and Elisaf, M., Reversible tubular dysfunction that mimicked Fanconi's syndrome in a patient with anorexia nervosa, *Int J Eat Disord* 30, 227–30, 2001.
62. Sheinin, J.C., Medical aspects of eating disorders, *Adolesc Psychiat* 13, 405–21, 1986.
63. Hall, R.C. and Beresford, T.P., Medical complications of anorexia and bulimia, *Psychiat Med* 7, 165–92, 1989.
64. Ishikawa, S., Kato, M., Tokuda, T., Momoi, H., Sekijima, Y., Higuchi, M. and Yanagisawa, N., Licorice-induced hypokalemic myopathy and hypokalemic renal tubular damage in anorexia nervosa, *Int J Eat Disord* 26, 111–4, 1999.
65. Silverman, J.A., Clinical and medical aspects of anorexia nervosa, *Int J Eat Disord* 2, 159, 1983.
66. Kiriike, N., Iketani, T., Nakanishi, S., Nagata, T., Inoue, K., Okuno, M., Ochi, H. and Kawakita, Y., Reduced bone density and major hormones regulating calcium metabolism in anorexia nervosa, *Acta Psychiat Scand* 86, 358–63, 1992.
67. Carmichael, K.A. and Carmichael, D.H., Bone metabolism and osteopenia in eating disorders, *Medicine (Baltimore)* 74, 254–67, 1995.
68. van Marken Lichtenbelt, W.D., Heidendal, G.A. and Westerterp, K.R., Energy expenditure and physical activity in relation to bone mineral density in women with anorexia nervosa, *Eur J Clin Nutr* 51, 826–30, 1997.
69. Ward, A., Brown, N. and Treasure, J., Persistent osteopenia after recovery from anorexia nervosa, *Int J Eat Disord* 22, 71–5, 1997.
70. Castro, J., Lazaro, L., Pons, F., Halperin, I. and Toro, J., Predictors of bone mineral density reduction in adolescents with anorexia nervosa, *J Am Acad Child Adolesc Psychiat* 39, 1365–70, 2000.
71. Carruth, B.R. and Skinner, J.D., Bone mineral status in adolescent girls: effects of eating disorders and exercise, *J Adolesc Health* 26, 322–9, 2000.
72. Andersen, A.E., Watson, T. and Schlechte, J., Osteoporosis and osteopenia in men with eating disorders, *Lancet* 355, 1967–8, 2000.
73. Seeman, E., Karlsson, M.K. and Duan, Y., On exposure to anorexia nervosa, the temporal variation in axial and appendicular skeletal development predisposes to site-specific deficits in bone size and density: A cross-sectional study, *J Bone Miner Res* 15, 2259–65, 2000.
74. Grinspoon, S., Thomas, E., Pitts, S., Gross, E., Mickley, D., Miller, K., Herzog, D. and Klibanski, A., Prevalence and predictive factors for regional osteopenia in women with anorexia nervosa, *Ann Intern Med* 133, 790–4, 2000.

75. Wong, J.C., Lewindon, P., Mortimer, R. and Shepherd, R., Bone mineral density in adolescent females with recently diagnosed anorexia nervosa, *Int J Eat Disord* 29, 11–6, 2001.

76. Zipfel, S., Seibel, M.J., Lowe, B., Beumont, P.J., Kasperk, C. and Herzog, W., Osteoporosis in eating disorders: A follow-up study of patients with anorexia and bulimia nervosa, *J Clin Endocrinol Metab* 86, 5227–33, 2001.

77. Turner, J.M., Bulsara, M.K., McDermott, B.M., Byrne, G.C., Prince, R.L. and Forbes, D.A., Predictors of low bone density in young adolescent females with anorexia nervosa and other dieting disorders, *Int J Eat Disord* 30, 245–51, 2001.

78. Jagielska, G., Wolanczyk, T., Komender, J., Tomaszewicz-Libudzic, C., Przedlacki, J. and Ostrowski, K., Bone mineral density in adolescent girls with anorexia nervosa — a cross-sectional study, *Eur Child Adolesc Psychiat* 11, 57–62, 2002.

79. Castro, J., Toro, J., Lazaro, L., Pons, F. and Halperin, I., Bone mineral density in male adolescents with anorexia nervosa, *J Am Acad Child Adolesc Psychiat* 41, 613–8, 2002.

80. Oliveri, B., Gomez Acotto, C. and Mautalen, C., Osteomalacia in a patient with severe anorexia nervosa, *Rev Rhum Engl Ed* 66, 505–8, 1999.

81. Jagielska, G., [Osteoporosis in anorexia nervosa: a literature review], *Psychiat Pol* 33, 887–96, 1999.

82. Lucas, A.R., Melton, L.J., 3rd, Crowson, C.S. and O'Fallon, W.M., Long-term fracture risk among women with anorexia nervosa: A population-based cohort study, *Mayo Clin Proc* 74, 972–7, 1999.

83. Hartman, D., Crisp, A., Rooney, B., Rackow, C., Atkinson, R. and Patel, S., Bone density of women who have recovered from anorexia nervosa, *Int J Eat Disord* 28, 107–12, 2000.

84. Newton, J.R., Freeman, C.P., Hannan, W.J. and Cowen, S., Osteoporosis and normal weight bulimia nervosa — which patients are at risk?, *J Psychosom Res* 37, 239–47, 1993.

85. Sundgot-Borgen, J., Bahr, R., Falch, J.A. and Schneider, L.S., Normal bone mass in bulimic women, *J Clin Endocrinol Metab* 83, 3144–9, 1998.

86. Goebel, G., Schweiger, U., Kruger, R. and Fichter, M.M., Predictors of bone mineral density in patients with eating disorders, *Int J Eat Disord* 25, 143–50, 1999.

87. Karlsson, M.K., Weigall, S.J., Duan, Y. and Seeman, E., Bone size and volumetric density in women with anorexia nervosa receiving estrogen replacement therapy and in women recovered from anorexia nervosa, *J Clin Endocrinol Metab* 85, 3177–82, 2000.

88. Bruni, V., Dei, M., Vicini, I., Beninato, L. and Magnani, L., Estrogen replacement therapy in the management of osteopenia related to eating disorders, *Ann N Y Acad Sci* 900, 416–21, 2000.

89. Munoz, M.T., Morande, G., Garcia-Centenera, J.A., Hervas, F., Pozo, J. and Argente, J., The effects of estrogen administration on bone mineral density in adolescents with anorexia nervosa, *Eur J Endocrinol* 146, 45–50, 2002.

90. Caillot-Augusseau, A., Lafage-Proust, M.H., Margaillan, P., Vergely, N., Faure, S., Paillet, S., Lang, F., Alexandre, C. and Estour, B., Weight gain reverses bone turnover and restores circadian variation of bone resorption in anorexic patients, *Clin Endocrinol (Oxf)* 52, 113–21, 2000.

91. Valla, A., Groenning, I.L., Syversen, U. and Hoeiseth, A., Anorexia nervosa: Slow regain of bone mass, *Osteoporos Int* 11, 141–5, 2000.

92. Nishizawa, K., Iijima, M., Tokita, A. and Yamashiro, Y., [Bone mineral density of eating disorder], *Nippon Rinsho* 59, 554–60, 2001.

93. Castro, J., Lazaro, L., Pons, F., Halperin, I. and Toro, J., Adolescent anorexia nervosa: the catch-up effect in bone mineral density after recovery, *J Am Acad Child Adolesc Psychiat* 40, 1215–21, 2001.

94. Heer, M., Mika, C., Grzella, I., Drummer, C. and Herpertz-Dahlmann, B., Changes in bone turnover in patients with anorexia nervosa during eleven weeks of inpatient dietary treatment, *Clin Chem* 48, 754–60, 2002.

95. Amano, K., Sakamoto, T., Hada, Y., Hasegawa, I., Takahashi, T., Suzuki, J. and Takahashi, H., [Association of anorexia nervosa and mitral valve prolapse], *J Cardiogr Suppl*, 141–7, 1986.

96. Moodie D.S., Anorexia and the heart. Results of studies to assess effects, *Postgrad Med* 81, 46–8, 51–2, 55 passim., 1987.

97. Lupoglazoff, J.M., Berkane, N., Denjoy, I., Maillard, G., Leheuzey, M.F., Mouren-Simeoni, M.C. and Casasoprana, A., [Cardiac consequences of adolescent anorexia nervosa], *Arch Mal Coeur Vaiss* 94, 494–8, 2001.

98. Biadi, O., Rossini, R., Musumeci, G., Frediani, L., Masullo, M., Ramacciotti, C.E., Dellosso, L., Paoli, R., Mariotti, R., Cassano, G.B. and Mariani, M., Cardiopulmonary exercise test in young women affected by anorexia nervosa, *Ital Heart J* 2, 462–7, 2001.

99. Kaysar, N., Kronenberg, J., Polliack, M. and Gaoni, B., Severe hypophosphataemia during binge eating in anorexia nervosa, *Arch Dis Child* 66, 138–9, 1991.

100. Winston, D., Treatment of severe malnutrition in anorexia nervosa with enteral tube feedings, *Nutr Supp Serv* 7, 24, 1987.

101. Schocken, D.D., Holloway, J.D. and Powers, P.S., Weight loss and the heart. Effects of anorexia nervosa and starvation, *Arch Intern Med* 149, 877–81, 1989.

102. Sanchez-Muniz, F.J., Marcos, A. and Varela, P., Serum lipids and apolipoprotein B values, blood pressure and pulse rate in anorexia nervosa, *Eur J Clin Nutr* 45, 33–6, 1991.

103. Sullivan, P.F., Gendall, K.A., Bulik, C.M., Carter, F.A. and Joyce, P.R., Elevated total cholesterol in bulimia nervosa, *Int J Eat Disord* 23, 425–32, 1998.

104. Feillet, F., Feillet-Coudray, C., Bard, J.M., Parra, H.J., Favre, E., Kabuth, B., Fruchart, J.C. and Vidailhet, M., Plasma cholesterol and endogenous cholesterol synthesis during refeeding in anorexia nervosa, *Clin Chim Acta* 294, 45–56, 2000.

105. Cravetto, C.A., Nejrotti, M. and Curtaz, G., [Hematological findings and blood coagulation tests in anorexia nervosa], *Arch Sci Med (Torino)* 134, 205–9, 1977.

106. Larrain, C., Ampuero, R. and Pumarino, H., [Hematologic changes in anorexia nervosa], *Rev Med Chil* 117, 534–43, 1989.

107. Bailly, D., Lambin, I., Garzon, G. and Parquet, P.J., Bone marrow hypoplasia in anorexia nervosa: A case report, *Int J Eat Disord* 16, 97–100, 1994.

108. Orlandi, E., Boselli, P., Covezzi, R., Bonaccorsi, G. and Guaraldi, G.P., Reversal of bone marrow hypoplasia in anorexia nervosa: A case report, *Int J Eat Disord* 27, 480–2, 2000.

109. Kaiser, U. and Barth, N., Haemolytic anaemia in a patient with anorexia nervosa, *Acta Haematol* 106, 133–5, 2001.

110. Gendall, K.A., Bulik, C.M. and Joyce, P.R., Visceral protein and hematological status of women with bulimia nervosa and depressed controls, *Physiol Behav* 66, 159–63, 1999.

111. Nova, E., Samartin, S., Gomez, S., Morande, G. and Marcos, A., The adaptive response of the immune system to the particular malnutrition of eating disorders, *Eur J Clin Nutr* 56, S34–7, 2002.

112. Marcos, A., Varela, P., Toro, O., Lopez-Vidriero, I., Nova, E., Madruga, D., Casas, J. and Morande, G., Interactions between nutrition and immunity in anorexia nervosa: a 1-y follow-up study, *Am J Clin Nutr* 66, 485S–490S, 1997.
113. Mustafa, A., Ward, A., Treasure, J. and Peakman, M., T lymphocyte subpopulations in anorexia nervosa and refeeding, *Clin Immunol Immunopathol* 82, 282–9, 1997.
114. Marcos, A., Varela, P., Santacruz, I., Munoz-Velez, A. and Morande, G., Nutritional status and immunocompetence in eating disorders. A comparative study, *Eur J Clin Nutr* 47, 787–93, 1993.
115. Marcos, A., Varela, P., Toro, O., Nova, E., Lopez-Vidriero, I. and Morande, G., Evaluation of nutritional status by immunologic assessment in bulimia nervosa: influence of body mass index and vomiting episodes, *Am J Clin Nutr* 66, 491S–497S, 1997.
116. Marcos, A., Varela, P., Santacruz, I. and Munoz-Velez, A., Evaluation of immuno-competence and nutritional status in patients with bulimia nervosa, *Am J Clin Nutr* 57, 65–9, 1993.
117. Staurenghi, A.H., Masera, R.G., Prolo, P., Griot, G., Sartori, M.L., Ravizza, L. and Angeli, A., Hypothalamic-pituitary-adrenal axis function, psychopathological traits and natural killer (NK) cell activity in anorexia nervosa, *Psychoneuroendocrinology* 22, 575–90, 1997.
118. Limone, P., Biglino, A., Bottino, F., Forno, B., Calvelli, P., Fassino, S., Berardi, C., Ajmone-Catt, P., Bertagna, A., Tarocco, R.P., Rovera, G.G. and Molinatti, G.M., Evidence for a positive correlation between serum cortisol levels and IL-1beta production by peripheral mononuclear cells in anorexia nervosa, *J Endocrinol Invest* 23, 422–7, 2000.
119. Nova, E., Gomez-Martinez, S., Morande, G. and Marcos, A., Cytokine production by blood mononuclear cells from in-patients with anorexia nervosa, *Br J Nutr* 88, 183–8, 2002.
120. Nagata, T., Tobitani, W., Kiriike, N., Iketani, T. and Yamagami, S., Capacity to produce cytokines during weight restoration in patients with anorexia nervosa, *Psychosom Med* 61, 371–7, 1999.
121. Pomeroy, C., Eckert, E., Hu, S., Eiken, B., Mentink, M., Crosby, R.D. and Chao, C.C., Role of interleukin-6 and transforming growth factor-beta in anorexia nervosa, *Biol Psychiat* 36, 836–9, 1994.
122. Monteleone, P., Luisi, M., Colurcio, B., Casarosa, E., Ioime, R., Genazzani, A.R. and Maj, M., Plasma levels of neuroactive steroids are increased in untreated women with anorexia nervosa or bulimia nervosa, *Psychosom Med* 63, 62–8, 2001.
123. Licinio, J., Wong, M.L. and Gold, P.W., The hypothalamic-pituitary-adrenal axis in anorexia nervosa, *Psychiat Res* 62, 75–83, 1996.
124. Berger, M., Pirke, K.M., Doerr, P., Krieg, C. and von Zerssen, D., Influence of weight loss on the dexamethasone suppression test, *Arch Gen Psychiat* 40, 585–6, 1983.
125. Gwirtsman, H.E., Kaye, W.H., George, D.T., Jimerson, D.C., Ebert, M.H. and Gold, P.W., Central and peripheral ACTH and cortisol levels in anorexia nervosa and bulimia, *Arch Gen Psychiat* 46, 61–9, 1989.
126. Stoving, R.K., Hangaard, J., Hansen-Nord, M. and Hagen, C., A review of endocrine changes in anorexia nervosa, *J Psychiat Res* 33, 139–52, 1999.
127. Katz, J.L., Weiner, H., Kream, J. and Zumoff, B., Cushing's disease in a young woman with anorexia nervosa: Pathophysiological implications, *Can J Psychiat* 31, 861–4, 1986.

128. Gniuli, D., Liverani, E., Capristo, E., Greco, A.V. and Mingrone, G., Blunted glucose metabolism in anorexia nervosa, *Metabolism* 50, 876–81, 2001.

129. Cuntz, U., Frank, G., Lehnert, P. and Fichter, M., Interrelationships between the size of the pancreas and the weight of patients with eating disorders, *Int J Eat Disord* 27, 297–303, 2000.

130. Nozaki, T., Tamai, H., Matsubayashi, S., Komaki, G., Kobayashi, N. and Nakagawa, T., Insulin response to intravenous glucose in patients with anorexia nervosa showing low insulin response to oral glucose, *J Clin Endocrinol Metab* 79, 217–22, 1994.

131. Gianotti, L., Broglio, F., Ramunni, J., Lanfranco, F., Gauna, C., Benso, A., Zanello, M., Arvat, E. and Ghigo, E., The activity of GH/IGF-1 axis in anorexia nervosa and in obesity: a comparison with normal subjects and patients with hypopituitarism or critical illness, *Eat Weight Disord* 3, 64–70, 1998.

132. Gianotti, L., Broglio, F., Aimaretti, G., Arvat, E., Colombo, S., Di Summa, M., Gallioli, G., Pittoni, G., Sardo, E., Stella, M., Zanello, M., Miola, C. and Ghigo, E., Low IGF-1 levels are often uncoupled with elevated GH levels in catabolic conditions, *J Endocrinol Invest* 21, 115–21, 1998.

133. Hotta, M., Fukuda, I., Sato, K., Hizuka, N., Shibasaki, T. and Takano, K., The relationship between bone turnover and body weight, serum insulin-like growth factor (IGF) I and serum IGF-binding protein levels in patients with anorexia nervosa, *J Clin Endocrinol Metab* 85, 200–6, 2000.

134. Monteleone, P., Fabrazzo, M., Tortorella, A., Fuschino, A. and Maj, M., Opposite modifications in circulating leptin and soluble leptin receptor across the eating disorder spectrum, *Mol Psychiat* 7, 641–6, 2002.

135. Monteleone, P., Di Lieto, A., Tortorella, A., Longobardi, N. and Maj, M., Circulating leptin in patients with anorexia nervosa, bulimia nervosa or binge-eating disorder: Relationship to body weight, eating patterns, psychopathology and endocrine changes, *Psychiat Res* 94, 121–9, 2000.

136. Svobodova, J., Haluzik, M., Papezova, H., Rosicka, M., Nedvidkova, J., Kotrlikova, E. and Kabrt, J., [The effect of partial refeeding on serum levels of leptin and resting energy expenditure in female patients with anorexia nervosa], *Cas Lek Cesk* 138, 748–52, 1999.

137. Pauly, R.P., Lear, S.A., Hastings, F.C. and Birmingham, C.L., Resting energy expenditure and plasma leptin levels in anorexia nervosa during acute refeeding, *Int J Eat Disord* 28, 231–4, 2000.

138. Polito, A., Fabbri, A., Ferro-Luzzi, A., Cuzzolaro, M., Censi, L., Ciarapica, D., Fabbrini, E. and Giannini, D., Basal metabolic rate in anorexia nervosa: Relation to body composition and leptin concentrations, *Am J Clin Nutr* 71, 1495–502, 2000.

139. Ferron, F., Considine, R.V., Peino, R., Lado, I.G., Dieguez, C. and Casanueva, F.F., Serum leptin concentrations in patients with anorexia nervosa, bulimia nervosa and non-specific eating disorders correlate with the body mass index but are independent of the respective disease, *Clin Endocrinol* (Oxford) 46, 289–93, 1997.

140. Nakai, Y., Hamagaki, S., Kato, S., Seino, Y., Takagi, R. and Kurimoto, F., Leptin in women with eating disorders, *Metabolism* 48, 217–20, 1999.

141. Eckert, E.D., Pomeroy, C., Raymond, N., Kohler, P.F., Thuras, P. and Bowers, C.Y., Leptin in anorexia nervosa, *J Clin Endocrinol Metab* 83, 791–5, 1998.

142. Di Carlo, C., Tommaselli, G.A., De Filippo, E., Pisano, G., Nasti, A., Bifulco, G., Contaldo, F. and Nappi, C., Menstrual status and serum leptin levels in anorectic and in menstruating women with low body mass indexes, *Fertil Steril* 78, 376–82, 2002.

143. Schulze, U.M., Pettke-Rank, C.V., Kreienkamp, M., Hamm, H., Brocker, E.B., Wewetzer, C., Trott, G.E. and Warnke, A., Dermatologic findings in anorexia and bulimia nervosa of childhood and adolescence, *Pediatr Dermatol* 16, 90–4, 1999.

144. Strumia, R., Varotti, E., Manzato, E. and Gualandi, M., Skin signs in anorexia nervosa, *Dermatology* 203, 314–7, 2001.

145. Hediger, C., Rost, B. and Itin, P., Cutaneous manifestations in anorexia nervosa, *Schweiz Med Wochenschr* 130, 565–75, 2000.

146. Tyler, I., Wiseman, M.C., Crawford, R.I. and Laird Birmingham, C., Cutaneous manifestations of eating disorders, *J Cutan Med Surg* 6, 345–53, 2002.

147. Taniguchi, S., Yamamoto, N., Kono, T. and Hamada, T., Generalized pruritus in anorexia nervosa, *Br J Dermatol* 134, 510–1, 1996.

148. Marshman, G.M., Hanna, M.J., Ben-Tovim, D.I. and Walker, M.K., Cutaneous abnormalities in anorexia nervosa, *Australas J Dermatol* 31, 9–12, 1990.

149. Morgan, J.F. and Lacey, J.H., Scratching and fasting: A study of pruritus and anorexia nervosa, *Br J Dermatol* 140, 453–6, 1999.

150. Evers, C.L., Dietary intake and symptoms of anorexia nervosa in female university dancers, *J Am Diet Assoc* 87, 66–8, 1987.

151. van der Ster Wallin, G., Norring, C., Lennernas, M.A. and Holmgren, S., Food selection in anorectics and bulimics: food items, nutrient content and nutrient density, *J Am Coll Nutr* 14, 271–7, 1995.

152. Gendall, K.A., Sullivan, P.E., Joyce, P.R., Carter, F.A. and Bulik, C.M., The nutrient intake of women with bulimia nervosa, *Int J Eat Disord* 21, 115–27, 1997.

153. Dempsey, D.T., Crosby, L.O., Pertschuk, M.J., Feurer, I.D., Buzby, G.P. and Mullen, J.L., Weight gain and nutritional efficacy in anorexia nervosa, *Am J Clin Nutr* 39, 236–42, 1984.

154. Walker, J., Roberts, S.L., Halmi, K.A. and Goldberg, S.C., Caloric requirements for weight gain in anorexia nervosa, *Am J Clin Nutr* 32, 1396–1400, 1979.

155. Kaye, W.H., Weltzin, T.E., McKee, M., McConaha, C., Hansen, D. and Hsu, L.K., Laboratory assessment of feeding behavior in bulimia nervosa and healthy women: Methods for developing a human-feeding laboratory, *Am J Clin Nutr* 55, 372–80, 1992.

156. Hsu, L.K., Rand, W., Sullivan, S., Liu, D.W., Mulliken, B., McDonagh, B. and Kaye, W.H., Cognitive therapy, nutritional therapy and their combination in the treatment of bulimia nervosa, *Psychol Med* 31, 871–9, 2001.

157. Unknown, www.anred.com, Anorexia Nervosa and Related Eating Disorders, Inc, 2002.

158. Yager, J., Practice guidelines for the treatment of patients with eating disorders (revision). *Am J Psychiat* 157, 1–39, 2000.

159. Bulik, C.M., Sullivan, P.F., Fear, J. and Pickering, A., Predictors of the development of bulimia nervosa in women with anorexia nervosa, *J Nerv Ment Dis* 185, 704–7, 1997.

160. Fisher, M., Simpser, E. and Schneider, M., Hypophosphatemia secondary to oral refeeding in anorexia nervosa, *Int J Eat Disord* 28, 181–7, 2000.

161. Adson, D.E., Mitchell, J.E. and Trenkner, S.W., The superior mesenteric artery syndrome and acute gastric dilatation in eating disorders: A report of two cases and a review of the literature, *Int J Eat Disord* 21, 103–14, 1997.

162. Robb, A.S., Silber, T.J., Orrell-Valente, J.K., Valadez-Meltzer, A., Ellis, N., Dadson, M.J. and Chatoor, I., Supplemental nocturnal nasogastric refeeding for better short-term outcome in hospitalized adolescent girls with anorexia nervosa, *Am J Psychiat* 159, 1347–53, 2002.

163. Solanto, M.V., Jacobson, M.S., Heller, L., Golden, N.H. and Hertz, S., Rate of weight gain of inpatients with anorexia nervosa under two behavioral contracts, *Pediatrics* 93, 989–91, 1994.

164. Foppiani, L., Luise, L., Rasore, E., Menichini, U. and Giusti, M., Frequency of recovery from anorexia nervosa of a cohort patients reevaluated on a long-term basis following intensive care, *Eat Weight Disord* 3, 90–4, 1998.

165. Baran, S.A., Weltzin, T.E. and Kaye, W.H., Low discharge weight and outcome in anorexia nervosa, *Am J Psychiat* 152, 1070–2, 1995.

166. Martinez-Olmos, M.A., Gomez-Candela, C., de Cos, A.I., Gonzalez-Fernandez, B., Iglesias, C., Hillman, N. and Castillo, R., [Results of nutritional treatment of anorexia nervosa: our experience (1989–1995)], *Nutr Hosp* 12, 160–6, 1997.

167. Bergh, C., Brodin, U., Lindberg, G. and Sodersten, P., Randomized controlled trial of a treatment for anorexia and bulimia nervosa, *Proc Natl Acad Sci USA* 99, 486–91, 2002.

168. Schebendach, J., Golden, N.H., Jacobson, M.S., Arden, M., Pettei, M., Hardoff, D., Bauman, N., Reichert, P., Copperman, N., Hertz, S. et al. Indirect calorimetry in the nutritional management of eating disorders, *Int J Eat Disord* 17, 59–66, 1995.

169. Leonard, T., Foulon, C., Samuel-Lajeunesse, B., Melchior, J.C., Rigaud, D. and Apfelbaum, M., High resting energy expenditure in normal-weight bulimics and its normalization with control of eating behaviour, *Appetite* 27, 223–33, 1996.

170. Russell, J., Baur, L.A., Beumont, P.J., Byrnes, S., Gross, G., Touyz, S., Abraham, S. and Zipfel, S., Altered energy metabolism in anorexia nervosa, *Psychoneuroendocrinology* 26, 51–63, 2001.

171. Scalfi, L., Marra, M., De Filippo, E., Caso, G., Pasanisi, F. and Contaldo, F., The prediction of basal metabolic rate in female patients with anorexia nervosa, *Int J Obes Relat Metab Disord* 25, 359–64, 2001.

172. Marra, M., Polito, A., De Filippo, E., Cuzzolaro, M., Ciarapica, D., Contaldo, F. and Scalfi, L., Are the general equations to predict BMR applicable to patients with anorexia nervosa? *Eat Weight Disord* 7, 53–9, 2002.

173. de Zwaan, M., Aslam, Z. and Mitchell, J.E., Research on energy expenditure in individuals with eating disorders: A review, *Int J Eat Disord* 32, 127–34, 2002.

174. Kotler, L.A., Devlin, M.J., Matthews, D.E. and Walsh, B.T., Total energy expenditure as measured by doubly labeled water in outpatients with bulimia nervosa, *Int J Eat Disord* 29, 470–6, 2001.

175. Pagliato, E., Corradi, E., Gentile, M.G. and Testolin, G., Changes in body composition and resting energy expenditure in anorectic patients after a weight gain of fifteen percent, *Ann N Y Acad Sci* 904, 617–20, 2000.

176. Rigaud, D., Hassid, J., Meulemans, A., Poupard, A.T. and Boulier, A., A paradoxical increase in resting energy expenditure in malnourished patients near death: The king penguin syndrome, *Am J Clin Nutr* 72, 355–60, 2000.

177. Van Binsbergen, C.J., Odink, J., Van den Berg, H., Koppeschaar, H. and Coelingh Bennink, H.J., Nutritional status in anorexia nervosa: Clinical chemistry, vitamins, iron and zinc, *Eur J Clin Nutr* 42, 929–37, 1988.

178. Mira, M., Stewart, P.M. and Abraham, S.F., Vitamin and trace element status of women with disordered eating, *Am J Clin Nutr* 50, 940–4, 1989.

179. Langan, S.M. and Farrell, P.M., Vitamin E, vitamin A and essential fatty acid status of patients hospitalized for anorexia nervosa, *Am J Clin Nutr* 41, 1054–60, 1985.

180. Vaisman, N., Wolfhart, D. and Sklan, D., Vitamin A metabolism in plasma of normal and anorectic women, *Eur J Clin Nutr* 46, 873–8, 1992.

181. Rock, C.L. and Vasantharajan, S., Vitamin status of ED patients: Relationship to clinical indices and effect of treatment, *Int J Eat Disord* 18, 257–62, 1995.

182. Moyano, D., Sierra, C., Brandi, N., Artuch, R., Mira, A., Garcia-Tornel, S. and Vilaseca, M.A., Antioxidant status in anorexia nervosa, *Int J Eat Disord* 25, 99–103, 1999.

183. Rock, C., Hunt, I., Swendseid, M.E. and Yager, J., Nutritional status and bone mineral density in patients with eating disorders, *Am J Clin Nutr* 46, 527, 1987.

184. Capo-chichi, C.D., Gueant, J.L., Lefebvre, E., Bennani, N., Lorentz, E., Vidailhet, C. and Vidailhet, M., Riboflavin and riboflavin-derived cofactors in adolescent girls with anorexia nervosa, *Am J Clin Nutr* 69, 672–8, 1999.

185. Hadigan, C.M., Anderson, E.J., Miller, K.K., Hubbard, J.L., Herzog, D.B., Klibanski, A. and Grinspoon, S.K., Assessment of macronutrient and micronutrient intake in women with anorexia nervosa, *Int J Eat Disord* 28, 284–92, 2000.

186. McClain, C.J., Stuart, M.A., Vivian, B., McClain, M., Talwalker, R., Snelling, L. and Humphries, L., Zinc status before and after zinc supplementation of ED patients, *J Am Coll Nutr* 11, 694–700, 1992.

187. Birmingham, C.L., Goldner, E.M. and Bakan, R., Controlled trial of zinc supplementation in anorexia nervosa, *Int J Eat Disord* 15, 251–5, 1994.

188. Su, J.C. and Birmingham, C.L., Zinc supplementation in the treatment of anorexia nervosa, *Eat Weight Disord* 7, 20–2, 2002.

189. Hill, K., Bucuvalas, J., McClain, C., Kryscio, R., Martini, R.T., Alfaro, M.P. and Maloney, M., Pilot study of growth hormone administration during the refeeding of malnourished anorexia nervosa patients, *J Child Adolesc Psychopharmacol* 10, 3–8, 2000.

190. Brambilla, F., Draisci, A., Peirone, A. and Brunetta, M., Combined cognitive-behavioral, psychopharmacological and nutritional therapy in eating disorders. 2. Anorexia nervosa — binge-eating/purging type, *Neuropsychobiology* 32, 64–7, 1995.

191. Brambilla, F., Draisci, A., Peirone, A. and Brunetta, M., Combined cognitive-behavioral, psychopharmacological and nutritional therapy in eating disorders. 1. Anorexia nervosa — restricted type, *Neuropsychobiology* 32, 59–63, 1995.

192. Casper, R.C., Kirschner, B., Sandstead, H.H., Jacob, R.A. and Davis, J.M., An evaluation of trace metals, vitamins and taste function in anorexia nervosa, *Am J Clin Nutr* 33, 1801–8, 1980.

193. Humphries, L., Vivian, B., Stuart, M. and McClain, C.J., Zinc deficiency and eating disorders, *J Clin Psychiat* 50, 456–9, 1989.

194. Varela, P., Marcos, A. and Navarro, M.P., Zinc status in anorexia nervosa, *Ann Nutr Metab* 36, 197–202, 1992.

195. Lask, B., Fosson, A., Rolfe, U. and Thomas, S., Zinc deficiency and childhood-onset anorexia nervosa, *J Clin Psychiat* 54, 63–6, 1993.

196. Winston, A.P., Jamieson, C.P., Madira, W., Gatward, N.M. and Palmer, R.L., Prevalence of thiamin deficiency in anorexia nervosa, *Int J Eat Disord* 28, 451–4, 2000.

197. Patchell, R.A., Fellows, H.A. and Humphries, L.L., Neurologic complications of anorexia nervosa, *Acta Neurol Scand* 89, 111–6, 1994.

198. Niiya, K., Kitagawa, T., Fujishita, M., Yoshimoto, S., Kobayashi, M., Kubonishi, I., Taguchi, H. and Miyoshi, I., Bulimia nervosa complicated by deficiency of vitamin K-dependent coagulation factors, *JAMA* 250, 792–3, 1983.

11 Nutritional Anemias

*Lisa M. Bodnar, Kelley S. Scanlon
and Mary E. Cogswell*

CONTENTS

0-8493-1337-6/03/$0.00+$1.50
© 2004 by CRC Press LLC

I. INTRODUCTION

Anemia is defined as a hemoglobin concentration or hematocrit lower than the reference cutoff value, traditionally less than the fifth percentile of the distribution of hemoglobin concentration in a reference population of healthy individuals of the same gender and age. Anemia is caused by decreased production of red blood cells (RBC) and hemoglobin, increased destruction of RBC (hemolysis), or excessive blood loss. Iron deficiency plays a major role in the occurrence of anemia, but other nutritional deficiencies, nonnutritional conditions and hereditary disorders also play a role.[1] In this chapter, we focus on nutritional causes of anemia.

Anemia is common throughout the world; the highest occurrences are in developing countries (Table 11.1) and among persons of low socioeconomic status.[2,3] Among adults, anemia disproportionately affects women of childbearing age, especially pregnant and postpartum women, primarily because women are more likely to have iron deficiency. Overall, anemia affects nearly 45% of women from the developing regions of the world and 13% of women from the developed regions.[3] Our focus in this chapter is on the United States. According to the third U.S. National Health and Nutrition Examination Survey (NHANES 1988–1994), 12% of nonpregnant women 15 to 49 years of age and 11% of pregnant women 15 to 49 years of age are anemic (L.M. Bodnar, unpublished 2002). Among low-income U.S. women who attend public assistance programs, 8% are anemic in the first, 12% are anemic in the second and 29% are anemic in the third trimester of pregnancy.[4] Postpartum anemia is also common, affecting approximately 10% of women up to 6 months after delivery.[5] Among low-income U.S. women, 22% are anemic up to 6 months postpartum.[5]

Mild anemia, defined as a hemoglobin concentration 1 to 2 g/dL below the reference threshold, has little clinical consequence. The underlying deficiency or disease is of greater concern and contributes to the more critical clinical

---

TABLE 11.1
Estimated Prevalence (%) Of Anemia In Women (ca. 1988)

	Pregnant	Nonpregnant
World	51	35
Developing countries	56	43
Developed countries	18	12
Africa	52	42
North America	17	10
Latin America	39	30
Asia	60	44
Europe	17	10
Oceania	71	66

Source: The Prevalence of Anemia in Women: A Tabulation of Available Information, 2nd ed. Geneva, Switzerland: World Health Organization, 1992.

manifestations. For example, in vitamin B_{12} deficiency anemia, the neurologic consequences of the vitamin deficiency are far more serious than the associated anemia. However, in severe anemia (hemoglobin less than 7 g/dL) from any cause, definite cardiovascular consequences are related to reduced oxygen delivery to tissues. Clinical pallor (paleness) where capillary beds are visible through skin or mucosa is useful in detecting severe anemia.[6] In extreme cases, very severe anemia (hemoglobin less than 4.0 g/dL) contributes to or directly causes childhood and maternal mortality.[7] In the United States, about 1.1% of childbearing-age women have hemoglobin less than 10 g/dL and 0.03% have hemoglobin less than 7 g/dL (L.M. Bodnar, NHANES III, unpublished 2002).

To properly prevent and treat anemia, determining the underlying cause is critical. If the cause is nutritional, assessment is performed to identify the nutrient or nutrients involved. Nutritional anemias can be caused by a deficiency of any nutrient essential to the production of hemoglobin.[8] Iron deficiency is by far the most common cause of nutritional anemia; folate and vitamin B_{12} deficiencies are the second and third most common causes.

In this chapter we discuss the stages of nutrient deficiency that lead to anemia, the clinical consequences of nutrient deficiency and anemia and the main factors that contribute to the underlying nutrient deficiencies. We also summarize the main parameters used to diagnose iron-, folate- and vitamin B_{12}-deficiency anemia as well as the recommendations for the prevention and treatment of each condition.

II. IRON DEFICIENCY ANEMIA

A. INTRODUCTION

Iron deficiency is the most common nutrient deficiency in the world and the single most common cause of nutritional anemia.[9] In countries where the prevalence of anemia is greater than 20%, the majority of cases are associated with a primary iron deficiency or iron deficiency in combination with other conditions.[10] Because iron deficiency without anemia is usually as common as anemia or more common than anemia, an even greater proportion of women usually have some degree of iron deficiency. Iron deficiency is not restricted to women in developing countries. In the United States, an estimated 11% of women 20 to 49 years of age have iron deficiency.[11] The prevalence is believed to be highest among pregnant women, but national estimates for pregnant women are not available. From 0 to 6 months postpartum, about 12% of women in the United States are iron deficient.[5] Iron deficiency is four times as common among low-income women up to 6 months postpartum (30%) as among their higher-income counterparts (7%).[5] In addition to disparities by socioeconomic status, data from national surveys and special studies suggest that the prevalence of iron deficiency is higher among women who are African American or Hispanic, are high parity, have a history of heavy menses and poor dietary intake and who donate blood more than three times per year.[12]

B. Iron and Anemia

Iron is an essential component of several body compounds. The approximate amount of iron present in the body of an average 55-kg (121-lb) woman is 2300 mg (Table 11.2).[13] Approximately 88% of this iron is found in functional iron compounds. Hemoglobin, the oxygen-carrying pigment of the RBC, is the main functional iron compound and contains approximately 85% of the functional iron in the body. Hemoglobin is made up of iron, protoporphyrin and globin, with iron composing one third the weight. In iron deficiency anemia, the supply of iron is insufficient for normal hemoglobin synthesis. Thus, the production of RBC is reduced and the cells that are produced are microcytic (small) and hypochromic (pale in color). The remaining 15% of functional iron is accounted for by myoglobin, the red iron-containing protein of muscle and the heme and nonheme enzymes.

Of the 12% of body iron not contained in functional compounds, less than 1% is found in transport iron as transferrin and the remainder is found in the storage compounds ferritin and hemosiderin. Iron is primarily stored in the liver, spleen and bone marrow. The stored iron is used for the production of essential iron compounds and for maintaining iron homeostasis by regulating iron absorption from the diet.[13]

The stages of iron deficiency that lead to anemia are summarized in Table 11.3.[14] In general, iron depletion is characterized by reduced iron stores, as reflected primarily by a decrease in the serum concentration of ferritin. Iron absorption increases as a result of a lower body iron content. As the deficiency progresses to iron deficient erythropoiesis (iron deficiency without anemia), the iron stores are exhausted and the production of hemoglobin and other iron compounds is impaired. Although a hemoglobin concentration above the cutoff that defines anemia is maintained, this stage is characterized by decreased transferrin saturation, indicating insufficient iron is being supplied to the bone marrow, and by increased free erythrocyte protoporphyrin concentration, marking the accumulation of protoporphyrin that occurs due to a lack of

TABLE 11.2
Approximate Amount Of Iron In a 55-Kg (121-lb) Woman By Compound

Purpose	Compound	Amount (mg)
Functional	Hemoglobin	1700
	Myoglobin	222
	Heme enzymes	50
	Nonheme enzymes	55
Transport	Transferrin	3
Storage	Ferritin	200
	Hemosiderin	70

Source: From Bothwell, T.H. and Charlton, R.W., Iron Deficiency in Women, A report of the International Nutritional Anemia Consultative Group (INACG), The Nutrition Foundation, Washington, D.C. 1981. With permission.

TABLE 11.3
Stages of Iron Deficiency

Measure	Iron overload	Normal	Iron depletion	Iron deficient erythropoiesis	Iron deficiency anemia
Serum ferritin concentration	elevated	normal	low	low	low
Transferrin saturation (%)	elevated	normal	normal	low	low
Free erythrocyte protoporphyrin concentration	normal	normal	normal	elevated	elevated
Erythrocytes	normal	normal	normal	normal	microcytic/ hypochromic
Mean cell volume	normal	normal	normal	normal	low

Source: From Herbert, V., The 1986 Herman Award Lecture, Nutrition Science as a continually unfolding story: The folate and vitamin B_{12} paradigm, *Amer. J. Clin. Nutr.*, 46, 387, 1987. With permission.

iron to form hemoglobin. In the final stage of iron deficiency, anemia is characterized by a hemoglobin concentration (or hematocrit) below the normal range.[11,15]

C. Consequences Of Iron Deficiency Anemia

The consequences of iron deficiency anemia in women are related to both the deficiency of iron and the anemia. The consequences of greatest concern, summarized here, are the potential effects on mortality, birth outcome, work capacity and cognition.

Very severe anemia (hemoglobin less than 4 g/dL) is associated with increased mortality.[3] Deaths associated with severe anemia generally occur at times of increased physiologic stress, such as during the peripartum period, when oxygen delivery and cardiovascular function are further compromised by worsening hemoglobin concentration.

Large observational studies in the United States have indicated an association between maternal hemoglobin concentration and infant birth weight or preterm delivery.[16] Because of the biases in previous randomized controlled trials that resulted in false-positive findings, at this time it is unknown whether supplementing women with iron, folate, or both increases birth weight and length of gestation.[16] Therefore, the association between anemia and adverse birth outcomes is clear, but the data are inconclusive for determining whether iron deficiency anemia causes these outcomes.

It is well established that iron deficiency anemia reduces work performance in women. In a well-controlled study of Chinese female cotton workers, Li and colleagues[17] reported a dose–response relationship between hemoglobin concentration and aerobic capacity, mirroring results from similar experiments in men.[18] Results from observational studies in women and in mixed groups of men and women support the causal relationship between anemia and impaired aerobic capacity.[18] Furthermore, research has consistently shown that women with iron deficiency anemia perform less voluntary activity and are less productive economically at their jobs than are nonanemic workers.[18] The effect of iron deficiency on work performance or energy expenditure appears to be mediated through a decreased oxygen-carrying capacity from the anemia and impaired muscle function related to the iron deficit. Studies have reported increased productivity and decreased energy expenditure at work when anemic female workers are supplemented with iron.[16,19]

Iron deficiency anemia is associated with altered behavior and impaired intellectual development in infants and children.[20] Less clear are the effects of iron deficiency anemia on adult cognition and behavior, although several studies have indicated a relationship between iron deficiency and aspects of brain functioning in women, including concentration and attention span,[21] verbal learning and memory[22] and intelligence.[23] In adults, iron deficiency is believed to affect cognition through a decreased activity of iron-containing enzymes in the brain[24] that alters neurotransmitter function and cellular oxidative processes.[25]

D. Factors Contributing To Iron Deficiency

The major causes of iron deficiency anemia among women are inadequate iron intake, increased physiologic requirements and excessive blood loss. Anemia caused by these factors occurs more rapidly when iron stores are already inadequate to compensate for increased need. Women of childbearing age are one of the groups at highest risk for anemia because they may not have adequate amounts of iron intake or stores relative to iron needs and losses. Among these women, at highest risk are pregnant women, postpartum women and women with excessive blood loss during menstruation. Among postmenopausal women with iron deficiency, gastrointestinal blood loss is usually the cause.

1. Inadequate Intake

Only about one fourth of childbearing-age women meet the recommended dietary allowance (RDA) for iron — 18 mg a day — through diet alone.[26,27] On average, women consume about 13 mg per day of iron through diet.[26] In 2002, supplemental iron, alone or in combination with other nutrients, was taken by 72% of pregnant women, 60% of lactating women, 9% of nonpregnant, nonlactating women aged 14 to 18 years and 23% of nonpregnant, nonlactating women aged 19 years and older.[28]

The adequacy of dietary iron intake is not only associated with the consumption of foods rich in iron (the richest sources of iron in the diet are meat, poultry and fish, eggs and whole, iron-enriched and iron-fortified grain products), but is strongly affected by the variation in absorption of iron.[29] Iron absorption varies with physiologic need: absorption increases when iron status is reduced and decreases when iron status is adequate. Iron absorption is also associated with the type of iron consumed and factors in the diet that enhance or inhibit absorption.

The type of iron consumed is far more important than the quantity of iron in the diet. [29,30] Heme iron, from the hemoglobin and myoglobin of animals, is generally well absorbed and unaffected by factors that inhibit iron absorption. Heme iron is taken up by the mucosal cell within the porphyrin ring, protecting the iron from ingredients in the diet that inhibit iron absorption. Nonheme iron, which makes up about 90% of the iron in the diet and is found in nonmeat food sources (including grains, vegetables, fruits, eggs, the nonheme iron of animals and iron supplements) is not well absorbed. In addition, the bioavailability of nonheme iron is generally affected by several factors that enhance or inhibit absorption. The effect of these factors is less pronounced when the entire composition of a diverse diet is considered. For example, Cook and colleagues[30] found a sixfold difference (13.5% vs. 2.3%) in iron absorption rates between a single iron absorption-enhancing meal and a single iron absorption-inhibitory meal, but only a 2.5-fold difference (8.0% vs. 3.2%) in iron absorption when an iron absorption-enhancing diet and an iron absorption-inhibitory diet were consumed for 2 consecutive weeks.

The main inhibitors of nonheme iron absorption are phytates and polyphenols.[31-34] Phytates are found primarily in cereal grains, nuts, legumes and some vegetables (e.g., spinach and beet greens). Polyphenols are found in coffee, tea, some vegetables and legumes. Meals that contain nonheme iron along with phytates and polyphenols can still contribute an important source of absorbable iron, however, especially if the meal also contains an enhancer of iron absorption.[34] The main enhancers of nonheme iron absorption are ascorbic acid and the "meat factor" — a protein found in fish, poultry and beef that contains amino acids that bind iron to increase its absorption.[34-36] These factors are relatively high in the diet of most Americans. Other organic acids (e.g., lactic acid) and alcohol are less powerful enhancers of iron absorption. [37]

2. Increased Physiologic Requirements

In 1998, the National Academy of Sciences' Institute of Medicine established the dietary reference intakes (DRIs), a series of reference values for each nutrient to be used for planning and assessing diets of healthy people.[38] Among the DRIs is the RDA, which is the average daily dietary intake level sufficient to meet the nutrient requirements of nearly all individuals in a particular life stage and gender group. Also established was the estimated average requirement (EAR), the value below which inadequate intake in a population may be a concern. The RDA is used to assess and plan diets of individuals, whereas the EAR should be used to assess diets of groups. The RDA (and EAR) for iron, which assumes a maximum absorption rate of 18%, is 18 mg/d for nonpregnant and nonlactating women aged 19 to 50 years (EAR = 8.1 mg/d) and 27 mg/d for pregnant women (EAR = 22 mg/d). [27] The requirement is lowest for lactating women aged 19 to 50 years who have not resumed menstruating (RDA, 9mg/d; EAR, 6.5 mg/d) because the amount of iron lost through breast milk is less than the iron lost in menstruation. [27]

The iron requirement is highest during pregnancy to meet the iron demands of an increased blood volume, to provide iron to the fetus and placenta and to compensate for blood loss during delivery (Table 11.4).[12,13,39] Iron deficiency ane-

Table 11.4
Iron Losses During Pregnancy and Iron Gains Postpartum in a 55 Kg Iron-Replete Woman.*

	Amount of iron (mg)
Gross Losses	1200
Fetus	280
Umbilical cord and placenta	90
Maternal blood loss	150
Obligatory losses from gut, etc. during gestation	230
Expansion of maternal red cell mass	450
Gain (contraction of maternal red cell mass after delivery)	450
Net Loss	750

*These represent average values. Considerable individual variations have been reported in different studies.

Source: From Bothwell, T.H. and Charlton, R.W., Iron Deficiency in Women, A report of the International Nutritional Anemia Consultative Group (INACG), The Nutrition Foundation, Washington, D.C., 1981 p. 8. With permission.

mia in pregnancy occurs when iron intake and stores are not adequate to meet these increased needs, which average about 1200 mg during the course of pregnancy.[13,39] Most women do not have this level of iron in stores; indeed, less than 5% of women have more than 400 mg of stored iron.[40] Increased iron absorption during the second half of pregnancy helps to make up the increased requirement, but the high iron requirement of 3 to 5 mg/d during this period cannot be easily met by increased absorption alone (Figure 11.1).[41] Increased intake and mobilization from stores are necessary. Because women generally begin pregnancy with low iron stores and because it is unlikely that food intake will supply the iron needed, iron supplementation during pregnancy is recommended to prevent the onset of iron deficiency.[42,43] Several studies have shown an association between iron supplementation and increased hemoglobin concentration in the third trimester of pregnancy,[44–50] but no published randomized controlled trials have clearly indicated that iron supplementation during pregnancy increases birth weight or gestational length.[16] Part of the reason for the lack of strong evidence is that physicians routinely prescribe supplements with iron to women during pregnancy. Thus, it would be difficult to conduct a proper evaluation of clinical outcomes with a control group not receiving iron.

As part of the DRIs, the Institute of Medicine also established tolerable upper intake levels (UL) for each nutrient, the highest level of daily nutrient intake likely to pose no risk of adverse health effects to almost all individuals in the general population.[38] The UL for iron was based on evidence of gastrointestinal side effects with high doses of iron. For adults, the UL was set at 45 mg/d.[27] The UL for pregnant and lactating women is the same as that for nonpregnant adults because limited data are available on the gastrointestinal effect in these women.[27]

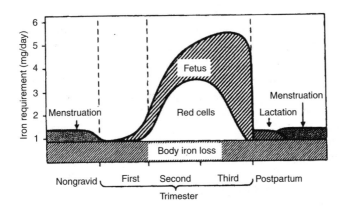

FIGURE 11.1 Daily iron requirements during pregnancy. From Bothwell, T.H., Charlton, R.W., Cook, J.D. and Finch, C.A., *Iron Metabolism in Man*, Blackwell, Oxford, 1979, 21. With permission.

3. Blood Loss

Blood loss can occur through trauma, disease or blood donation. Among women, physiologic blood loss occurs through menstruation. Pregnant women also lose blood during and after delivery. The effect of any blood loss on iron status depends on the quantity of blood lost and the iron stores of the individual.

Women lose an average of 27 ml of blood per 28-day cycle in menses;[27] approximately 10% of women lose more than 80 ml per month.[41,51–53] This excessive blood loss can contribute to the development of iron deficiency anemia, because women generally do not have adequate stored iron to compensate for the iron lost in heavy menses and because increased iron absorption cannot compensate for such high losses. The amount of iron lost through menstruation also varies with the type of contraception used. Intrauterine devices can cause a twofold increase in blood loss, whereas the contraceptive pill can reduce blood loss by one half. [13]

Pregnancy complications that can lead to intrapartum or postpartum blood loss have been associated with increased risk of anemia. Because of their association with intrapartum bleeding, placenta previa and placental abruption are independent risk factors for anemia immediately after delivery. [54] During a normal vaginal delivery, women on average lose about 500 ml of blood — the equivalent of 200 mg of iron. Blood loss can increase twofold during a cesarean delivery. [55] Cesarean delivery, uterine atony and lacerations of the vagina and cervix are the most common causes of postpartum hemorrhage, which is classically defined as the loss of 500 ml or more of blood from the reproductive tract after the third stage of labor.[55] Postpartum hemorrhage is a risk factor for anemia immediately following delivery.[54,56]

Another route of blood loss related to childbirth is lochia, the vaginal discharge of blood following childbirth. Lochia lasts approximately 27 to 33 days, but sometimes much longer.[57–59] Blood loss from lochia has not yet been quantified by researchers and thus its contribution to anemia cannot be determined.

Exclusive breastfeeding lengthens postpartum amenorrhea,[60–62] thereby reducing bodily iron losses, and may protect breastfeeding women from developing iron deficiency anemia. Not exclusively breastfeeding has previously been shown to be a predictor of postpartum anemia,[63,64] but it is unknown whether the protective effect of breastfeeding is due to amenorrhea or to healthy behaviors associated with breastfeeding, such as iron supplement use or adequate iron intake.

Pathological blood loss from parasitic infection and gastrointestinal lesions can be significant and contribute to iron deficiency anemia. Hookworm infestation is extremely rare in the United States, but it is a significant burden for women in developing countries. Although iron deficiency anemia is relatively uncommon among postmenopausal women, when detected, it is most often due to gastrointestinal blood loss associated with lesions of the gastrointesinal tract.[65] Gastritis, ulcers, colonic carcinoma and colonic polyps are among the common lesions. Increased blood loss can also result from the ingestion of certain medications. For example, adrenocorticosteroids or nonsteroidal anti-inflammatory agents may cause some gastrointestinal bleeding. Aspirin, especially when taken with alcohol, may cause hemorrhage, gastritis and subsequent blood loss.

Blood donation is a nonpathological reason for significant blood loss. Iron deficiency as a result of blood donation is not a concern when donations are made infrequently or when the donor has adequate iron stores that can easily be replenished. Because women generally have low stores of iron, however, donating blood more than three times per year increases a woman's risk for iron deficiency if she does not regularly use iron supplements.[12]

E. DIAGNOSIS OF IRON DEFICIENCY ANEMIA

Iron deficiency is one of the most common causes of anemia in women. Thus, a diagnosis of anemia alone is often used as the screening test for iron deficiency anemia. Anemia is commonly diagnosed on the basis of a hemoglobin concentration or hematocrit level that is below a sex- and age-specific cutoff value for the population under study. The anemia criteria for women of childbearing age proposed by the U.S. Centers for Disease Control and Prevention (CDC) are based on population data from NHANES III (Table 11.5).[43] Cutoff values for anemia during pregnancy were based on results from studies of women who were adequately supplemented throughout pregnancy.[45–47,66]

In assessing whether iron deficiency is the actual cause of the anemia, the most common follow-up tests are the hemoglobin response to iron supplementation and abnormal results on laboratory measures of iron status. Observing an individual's response to iron therapy is one of the more specific tests. If hemoglobin concentrations increase at least 1.0 g/dl after 1 month of iron treatment, then iron deficiency is the most likely etiology of the anemia. Iron supplementation can also be done at the population level. The hemoglobin distribution for the population is then compared for pre- and post-supplementation. Supplementation of the population may be preferred over individual supplementation when the prevalence of anemia is high and it can be assumed that most persons in the population have some level of iron deficiency.[10]

TABLE 11.5
Anemia Criteria for U.S. Women

Anemia criteria	Hemoglobin concentration (g/dL)	Hematocrit value (%)
Nonpregnant women and lactating women (age, in years)		
12–<15	< 11.8	< 35.7
≥15	< 12.0	< 35.9
Pregnant		
1st trimester	< 11.0	< 33.0
2nd trimester	< 10.5	< 32.0
3rd trimester	< 11.0	< 33.0

Source: From Centers for Disease Control and Prevention, Recommendation to prevent and control iron deficiency in the United States. *Morb. Mortal. Wkly. Rep.*, 47 (RR-3), 1998. With permission.

The common biochemical measures of iron status are mean corpuscular volume (MCV), serum ferritin concentration, transferrin saturation, free erythrocyte protoporphyrin concentration and transferrin receptor concentration (Table11.6). A diagnosis of anemia accompanied by abnormal results on at least two of these iron status measures is an established method of confirming iron deficiency anemia for population-based assessment.[67] For individual assessment, a single biochemical test other than hemoglobin or hematocrit is helpful in confirming iron deficiency. Other causes of mild anemia can interfere with the test results, however. For example, a low MCV can also be the result of infection, chronic inflammatory conditions, or mild hereditary anemia such as α- or β-thalassemia traits. Inflammatory conditions can also depress transferrin saturation and elevate erythrocyte protoporphyrin concentrations. Among the battery of common iron tests listed in Table 11.6, serum ferritin concentration appears to be the most specific indicator of iron deficiency when levels of iron are low. But because serum ferritin is an acute-phase reactant and becomes elevated with infection and chronic inflammatory conditions, the absence of a low serum ferritin concentration does not rule out iron deficiency. Transferrin receptor concentration, on the other hand, is not affected by inflammatory conditions, but is less sensitive to changes in iron status than is serum ferritin concentration because it is an indicator of iron deficient erythropoesis rather than iron depletion.[68,69]

F. PREVENTION AND TREATMENT

1. Prevention

Iron deficiency anemia is prevented by maintaining a balance between iron intake and iron requirement and loss. The amount of iron necessary to maintain this balance varies from one woman to another, depending on her reproductive history and the quantity of blood lost during menstruation.

TABLE 11.6
Common Biochemical Measures Taken To Confirm Iron Deficiency

Measure	Meaning of the test	Common cutoffs used for identifying iron deficiency in adult women	Comments
Mean cell volume	Reflects the average size of the red blood cell.	< 80 fL	Decreased in iron deficiency anemia. May also decrease in the anemias of infection, chronic inflammatory disease, thalassemia minor and lead poisoning.
Serum ferritin concentration	Reflects the amount of iron in storage.	< 12 ng/mL	Decreased during the early stage of iron depletion. Increased by infection, chronic inflammatory diseases, acute and chronic liver disease, leukemia, Hodgkin's disease and the decreased erythropoiesis associated with vitamin B_{12} and folate deficiency.
Transferrin saturation	Reflects the amount of iron in transit from the reticuloendothelial system to the bone marrow. Percent transferrin saturation = serum iron concentration/total iron binding capacity (TIBC).	< 16%	Decreased in iron deficiency, as serum iron concentration decreases and TIBC increases. In chronic inflammatory disease, serum iron concentration and TIBC decrease, resulting in a low normal transferrin saturation.
Free erythrocyte protoporphyrin concentration	Reflects the accumulation of protoporphyrin in the red blood cell that results from decreased heme synthesis.	> 70 µg/dL	Increased in early iron deficiency. Also increased in chronic inflammatory disease and lead poisoning.
Transferrin receptor concentration	Reflects the increase in transferrin receptors on cells with increased erythrocyte production after a depletion of body iron.	Test dependent	Increased in early iron deficiency. Not influenced by most acute or chronic inflammatory conditions.

To prevent iron deficiency anemia caused by increased blood loss, medications and contraceptive practices that increase blood loss should be avoided and the patient must be clinically evaluated for possible sources of gastrointestinal blood loss. Also, reducing the frequency with which women donate blood can prevent iron deficiency anemia.

Increasing iron intake to meet iron requirements is accomplished through improved dietary choices. A diet that provides adequate iron should emphasize foods that contain heme iron and foods that contain factors that enhance the absorption of nonheme iron and minimize foods that contain factors that inhibit absorption. If the iron requirement exceeds usual dietary intake, then iron intake can be improved by taking iron supplements. Supplementation may be an especially important strategy for high-risk women, specifically pregnant and postpartum women. The CDC and the American College of Obstetricians and Gynecologists recommend that all pregnant women receive a low-dose supplement (30 mg/d) throughout pregnancy as well as counseling about iron-rich foods and foods that enhance iron absorption.[42,43] If a positive anemia screening result is obtained during pregnancy, treatment with 60 to 120 mg/d of iron is suggested.

Iron supplementation as a strategy to increase iron intake can be successful only if the individual complies with supplement use. Many factors contribute to poor compliance, such as personal difficulty in remembering to take the supplement each day, financial difficulty in purchasing the supplements regularly and unpleasant side effects from the iron (specifically, gastrointestinal disturbances). Capsules made by packing iron sulfate with a "gastric delivery system" appear to improve tolerance for iron supplements by minimizing these adverse gastrointestinal effects while simultaneously improving the pill's iron absorption.[70] Microencapsulated ferrous fumarate plus ascorbic acid in powdered form, to be sprinkled onto any complementary food eaten, is easy to use and has been shown to be effective in treatment of anemia.[71] Other strategies to improve compliance with iron supplementation include educating women on the importance of supplements and advising on the common side effects.[72]

Iron fortification of cereal and grain products is an inexpensive strategy for improving the iron intake of a population. In the United States, grain products are only partially fortified. Although the impact of this fortification program on the iron status of women has not been formally evaluated, national data suggest that iron-fortified ready-to-eat cereals and yeast breads are the highest contributors to total iron intake in the United States, supplying 19% and 14% of dietary iron, respectively.[73] In Sweden, where highly fortified grain products supplied up to 40% of dietary iron before 1995,[74] the fortification program contributed significantly to the decline in iron deficiency among women of childbearing age.[75] Nonetheless, this program, which was the highest level of fortification in the world, was discontinued in 1995 because of concerns that such high levels of iron in the diet increased the risk for iron overload and related illness among persons with undiagnosed hemochromatosis. The evidence supporting this relationship is based mainly on absorption studies and theoretical modeling, but one Swedish study showed that withdrawing fortification has lowered the amount of iron absorbed per day among men with hemochromatosis and extended the interval between their phlebotomies.[76] These findings and others are the basis for the strong opposition to increasing the amount of iron added to grain products in the U.S. diet.

2. Screening and Treatment

Although iron deficiency anemia is associated with serious functional consequences, these adverse outcomes may be subtle and rarely would they be reason for seeking medical attention. Screening, therefore, is necessary to identify which women should be treated to reduce anemia-related morbidity.

The CDC[43] recommends that all adolescent girls and nonpregnant women of childbearing age should be screened for anemia every 5 to 10 years during routine health examinations if no risk factors for anemia are present. If risk factors are present (e.g., high menstrual or other blood loss, previous diagnosis of iron deficiency anemia, or low iron intake), screening should be annual. Those with anemia should be treated with an oral dose of 60 to 120 mg/d of iron and counseled on increased dietary iron intake; in 4 weeks, a repeat anemia screening should be done. Iron deficiency anemia is confirmed if the repeat screen shows an increase in hemoglobin concentration of at least 1 g/dl or in hematocrit of at least 3%; treatment should continue for 2 to 3 months.

For pregnant women the CDC recommends universal screening at the first prenatal visit,[43] whereas the Institute of Medicine[77] and the American College of Obstetricians and Gynecologists[42] recommend screening once during each trimester of pregnancy. The Institute of Medicine also recommends the determination of serum ferritin concentration in addition to hemoglobin concentration and suggests supplementation if a lower than normal serum ferritin concentration accompanies the anemia.

All three groups agree that women identified as mildly anemic should be given an oral dose of 60 to 120 mg/d of iron; the dose should be decreased to 30 mg/d when the hemoglobin concentration or hematocrit becomes normal for the stage of gestation. Women whose hemoglobin concentration at screening is 9.0 g/dL or lower or hematocrit is less than 27.0% should be referred for further medical evaluation.

Currently, the CDC and the Institute of Medicine recommend anemia screening at 4 to 6 weeks postpartum for women who had anemia through the third trimester of pregnancy, a multiple birth, or excessive blood loss at delivery.[43,77] In the only evaluation of these selective screening criteria, the CDC risk assessment algorithm correctly identified 79% of postpartum anemia cases and correctly identified 53% of noncases in a population of single gestations where 19% of women had postpartum anemia.[64] This study identified three additional independent risk markers of postpartum anemia: multiparity, prepregnancy obesity and not exclusively breastfeeding.[64] The results of this analysis indicated that, if clinic resources cannot support universal screening, consideration of clinic postpartum anemia prevalence and a selective screening algorithm provide a useful approach. [64]

III. FOLATE AND VITAMIN B$_{12}$ DEFICIENCY ANEMIA

A. INTRODUCTION

In the United States, anemia is caused mainly by iron deficiency; the remainder of nutritional anemia is due almost exclusively to advanced folate (vitamin B$_9$) or colbalamin (vitamin B$_{12}$) deficiency. The type of anemia caused by folate and cobalamin deficiency is called nutritional megaloblastic anemia.

Folate deficiency anemia is the second most common nutritional anemia in the world. Although data on its prevalence in the United States are unavailable, data from NHANES III indicate that 13% of women 15 to 44 years of age have low RBC folate concentrations (less than 140 ng/mL) and 6% have both low RBC concentrations and low serum folate concentrations (less than 3 ng/mL).[78] Since food fortification began in 1998, serum and RBC levels have risen and the proportion of women with low levels appears to have decreased substantially,[79] although the exact proportions of women with low serum or RBC folate concentrations are not currently available. Data from small studies suggest that women at increased risk of folate deficiency include low-income pregnant women, particularly adolescents and women who abuse alcohol.[80–82]

Vitamin B$_{12}$ deficiency anemia is relatively rare, occurring primarily in elderly persons who have inadequate levels of intrinsic factor, which is necessary for the intestinal absorption of vitamin B$_{12}$, a condition referred to as pernicious anemia. The prevalence of pernicious anemia is highest among persons over 50 years of age and increases with age. An estimated 2% of persons over 60 years of age have this condition.[83] Vitamin B$_{12}$ deficiency without anemia is more common among the elderly, affecting between 10% and 15% of elderly persons.[84,85] Pernicious anemia may also be more prevalent among younger African-American women than younger women of other racial and ethnic backgrounds; however, these data are limited and further study is warranted.[86] Among vegetarians who consume no animal products, a group at risk for vitamin B$_{12}$ depletion, the advanced stage of vitamin B$_{12}$ deficiency that characterizes megaloblastic anemia is extremely rare.

B. THE B VITAMINS AND ANEMIA

The hematologic manifestations of folate and vitamin B$_{12}$ deficiencies are indistinguishable because both vitamins are involved in DNA synthesis. Specifically, vitamin B$_{12}$ is an essential coenzyme in the transfer of a methyl group from methyl folate to homocysteine, an important step in regenerating tetrahydrofolic acid, which is involved in DNA synthesis. In folate deficiency, the supply of folate is inadequate for conversion to tetrahydrofolic acid. In vitamin B$_{12}$ deficiency, folate is "trapped" as metabolically inactive methyl folate. In both deficiencies, DNA synthesis is impaired, leading to abnormal cell replication, hypersegmentation of neutrophils, macrocytosis and megaloblastosis.

C. CONSEQUENCES OF FOLATE AND VITAMIN B$_{12}$ DEFICIENCY

1. Folate

A dramatic consequence of the impaired DNA synthesis that accompanies folate deficiency is an increased risk of neural tube defects (NTDs) among women genetically susceptible to delivering infants with NTDs.[83] NTDs are the most common major congenital malformations of the central nervous system. Observational studies have shown a 50% reduction in NTD risk among women consuming 400 µg/d of folic acid before and during pregnancy.[87] Furthermore, randomized trials have shown that folic acid supplementation before conception and during the first trimester of pregnancy reduce the incidence of an NTD-infected pregnancy by 70% to 100%.[88,89] During pregnancy, inadequate folate intake and low concentrations of serum folate have also been associated with preterm birth and low birth weight.[90,91]

Folate deficiency is also associated with elevated blood concentrations of the amino acid homocysteine. The relationship between folate and homocysteine metabolism is important because elevated homocysteine concentration is an independent risk factor for cardiovascular disease.[92] Several clinical trials are currently being conducted to determine whether folic acid supplements can reduce the risk of cardiovascular disease.

The stages of folate deficiency leading to folate deficiency anemia are summarized in Table 11.7. Initially, serum folate concentration drops, which can occur after only 2 to 3 weeks of negative folate balance. As the deficiency progresses, the RBC folate concentration also falls, indicating folate depletion. Folate deficient erythropoiesis is characterized by an abnormal diagnostic deoxyuridine suppression test corrected *in vitro* by folate, which is indicative of defective DNA synthesis, by decreased liver stores of folate (less than 1.2 µg/g) and by hypersegmentation of the neutrophils (lobe average greater than 3.5). When stores are severely depleted, folate deficiency anemia is observed. At this final stage of deficiency, macrocytic RBC can be observed in the circulating blood, MCV is elevated, hemoglobin is decreased and megaloblasts are observed in the bone marrow. The anemia may occur months after the initial folate depletion. In a severe folate deficiency of very short duration, the anemia may occur sooner, even before RBC folate concentration has a chance to decrease.

2. Vitamin B$_{12}$

In addition to its essential role in DNA synthesis, vitamin B$_{12}$ is essential to myelin synthesis. Thus, deficiency of vitamin B$_{12}$, but not folate, can also lead to impaired nerve function. The neurologic abnormalities of vitamin B$_{12}$ deficiency include paresthesias, impaired vibration sense, impaired touch or pain perception, ataxia, abnormal gait, memory loss, decreased reflexes and muscle strength, psychiatric disorders, disorientation, spasticity and decreased vision or optic atrophy.[93,94] Inappropriate treatment of a vitamin B$_{12}$ deficiency anemia with folic acid will correct the megaloblastic anemia, leading a health care professional to believe that the problem is remedied. However, vitamin B$_{12}$ deficiency will remain, allowing neurologic manifestations to progress unnoticed and sometimes lead to permanent

TABLE 11.7
Stages of Folate Deficiency

	Normal	Negative folate balance	Folate depletion	Folate deficient erythropoiesis	Folate deficiency anemia
Serum folate concentration	normal	low	low	low	low
Red blood cell folate concentration	normal	normal	low	low	low
Deoxyuridine suppression	normal	normal	normal	abnormal	abnormal
Hyper-segmentation	no	no	no	yes	yes
Liver folate concentration	normal	normal	low normal	low	low
Erythrocytes	normal	normal	normal	normal	macro-ovalocytic
Mean cell volume	normal	normal	normal	normal	elevated
Hemoglobin concentration	normal	normal	normal	normal	low

Source: From Herbert, V., The 1986 Herman Award Lecture, Nutrition Science as a continually unfolding story: The folate and vitamin B_{12} paradigm, *Amer. J. Clin. Nutr.*, 46, 387, 1987. With permission.

neurologic damage.[93,94] It is therefore critical to determine the nutritional cause of megaloblastic anemia before treatment is initiated.

The stages of vitamin B_{12} deficiency that lead to anemia are summarized in Table 11.8. Initially, the amount of vitamin B_{12} absorbed is decreased, resulting in a lower level of the vitamin B_{12} transport protein transcobalamin II with attached vitamin B_{12} (holotranscobalamin II) and reduced saturation of transcobalamin II. If the negative balance continues, serum vitamin B_{12} concentrations are depressed, indicating vitamin B_{12} depletion. The third stage of deficiency, vitamin B_{12} deficient erythropoiesis, is marked by further reductions in the vitamin B_{12} transport protein measures and serum vitamin B_{12} concentration, an abnormal deoxyuridine suppression test and hypersegmentation of the neutrophils. Because of vitamin B_{12}'s role in the transport and uptake of folate by the cells, RBC folate concentration is also decreased during this stage. The final stage of deficiency is characterized by the presence of megaloblastic anemia.

D. FACTORS CONTRIBUTING TO FOLATE DEFICIENCY ANEMIA

The main cause of folate deficiency among U.S. women is inadequate dietary intake of the vitamin. Additional important causes include poor absorption of dietary folate and increased physiologic requirement for the nutrient. Less common causes of

TABLE 11.8
Stages of Vitamin B$_{12}$ Deficiency

	Normal	Negative vitamin B$_{12}$ balance	Vitamin B$_{12}$ depletion	Vitamin B$_{12}$ deficient erythro-poiesis	Vitamin B$_{12}$ deficiency anemia
Holotrans-cobalamin II	normal	low	low	low	low
transcobalamin II % saturation	normal	low	low	low	low
Serum vitamin B$_{12}$ concentration	normal	normal	normal	low	low
Deoxyuridine suppression	normal	normal	normal	abnormal	abnormal
Hypersegmentation	no	no	no	yes	yes
Red blood cell folate concentration	normal	normal	normal	low	low
Erythrocytes	normal	normal	normal	normal	macro-ovalocytic
Mean cell volume	normal	normal	normal	normal	elevated
Hemoglobin concentration	normal	normal	normal	normal	low

Source: From Herbert, V., The 1986 Herman Award Lecture, Nutrition Science as a continually unfolding story: The folate and vitamin B$_{12}$ paradigm, *Amer. J. Clin. Nutr.*, 46, 387, 1987. With permission.

folate deficiency are folate antagonists (e.g., methotrexate), congenital or acquired enzyme deficiencies (inadequate folate utilization), renal dialysis (increased folate loss) and specific disease states and drugs.[95–97]

1. Inadequate Intake

Folate is the generic term to describe the B-complex vitamin that exists in many forms. Naturally occurring folate (pteroylpolyglutamate) is often called food folate. Food folate is widely distributed in the food supply and the main sources are liver, yeast, fresh leafy vegetables, some fresh fruits and legumes. Folic acid (pteroylglutamic acid) is rarely found in food naturally, but is used in vitamin supplements and to fortify food products. To account for the greater bioavailability of folic acid from fortified foods and supplements than the same amount of food folate the Institute of Medicine expresses the RDA, EAR and UL for folate in terms of dietary folate equivalents (DFE).[83] To estimate DFE, units of folic acid from diet and supplements are multiplied by a factor of 1.7 and then added to units of food folate.[83] National food consumption surveys indicate that the average folate intake of U.S. women before fortification (prior to 1998) was approximately 240 µg/d.[98] In an analysis to adjust folate intakes to reflect increased folic acid in foods due to fortification, median intake was estimated to be about 455 µg DFE/d.[99] About 15% of women were estimated to consume less than the 320 µg DFE/d EAR for folate,[99] suggesting that 15% of women are at high risk of inadequacy. In addition to poor food choices, overprocessing of foods contributes to inadequate folate ingestion because 50% to 95% of the folate in food may be destroyed by food processing and cooking.[95]

2. Poor Absorption

Owing to their distinct chemical structures, food folate and folic acid have different bioavailabilities. Folic acid from supplements is thought to be 100% bioavailable when taken on an empty stomach and 85% bioavailable when consumed with food.[83,100] On the other hand, food folate has about 50% the bioavailablilty of folic acid.[101] The bioavailability of food folate is compromised by specific factors in the foods, such as a factor found in yeast and legumes. In general, folate malabsorption occurs under conditions that create an acidic pH of the intestinal environment. Folate absorption is also impaired in malabsorption syndromes such as gluten-induced enteropathy and tropical sprue and as a result of ingestion of certain drugs (e.g., salicylazosulfapyridine and diphenylhydantoin) and alcohol.[102]

3. Increased Physiologic Requirements

The Institute of Medicine recommends that 320 µg DFE/d are needed to prevent inadequacy in about half of the population of nonpregnant women; individual women should be counseled to consume 400 µg DFE/d.[83] Because literature has shown that 400 µg/d of folic acid reduces risk of NTDs,[87] the U.S. Public Health Service and the Institute of Medicine recommend that women capable of becoming pregnant should consume 400 µg/d of folic acid from supplements or fortified foods in addition to folate from a healthy diet.[83,87] Folate requirements also may be increased for individuals with chronic heavy alcohol intake and individuals on chronic anti-convulsant or methotrexate therapy.[83]

The folate requirement for pregnant women is higher because of the acceleration of single-carbon transfer reactions in cell division associated with uterine enlarge-ment, placental development, expansion of maternal RBC mass and fetal growth.[103] Folate is also actively transferred to the fetus. The EAR for pregnancy is 520 µg DFE/d and the RDA is 600 µg DFE/d.[83] Requirements are also high during lactation to provide approximately 85 µg of folate per liter of breast milk and to maintain maternal folate status; the EAR for lactating women is 450 µg DFE/d and the RDA is 500 µg DFE/d.[83]

Prior to fortification, it could be difficult for individuals to consume the required amount of folate through diet alone and oral folate supplements were recommended for those at high risk of deficiency, particularly pregnant women. Now that the food supply is more highly fortified, national nutrition surveys are needed to determine whether folate supplementation is necessary.

D. Factors Contributing To Vitamin B$_{12}$ Deficiency Anemia

The main cause of vitamin B$_{12}$ deficiency anemia in the United States is impaired absorption of the nutrient. Much less common causes of vitamin B$_{12}$ deficiency, including intake of vitamin B_{12} antagonists, congenital or acquired enzyme deficiencies or deletions, abnormalities in binding proteins and specific diseases and drugs, are reviewed elsewhere.[95–97]

Absorption of vitamin B_{12} occurs in multiple stages. Initially, gastric acid and gastric and intestinal enzymes release ingested vitamin B_{12} from polypeptide links in food. The vitamin then attaches to salivary R binder polypeptides, a link later broken when the R binders are destroyed in the intestine by pancreatic trypsin. This separation allows the vitamin B_{12} to combine with a protein called intrinsic factor; the vitamin-intrinsic factor complex is absorbed through the wall of the ileum.[95,104]

Vitamin B_{12} absorption is impaired under conditions that affect the function of intrinsic factor or alter the state of the ileum. Pancreatic disease affects absorption. Specific drugs, including para-aminosalicylic acid, colchicine, neomycin, ethanol and metformin, are known to decrease vitamin B_{12} take-up. Oral contraceptive agents may also impair absorption. A deficiency of the vitamin itself can produce poor vitamin B_{12} absorption. Specifically, the megaloblastosis that occurs in vitamin B_{12} and folate deficiencies affects all cells, including those of the intestinal lumen, causing atrophy of the intestinal absorptive cells.[104] Deficiency as a result of poor absorption can occur 3 to 6 years after vitamin B_{12} absorption is impaired.[104] Vitamin B_{12} deficiency anemia due to poor absorption as a result of insufficient secretion of intrinsic factor is specifically referred to as pernicious anemia. Approximately half of all cases of pernicious anemia among adults result from acquired gastric atrophy as an end result of inflammatory gastritis.[74] The condition is diagnosed with the Schilling test.[96,105] If the first part of the test indicates vitamin B_{12} malabsorption, which is corrected by the addition of intrinsic factor in the follow-up test, pernicious anemia is indicated. If the malabsorption is not corrected, other etiologies of the malabsorption are suspected, such as an ileal or pancreatic defect or parasitic infestation (e.g., fish tapeworm). For the elderly, who lose their ability to split vitamin B_{12} off from food as they age, the first part of the test must be performed with food rather than crystalline vitamin B_{12}.

Vitamin B_{12} deficiency caused by inadequate intake of the nutrient is very rare but can occur in strict vegetarians who consume no foods of animal origin and no supplemental source of vitamin B_{12}.[106,107] Among such persons, vitamin B_{12} depletion occurs slowly because the body recycles any vitamin B_{12} ingested, including the small amount found in foods contaminated by microorganisms.

E. ASSESSING THE ETIOLOGY OF NUTRITIONAL MEGALOBLASTIC ANEMIA

When it is apparent from initial studies of cell morphology or other laboratory measures that an observed anemia is not due to iron deficiency, an inquiry into other possible causes of anemia is undertaken. Inquiry should also be done in the presence of iron deficiency because the macrocytosis of folate and vitamin B_{12} deficiency could be masked by a concurrent iron deficiency.

If abnormally large RBC or if hypersegmentation of neutrophils are observed on the peripheral blood smear, folate or vitamin B_{12} deficiency anemia is suspected. The evaluation of neutrophil hypersegmentation is useful (in nonpregnant populations)

TABLE 11.9
Three Common Assays Used In Differentiating Folate and Vitamin B$_{12}$ Deficiency Anemia

Clinical situation	Serum folate concentration	Red blood cell folate concentration	Serum vitamin B$_{12}$ concentration
Folate deficiency anemia	low	low	generally normal, but may be low
Vitamin B$_{12}$ deficiency anemia	generally normal, but may be high	low	low
Both folate and vitamin B$_{12}$ deficiency anemia	low	low	low

Source: Herbert, V. Anemias, in *Clinical Nutrition*, 2nd ed., Paige, D., Ed., C.V. Mosby, St. Louis, 1988, 593. With permission

because it is apparent even if the macrocytosis is masked by iron deficiency. If the diet of the individual or the population contains no animal foods, vitamin B$_{12}$ deficiency would be suspected. Because a concurrent folate deficiency could also be present, however, diagnostic tests for both deficiencies should still be undertaken. Macrocytosis is confirmed by measuring MCV (see Table 11.6). If this measure is elevated, a biopsy can be performed to confirm the presence of megaloblasts (abnormally large RBC precursors) in the bone marrow. Once megaloblastic anemia is confirmed, additional laboratory tests are performed to determine whether the etiology of the anemia is folate or vitamin B$_{12}$ deficiency.[108]

Serum and RBC folate concentrations and serum vitamin B$_{12}$ concentration are routinely measured as a battery to differentiate between folate and vitamin B$_{12}$ deficiency as the nutritional cause of the megaloblastic anemia (Table 11.9). In general, serum folate concentrations are low (usually less than 3.0 ng/mL) in folate deficiency anemia, but can also be low in the absence of deficiency because serum concentrations of folate are very sensitive to recent changes in folate intake and metabolism.[109] Serum folate concentration is also lowered by alcohol consumption[88] and cigarette smoking.[110] Contrary to older investigations,[111–112] large population-based studies[82] and well-controlled metabolic studies[113] reported that folate status is not affected by the use of oral contraceptives.

RBC folate concentration, a more stable measure that reflects liver stores of the nutrient, is usually low (less than 140 ng/mL) in folate deficiency anemia[95,109] unless the progression was very rapid, which may occur in the megaloblastic anemia of pregnancy. In addition, RBC folate concentration is depressed in vitamin B$_{12}$ deficiency because vitamin B$_{12}$ is involved in the transport and storage of folate in cells.[114,115]

A low serum vitamin B$_{12}$ concentration alone is insufficient evidence to conclude that a megaloblastic anemia is due to vitamin B$_{12}$ deficiency alone. Additional evidence is necessary. A normal vitamin B$_{12}$ concentration (more than 100 pg/mL) in the presence of low serum or RBC folate concentrations suggests a primary folate deficiency; however, low levels on all three vitamin assays do not rule out a primary folate deficiency. Approximately one third of individuals with megaloblastic anemia due to primary folate deficiency have low serum vitamin B_{12} concentrations that are restored in 7 to 10 days of folate treatment.[96] The reason for this finding is unknown.

The *in vitro* deoxyuridine suppression test is a more precise assay to distinguish between folate and vitamin B_{12} deficient anemia.[104,109,116] The test is designed to assess defective DNA synthesis in cultured bone marrow cells. The general principle is that normal folate metabolism is necessary in the methylation of deoxyuridine to thymidine. Folate or vitamin B_{12} are added to separate cell cultures to determine which vitamin corrects the results. The addition of folate corrects the test results for folate and vitamin B_{12}-deficient cultures; the addition of vitamin B_{12} partially corrects the results in the vitamin B_{12} deficient-culture and does not correct the results in the folate-deficient culture. An advantage of this test is that the results are not affected by a concurrent iron deficiency or other confounding disease states; however, the difficulty of the test makes it impractical for routine use.

Measurement of serum or urinary methylmalonic acid (MMA) is particularly useful because the test is specific to vitamin B_{12} deficiency. A vitamin B_{12}-containing coenzyme is essential for the conversion of methylmalonyl coenzyme A to succinyl coenzyme A. Thus, an inadequate supply of vitamin B_{12} results in the accumulation of MMA in the serum. Elevated serum MMA is found in more than 90% of persons with vitamin B_{12} deficiency.[84,117,118] A disadvantage of the test is that the laboratory procedures involved are not practical for all settings.

Additional laboratory measures of interest in assessing folate and vitamin B_{12} deficiency include the FIGLU test, which measures urinary excretion of formiminoglutamic acid and serum homocysteine concentrations.[117,118] These measures are of limited use in differentiating between the two vitamin deficiencies that cause megaloblastic anemia, however, because levels of both metabolites are elevated in both folate and vitamin B_{12} deficiency.

F. PREVENTION AND TREATMENT

Treatment for megaloblastic anemia due to folate and vitamin B_{12} deficiencies will vary according to the cause of the underlying deficiency and to the presence of concurrent illnesses and nutrient deficiencies. The appropriate treatment should be administered under the care of a clinician.

1. Folate

Folate deficiency and folate deficiency anemia are prevented by providing adequate dietary folate to meet requirements. This is accomplished through a choice of folic acid-fortified foods and foods rich in naturally occurring folate with minimal processing of the foods before consumption. High-risk women, specifically pregnant women, should be counseled on how to improve their folate intake through diet and supplements.

Meeting dietary requirements for folate has been made easier by the United States Food and Drug Administration's mandate that by January 1, 1998, all enriched cereal grains had to be fortified with 140 μg of folic acid per 100 g of grain.[119] The agency anticipated that fortification would add approximately 100 μg of folic acid to the daily diet of the average individual and would result in about 50% of child-bearing-aged women receiving 400 μg of folate from all sources,[119,120] thereby reducing the occurrence of NTDs in the population. Thus far, data suggest that since fortification began, the folate status of childbearing-aged women has greatly improved.[79,121–123] Moreover, since 1998, the prevalence of NTDs has declined by 19%.[124] Also, significant declines in plasma homocysteine concentrations have been observed after grain and cereal fortification,[125] an important finding since elevated homocysteine concentration is associated with cardiovascular disease.[92]

Despite evidence that fortification may be a primary preventive mechanism for NTDs, the issue is controversial. Some scientists believe that higher levels of fortification would be more effective in preventing NTDs.[126,127] Others argue that because high intakes of folic acid correct vitamin B_{12} anemia, fortification may prevent identification of vitamin B_{12} deficiency.[128] Masking of vitamin B_{12} deficiency due to fortification has not been studied directly. The lack of detailed data on the topic and the potential interaction of folic acid and vitamin B_{12}, led the Institute of Medicine to recommend a tolerable UL of 1000 μg DFE/d for adults.[83]

2.   Vitamin B_{12}

Prevention of vitamin B_{12} deficiency among women who absorb adequate amounts of the vitamin can be accomplished by consuming foods of animal origin, including meat, fish, poultry, eggs, milk and cheese. Women of childbearing age should consume 2.4 μg/d of vitamin B_{12}.[83] Women who consume no animal products, especially pregnant and lactating women, should be advised to take supplemental vitamin B_{12}. Women who do not absorb adequate amounts of vitamin B_{12} should receive periodic injections of the vitamin.

IV. SUMMARY AND CONCLUSIONS

Anemia is common in the United States, particularly among pregnant and postpartum women and women of low socioeconomic status. Iron deficiency is by far the most common cause of nutritional anemia in women of childbearing age because there is often an imbalance between iron intake and iron requirements and loss. Iron deficiency anemia is more than a blood disorder; it has been associated with reduced work capacity, impaired cognition and adverse birth outcomes. Nonetheless, more research is needed to study functional consequences in women of childbearing age in order to determine if prevention strategies are cost effective.

Megaloblastic anemia caused by folate and vitamin B_{12} deficiency is less common, but has serious consequences. Folate deficiency increases risk of NTDs and is associated with elevated blood concentrations of homocysteine (a risk factor for cardiovascular disease). Vitamin B_{12} deficiency can lead to impaired nerve function, which if untreated, can result in permanent neurologic damage. Unlike folate deficiency, vitamin B_{12} deficiency rarely is a problem for women of childbearing age, so as long as animal products are consumed. Folate fortification of the food supply

has significantly improved folate status of women, but at the current level of fortification is unlikely to further decrease prevalence of NTDs beyond 19%. Future
research is needed to determine effective ways to reduce functional outcomes of
folate deficiency without compromising the population's vitamin B_{12} status.

REFERENCES

1. Beutler, E., The common anemias, *J. Amer. Med. Assoc.*, 259, 2433, 1988.
2. De Maeyer, E. and Adiels-Tegman, M., The prevalence of anaemia in the world, *Wld. Health Stat. Q.*, 38, 302, 1985.
3. World Health Organization, *The Prevalence of Anemia in Women: A Tabulation of Available Information*, 2nd ed., WHO, Geneva, 1992, 1.
4. Centers for Disease Control and Prevention, *Pregnancy Nutrition Surveillance, 1996 Full Report*, U.S. Department of Health and Human Services, Centers for Disease Control and Prevention, Atlanta, 1998.
5. Bodnar, L.M., Cogswell, M.E., Scanlon, K.S., Low-income postpartum women are at risk of iron deficiency, *J. Nutr.*, 132, 2298, 2002.
6. Stoltzfus, R.J., Edward-Raj, A., Dreyfuss, M.L., Albonico, M., Montresor, A., Thapa, M.D., West, K.P., Chwaya, H.M., Savioli, L., Tielsch, J., Clinical pallor is useful to detect severe anemia in populations where anemia is prevalent and severe, *J. Nutr.*, 129, 1675, 1999.
7. Brabin, B.J., Hakimi, M., Pelletier, D., Analysis of anemia and pregnancy-related maternal mortality, *J. Nutr.*, 131, 604S, 2001.
8. Oski, F.A., Anemia related to nutritional deficiencies other than vitamin B_{12} and folic acid, in *Hematology*, 3rd ed., Willams, W.J., Beutler, E., Erslev, A.J. and Lichtman, M.A., Eds., McGraw-Hill Book Company, New York, 1983.
9. United Nations ACC/SCN, *Second Report on the World Nutrition Situation, Vol 1: Global and Regional Results*, ACC/SCN, Geneva, 1992.
10. Binkin, N.J. and Yip, R., When is anemia screening of value in detecting iron deficiency? in *Recent Knowledge On Iron and Folate Deficiencies In the World*, Vol. 197, Hercberg, S., Galan, P., Dupin, H., Eds., L'Institut National de la Santé et de la Recherché Medicale, Paris, 1990, 137.
11. Looker, A.C., Dallman, P.R., Carroll, M.D., Gunter, E.W., Johnson, C.L., Prevalence of iron deficiency in the United States, *J. Amer. Med. Assoc.*, 277, 973, 1997.
12. Institute of Medicine, National Academy of Sciences, *Nutrition during Pregnancy*, National Academy Press, Washington, D.C., 1990, 272.
13. Bothwell, T.H. and Charlton, R.W., *Iron Deficiency In Women, a Report of the International Nutritional Anemia Consultative Group (INACG)*, The Nutrition Foundation, Washington, D.C., 1981.
14. Herbert, V., The 1986 Herman Award Lecture, Nutrition Science as a continually unfolding story: The folate and vitamin B_{12} paradigm, *Am. J. Clin. Nutr.*, 46, 387, 1987.
15. Centers for Disease Control, CDC criteria for anemia in children and childbearing-aged women, *Morb. Mortal. Wkly. Rep.*, 38, 400, 1989.
16. Rasmussen, K.M., Is there a causal relationship between iron deficiency or iron-deficiency anemia and weight at birth, length of gestation and perinatal mortality?, *J. Nutr.*, 131, 590S, 2001.

17. Li, R., Chen, X., Yan, H., Deurenberg, P., Garby, L., Hautvast, J.G., Functional consequences of iron supplementation in iron-deficient female cotton workers in Beijing, China, *Am. J. Clin. Nutr.*, 59, 908, 1994.

18. Haas, J.D. and Brownlie T., Iron deficiency and reduced work capacity: A critical review of the research to determine a causal relationship. *J. Nutr.*, 131, 676S, 2001.

19. Li, R., Functional Consequences of Iron Deficiency in Chinese Female Workers [dissertation], Wageningen Agricultural University, Wageningen, The Netherlands, 1993.

20. Grantham-McGregor, S. and Ani, C., A review of studies on the effect of iron deficiency on cognitive development in children, *J. Nutr.*, 131, 649S, 2001.

21. Ballin, A., Berar, M., Rubinstein, U., Kleter, Y., Hershkovitz, A., Meytes, D., Iron state in female adolescents. *Am. J. Dis. Child.*, 146, 803, 1992.

22. Bruner, A.B., Joffe, A., Duggan, A.K., Casella, J.F., Brandt, J., Randomised study of cognitive effects of iron supplemenation in non-anaemic iron-deficient adolescent girls, *Lancet*, 348, 992, 1996.

23. Lynn, R. and Harland, E.P., A positive effect of iron supplemenation on the IQs of iron deficient children, *Pers. Individ. Differ.*, 24, 883, 1998.

24. Oski, F.A., The nonhematologic manifestations of iron deficiency, *Am. J. Dis. Child.*, 133, 315, 1979.

25. Beard, J.L., One person's view of iron deficiency, development and cognitive function, *Am. J. Clin. Nutr.*, 62, 709, 1995.

26. United States Department of Agriculture, Agriculture Research Service. Data tables: Results from USDA's 1994–96 Continuing Survey of Food Intakes by Individuals and 1994–96 Diet and Health Knowledge Survey. USDA, ARS, Beltsville Human Nutrition Research Center, Riverdale, MD; December 1997. <http://www.barc.usda.gov/bhnrc/foodsurvey/home.htm>. March 1, 2002.

27. Institute of Medicine, Food and Nutrition Board, Dietary Reference Intakes for Vitamin A, Vitamin K, Arsenic, Boron, Chromium, Copper, Iodine, Iron, Manganese, Molybdenum, Nickel, Silicon, Vanadium and Zinc, National Academy Press, Washington, D.C., 2001.

28. Cogswell, M.E., Ramakrishnan, U., Iron supplement use among women: Science, policy and practice, Conference on Dietary Supplement Use in Women, Current Status and Future Directions, Washington, D.C.: January 28-29, 2002.

29. Bothwell, T.H., Baynes, R.D., MacFarlane, B.J. and MacPhail, A.P., Nutritional iron requirements and food iron absorption, *J. Intern. Med.*, 226, 357, 1989.

30. Cook, J.D., Dassenki, S.A. and Lynch, S.R., Assessment of the role of nonheme iron availability in iron balance, *Am. J. Clin. Nutr.*, 54, 717, 1991.

31. Hallberg, L., Brune, M. and Rossander L., Iron absorption in man: ascorbic acid and dose-dependent inhibition by phytate, *Am. J. Clin. Nutr.*, 49, 140, 1989.

32. Morck, T.A. and Cook, J.D., Factors affecting the bioavailability of dietary iron, *Cereal Foods World*, 26, 667, 1981.

33. Gillooly, M., Bothwell, T.H., Torrance, J.D., MacPhail, A.P., Derman, D.P., Bezwoda, W.R., Mills, W. and Charlton, R.W., The effects of organic acids, phytates and polyphenols on the absorption of iron from vegetables, *Br. J. Nutr.*, 49, 331, 1983.

34. Siegenberg, D., Baynes, R.D., Bothwell, T.H., Macfarlane, B.J., Lamparelli, R.D., Car, N.G., MacPhail, P., Schmidt, U., Tal, A. and Mayet, F., Ascorbic acid prevents the dose-dependent inhibitory effects of phenols and phytates on nonheme iron absorption, *Am. J. Clin. Nutr.*, 53, 537, 1991.

35. Hallberg, L., Brune, M. and Rossander L., Effect of ascorbic acid on iron absorption from different types of meals. Studies with ascorbic acid given in different amounts with different meals, *Ann. Nutr. Appl. Nutr.*, 40A, 97, 1986.

36. Charlton, R.W. and Bothwell, T.H., Iron absorption, *Ann. Rev. Med.*, 34, 55, 1983.

37. MacPhail, P. and Bothwell, T.H., The prevalence and causes of nutritional iron deficiency anemia, in *Nutritional Anemias*, Fomon, S.J. and Zlotkin, S., Eds., Nestle Nutrition Workshop Series, Vol. 30, Nestec and Raven Press, New York, 1992, 1.

38. Institute of Medicine, Food and Nutrition Board, Dietary Reference Intakes: Applications in Dietary Assessment, National Academy Press, Washington, D.C., 2000.

39. Hallberg, L., Iron balance in pregnancy, in *Vitamins and Minerals in Pregnancy and Lactation*, Berger, H., Ed., Raven Press, New York, 1988, 115.

40. Cook, J.D., Skikne, B.S. and Reussner, M.E., Estimates of iron sufficiency in the U.S. population, *Blood*, 68, 726, 1986.

41. Bothwell, T.H., Charlton, R.W., Cook, J.D. and Finch, C.A., *Iron Metabolism in Man*, Blackwell, Oxford, 1979, 21.

42. American Academy of Pediatrics, The American College of Obstetricians and Gynecologists, *Guidelines for Perinatal Care*, 4th ed., American Academy of Pediatrics, Elk Grove Village, IL, 1997.

43. Centers for Disease Control and Prevention, Recommendation to prevent and control iron deficiency in the United States, *Morbid. Mort. Wkly. Rep.*, 47(RR-3), 1998.

44. Chanarin, I. and Rothman, D., Further observations on the relation between iron and folate status in pregnancy, *Br. Med. J.,* 2, 81, 1971.

45. Svanberg, B., Arvidsson, B., Norrby, A., Rybo, G. and Sölvell, L., Absorption of supplemental iron during pregnancy — A longitudinal study with repeated bone-marrow studies and absorption measurements, *Acta Obstet. Gynecol. Scand. Suppl.*, 48, 87, 1976.

46. Puolakka, J., Jänne, O., Pakarinen, A. and Vihko, R., Serum ferritin as a measure of stores during and after normal pregnancy with and without iron supplements, *Acta Obstet. Gynecol. Scand. Suppl.*, 95, 43, 1980.

47. Taylor, D.J., Mallen, C., McDougall, N. and Lind, T., Effect of iron supplementation on serum ferritin levels during and after pregnancy, *Br. J. Obstet. Gynecol.*, 89, 1011, 1982.

48. Romslo, I., Haram, K., Sagen, N. and Augensen, K., Iron requirements in normal pregnancy as assessed by serum ferritin, serum transferrin saturation and erythrocyte protoporphyrin determinations, *Br. J. Obstet. Gynaecol.*, 90, 101, 1983.

49. Wallenburg, H.C.S. and van Eijk, H.G., Effect of oral iron supplementation during pregnancy on maternal and fetal iron status, *J. Perinat. Med.*, 12, 7, 1984.

50. Dawson, E.B. and McGanity, W.J., Protection of maternal iron stores in pregnancy, *J. Reprod. Med.*, 32, 478, 1987.

51. Hallberg, L., Högdahl, A.M., Nilsson, L. and Rybo, G., Menstrual blood loss — a population study. Variation at different ages and attempts to define normality, *Acta Obstet. Gynecol. Scand.*, 45, 320, 1966.

52. Cole, S.K., Billewicz, W.Z. and Thompson, A.M., Sources of variation in blood loss, *J. Obstet. Gynaecol. Brit. Commonwealth*, 78, 933, 1971.

53. Göltner, E., Iron requirement and deficiency in menstruating and pregnant women, in *Iron Metabolism and Its Disorders*, Kief, H., Ed., Exerpta Medica, Amsterdam, 1975, 159.

54. Nicol, B., Croughan-Minihane, M., Kilpatrick, S.J., Lack of value of routine postpartum hematocrit determination after vaginal delivery, *Obstet. Gynecol.*, 90, 514, 1997.

55. ACOG, Postpartum Hemorrhage, educational bulletin Number 243, January, 1998, American College of Obstetricians and Gynecologists. *Int. J. Gynaecol. Obstet.*, 61, 79, 1998.

56. Lao, T.T., Lee, C., Mak, W., Postpartum anemia is not related to maternal iron status in the third trimester, *Eur. J. Obstet. Gynecol. Reprod. Biol.,* 64, 7, 1996.
57. Oppenheimer, L.W., Sherriff, E.A., Goodman, J.D., Shah, D., James, C.E., The duration of lochia, *Br. J. Obstet. Gynaecol.,* 93, 754, 1986.
58. Visness, C.M., Kennedy, K.I., Ramos, R., The duration and character of postpartum bleeding among breastfeeding women, *Obstet. Gynecol.,* 89, 159, 1997.
59. World Health Organization Task Force on Methods for the Natural Regulation of Fertility, The World Health Organization multinational study of breastfeeding and lactational amenorrhea IV, Postpartum bleeding and lochia in breastfeeding women, *Fertil. Steril.,* 72, 441, 1999.
60. Cronin, T.M., Influence of lactation upon ovulation. *Lancet,* 2, 422, 1968.
61. Kava, H.W., Klinger, H.P., Molnar, J.J., Romney, S.L., Resumption of ovulation postpartum, *Am. J. Obstet. Gynecol.,* 102, 122, 1968.
62. Lyon, R.A. and Stamm, M.J., The onset of ovulation during the puerperium, *Calif. Med.,* 65, 99, 1946.
63. Bodnar, L.M., Scanlon, K.S., Freedman, D.S., Siega-Riz, A.M., Cogswell, M.E., High prevalence of postpartum anemia among low-income women in the United States, *Am. J. Obstet. Gynecol.,* 185, 438, 2001.
64. Bodnar, L.M., Siega-Riz, A.M., Miller, W.C., Cogswell, M.E., McDonald T., Who should be screened for postpartum anemia? An evaluation of current recommendations, *Am. J. Epidemiol.,* 156, 10, 903, 2002.
65. Rockey, D.C. and Cello, J.P., Evaluation of the gastrointestinal tract in patients with iron-deficiency anemia, *New Engl. J. Med.,* 329, 1691, 1993.
66. Sjostedt, J.E., Manner, P., Nummi, S., Ekenved, G., Oral iron prophylaxis during pregnancy: A comparative study on different dosage regimens, *Acta. Obstet. Gynecol. Scand. Suppl.,* 50, 3, 1977.
67. Cook, J.D. and Finch, C.A., Assessing iron status of a population, *Am. J. Clin. Nutr.,* 32, 2115, 1979.
68. Herbert, V., Everyone should be tested for iron disorders, *J. Am. Diet. Assoc.,* 92, 1501, 1992.
69. Baynes, R.D., Iron deficiency, in *Iron Metabolism In Health and Disease,* Brock, J.H., Halliday, J.W., Pippard, M.J., Powell, L.W., Eds., WB Saunders, London, 1994, 189.
70. Cook, J.D., Garriaga, M., Kahn, S.G., Schalch, W. and Skikne, B., Gastric delivery system for iron supplementation, *Lancet,* 335, 1136, 1990.
71. Zlotkin, S., Arthur, P., Antwi, K.Y., Yeung, G., Treatment of anemia with microencapsulated ferrous fumarate plus ascorbic acid supplied as sprinkles to complementary (weaning) foods, *Am. J. Clin. Nutr.,* 74, 791, 2001.
72. Galloway, R., Supplies, Side Effects or Psychology? Determinants of Compliance with Iron Supplementation in Pregnancy, World Bank, Washington, D.C., 1991, p. 1.
73. Subar, A.F., Krebs-Smith, S.M., Cook, A., Kahle, L.L., Dietary sources of nutrients among US adults, 1989-91, *J. Am. Diet. Assoc.,* 98, 537, 1998.
74. Hallberg L., Iron balance in pregnancy and lactation, in *Nutritional Anemias,* Fomon S.J. and Zlotkin S., Eds., Nestle Nutrition Workshop Series, Vol. 30, Nestec Ltd., Raven Press, Ltd., New York, 1992, 13.
75. Hurrell, R.F., Prospects for improving the iron fortification of foods, in *Nutritional Anemias,* Forman, S.J. and Zlotkin, S., Eds., Nestle Nutrition Workshop Series, Vol. 30, Nestec and Raven Press, New York, 1992, 193.

76. Olsson, K.S., Vaisanen, M., Konar, J., Bruce, A., The effect of withdrawal of food iron fortification in Sweden as studied with phlebotomy in subjects with genetic hemochromatosis, *Euro. J. Clin. Nutr.*, 51, 782, 1997.

77. Institute of Medicine, *Iron Deficiency Anemia: Recommended Guidelines for the Prevention, Detection and Management among U.S. Children and Women of Child-bearing Age*, Earl, R. and Woteki, C. E., Eds., National Academy Press, Washington, D.C., 1993, 1.

78. Senti, F.R. and Pilch, S.M., Eds., Assessment of the Folate Nutritional Status of the U.S. Population Based on Data Collected in the Second National Health and Nutrition Examination Survey, 1976-1980, Life Sciences Research Office, Federation of American Societies for Experimental Biology, Bethesda, MD, 1984. 1.

79. Centers for Disease Control and Prevention, Folate status in women of childbearing age — United States, 1999, *Morbid. Mortal. Wkly. Rep.,* 49, 962, 2000.

80. Shojania, A.M., Folic acid and vitamin B_{12} deficiency in pregnancy and in the neonatal period, *Clin. Perinatol.*, 11, 433, 1984.

81. Bailey, L.B., Mahan, C.S. and Dimperio, D., Folacin and iron status in low-income pregnant adolescent and mature women, *Am. J. Clin. Nutr.*, 33, 1997, 1980.

82. Savage, D. and Lindenbaum, J., Anemia in alcoholics, *Medicine*, 65, 322, 1986.

83. Institute of Medicine, *Dietary Reference Intakes For Thiamin, Riboflavin, Niacin, Vitamin B_6, Folate, Vitamin B_{12}, Pantothenic Acid, Biotin and Choline*, National Academy Press, Washington, 1998.

84. Lindenbaum, J., Rosenberg, I.H., Wilson, P.W.F., Stabler, S.P. and Allen, R.H., Prevalence of cobalamin deficiency in the Framingham elderly population, *Am. J. Clin. Nutr.*, 60, 2, 1994.

85. Pennypacker, L.C., Alen, R.H., Kelly, J.P., Matthews, L.M., Grigsby, J., Kaye, K., Lindenbaum, J., Stabler, S.P., High prevalence of cobalamin deficiency in elderly outpatients, *J. Am. Geriatr. Soc.*, 40, 1197, 1992.

86. Carmel, R. and Johnson, C.S., Racial patterns in pernicious anemia: Early age at onset and increased frequency of intrinsic-factor antibody in black women, *New Engl. J. Med.*, 298, 647, 1978.

87. Centers for Disease Control, Recommendations for the use of folic acid to reduce the number of cases of spina bifida and other neural tube defects, *Morb. Mortal. Wkly. Rep.*, 41 (RR-14), 1992.

88. Czeisel, A.E. and Dudas, I., Prevention of the first occurrence of neural tube defects by periconceptional vitamin supplementation, *New Engl. J. Med.*, 327:1832, 1992.

89. MRC Vitamin Study Research Group, Prevention of neural tube defects, *Lancet,* 338, 131, 1991.

90. Scholl, T.O., Hediger, M.L., Schall, J.I., Khoo, C., Fisher, R.L., Dietary and serum folate: Their influence on the outcome of pregnancy, *Am. J. Clin. Nutr.,* 63, 520, 1996.

91. Tamura, T., Goldenberg, R.L., Freeberg, L.E., Cliver, S.P., Cutter, G.R., Hoffman, H.J., Maternal serum folate and zinc concentrations and their relationships to pregnancy outcome, *Am. J. Clin. Nutr.*, 56, 365, 1992.

92. Ueland, P.M., Refsum, H., Beresford, S.A.A., Vollset, S.E., The controversy over homocysteine and cardiovascular risk, *Am. J. Clin. Nutr.*, 72, 324, 2000.

93. Lindenbaum, J., Healton, E.B., Savage, D.G., Brust, J.C.M., Garrett, T.J., Podell, E.R., Marcell, P.D., Stabler, S.P. and Allen, R.H., Neuropsychiatric disorders caused by cobalamin deficiency in the absence of anemia or macrocytosis, *New Engl. J. Med.*, 318, 1720, 1988.

94. Healton, E.B., Savage, D.G., Brust, J.C.M., Garrett, T.J. and Lindenbaum, J., Neurologic aspects of cobalamin deficiency, *Medicine*, 70, 229, 1991.

95. Herbert, V. and Das, K.C., Folic acid and vitamin B_{12}, in *Modern Nutrition in Health and Disease*, 8th ed., Shils, M.E., Olson, J.A. and Shike, M., Eds., Lea & Febiger, Philadelphia, 1994, 402.

96. Chanarin, I., *The Megaloblastic Anemias*, 3rd ed., Blackwell Scientific, Oxford, 1990.

97. Beck, W. S., Megaloblastic anemias, in *Cecil Textbook of Medicine*, 18th ed., Wyngaarden, J.B. and Smith, L.H., Eds., W.B. Saunders Co., Philadelphia, 1988, 900.

98. Alaimo, K., McDowell, M.A., Briefel, R.R., Bischof, A.M., Caughman, C.R., Loria, C.M. and Johnson, C.L., Dietary intake of vitamins, minerals and fiber of persons ages 2 months and over in the United States: Third National Health and Nutrition Examination Survey, Phase 1, 1988-91, Advance Data from Vital and Health Statistics, No. 258, National Center for Health Statistics, Hyattsville, MD, 1994.

99. Lewis, C.J., Crane, N.T., Wilson, D.B., Yetley, E.A., Estimated folate intakes: Data updated to reflect food fortification, increased bioavailability and dietary supplement use, *Am. J. Clin. Nutr.*, 70, 198, 1999.

100. Gregory, J.F., Bioavailability of folate, *Eur. J. Clin. Nutr.*, 51, S54, 1997.

101. Sauberlich, H.E., Kretsch, M.J., Skala, J.H., Johnson, H.L. and Taylor, P.C., Folate requirement and metabolism in nonpregnant women, *Am. J. Clin. Nutr*, 46, 1016, 1987.

102. Halsted, C.H., Intestinal absorption of dietary folates, in *Folic Acid Metabolism in Health and Disease*, Picciano, M.F., Stokstad, E.L.R. and Gregory, J.F., III, Eds., Wiley-Liss, New York, 1990, 23.

103. Cunningham, F.G., MacDonald, P.C., Grant, N.F., *Williams Obstetrics*, Appleton & Lange, Norwalk, CT, 1989.

104. Herbert, V. Anemias, in *Clinical Nutrition*, 2nd ed., Paige, D., Ed., C.V. Mosby, St. Louis, 1988, 593.

105. Schilling, R.F., Intrinsic factor studies II. The effect of gastric juice on the urinary excretion of radioactivity after oral administration of radioactive vitamin B_{12}, *J. Lab. Clin. Med.*, 42, 860, 1953.

106. Rose, M., Vitamin B_{12} deficiency in Asian immigrants [letter], *Lancet*, 2, 681, 1976.

107. Chanarin, I., Malkowska, V., O'Hea, A-M., Rinsler, M.G. and Price, A.B., Megaloblastic anemia in a vegetarian Hindu community, *Lancet*, 2, 1168, 1985.

108. Gibson, R.S., *Principles of Nutritional Assessment*, Oxford University Press, New York, 1990.

109. Herbert, V., Making sense of laboratory tests of folate status: Folate requirements to sustain normality, *Am. J. Hematol.*, 26, 199, 1987.

110. Hillman, R.S., McGuffin, R. and Campbell, C., Alcohol interference with the folate enterohepatic cycle, *Trans. Assoc. Am. Physicians*, 90, 145, 1977.

111. Shojania, A.M., Hornady, G.J., Barnes, P.H., The effect of oral contraceptives on folate metabolism, *Am. J. Obstet. Gynecol.*, 111, 782, 1971.

112. Smith, J.L., Goldsmith, G.A., Lawrence, J.D., Effect of oral contraceptive steroids on vitamin and lipid levels in serum, *Am. J. Clin. Nutr.*, 28, 371, 1975.

113. Rhode, B.M., Cooper, B.A., Farmer, F.A., Effect of orange juice, folic acid and oral contraceptives on serum folate in women taking a folate-restricted diet, *J. Am. Coll. Nutr.*, 2, 221, 1983.

114. Tisman, G. and Herbert, V., B_{12} dependence of cell uptake of serum folate: an explanation for high serum folate and cell folate depletion in B_{12} deficiency, *Blood*, 41, 465, 1973.

115. Allen, R.H., Human vitamin B_{12} transport proteins, *Prog. Hematol.*, 9, 57, 1975.

116. Das, K.C. and Herbert, V., *In vitro* DNA synthesis by megaloblastic bone marrow, effect of folates and cobalamin on thymidine incorporation and de novo thymidylate synthesis, *Am. J. Hematol.*, 31, 11, 1989.

117. Allen, R.H., Stabler, S.P., Savage, D.G. and Lindenbaum, J., Diagnosis of cobalamin deficiency. I. Usefulness of serum methylmalonic acid and total homocysteine concentrations, *Am. J. Hematol.*, 34, 90, 1990.

118. Lindenbaum, J., Savage, D.G., Stabler, S.P. and Allen, R.H., Diagnosis of cobalamin deficiency. II. Sensitivity of serum cobalamin, methylmalonic acid and total homocysteine concentrations, *Am. J. Hematol.*, 34, 99, 1990.

119. Food and Drug Administration, Food standards: Amendments of standards of identity for enriched grain products to require addition of folic acid, *Fed. Re.g.*, 61, 8781, 1996.

120. Romano, P.S., Waitzman, N.J., Scheffler, R.M., Pi, R.D., Folic acid fortification of grain, *Am. J. Pub. Hlth.*, 85, 667, 1995.

121. Lawrence, J.M., Chiu, V., Petitti, D.B., Fortification of foods with folic acid, *New Engl. J. Med.*, 343, 970, 2000.

122. Lawrence, J.M., Petitti, D.B., Watkins, M., Umekubo, M., Trends in serum folate after food fortification, *Lancet*, 354, 915, 1999.

123. Caudill, M.A., Thia, L., Sheniz, M.A., Esfahani, S.T., Cogger, E.A., Folate status in women of childbearing age residing in southern California after folic acid fortification, *J. Am. Coll. Nutr.*, 20 (2 suppl), 129, 2001.

124. Honein, M.A., Paulozzi, L.J., Mathews, T.J., Erickson, J.D., Wong, L.C., Impact of folic acid fortification of the US food supply on the occurrence of neural tube defects, *J. Amer. Med. Assoc.*, 285, 2981, 2001.

125. Selhub, J., Jacques, P.F., Bostom, A.G., Wilson, P.W., Rosenberg, I.H., Relationship between plasma homocysteine and vitamin status in the Framingham study population. Impact of folic acid fortification, *Pub. Hlth. Rev.*, 28, 117, 2000.

126. Bower, C., Wald, N.J., Vitamin B_{12} deficiency and the fortification of food with folic acid, *Eur. J. Clin. Nutr.*, 49, 787, 1995.

127. Oakley, G.P. Jr., Let's increase folic acid fortification and include vitamin B_{12}, *Am. J. Clin. Nutr.*, 65, 1889, 1997.

128. Savage, D.G. and Lindenbaum, J., Folate-cobalamin interactions, in *Folate in Health and Disease*, Bailey, L.B. Ed., Marcel Dekker, New York, 1995, 237.

129. Rasmussen, S.A., Fernhoff, P.M., Scanlon, K.S., Vitamin B_{12} deficiency in children and adolescents, *J. Pediatr.*, 138, 10, 2001.

12 Diet and Osteoporosis

John J.B. Anderson

CONTENTS

I. INTRODUCTION

The major concern about the skeleton for women is a fracture, especially fractures of the proximal femur (hip) in old age. The gains of bone mass, however, occur early in life — within the first 15 to 20 years or so. Therefore, if a woman is to accrue an optimal amount of skeletal mass, she needs to start early, i.e., within the first decade, but not many young girls are able to think ahead six or seven decades and make appropriate behavior changes. In this sense, females are placed in a catch-22 situation. The only obvious ways to overcome this potentially adverse scenario is to consume optimal amounts of nutrients *and* to be physically active in sports, dance, or other activities that place strains (forces) on the skeleton while the bones are most plastic. Aside from heredity, these two variables probably have the greatest impacts on the skeleton when it is most susceptible to gains in mass and to establishing microarchitectural quality of bone tissue. Osteoporosis results from declines in bone mineral content (BMC) or bone mineral density (BMD) and from deterioration of the microarchitectural structure (and stability) of bone tissue.

This chapter reviews the following topics:

- The etiology of osteoporosis
- The structural aspects of bone tissue
- The nutrient needs for growth and maintenance of the skeleton throughout the life cycle

The two current thrusts of osteoporosis prevention are the use of nutrition to enhance early life skeletal development, i.e., optimize peak bone mass, and the use of drugs in combination with additional nutrients to maintain bone later in life. These two segments of the life cycle provide the focus of this review.[1-3]

II. DEFINITIONS

Definitions of selected terms used in this chapter are given in relation to changes of bone across the life cycle.

Bone   a mineralized tissue containing an organic matrix (osteoid) that forms hydroxyapatite crystals.

Bone as a tissue   mature bone tissue exists as cancellous (trabecular) and cortical (compact) tissue in the *same* bone.

Bone as an organ   individual bones, e.g., femur and 4th lumbar vertebra that make up the skeleton.

Bone measurements using dual-energy x-ray absorptiometry (DXA)   DXA devices used to measure bone parameters permit good diagnostic precision of patients with osteopenia or osteoporosis by assessing bone mass or density of the entire skeleton or of regions of interest.

Bone mass or bone mineral content (BMC)   BMC is measured in units g/cm for a planar cross-section of bone at a given site.

Bone density (BMD)   planar or areal bone density in g/cm^2 is calculated by dividing BMC by the length of the bone site being measured.

Bone modeling   the development (building) of a bone from a genetic program; osteoblasts that form bone dominate over osteoclasts that degrade (resorb) bone.

Bone remodeling   the restructuring of a bone (or tissue) after the cessation of growth that occurs throughout adulthood, including late life; the normal sequence is activation of the osteoclasts, which degrade bone, and then osteoblastic formation of new bone to replace what was lost during resorption; in older individuals, the amount of new bone is typically not sufficient to replace all the bone lost, which results in a net decrement of both bone mass and density.

Bone turnover   the rates of resorption by osteoclasts and formation by osteoblasts that result in a net gain or loss or no change in bone mass or density; the rates of resorption and formation vary throughout the life cycle, being higher during the early growth phases and lower after this period, until the pre-menopause and early menopausal years when turnover increases again; bone turnover markers are used to assess the rates of activities of bone cells.

Fracture   the event of a fracture, whatever the cause.

Minimal trauma (fragility) fracture   fracture that results from minor trauma, such as from falling, coughing or other activities

Traumatic fracture   fracture that results from a large external force (strain), such as being thrown from a horse or banged in an auto accident or other high-impact collision.

Osteopenia   low bone density (between 1.0 and 2.5 standard deviations (SDs) below the healthy mean BMDs); a precedent of osteoporosis.

Osteoporosis   low bone density (>2.5 SDs below the mean BMDs for healthy young adults); also characterized by poor bone quality at the microscopic level.

Primary osteoporosis of Type I and Type 2   classes of osteoporosis related to low or deficient gonadal hormones (Type I) or ages of late life (Type 2); postmenopausal osteoporosis (Type I); senile osteoporosis (Type 2).

Secondary osteoporosis   osteoporosis associated with drug therapy or another disease.

Idiopathic osteoporosis   osteoporosis of unknown etiology.

Peak bone mass (PBM) and density (PBD)   the greatest amount of bone mass (mineral content) or density at any time during the lifecycle; typically PBM is achieved by age 30, although most bone mass accrues by age 18 in females and age 22 in males; PBM is achieved by about age 16 by both females and males.

III. EPIDEMIOLOGY OF OSTEOPOROSIS

Multiple factors contribute to the development of osteoporosis, but it remains that too much resorption of bone tissue results over time in first osteopenia (too little bone mass) and later osteoporosis (too little bone mass plus microarchitectural deterioration). World Health Organization (WHO) definitions of osteopenia (between 1.0 and 2.5 SDs below the mean of healthy 20–29 year olds by DXA measurement) and osteoporosis (>2.5 SDs) are used now to determine the bone status of postmenopausal women. Because of the greater average longevity of women, more fractures are occuring, but the age-adjusted rates in the U.S. are remaining fairly constant. The same is considered to hold for developed nations, but not for developing nations, where the rates of osteoporotic fractures are rising.[4]

IV. MULTIPLE RISK FACTORS FOR OSTEOPOROSIS

"Risk factor" typically means a variable that has a deleterious effect on the host (individual), but it also includes the flip-side meaning, a positive effect. Variable, a neutral term for a positive or negative risk, is often employed instead of the term risk factor.

The causation or etiology of osteoporosis is complex; many variables may contribute to low bone mass, low bone density, and microanatomic deterioration of bone tissue.[5] A variety of inherited and acquired factors, therefore, serve as determinants of osteoporosis. Some of the most common risk factors are summarized in Sections V and VI. Osteoporosis results when too much bone resorption occurs, too little formation exists, or a combination of both coexists. Two major types of osteoporosis have been established (Table 12.1).

A common cause of increased bone resorption (often termed "Type 1" osteoporosis) results from the estrogen deficiency associated with menopause in normal women. An early menopause is associated with increased risk for osteoporosis since the woman will likely live to approximately 80, but her postmenopausal life will be extended by additional years or decades, which increases her odds of having a hip fracture. Accelerated bone loss continues for about 10 years after menopause at a rate of close to 2% per year, then the rate of decline subsides to near the rate that exists for normal aging, i.e., 1% per year. Thus, an 80-year-old woman who had a "normal" menopause at age 50 would have lost approximately 40–50% of her skeletal mass over the 30-year period. Type 2 osteoporosis, which is associated with late life, is common in both men and women. Table 12.1 distinguishes between Types 1 and 2 osteoporosis.

Table 12.2 shows the approximate changes — gains or losses — in bone mass over the life cycle of a woman. Both types of osteoporosis that occur after approximately age 50 (or the menopause) result in bone loss, whereas bone gain or maintenance accompanies the years before menopause. A similar pattern occurs for men, except that the major loss phase begins after age 60 years or later. The early life gains of bone and the later life losses are illustrated in Figure 12.1.

Estrogen replacement in the postmenopausal period reduces the rate of resorption and stabilizes bone mass so that little loss occurs. Men with hypogonadism have accelerated bone loss similar to that of postmenopausal women. Other conditions that cause increased bone resorption include hyperparathyroidism and hyperthyroidism.

Age-related bone loss (also known as "Type 2" osteoporosis) is characterized by low rates of bone formation. This type of osteoporosis affects both men and women. Although the causation of age-related bone loss is poorly understood, it may be related to decreased intestinal absorption of calcium. Other factors besides advanced age that may cause impaired bone formation include exposure to certain drugs, such as glucocorticoids, and immobilization or lack of mechanical stress on bone itself.

Genetic factors undoubtedly play a major role in determining both the peak bone mass of young adults and the rate of bone loss in older individuals. In population-based studies, natural variations (polymorphisms) in genes for the vitamin D receptor, the estrogen receptor and for type I collagen matrix protein all appear to affect bone mass.

V. NONDIETARY RISK FACTORS FOR OSTEOPOROSIS

In addition to hereditary determinants, several nondietary factors are involved in the determination of osteoporosis. These are: thinness with low lean body mass (LBM); cigarette smoking; excessive alcohol consumption; insufficient physical activity;

TABLE 12.1
Major Types of Osteoporosis

	Type 1	Type 2
Period	Postmenopausal	Senescent or senile
Gender	Female[a]	Female and male
Bone Tissue	Cancellous	Cortical and cancellous
Fractures	Vertebrae and wrist[b]	Hips, vertebrae, other sites
Etiology	Loss of estrogens[c] (ovarian)	Declining activity, falls, other

[a]Rarely, males with low gonadal activity

[b]Proximal forearm — radius or ulna

[c]Natural or surgical menopause and amenorrhea from any cause

TABLE 12.2
Changes in Bone Mass across the Life Cycle of Females: The Approximate Quantitative Changes, Gains or Losses of Bone Mass

Age (years)	Years Relative Gain,%	Relative Loss,%
0–8	45	—
8–16	45	—
17–30	10	—
30–50[a]	—	0–5
50–60[b]	—	10–20
60–80[c]	—	20–30
Totals	100%	30–55%

[a] Menopause is assumed to begin at approximately 50 years of age, but some bone loss may occur in the decade prior to menopause.

[b] Bone loss in the first postmenopausal decade is related to Type I osteoporosis.

[c] Bone loss in the later decades is related to Type 2 osteoporosis.

drug usage, including over-the-counter and prescription; declines of sensory perceptions, especially visual; and falls, typically associated with poor balance. Other variables may also contribute to osteoporosis, but these seven nondietary risk factors are the most common.

VI. DIETARY RISK FACTORS FOR OSTEOPOROSIS

In addition to adverse environmental and lifestyle factors, numerous dietary factors may also have adverse effects on skeletal tissue. These deleterious factors are thought to operate throughout the life cycle, not just during late life. The major

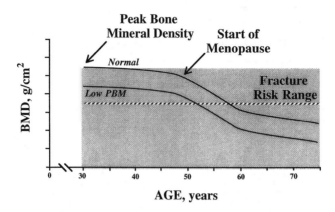

FIGURE 12.1 Early Gains and Later Losses of Bone. Adapted from Anderson, J.J.B. and Garner, S.C., Eds. *Calcium and Phosphorus in Health and Disease*. CRC Press, Boca Raton, FL, 1995.

variables are as follows: low calcium intake; high phosphorus intake (most of life); low vitamin D intake; High vitamin A intake; high animal protein, which generates an acid load; high salt (sodium) intake, especially from snack foods; vegetarian (vegan) dietary pattern; and poor diet in general (see below).

Recommendations of nutrient intakes for bone health have been prepared by the Food and Nutrition Board of the Institute of Medicine (1997), but mean (or median) intakes are generally below the recommendations for several nutrients, including calcium, vitamin D and magnesium.[6] Table 12.3 lists the recommended intakes of calcium (and other nutrients critical for bone health).

TABLE 12.3
Recommended Intakes of Calcium and Other Bone-Related Nutrients

Age, Years	Calcium mg/d AI	Phosphorus mg/d RDA	Magnesium mg/d RDA		Vitamin D mg/d AI	Fluoride mg/d AI	
			M	F		M	F
1–3	500	460	80		5	0.7	
4–8	800	500	130		5	1.1	
9–13	1300	1250	240	240	5	2.0	2.0
14–18	1300	1250	410	360	5	3.2	3.9
19–30	1000	700	400	310	5	3.8	3.1
31–50	1000	700	420	320	5	3.8	3.1
51–70	1200	700	420	320	10	3.8	3.1
>70	1200	700	420	320	15	3.8	3.1

Source: Food and Nutrition Board, 1997
AI = Adequate Intake
RDA = Recommended Dietary Allowance

VII. BONE AS TISSUE AND ORGAN

The skeleton consists of many bones, such as the femur, which serve different roles as organs. In addition, each individual bone contains two types of bone tissue: trabecular (cancellous) and cortical (compact). Trabecular tissue is the more metabolically active because it has approximately 8–10 times greater total surface area than a similar mass of cortical tissue. These surfaces are almost totally covered by bone cells, including osteoblasts and osteoclasts. Osteoblasts are responsible for new bone formation and osteoclasts are involved in resorption of existing bone. Each specific bone contains both types of bone tissue, but the proportions of each tissue type are different. For example, long bones, such as the femur, contain mostly cortical bone tissue, but relatively much more trabecular tissue exists at either end, e.g., near the hip joint or knee joint; a much greater proportion of cortical bone is found in the shaft that connects the two ends. For the lumbar vertebrae, a common site of fractures, trabecular bone is located within much of the body of each vertebra, whereas more cortical bone is located in the outer shell, i.e., just beneath the periosteal surface. This distinction between types of bone tissue is important because most fractures occur where metabolically active trabecular bone tissue predominates.

The chemical nature of bone tissue consists of an organic matrix, made primarily of collagen fibers and mineral, formed as hydroxyapatite crystals that associate in a unique way with the matrix. The synthesis of matrix proteins requires the same cell organelles and metabolic pathways as in most other cells of the body, but mineralization requires primarily calcium and inorganic phosphate for the formation of calcium hydroxapatite. Both matrix formation and mineralization occur within osteoblasts. Further maturation of molecules also occurs in the extracellular matrix.

VIII. NUTRITION, BONE DEVELOPMENT AND BONE CONSOLIDATION

The development of bones (organs) early in life involves the process of modeling, i.e., formation first and resorption second, as the bones enlarge and re-shape during growth. Bone mass accrues as a result of this process. The late-life changes in bone involve re-modeling, i.e., resorption followed by formation, which usually results in a loss of bone mass because the formation never generates enough bone to equal what is lost in resorption.

In early life, during the growth phases of the skeleton, bone acquisition through new bone formation dominates.[7-9] This phase represents the making of the skeletal model, i.e., modeling, and it typically ends by 16–18 years in females and 18–22 years in males. Modeling is characterized by greater formation than resorption and results in a net gain of bone mass or BMC by the end of the growth phase. Modeling is completed at the end of linear growth. In remodeling of the skeleton, resorption of bone equals formation. In this phase, the net amount of bone mass remains fairly constant, though some modest gain may still occur until the mid

20s or beyond. At the end of the modeling phase, fusion of the epiphyses of the long bones causes cessation of growth in length. By age 30, most individuals have achieved maximum bone mass that will serve as a "healthy norm" for the rest of life. Beyond age 30, a very slow loss of bone mass typically occurs with normal aging. In the definitions of osteopenia and osteoporosis, the mean bone density measurements of a population of 20- to 29-year-old males or females are taken as the standards of comparison for determining whether osteoporosis is present later in life.

Bone consolidation in early adult life, possibly as late as 30 years, means that the skeleton has practically finished adding mineral so that peak bone mass (PBM) is fully achieved. (Peak bone density is typically achieved by ages 15–16 or by the end of puberty in girls.) BMC and BMD values remain fairly constant until the 40s, when estrogen production begins to decline. If an early menopause (surgical or other) occurs, the woman would need a bone-conserving drug to help maintain her bone mass and density.

In late life, i.e., after the menopause in women and a decade or so later in men, imbalances in the remodeling of the skeleton result in more rapid bone losses, so that reductions in BMC and BMD occur. The loss of estrogens after menopause and probably the later decline of androgens in both women and men contribute to the increase in resorption, the reduction of formation, or both. The increase in resorption is triggered by increased activity of osteoclasts, and the decline in formation is directly related to decreased activity of osteoblasts. An increase in bone turnover, i.e., increased rates of resorption and formation with resorption dominating formation, greatly accelerates the rate of bone loss. Most individuals are slow or moderate losers of bone, while only a small fraction are "fast losers." Bone turnover is assessed by measurement of chemical markers of degraded matrix proteins, such as collagen, resulting from bone resorption and of hormones, especially parathyroid hormone, involved in calcium homeostasis.

Nutritional needs during the early phases of the life cycle are typically not met by diets of young girls because of poor food choices, including sodas containing phosphoric acid.[10,11] By age 11 years in the U.S., the mean intakes for calcium begin to fall substantially below the recommended amounts. Figure 12.2 shows the disparities between mean calcium intakes and the recommended amounts (Adequate Intakes or AIs) for women across the life cycle.[12] Adequate calcium intakes, either from foods or a combination of foods and supplements, support the accumulation of bone mass and maximize skeletal health.[7,9] Vitamin D is also important early in life to assure adequate calcium absorption, especially when calcium intake is low. The adaptational role of this vitamin as a hormone has probably been under appreciated (see sections below).

Physical activity early in life is now considered to be the more important contributor to bone mass accrual during bone development than calcium,[13–18] although having adequate amounts of calcium is still essential for the gains in bone mass.[19–22] Pre-adolescent girls (and boys) with poor bone development are thought to be at increased risk for fractures, especially when calcium intakes are not adequate.[23] A high phosphate intake relative to calcium has also been implicated as a risk factor for fractures in adolescents.[24]

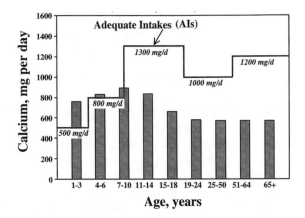

FIGURE 12.2 Disparities between Mean Calcium Intakes and AIs of Females across the Life Cycle. Data from USDA, Household Food Consumption Survey of Food Intakes of Individuals (HFCS II).

IX. NUTRIENT NEEDS FOR BONE HEALTH DURING EARLY POSTMENOPAUSE

The first 5–10 years following the menopause, e.g., from 50 to 60 years of age, women undergo a high rate of bone loss, i.e., approximately 2% per year. The loss of estrogens is so powerful that adding extra quantities of nutrients, such as calcium and vitamin D supplements, to the diet has little effect on the retention of calcium, as indicated by measurements of bone mass or density.[25]

Good nutrition and physical activity practices typically are not sufficient to prevent bone loss during this period of adjustment to the loss of ovarian estrogens. Drug therapy may be necessary for practically all women (see below).

X. NUTRITION AND BONE MAINTENANCE IN LATE LIFE

The changes in the skeleton over the life cycle reflect early-life gains and late-life losses. When the losses become sufficient to deteriorate to the state of osteoporosis, an individual becomes at risk of fragility fractures of bones such as the lumbar vertebrae and proximal femur (hip). The hip fractures are the most severe and debilitating and many individuals never recover.

Undernutrition of practically all nutrients among the elderly may promote continuous loss of lean body mass, especially muscle and bone mass, because of the body's need for more energy, protein and other nutrients. A decline in caloric intake — with accompanying deficits of micronutrients — is especially common in individuals with very little physical activity in daily life. Too little protein of high quality, including practically all animal products, may also contribute to the loss of lean body mass and skeletal mass. In essence, elderly individuals need to maintain reasonable activities each day so that they have better appetites and consume greater

amounts of total energy and protein. Such a higher intake also provides more of the essential micronutrients, i.e., vitamins and minerals, as well.

Nutritional needs of the elderly remain varied, as during other phases of the life cycle. Calcium, vitamin D and other bone-related nutrients need to be consumed in sufficient amounts, as recommended (DRIs). An important role for additional calcium, as a supplement, is that the serum calcium has an inhibitory effect on the secretion of parathyroid hormone by the parathyroid glands. The actual amount of total calcium — from both diet and supplements — may not need to exceed 1000 mg a day if physical activity is at good level and diet, in general, is good. In reality, most elderly women find it difficult to consume much more than 500 mg a day because of low total caloric intakes. Low vitamin D intakes are also common among the elderly and deficiency seems to be widespread among elderly shut-ins. Even phosphorus intakes may become so low that bone mineralization may be compromised. In general, low-energy intakes almost certainly assure inadequate intakes of calcium, vitamin D and other bone-requiring nutrients. Under this low-energy scenario, nutrient supplements are required.

Nutritional needs of women later in life also are important,[26] but, for a variety of reasons, even high calcium intakes may be less beneficial than is desirable.[27] One of the main reasons for this statement is that the relative elevation of parathyroid hormone in older age can be suppressed only in part by additional dietary calcium, especially in supplements, that meets or exceeds the AI.[28]

Two major supplement studies using calcium and vitamin D have conclusively shown improved BMD in elderly women[29–30] and in men;[30] a reduction in nonvertebral fractures was highly significant in the women over age 80.[29] The results of these two studies[29–30] suggest that many elderly have insufficient intakes of calcium and vitamin D from foods, low sunlight exposure for skin biosynthesis of vitamin D and little or no use of supplemental nutrients.

Drug therapy, therefore, has become a much more significant approach for the secondary prevention of osteoporosis following the menopause. The use of hormone replacement therapy (or simply estrogen replacement therapy) has declined greatly because of the fear of breast cancer, even though estrogens may still have important bone-conserving effects following the menopause.[31] Beyond a decade or so of the menopause, other drugs have become the main tools to prevent osteoporosis. For example, bisphosphonates and selective estrogen receptor modulators (SERMs) are now prescribed, often in combination, for the prevention of bone loss by postmenopausal women. These drugs and also estrogens are recommended along with 500–1000 mg of calcium and 400–800 IU of vitamin D so that any new bone formation will have sufficient calcium for mineralization. Intermittent parathyroid hormone, a new drug not yet approved by the FDA, holds great promise for the prevention and treatment of postmenopausal osteoporosis because it increases new bone formation.

XI. SUMMARY AND CONCLUSIONS

The IOM recommendations for the bone-related nutrients across the life cycle, as shown in Table 12.3, are as well considered and balanced as possible with our current knowledge. Yet these recommendations reflect an incomplete understanding of the

requirements of several nutrients critical for bone health, especially for vitamin D. Several other nutrients, especially trace minerals, have less well established but potentially important roles in bone development or maintenance or both, even though their quantitative needs and allowances (DRIs) may be low. Much remains to be learned about many of the specific nutrients required for optimal bone health across the life cycle. Our knowledge of a few of the critical nutrient–bone linkages, such as the connection between excessive vitamin A and hip fractures in the elderly,[32] has been advanced by epidemiological investigations. Laboratory and clinical investigators have also made important contributions to our knowledge base because of the clues of linkages found by epidemiological investigations. Finally, specific drug therapies, accompanied by calcium and vitamin D supplements, have been found to be much more effective in reducing bone losses than nutrient supplements alone. Nevertheless, adequate amounts of nutrients still are needed to maintain both the matrix and mineral phases of bone tissue, whether in conjunction with drug therapy or not. Because the consumption of bone-conserving drugs is becoming an increasing phenomenon among postmenopausal women and men in the U.S., care needs to be taken to assure that the elderly also take nutrient supplements for bone maintenance.

The major concern regarding osteoporosis is the high prevalence of hip fractures that result in late life from low bone mineral density. Women who reach their 80s are at high risk of a hip fracture, or even a second fracture, because of low BMD that is typically associated with microarchitectural defects of the proximal femur. The morbidity and mortality relating to hip fractures is very high at the superannuated ages. Technologically advanced societies, which are both westernized and urbanized, are now feeling the crunch of hip fractures and demand for hospital beds, but implementation of preventive strategies remain abysmal. Women need to take greater control of their own fates to prevent or delay osteoporosis.

REFERENCES

1. Anderson, J.J.B. and Garner, S.C., Eds. *Calcium and Phosphorus in Health and Disease*. CRC Press, Boca Raton, FL, 1995.
2. Weaver, C. Calcium, in *Present Knowledge of Nutrition*, 8th ed., Bowman, B.A. and Russell, R.M., Eds., ILSI Press, Washington, D.C., 300, 2001.
3. Anderson, J.J.B., Sell, M.L., Garner, S.C. and Calvo, M.S. Phosphorus, in *Present Knowledge of Nutrition*, 8th ed., Bowman, B.A. and Russell, R.M., Eds., ILSI Press, Washington, D.C., 300, 2001.
4. Riggs, B.L. and Melton, L.J., III. The worldwide problem of osteoporosis: Insights afforded by epidemiology. *Bone,* 17, 505s, 1995.
5. Riggs, B.L. and Melton, L.J., III. Involutional osteoporosis. *New Engl J Med*, 314, 1676–1686, 1986.
6. Committee on Dietary Allowances, Institute of Medicine. *Dietary Reference Intakes for Calcium, Phosphorus, Magnesium, Vitamin D and Fluoride*. National Academy Press, Washington, D.C., 1997.
7. Bonjour, J.P., Theintz, G., Buchs, B., Slosman, D. and Rizzoli, R. Critical years and stages of puberty for spinal and femoral bone mass accumulation during adolescence. *J Clin Endocrinol Metab*, 73, 555–563, 1991.

8. Bachrach, L. Acquisition of optimal bone mass in childhood and adolescence. *Trends Endocrinol Metab,* 12, 22–28, 2000.

9. Anderson, J.J.B. Calcium requirements during adolescence to maximize bone health. *J Am Coll Nutr,* 20, 1–6, 2001.

10. Harnack, L., Stang, J. and Story, M. Soft drink consumption among U.S. children and adolescents: Nutritional consequences. *J Am Diet Assoc,* 99, 436–441, 1999.

11. Cavadini, C., Siega-Riz, A.M. and Popkin, B.M. U.S. adolescent's food intake trends from 1965–1996. *Arch Dis Childh,* 83, 18–24, 2000.

12. USDA, Agricultural Research Service. Household Consumption Survey of Food Intakes of Individuals (HCSFII). Washington, D.C., 1995.

13. Welten, D.C., Kempner, H.C.G., Post, G.B., van Mechelen, W., Twisk, J., Lips. P. and Teule, G.J. Weight-bearing activity during youth is a more important factor for peak bone mass than calcium intake. *J Bone Miner Res,* 9, 1089–1096, 1994.

14. Bass, S., Pearce, G., Bradney, M., Hendrich, E., Delmas, P.D., Harding, A. and Seeman, E. Exercise before puberty may confer residual benefits in bone density in adulthood: Studies in active prepubertal and retired female gymnasts. *J Bone Miner Res,* 13, 500–507, 1998.

15. Wosje, K.S., Binkley, T.L., Fahrenwald, N.L. and Specker, B.L. High bone mass in a female Hutterite population. *J Bone Miner Res,* 15, 1429–1436, 2000.

16. Anderson, J.J.B. Exercise, dietary calcium and bone gain in girls and young adult women. *J Bone Miner Res,* 15, 1437–1439, 2000.

17. Specker, B. Are activity and diet really important for children's bones? *Nutr Today,* 37 (No. 2), 44–49, 2002.

18. Tylavsky, F.A., Anderson, J.J.B., Talmage, R.V. and Taft, T.N. Are calcium intakes and physical activity patterns during adolescence related to radial bone mass of white college-age females? *Osteopor Int,* 2, 232–240, 1992.

19. Cadogan, J., Eastell, R., Jones, N. and Barker, M.E. Milk intake and bone mineral acquisition in adolescent girls: Randomized, controlled intervention trial. *Br Med J,* 315, 1255–1258, 1997.

20. Bonjour, J.P., Carrie, A.L., Ferrari, S., Clavien, H., Slosman, D., Theintz, G. and Rizzoli, R. Calcium-enriched foods and bone mass growth in prepubertal girls: A randomized, double-blind, placebo-controlled trial. *J Clin Invest,* 99, 1287–1294, 1997.

21. Teegarden, D., Lyle, R.M., McCabe, G.P., McCabe, L.B., Proulx, W.R., Michon, K., Knight, A.P., Johnston, C.C. and Weaver, C.M. Dietary calcium, protein and phosphorus are related to bone mineral density in young women. *Am J Clin Nutr,* 68, 749–754, 1998.

22. Abrams, S.A. and Stuff, J.E. Calcium metabolism in girls: Current dietary intakes lead to low rates of calcium absorption and retention during puberty. *Am J Clin Nutr,* 60, 739–746, 1994.

23. Goulding, A., Cannan, R., Williams, S.M., Gold, E.J., Taylor, R.W. and Lewis-Barned, N.J. Bone mineral density in girls with forearm fractures. *J Bone Miner Res,* 13, 1143–148, 1998.

24. Wyshak, G. and Frisch, R.E. Carbonated beverages, dietary calcium, the dietary calcium/phosphorus ratio and bone fractures in girls and boys. *J Adolesc Health,* 15, 210–215, 1994.

25. Dawson-Hughes, B., Dallal, G.E., Krall, E.A., Sadowski, L., Sahyoun, N. and Tannenbaum, S. A controlled trial of the effect of calcium supplementation on bone density in postmenopausal women. *New Engl J Med,* 332, 878–885, 1990.

26. Heaney, R.P. Calcium needs of the elderly to reduce fracture risk. *J Am Coll Nutr,* 20, 192S–197S, 2001.

27. Anderson, J.J.B. and Sjoberg, H.E. Dietary calcium and bone health in the elderly: Uncertainties about recommendations. *Nutr Res,* 21, 263–268, 2001.

28. McKane, W.R., Khosla, S., Egan, K.S., Robins, S.P., Burritt, M.F. and Riggs, B.L. Role of calcium intake in modulating age-related increases in parathyroid function and bone resorption. *J Clin Endocrinol Metab,* 81, 1699–1706, 1996.

29. Chapuy, M.C., Arlot, M.E., Duboeuf, F., Brun, J., Crouzet, B., Arnaud, S., Delmas, P.D. and Meunier, P.J. Vitamin D3 and calcium to prevent hip fractures in elderly women. *New Eng J Med,* 327, 1637–1642, 1992.

30. Dawson-Hughes, B., Harris, S.S., Krall, E.A. and Dallal, G.E. Effect of calcium and vitamin D supplementation on bone density in men and women 65 years of age or older. *New Eng J Med,* 337, 670–676, 1997.

31. Women's Health Initiative Investigators. Risks and benefits of estrogen plus progestin in healthy postmenopausal women: Principal results from the Women's Health Initiative randomized controlled trial. *JAMA,* 288, 321–333, 2002.

32. Anderson, J.J.B. Oversupplementation of vitamin A and osteoporotic fractures in the elderly: To supplement or not to supplement with vitamin A. *J Bone Miner Res,* 17, 1359–1361, 2002.

13 Nutritional Issues of Cardiovascular Disease in Women

Dorothy Klimis-Zacas, Anastasia Z. Kalea and Ira Wolinsky

CONTENTS

I. INTRODUCTION

Over the last decades there has been recognition of the differences that occur among men and women with regard to the function of the cardiovascular system. Epidemiological data and clinical findings have suggested many differences, as far as the physiology of cardiovascular disease (CVD) is concerned.

Until recently, women were excluded from epidemiological studies because:

- The results would be confounded by women's cyclical hormonal changes.
- The study populations would be less homogenous.
- The sex-specific hypotheses or analyses require larger and more costly studies.
- Legal and ethical issues surmount potential risk to a fetus.
- Recruitment of women is more difficult.[1]

As a result, physicians do not have adequate information on which to base clinical decisions and these must be made by using data and knowledge that are based on studies that include mostly men. Recently, with the establishment of the Office of Research on Women's Health by the National Institute of Health, inclusion of females in studies has increased. Female subjects have only been between a fifth and a quarter of the cohort in most of the trials. Thus, the findings of these studies are too recent to affect the national policies of disease prevention and the therapeutic procedures.[2]

Despite the enormous expenditures in the U.S. on CVD prevention programs, heart disease still remains the first — and stroke the third — cause of death for the last 50 years.[3] The fact that the prevalence of CVD in women has been decreasing at a much slower rate than in men suggests that the prevention of the same CVD risk factors is not as effective for both genders. It is very important that future trials focusing on therapeutic procedures recruit sufficient numbers of women to allow meaningful conclusions to be drawn.[2,3]

II. EPIDEMIOLOGY

Heart disease and stroke are the most common causes of death from CVD for U.S. women.[4,5] In the vital health statistics data, collected in 1991 by the National Center for Health Statistics, 474,653 women died from CVD, which represents 45.3% of all deaths among women. Unfortunately, the focus of CVD research on males has given the impression that CVD is basically a male affliction, yet it is the leading cause of death among American women.[4,6–12] Furthermore, it is a misapprehension that coronary heart disease (CHD) is a male issue, a mistaken belief that stems from the fact that the manifestations of the disease are delayed in women when compared with men.[13] The causes for this delay remain a matter of debate, but are probably related to the beneficial effects of endogenous sex steroid hormones, particularly estrogens, in premenopausal females.[2]

Although overall mortality for CVD has decreased, the decline has been greater for men than for women.[5,6] Additionally, CHD and stroke still rank first and third as the causes of death for older and middle aged women. With each decade of life the death rate from CVD increases three- to fivefold.[7] Although women develop heart disease about 10 years later than men, the average 55-year-old woman can have the same risk of a heart attack as the average 55-year-old man.[7] Compared with men, women generally have a lower referral rate, more advanced disease at the time of diagnosis, poorer prognosis [12] and are more likely to receive less aggressive treatment.[6–8,14–17] Specific CVD manifestations, such as congestive heart failure with systolic dysfunction, have increased prevalence in women compared with men, especially in older women.[18]

In the Rochester Epidemiology Project, it was reported that women experienced 51% of the total number of heart disease deaths and 71% of these deaths were attributed to CVD. Postmortem examination indicated higher prevalence and severity of atherosclerosis in the female population than in the male population. Additionally, the decline in heart disease mortality for men was higher than the decline for women (4.2% vs. 2.5% per year, from 1979 to 1994).[19] Women seem to worry less about their cardiovascular health or to identify their symptoms as stress related.[20]

The occurrence of clinical manifestations of CVD increases suddenly when examining the geographic patterns of heart disease mortality. CVD rates for both men and women are higher in the southern U.S. states, while death rates from CVD are higher in the Mid-Atlantic states (New York, New Jersey, Pennsylvania, Kentucky and West Virginia). The western mountain states rank in the lowest quartile for both genders.[21] In spite of the observed decline in heart disease and stroke on a national level in the U.S. in the last years, there was no improvement in risk factors for the female population in several states.[22] Risk factors such as unhealthy dietary choices and physical inactivity still need to be eliminated since they have a direct effect on CVD mortality and morbidity.[23] Different statistics between men and women by geographic area are essential for designing intervention programs.

Diabetes is associated with high risk of CVD complications, particularly among women. Black women compared with white women are reported to be more physically inactive and obese, having high blood pressure and lower prevalence of high non-HDL cholesterol (HDL-C), all risk factors for CVD.[24] Mexican-American women, especially those who speak Spanish at home, appeared to be less likely to ask for treatment for diabetes, less willing to lose weight or comply with the doctor's recommendations to receive medication for the treatment of hypertension or hypercholesterolemia.

III. RISK FACTORS

A variety of risk factors for CVD have been identified in women.[25,26] Risk factors for definite coronary disease for women included glucose intolerance, elevated systolic or diastolic blood pressure, cigarette smoking, increased total serum cholesterol (TSC) and low-density lipoprotein levels (LDL-C), decreased high-density lipoprotein cholesterol levels (HDL-C) and deprivation of estrogen after natural or surgical menopause.[27–29]

A. GENDER-RELATED FACTORS AND CARDIOVASCULAR DISEASE RISK

It is generally agreed that genetic factors are important determinants of CVD risk in both men and women.[30–33] In the Framingham Study, the presence of Apo-E4 allele had a stronger effect in increasing LDL-C levels in females compared with males.[34] The Nurses' Health Study Cohort [35] reported that women who had a parental history of myocardial infarction prior to age 50 were five times more likely to develop CVD. It is interesting that the survival after the acute manifestation of symptoms of cardiomyopathy in women is higher than men's.[36] Although the underlying pathophysiological processes are similar for both sexes, there are differences in the functional and pharmacodynamic characteristics of the vessels, due to the different hormonal profile of females, which affects their cardiovascular electrophysiology and the vascular responses.[37–39]

Clinical manifestations of the disease and its end points appear significantly later in women, although they might demonstrate subclinical symptoms for a long time.[40] Cardiovascular disease manifestations are extremely rare in premenopausal women but increase after menopause, which suggests that the reason for this sex-related delay in the expression of vascular disease may be largely attributable to the actions of endogenous estrogens.[13] Estrogens are reported to have a favorable impact on plasma lipids and platelets, while they preserve endothelium-mediated vasodilatation, having antioxidant effects at the same time.[41] Women who have used hormone replacement therapy (HRT) but not oral contraceptives have a lower risk for CVD manifestations (e.g., aneurismal subarachnoid hemorrhage), suggesting an etiologic role of estrogens in the pathogenesis of hemorrhage.[42]

In midlife, significant increases in absolute risk for CVD occur as women experience menopause. The changes in lipids are more substantial between the premenopausal and beginning-postmenopausal year than between the first and fifth postmenopausal years.[43] Estrogen replacement therapy in postmenopausal women is associated with a 15% lowering of LDL-C and an increase in HDL-C of the same extent, especially of the protective HDL-2 fraction. Estrogens lower the levels of Lp(a), but, at the same time, they might increase TG levels and the proportion of the small more atherogenic LDL-C particles.[2,44] As a result, endogenous female hormones also affect qualitative characteristics of lipoproteins, such as their size. It has been reported that premenopausal women have larger LDL particles than do postmenopausal women or men.[45] In the Healthy Women's Study, the increase in LDL-C levels from baseline was twice as great in the women who became menopausal compared with controls. Combining the alterations in HDL-C and LDL-C only, these changes are equal to a 25% increase in CVD risk.[46] Hypertension, dyslipidemia, smoking, insulin resistance, age, family history, obesity and physical inactivity, all of the traditional CVD risk factors seem to be as important risk factors for women as for men.[2]

Very often, certain risk factors might affect women differently from men. Low levels of HDL-C, hypertriglyceridemia, diabetes and hyperuricemia appear to be stronger risk factors for women than for men.[26,47–54] Obesity and sedentary lifestyle are also important risk factors of CVD in women,[55–57] while all types of exercise seem to reduce CVD risk.[58] Truncal obesity (waist:hip ratio) has also been recently recognized as a risk factor for CVD in women.[59] Untreated diseases such as diabetes, polycystic ovary syndrome or other endocrine disorders may also increase CVD risk.[60]

Other risk factors associated with the changing role(s) of women in society deal with several psycho-social factors [61] that include type A behavior,[62] suppressed anger,[63] stress, tension and anxiety, [20,64] working in clerical jobs,[65] subordinate status,[66] social isolation and loneliness,[67] being unmarried,[68] bereaved[69]or childless,[70,71] or having more than six pregnancies.[72] Higher levels of depression, fatigue and exhaustion have also been associated with increased risk for CVD.[73] Recent studies [74] indicate that employment in middle-aged women resulted in significantly lower TSC and fasting plasma glucose than in unemployed women. Finally, lower levels of education[75,76] and low socioeconomic status in the Project-Monitoring of Cardiovascular disease (MONICA)[77] were associated with higher incidence of CVD and higher fatal coronary events in women.

B. DIET RELATED RISK FACTORS

1. Hyperlipidemia

About one third of women in the U.S. and 50% of women older than 55 years of age are hypercholesterolemic.[47] Lowering the concentration of TSC and LDL-C decreases the risk of CVD in men.[46,78] However, in women, it is the concentration of HDL-C that protects against coronary deaths.[48,79]

The lipoprotein concentrations between men and women are different over the life span.[45,80] In childhood, LDL-C and HDL-C levels are similar. Beginning at puberty, HDL-C levels fall in boys, while LDL-C levels are maintained into old age. Premenopausal women have lower TSC, higher HDL-C and lower LDL-C than men of the same age.[2,81] The difference in HDL-C resides principally in the HDL-2 subclass, the fraction most strongly associated with atherosclerosis.[82] Longitudinal data from the Framingham Heart Study report that TSC levels increase in women following menopause [82] except for women who take exogenous estrogens,[2] coming primarily from an increase in LDL-C levels,[83] high HDL-3 subfraction [84] and triglycerides and decreased concentration of HDL-2 cholesterol. High-density lipoprotein cholesterol levels increase slightly with age in both sexes and are higher in both white and black women ages 45 to 65 years than in men.[85] Premature cardiovascular disease in women is associated with additional risk factors, whereas atherosclerosis in men is primarily associated with simple hypercholesterolemia. Additionally, the accumulation of lipoprotein in women is greater when insulin effectiveness is impaired.[44]

The same observations are made for apolipoprotein A-I (Apo-A-I).[2,86] Women as a group have lower LDL-C and apolipoprotein B (Apo-B) levels than do men in midlife. After the age of 55 years, women's levels of LDL-C and Apo-B exceed those of men.[87] With increasing age, triglyceride (TG) levels increase in women and remain stable in men.[45,88] The Apo B:Apo A-I ratio after age adjustment is lower in premenopausal women, intermediate in postmenopausal women and higher in men.[83] These changes after menopause are associated with increased incidence of CVD.[85] It has been reported that the LDL particle size distribution in premenopausal women is skewed toward larger particles as compared with men, who have more symmetrical distribution.[45,89] Smaller LDL particle size has been associated with increased risk of CVD.[90,91] Thus, the premenopausal female profile is cardioprotective due to the hormonal background, but after menopause, all the modest hormonal changes lead to the increase in LDL-C, apo-B and Lp(a) levels.[88]

It is interesting that these changes and sex differences are observed in populations that have high CVD risk, such as in North America. Gender differences in lipoprotein levels in societies with low incidence of CVD appear to be insignificant compared with societies where CVD is a public health problem. It is questionable whether the interaction of gender with perhaps socioeconomic status is able to explain gender differences in lipoprotein profiles observed in societies with high prevalence of CVD.[82] It appears that there is also a racial difference in postmenopausal hyperlipidemia (increase in TSC and DL-C levels), since the cholesterol–coronary heart disease relationship is less prominent in postmenopausal black women than in postmenopausal white women.[47,92]

The rate of formation of vascular atherosclerotic lesions accelerates when men are 25–30 years of age and women 40–45. Even though the process of lipid accumulation and oxidation of LDL particles leading to endothelial dysfunction and plaque rupture is the same for both genders, there is a difference between men and women in the nature of the distribution of atherosclerotic plaques.[2] Women have more fatty lesions localized in the aorta than the coronary arteries.[93] Whether the gender factor affects the peripheral disposition of atherosclerotic plaques in the presence of hyperlipidemia is not known.[44]

Triglyceride (TG) levels, when associated with high TSC and low HDL-C levels, are often reported to be a risk factor in women.[45] A significant association was detected between CVD and elevated fasting TGs, as well as with the high ratio of triglycerides to HDL-C. As expected, this relationship remained statistically significant, even after adjusting for HDL-C, indicating that high fasting TG may provide valuable information about the potential of atherogenesis, particularly when low HDL-C levels co-exist.[94,95]

It seems probable that when low HDL-C levels and high TG levels are combined, there is a greater risk of CVD in women as compared with men.[47,96,97] Thus, given the greater predictive value for HDL-C in women and the higher average TSC and LDL-C at most ages, screening for CVD risk in women should be done by measuring the HDL-C and TSC levels before any diagnosis for hyperlipidemia.[98,99]

2. Obesity

Obesity is an independent risk factor for CVD in women.[100] The so-called deadly quartet includes hypertension, high TG levels, carbohydrate intolerance and high waist-to-hip ratios.[45] The increasing prevalence of overweight among U.S. citizens (BMI> $27.3 kg/m^2$ for women) is a problem especially for women, with black non-Hispanic and Mexican-origin females in the highest risk groups for diet-related mortality and morbidity.[5] High Body Mass Index (BMI) and obesity appear to increase the incidence of all CVD events in many studies.[48] The interaction of genetic and environmental factors is responsible for the formation of subcutaneous fat, fat mass and regional fat distribution, as well as for the response of increasing body weight following overfeeding and physical inactivity.[101]

In the National Heart, Lung and Blood Institute study, black females appeared to have three times higher BMI than white females, even from the age of 9–10 years old, while adiposity becomes significantly higher after 12 years of age, when they enter puberty.[102] Obesity is associated with an atherogenic lipid and lipoprotein profile in both men and women, including increases in TSC and LDL-C and decreases in HDL-C and in particular HDL2-C, and it appears to be independent of exogenous estrogen use, alcohol consumption or smoking. National surveys report that women with high BMI have TSC concentrations 189% higher than women with low BMI.[103]

Data from the Framingham and LRC prevalence studies[103] indicate that increased relative body weight is an independent risk factor for CVD and also contributes to hypertension, low HDL-C concentrations, decreased glucose tolerance and elevated plasma cholesterol and TG concentrations. Obese subjects have increased VLDL synthesis that is associated with hypertriglyceridemia, decreased plasma HDL-C and increased LDL production.[104] In the CARDIA study,[105] which included women 18–30 years of age, BMI was positively correlated with TSC and LDL-C levels and inversely correlated with HDL-C. Hormonal fluctuations in women during their lifetime (menarche, pregnancy, menstrual cycle, menopause) may increase the risk for obesity.[106]

The distribution of body fat is an additional important determinant of lipoprotein concentrations and CVD.[107,108] Women with upper-body obesity, which is a pattern usually seen in men, are more prone to diabetes and atherosclerosis than women with low-body obesity.[109–111] The waist:hip circumference is associated with adverse lipid and lipoprotein levels, is predictive of CVD and may be able to explain the sex differences observed in TG levels, HDL-C and apolipoproteins B and A-I.[112–113] The "apple-shaped" body-type, also observed in female smokers, predisposes them to CVD.[107,114]

Age plays an important role in both genders. Before and after the age of 45, the annual changes in TSC and LDL-C are correlated with annual changes in adiposity. In the Fels Longitudinal Study the correlation of BMI with changes in TSC, LDL-C, TGs and HDL-C in younger men was generally greater than in younger women, but was similar in both genders in older age.[115]

Women with normal TSC levels and body weight greater than 130% of recommended weight seem to be three times more likely to have a myocardial infarction than lean women, while the risk increases to about eight times for hypercholesterolemic women.[47] Thus, obesity is one of the factors that contribute to the increased LDL-C concentrations and weight control can improve both the lipid and the cardiovascular risk profile.

3. Hypertension

One half of white women in U.S. and almost 80% of black women older than 45 years of age are hypertensive. Black women develop more severe hypertension. Hypertension is an independent risk factor for CVD among both normotensive and hypertensive women.[116] Women aged 30–64 years with inadequately controlled blood pressure were at high CVD risk, followed by untreated hypertensives, women with adequately controlled blood pressure and normotensives. More than twice as many women as men develop hypertension after the age of 50 years.[36,47] Women are more likely than men to have hypertension and its complications, especially over the age of 65 years of age, when 70% of the female population of elderly individuals suffers from high blood pressure. In population studies of women, systolic blood pressure continues to rise until at least 80 years of age, though in men it tends to peak in middle age.[48] In both genders, control of isolated systolic hypertension lessens the risk of both stroke and fatal and nonfatal cardiovascular events.[47]

4. Glucose Intolerance and Diabetes

Almost 50% of people who die each year from diabetes and its complications are women.[118] The prevalence of diabetes and especially type 2 diabetes after the age of 45 tends to be greater in women than in men, even after adjusting for the fact that the female population is larger than the male population.[119,120] Overall, diabetes mellitus is the seventh leading cause of death in the U.S., with 61,767 deaths in 1996 attributed to severe complications of the disease such as cardiovascular and cerebrovascular disease, and men are more likely to die from diabetes than women.[5] In the Framingham Heart Study, women with diabetes mellitus were more prone to develop CVD than women without diabetes.[36]

Diabetes is associated with a three- to sevenfold elevation in CVD risk among women, compared with a two- to threefold elevation among men; the effect of diabetes on lipids and blood pressure possibly explains the observed gender differences.[36,48,121]

Hyperlipidemia is a typical and maybe more marked sign in diabetic women as compared with men. It is observed that diabetic women have higher levels of TG and VLDL compared with controls and higher levels of VLDL and LDL compared with diabetic men.[122] Finally, HDL-C levels are more severely depressed in diabetic women as compared with men in general.[44,123–125]

High oxidative and osmotic stress due to hyperglycemia in diabetes results in endothelial dysfunction of similar degree in both diabetic women and men, increasing significantly the risk of cardiovascular disease.[102,126] Falkner et al.[127] reported that black women with normal or borderline blood pressure have lower insulin sensitivity than black men. However, when this value was corrected for adiposity, in each subject, by expressing insulin-stimulated glucose utilization in mg/kg fat free mass, the gender differences disappeared.

5. Other Nutritional Factors

a. Homocysteine

Homocysteine is reported to be an independent and modifiable risk factor for CVD, affecting the atherothrombotic process. The Third National Health and Nutrition Examination Survey reported that high levels of plasma homocysteine are associated with high prevalence of nonfatal stroke.[128] Whether high hyperhomocysteinemia is an effect or a cause for acute vascular occlusion or whether it is a short-term or a long-term risk factor, are still under question.[79,129,130]

Prospective studies[131] for postmenopausal women showed that high concentrations of plasma homocysteine increase the risk of cardiovascular disease, regardless of any other coexisting CVD risk factors. Increased dietary folate was associated with lower relative risk for stroke and CVD events.[132] Supplementation with multivitamins eliminates this risk, justified by the ability of B_6, B_{12} and folic acid to reduce high concentrations of homocysteine.[129–131,133–139]

Hyperhomocysteinemia may be caused by factors such as heredity,[131] age, gender, physiological abnormalities and medications, as well as nutrition.[129] Although women usually have lower homocysteine levels than men of the same age, menopausal status is strongly related to fasting homocysteine levels. Natural menopause increases plasma homocysteine levels by 7%, which lasts from up to 4–8 years after menopause. Whether estrogens affect homocysteine levels in pre-menopausal women is still unknown.[130]

b.   Vitamins and Minerals

Low intake of fruits and vegetables, as well as low total vitamin intake in women has been associated with higher CVD risk in epidemiological studies.[140–142] Observational data from other women's studies showed that high folate and vitamin B_6 dietary intakes from food sources and supplements are associated with lower CVD risk.[143,144] There has not been much research on how the specific carotenoids are related to CVD risk. In the Antioxidant Supplementation in Atherosclerosis Prevention (ASAP) Study, it was reported that low levels of plasma lycopene in Finnish men is associated with increased thickness of arterial wall and early atherosclerosis, an association that does not exist for women.[145]

Theoretically, by scavenging free radicals, vitamin E is able to increase the resistance of the LDL molecules to oxidation. In epidemiological studies and clinical trials, the use of vitamin E supplementation was associated with a significant reduction of CVD risk, described by an increase in arterial compliance, which depicts the improvement in structural and functional properties of the artery.[146,147] In other studies on postmenopausal women, the protective effect of vitamin E was attributed only to food sources of this nutrient.[148,149]

Many associations of one or more micronutrients and trace elements with high risk of CVD events have been reported.[150–153] Low dietary potassium increased risk of stroke and low calcium intake increased risk of ischemic stroke in middle-aged American women. The relationship of dietary potassium to sodium-induced hypertension can explain its implication in the process of CVD. Studies in Belgian women revealed that protein-corrected calcium intake is associated with high TSC and HDL-C levels.[154]

Moderately excessive iron may be responsible for oxygen free radical formation, which may easily oxidize LDL-particles and form fatty streaks. As a result, there has been much interest in iron overload, which, due to cessation of menstrual blood loss after menopause, may be an important risk factor of CVD. Berge et al.[155] reported a parallel rise in serum ferritin, TC and LDL-C, which might contribute to the increased risk of CVD among postmenopausal women. In the Atherosclerosis Risk in Communities (ARIC) Study,[156] ferritin was significantly and positively correlated with BMI in both sexes and with waist:hip ratio in women. Dietary iron was independent from all indicators for LDL oxidation or from ferritin level. These findings are in accordance with other studies[40,106,157–160]that either do not support a special role of body iron stores in promoting LDL-C oxidation or suggest that more studies need to be conducted on higher numbers of female subjects. Other minerals such as magnesium deficiency may be involved in many cardiovascular disorders, such as high blood pressure and coronary heart disease.[153]

Even though observational studies are able to provide evidence for an association between a nutrient and increased incidence of a disease, randomized controlled trials are necessary to detect and describe any cause–effect association.[150,161] Studies for micronutrient and trace mineral metabolism in women are necessary to detect any differences in the physiologic pathways that might be influenced by the presence of estrogens and, thus, affect CVD risk.[145,151]

c.   Fiber

Epidemiological studies in men have shown that dietary fiber or foods rich in fiber, especially fruits, vegetables and cereal products, protect against CVD, but data on women are limited.[140] It is well known that whole grain cereal products are a main source of phytoestrogens in an average Western diet, in which soy products are not usually consumed.[162] Evidence from the Nurses' Heart Study[162] support that higher fiber intake, particularly from cereal sources, reduces the risk of CVD in middle-aged women by 34% compared with those in the lowest quartile for fiber consumption. This inverse association could not be attributed just to the higher dietary intakes of vitamin E, folate, vitamin B_6 and magnesium, nor from higher consumption of vegetables and fruits.[163] Among different sources of dietary fiber (e.g., vegetables, cereals, fruit), only cereal fiber was significantly associated with a reduced incidence of coronary death. Higher intake of whole grains in general was related just to lower risk of ischemic stroke in women.[164] Lower CVD risk with cereal fiber was strongest among nonsmoking women, eliminating the possibility that unmeasured aspects of smoking could account for the findings.[162]

IV. EFFECT OF DIET ON CARDIOVASCULAR DISEASE RISK FACTORS

A.   FAT, CHOLESTEROL AND FATTY ACIDS

Evidence suggests that blood lipid levels in women respond to dietary intervention, but not as strongly or consistently as in men. The influence of specific dietary factors including type of fat, cholesterol, fiber and carbohydrates on the process of CVD in women has not been completely defined.

Data from the 1987/88 Nationwide Food Consumption Survey indicated that women consumed approximately 37% of kilocalories from fat.[165] Fifteen to 18% of women aged 30–49 years met the recommendation for fat calories. Fourteen to 23% of women met the recommendation for saturated fatty acid calories and 70–72% of women met the recommendation for dietary cholesterol. Thus, most women don't meet the dietary recommendations set by the National Academy of Sciences and the National Cholesterol Education Program.[166,167]

High intakes of cholesterol have been associated with hypercholesterolemia in human and nonhuman primates. High intakes of total animal fat, saturated fat and dietary cholesterol were associated with increased mortality from ischemic heart disease and its complications.[168,169] In humans, high variability in their response to dietary cholesterol has been reported to result in "hyper-responders" and "hypo-responders" and postulated a genetic basis (Apo E genotype) for that response.[170] Shekelle and Stamler[171] reported that more than 12% of all CVD could be attributed to excess consumption of cholesterol. Investigators concluded that the level of dietary cholesterol has an independent serum-cholesterol-raising effect[172–176] that is exaggerated when the diet is high in saturated fat.[177]

Keys et al.,[178] working with white men, reported that the response of serum cholesterol is in proportion to baseline serum cholesterol levels. A similar relationship has also been observed in a randomized controlled dietary trial with postmenopausal women[179] and has been confirmed by studies conducted by Katan et al. with nuns in Dutch and Belgian Trappist monasteries.[180,181]

The qualitative effects of blood lipids in response to different dietary fatty acids are similar in men and women,[177] but their quantitative effects have not been adequately researched. A number of studies[182,183] have reported responses of plasma lipids in men and women fed controlled diets. Results from these studies are inconclusive since most studies have not been well controlled for factors such as sample size,[184] hormonal premenopausal status, menstrual cycle, HRT, oral contraceptive use vs. postmenopausal status,[182,185] hyperlipidemia,[186] weight loss during the study[187,188] decreasing total dietary fat[185] vs. modifying the fatty acid composition of the diet and not decreasing total dietary fat.

The first epidemiological study to examine the associations between intakes of individual saturated fatty acids and their food sources in relation to the risk for CVD, was based on the food frequency questionnaires that were completed by 80,082 women in the Nurses' Health Study in 1980, followed by a 14-year follow-up. When the intake of SFAs in women increased by 5%, there was a 17% increase in CHD risk. Total fat intake was not significantly associated with CVD risk, while intakes of longer chain fatty acids (12:0–18:0) were associated with a small but significant increase in risk.[113,186]

Epidemiological studies have shown that saturated fat raises HDL-C levels in both men and women, whereas a high polyunsaturated:saturated fatty acid (P/S) ratio decreases the HDL-C level.[189,190] Dietary cholesterol increases HDL-C, but in women only.[189] When the Food and Agricultural Organization (FAO) of the United Nations examined the relationship between fat intake and HDL-C levels using food balance sheets, the HDL-C in women significantly correlated with the intake of monounsaturated fatty acids (MUFA). Saturated fatty acids (SFA) and MUFA correlated highly with female:male HDL-C ratio. Only MUFA correlated significantly with HDL-C levels in women. Thus, significant correlations with dietary SFA and MUFA, dietary cholesterol and the female:male HDL-C ratio were observed.[191] Krummel et al.[192] reported that, in premenopausal women, SFA intake was positively related to TSC, LDL-C and HDL-C. Other studies support the relationships described above.[193,194]

Kesteloot and Sasaki[191] reported that Western women show an inborn resistance to atherosclerosis, probably attributable to their ability to increase their HDL-C on a high-in-MUFA diet. Both SFA and MUFA and dietary cholesterol increase the female:male HDL-C ratio significantly, but MUFA appears to exert the major effect. Several short-term studies [95,196] have shown that a high fat intake increases HDL2-C and Apo-A-I levels more in women than in men. A high SFA and cholesterol diet increased HDL2-C by 0.09 mmol/l in women as compared with 0.03 mmol/l in men.[195]

A gender–diet interaction likely exists in countries where fat intake is high. Women have higher HDL-C levels (8–10 mg/dl) than those of men, whereas in countries where fat intake is low, women have HDL-C levels only 4–5 mg/dl higher than those of men.[183,191] Some countries with low fat diets have lower rates of CVD and diet-induced HDL-C lowering may not confer an increase in CVD risk. A change in LDL-C:HDL-C ratio induced by a change in total fat intake may underestimate a true reduction in CVD risk. Thus, women differ from men in their lipid and lipoprotein responses to these lifestyle changes.

Denke [197]studied the effect of Step I low fat diet on 41 moderately hypercho-lesterolemic, postmenopausal women and reported significant LDL-C and TSC reductions, a nonsignificant reduction in HDL-C levels and no improvement in the LDL-C:HDL-C ratio. A decrease in HDL-C has been described in women on a diet with a high P/S ratio and low in saturated fat. Their HDL-C levels were reduced to the same level as in men. This is in agreement with epidemiologic studies showing similar HDL-C levels between men and women with low saturated fat and high P/S ratio diets.[198] It seems that, on a low fat diet, both estradiol and HDL-C levels markedly decrease in postmenopausal Western women. On a low fat diet, the estra-diol levels were halved and the HDL-C levels decreased from a mean of 55–42 mg/dl.[199] In a small cross-sectional study[189]of healthy young women and men (18–35 years of age) that examined the association between P/S ratio and serum lipid responses, it was found that the correlation between P/S ratio and LDL-C and VLDL-C concentrations was stronger for men than for women. However, in other studies, no such association was found in either men or women.[200,201]

Ernst et al.[202] studied the effect of an isocaloric diet with a high P/S ratio and low dietary cholesterol levels on normal and type II hyperlipoproteinemic women and men. In women with type II hyperlipidemia, a 9% reduction was observed in both TSC and LDL-C, while an HDL-C was reduced by 10%. Hyperlipidemic men experienced higher reductions in TSC, LDL-C and HDL-C, of 13, 11 and 25%, respectively. The greater response of men to the modified diet was also observed in normolipidemic men.

An intervention study[203] of premenopausal, normocholesterolemic women who were fed a high fat diet (40% of total calories) and were then switched to a low fat diet (20% of total calories) showed that even though there was only a 7% decrease in TSC, the HDL-C response was influenced by the P:S ratio. Women who consumed a low P:S ratio diet (1.0) showed no change in HDL-C. This is in agreement with studies conducted by Brussard et al.[204] and Weisweiler et al.[205] Thus, for healthy premenopausal women with low baseline plasma cholesterol levels, a marked decrease in intake on a weight maintenance diet is not accompanied by statistically significant changes in plasma cholesterol.

A diet rich in complex carbohydrates and olive oil is able to increase HDL-C more in healthy men than in healthy women, although TSC and LDL-C responses are similarly affected in both sexes.[182] Masarei et al.[206] placed normolipidemic men and women on a vegetarian diet and observed significant reductions in TSC, LDL-C and HDL-C in men only. Cole et al.[207] evaluated the long-term efficacy of the American Heart Association phase III diet (39% kilocalories from carbohydrates, 21% kilocalories from fat, 96 mg cholesterol and P:S = 1.8) in premenopausal women, who had moderately elevated serum cholesterol. Obese women had a smaller reduction in their TSC and reported higher TG-raising response to the above dietary modifications than did their lean counterparts. That questions whether dietary rec-ommendations are appropriate for all subgroups even in the same population.

The DELTA-1 study was designed specifically to examine the efficacy of the Step I diet and another diet with further reductions in saturated fat in pre- and postmenopausal women. It was reported that both Step I and low-saturated fatty acid diets were able to reduce TSC and LDL-C in women after 8 weeks by 9.3 and 5.5 mg/dl in the two diet groups respectively. These results agree with those reported by Denke et al.[197] for postmenopausal women. Total and LDL-C levels were reduced by 5.6% and 7.4% respectively during consumption of the Step I diet in the group of pre- and postmenopausal women. Step I and Low-SFA diets reduced HDL-C and plasma Apo-A-I concentrations in both groups, when compared with the average American diet.[208]

High PUFA diets reduce both HDL-C and LDL-C concentration.[187] The ideal diet would be one that would reduce LDL-C levels and increase HDL-C levels or keep them unchanged. Mata et al.[187] studied the effects of a diet enriched in MUFA and one enriched in PUFA for 12 weeks (37% of total energy came from fat calories) in men and premenopausal women. The MUFA diet did not change TSC levels in men, but caused a rise of 9% in women. The atherogenic index fell significantly in both sexes, without any significant changes in LDL-C or TG.

Mata et al.[184] also studied the effect of a saturated fat diet followed by a monounsaturated fat diet rich in olive oil, followed by a sunflower oil-rich diet in pre- and postmenopausal, normolipidemic women. A diet rich in MUFA not only lowered TSC and LDL-C but increased HDL-C and Apo-A-I when compared with the poly and saturated fatty acid-rich diets. These effects were independent of menopausal status. In short term dietary studies with men and premenopausal women, Mensink et al.[209] reported that, in men that followed diets enriched in MUFA or PUFA, HDL-C levels fell slightly, but not significantly, but the same pattern was not observed in women.

Trans-fatty acids increase LDL-C levels to the same extent when compared with saturated fatty acids, while at the same time they decrease HDL-C levels.[210] In a metabolic study conducted in men and women, a diet rich in transhydrogenated fatty acids levels increased Lp(a) levels in both sexes, an important CVD risk factor.[211] Metabolic and clinical studies conducted in female populations are necessary to detect the exact mechanism by which trans-fatty acids lower HDL-C levels, a significant CVD risk factor for females.[212] It is interesting to mention that if we replace 2% of the energy from trans-fatty acids with energy from nonhydrogenated, unsaturated fat, the CVD risk for women will be reduced by 53%, as reported in the Nurses' Health Study Cohort.[186]

The concentration of TSC and TG were found to be lower in fish-eating populations than in nonfish-eating.[213] When 79,839 women were followed up for 14 years, in the Nurses' Heath Study cohort, fish and omega-3 PUFA intake reduced significantly the risk of thrombotic infraction among women that ate fish two or more times per week. Women in the highest quintile of long chain omega-3 PUFA intake had reduced risk of total stroke and thrombotic infraction.[214] Fish oils seem to reduce the susceptibility of LDL-C to oxidation, while they are likely to increase the LDL molecular size.[215]

The fact that oxidative susceptibility increases with the number of double bonds in a fatty acid *in vitro* made many scientists question the real effect of higher PUFAs consumption. However, there was no evidence of increased lipid peroxidation with fish oil supplementation in postmenopausal women when they were supplemented with oleate (12.3g/d from sunflower oil), linoleate (10.5g/d from safflower oil) and both eicosapentanoic and docosahexanoic acids (2.0g/d EPA and 1.4g/d DHA from fish oil) in a three-treatment crossover trial for 5 weeks with a 7-week washout interval.[216,217] A placebo-controlled double-blind trial evaluated the effects of omega-3 fatty acid supplementation on serum lipids in postmenopausal women who were either receiving or not receiving HRT. The omega-3 fatty acid supplement used (fish-oil-derived from EPA and DHA concentrate), significantly lowered TG concentrations in both groups of women to the same extent without affecting other lipid levels. The ratio of TG:HDL-C also decreased in all subjects who took the omega-3 fatty acid supplement, but the reduction was higher in women who were not under any hormonal treatment.[218] It was estimated by the researchers that this approach could reduce the risk of CVD in postmenopausal women by 27%.

Thus, a habitual diet rich in monounsaturated fatty acids with a relatively low P:S ratio has essentially the same effects on plasma LDL-C concentration as does a diet high in polyunsaturated fatty acids. This diet also increases HDL-C concentration, which may be of greater benefit to women than men in Western countries who tend to have relatively high fat intakes.

In summary, the data suggest that dietary intake (diets of high P:S and low cholesterol) affects serum lipids and lipoprotein concentrations in women, but the magnitude of lipid reductions appears to be less than in men, with a less detrimental decrease of HDL-C in women. It may be that endogenous hormone secretion in women modifies or overrides the modifying effect on diet. Thus, since gender[219] differences exist in HDL-C response and HDL-C predicts CVD risk for women, well-controlled studies are needed to determine gender differences in dietary responsiveness and their applications to the general population of U.S. women.

B. PROTEIN

Not many women's studies concerning protein intake as related to CVD are available. As far as specific types of protein are concerned, in a Scandinavian population, animal protein from meat did not appear to be related to high CVD risk.[220] Fat derived from meat contributed a small part to the total fat intake. High consumers of meat were reported to have the same intake of atherogenic substances such as SFAs, as low consumers of meat. Dairy products were usually the main contributors of SFAs.[220]

Soy protein, which is consumed in higher amounts by Asian populations, has been found to decrease blood lipids.[221] Due to variations in human study designs, there have been controversial data on the effect of soy protein on lipoprotein profile and the exact mechanism by which it acts.[222] Compliance with the diets that contain high amounts of soy has been the main problem for all the intervention trials, especially in non-Asian populations. Studies with isolated soy protein (which does not contain isoflavones), reported that 30–50 gm of soy protein is able to decrease TSC, LDL-C and plasma homocysteine, having no effect on Lp(a).[223] Gardner et al.[224] compared soy protein with milk protein in postmenopausal, mildly hypercholesterolemic females and reported no significant lipid-lowering effects in the soy group. The mechanisms by which soy might influence lipid metabolism are under study. Genetic studies have suggested that, in genetically engineered mice, soy protein seems to have a direct effect on the process of atherosclerosis that is independent from LDL- receptor-mediated pathways and lipoprotein metabolic sequences.[225]

Although soy protein seems to have a significant lipid lowering effect, in normotensive postmenopausal women it is not always followed by an obvious immediate improvement in vascular function.[226,227] Furthermore, one of the main outcomes of soy protein supplementation of perimenopausal women was the beneficial significant increase in the total antioxidant status. Isolated soy protein increases the total plasma antioxidant concentrations in perimenopausal women, indicating a strong antioxidant effect of the soy protein moiety, which prevents oxidative stress, a CVD risk factor.[228]

In October, 1999, the U.S. Food and Drug Administration (FDA) supported the recommendation that 25g/d of soy protein, as part of a diet low in saturated fat and cholesterol, may reduce the risk for CVD.[220,227]

C. OTHER FOOD COMPOUNDS

1. Phytoestrogens

There has been increased interest over the last decade in the role of phytoestrogens in alleviating menopausal symptoms, especially after the debate and controversial data on the effect of oral contraceptives in young women and on ERT for postmenopausal women CVD risk.[228–235] Most of phytoestrogenic compounds, such as genistein, act similar to selective estrogen receptor modulators (SERMS).[236] These affect the blood vessel wall to inhibit atherosclerosis by binding to hormone receptors.[42] Thus, phytoestrogens are also likely to lower cholesterol and therefore cardiovascular risk.[237–239] The low rates of cardiovascular disease and the high intakes of dietary phytoestrogens in Asian populations, especially in women, are consistent with a potential protective effect on phytoestrogens.[221] However, many other concomitant dietary differences (e.g., low saturated fat intake in Asian populations) do not allow scientists to attribute the observed differences in disease rates to phytoestrogen intake.[238] The dispute whether it is soy protein or phytoestrogens that contribute to the beneficial effects of soy on cardiovascular health still remains unresolved.[240]

The theories that attempt to explain the effect of phytoestrogens on CVD suggest that, since these molecules inhibit the activity of cholesterol-7a-hydroxylase, the rate-limiting enzyme in the formation of primary bile acids from cholesterol, they might inhibit the endogenous cholesterol synthesis or regulate the LDL-receptor molecules.[13,238] The possible effect of phytoestrogens on lowering Lp(a), an independent risk factor of CVD, remains to be investigated.[238]

Natural estrogens are handled by the body in a similar way to ovarian estrogenic steroids. These plant-derived estrogens may exert both estrogenic and antiestrogenic effects on metabolism, depending on their type, their concentration, the concentrations of endogenous estrogens and individual characteristics, such as gender and menopausal status.[237,241]

Soy is generally considered one of the major dietary sources of the most active phytoestrogens in humans. The high content of phytoestrogens in soy might help in preventing CVD in asymptomatic postmenopausal women and replace hormonal therapies that might have negative effects on the endometrium.[242] Increase in soy consumption led to an improved ratio of TSC:HDL-C, an important risk factor for women. Soy isoflavones, unlike HRTs, do not decrease HDL-C levels.[237,243] However, when mildly hypercholesterolemic postmenopausal women were supplemented with different amounts of soy isoflavones as isolated soy protein, there was an improvement in their lipid profile, described by a decrease of TSC, LDL-C and improved LDL-C:HDL-C ratio, which was attributed just to the soy protein itself.[244] Isoflavones did not seem to have any effect at all.[245] Studies in postmenopausal women, testing the effect of phytoestrogens from other sources such as flaxseed or red clover extract, reported a small lipid lowering effect.[239]

Most of the potential health benefits of phytoestrogens, such as isoflavones, are not attributable to metabolic properties that involve estrogen receptors.[238] Genistein and daidzein, as well as their glycones, are the main isoflavones of soy products and both of them, as well as their main metabolite equal, seem to protect against the oxidative damage of membrane lipids and lipoproteins.[246] One hypothesis for their action is the possibility that they reduce the formation of lipid hydroperoxides, which are responsible for the oxidation process.[247] The reduction of cardiovascular risk that is attributed to isoflavones is important, though not related to lipid lowering mechanisms.[240] Isoflavones have significant antioxidant properties, that lower oxidative stress and reduce lipid peroxidation, while, at the same time, they increase the resistance of LDL-particles to oxidation.[247,248]

The bioavailability of different phytoestrogens and the different mechanisms of action that these molecules share in cells and tissues may explain the controversial findings of the above studies.

2. PHENOLS

Experimental and epidemiologic evidence during the last decades has documented that polyphenol antioxidants are able to prevent degenerative disease such as cancer and cardiovascular disease. Green and black tea, red wine and beer consumption, as well as olive oil have been reported to lower the risk for CVD.[249-252]

Alcohol consumption differs between genders.[48] In women, the large group of abstainers presented higher risk for CVD events, while alcohol was related with cardioprotective effect for both sexes.[253] Moderate red wine consumption, described as one to two glasses of wine per day (30g of alcohol), was able to increase HDL-C and Apo A-I, while it reduced plasma LDL-C, Apo-B and TGs in postmenopausal women who participated in an intervention study.[144,252-258] Moderate consumption of red wine or red grape juice with evening dinner had a small effect in premenopausal women using oral contraceptives, whereas in postmenopausal women, fibrinolytic activity decreased directly after alcohol consumption.[92] Moderate alcohol consumption in postmenopausal women was as beneficial as for middle-aged men, as far as the response of fibrinolytic activity is concerned.

Anthocyanins, stilbenes, flavanols and flavonols present in red wine are responsible for its antioxidant and free-radical scavenging properties.[259–263] Wine phenols not only have antioxidant properties but, additionally, they act in an indirect way, working as co-factors of selenium, vitamin E or C enzymes, thus preventing endothelial damage.[250,264–267]

Studies for tea consumption and its effect on the cardiovascular system have, so far, been inconsistent.[268,269] Tea polyphenols, present mainly in black tea, are potential inhibitors of lipoprotein oxidation and thus may be considered as cardioprotective food components. Population studies reported lower CVD risk for tea consumers.[270] However, in a Japanese population, green tea consumption was associated with a lower CVD risk for men but not for women.[269] Studies on *in vivo* or *ex vivo* lipid peroxidation, revealed a mild[270] or no effect of tea polyphenols.[268]

Polyphenols found in high concentrations in nuts might be the reason for the association of high nut consumption and lower CVD risk, as well as lower all-cause mortality.[271] Epidemiological observations, mainly in vegetarian populations, reported that nut consumption was associated with lower risk of myocardial infarction and lower death risk from ischemic heart disease. Isolated walnut polyphenolics were able to inhibit LDL oxidation *in vitro* in human plasma, thus blocking one of the main initiating pathways of atherosclerosis.[272] It is this property of nuts, in addition to their effect on the lipid profile, that increases the need for more intervention trials to detect any possible cardioprotective effect they may have.

V. PUBLIC HEALTH PROGRAMS FOR CARDIOVASCULAR DISEASE

The baseline findings of the WISEWOMAN project,[107] which included 4842 financially disadvantaged women, revealed a high prevalence of cardiovascular risk factors. High TSC was found in 40% of the women in North Carolina and Massachusetts, hypertension was found among 63% of the women in North Carolina and 83% of the women in Arizona were overweight.[107] When the 2148 women in North Carolina who participated in the program followed the intervention, which was composed of specially constructed counseling sessions spanning 6 months, beneficial changes in TSC-C levels, HDL-C, diastolic blood pressure and BMI were observed, showing that intervention was feasible among low-income women without unreasonably expensive prevention programs.[273] Thus, general dietary guidelines such as the Dietary Guidelines for Americans do not seem to be effective enough to lead women to undertake major dietary changes to minimize their CVD risk factors and optimize their health.[274] Population intervention studies focusing on lifestyle changes, such as changes in the saturated fat content of cooking fats, or increasing dietary fiber intake through nutrition education may result in decline in CVD risk factors.[275,276]

Counseling sessions with experienced dietitians or health educators can be very successful, as long as there is a long-term follow-up for the population at high risk.[277] It could be argued that intensive counseling sessions such as those used in many studies such as Trials of Hypertension Prevention Phase II (TOHP II) are not cost effective and third-party players do not reimburse them, but, in the long run, they will prove to be cost effective for the U.S. population. Community prevention programs designed primarily for female populations can produce long-standing effects on CVD-risk-factor patterns.[275] A prevention program includes action at several levels such as policy, quality of care, well-trained educators and incorporating a team approach to patient care that involves dietitians and health educators.[277,278]

Additionally, presenting consumers with better food choices by encouraging manufacturers to reformulate foods has been neglected as a policy tool in the U.S. and it should be used to formulate policy to encourage positive development of these foods.[5]

Some of the recent changes in the typical "American diet," such as dietary saturated fat reduction or higher fruit and vegetable consumption have increased the proportion of people in the U.S. or other countries that meet the average daily goals of the Dietary Guidelines for fat and saturated fat.[140] According to the review of Healthy People 2000 goals, approximately one third of the population consume less than 30% of calories from fat and less than 10% of calories from saturated fat and the number of servings of fruits, vegetables and grains has increased since the beginning of the decade, but there is still work to be done.[51,40,279,280] Obesity is seriously increasing in the U.S. and public health authorities should consider, for instance, the strong relationship of the increasing food portion size in the U.S. to caloric intake, obesity and diseases such as CVD and diabetes.[281]

VI. RECOMMENDATIONS FOR DIETARY CHANGE

In U.S. women, total fat intake decreased significantly from 1980 to 1990.[282] The consumption of fruits, vegetables, whole grains, low-fat dairy products and lean meat are associated with lower mortality from all causes and generally improve health.[283] It is impressive that nonsmoking, normal-weight, physically active females with moderate alcohol consumption have been reported in the Nurses' Health Study to have 80% lower CVD risk compared with the rest of the female population.[26,284–288]

The recently published National Institute of Public Health third report of the National Cholesterol Education Program "Adult Treatment Panel III" recommends a multifaceted lifestyle approach to reduce CVD risk. This approach is designated as therapeutic lifestyle changes (TLC) and includes reducing saturated fat intake to 7% of total calories and cholesterol to <200 mg per day, with total fat between 25–35% of total calories and monounsaturated fat up to 20% of total calories. Lowering LDL seems to be the primary target either by plant sterols or stanols (2 g/day) and increased soluble fiber (20–35 g/day). Managing weight by balancing energy intake and expenditure (regular physical activity 30 min on most days) to prevent weight gain is critical. No distinction is made in the diet therapy between men and women.[22]

Enriching the diets with monounsaturated fatty acids may be beneficial, since they do decrease HDL-C, a change observed in increased polyunsaturated fatty acid or restricted total fat kilocalorie diets. In women, the desirable level of HDL-C would be more than 45 mg/dL, to be in low risk for CVD.[120]

There is little evidence that reducing LDL-C levels in most women will reduce their CVD risk. LDL-C is not a strong predictor of CVD risk in women, as it is in men. When hypercholesterolemic women followed a Step II diet for 1 year, with further decreases in dietary saturated fat and cholesterol, there was a greater decrease in HDL-C, HDL2-C and apolipoprotein A-I levels, compared with men, while differences in LDL-C decrease were similar.[289] Since HDL-C is a stronger predictor of CVD risk in low-risk women, the present dietary advice for women needs to be reexamined.[120]

Recognizing the vulnerability of diabetic women to CVD, it is essential to control diabetes, since it puts even younger women at a higher risk.[290] The fact that women appear to be more insulin sensitive than men suggests that diabetic women are more able to succeed in controlling their blood glucose.[126,291] Recent data[253,264,292] suggest that in the therapeutic options for glucose control (weight loss, exercise and cessation of smoking), one could probably add controlled moderate alcohol consumption (preferably red wine), which is able to enhance insulin sensitivity and at the same time improve HDL-C metabolism.[293]

In the Dietary Approaches to Stop Hypertension (DASH), the increase in fruit and vegetable consumption in combination with low-fat dairy products and low-in-saturated-fat foods was very effective in regulating blood pressure and subjects showed great compliance to the diet.[294] Replacing red meat and high-fat dairy products with poultry, fish and low-fat dairy products substantially reduced the risk for CVD.[295,296] Modification of risk factors such as obesity, smoking, sedentary lifestyle and poor lipid profile should always be considered.[286,297–300] Women should follow the time-tested recommendation of reducing dietary fat to 25–30% of calories and they should maintain low intakes of saturated fat and dietary cholesterol while increasing their monounsaturated fatty acid intake.[22,294]

VII. CONCLUSION

Current therapeutic treatments of CVD are based on studies that have involved few women. This gender bias is probably enough to explain the reason that the prevalence of CVD in women has decreased in a smaller degree compared with men. Designing studies that are going to enable scientists to generalize their results to the population as a whole is warranted. Furthermore, educating the medical profession about the different manifestations of CVD in women along with the response of the blood lipid profile to different dietary treatments and medications is crucial for the progression and outcomes of CVD in women.

Even though progress has been made, more research is needed in exploring the risk factors — especially nontraditional — and setting dietary guidelines and drug treatments specifically targeted for women. Thus, the need for separate medical nutrition therapy for women is warranted.

REFERENCES

1. Kumanyika, S.K., Women and health research: Rewriting the rules, *Perspect. Appl. Nutr.*, 2, 10, 1994.
2. Maxwell, S.R.J., Women and heart disease, *Bas. Res. Cardiol.*, 93S, 79, 1998.
3. Mosca, L., Manson, J.E., Sutherland, S.E., Langer, R.D., Manolio, T. and Barrett-Connor, E., Cardiovascular disease in women: A statement for healthcare professionals from the American Heart Association, *Circulation*, 96, 2468, 1997.
4. Heart Memo, The cardiovascular health of women, special ed., National Heart, Lung and Blood Institute, National Institutes of Health, Bethesda, M.D., 1994.
5. Bush, L.M. and Williams, R.A., Diet and health: New problems, new solutions, *Food Policy*, 24, 135, 1999.
6. National Cholesterol Education Program (NCEP), Report of the Expert Panel on Population Strategies for Blood Cholesterol Reduction, N.I.H. Publ., U.S. Department of Health and Human Services, Public Health Service, National Heart, Lung and Blood Institute, National Institutes of Health, Bethesda, M.D., 3046, 1990.
7. Sempos, C.T., Cleeman, J.I., Carroll, M.D., Johnson, C.L., Bachoric, P.S., Gordon, D.J., Burt, V.L., Briefel, R.R., Brown, C.D., Lippel, K. and Rifkind, B.M. Prevalence of high blood cholesterol among U.S. adults: An update based on guidelines from the second report of the national cholesterol education program adult treatment panel, *JAMA*, 269, 3009, 1993.
8. U.S. Senate Special Committee on Aging, Aging America: Trends and Projections, U.S. Department of Health and Human Services, Washington, D.C., 1988.
9. Langer, R.D. and Barrett-Connor, E., Coronary heart disease prevention in women, *Pract. Cardiol.*, 17, 45, 1991.
10. Keil, J.E., Gazes, P.C., Loadholt, C.B., Tyrolen, H.A., Sutherland, S., Gross, A.J., Knowles, M. and Rust, P.F., Coronary heart disease mortality and its predictors among women in Charleston, SC, in *Coronary Heart Disease in Women*, Eaker, E.D., Packard, B., Wenger, N.K., Clarkson, T.B. and Tyroler, H.A., Eds., Haymarket Doyma Inc., New York, 1987.
11. Steingart, R.M., Packer, M., Hamm, P., Goglianese, M.E., Gersh, B., Geltman, E.M., Sollano, J., Katz, S., Moye, L., Basta, L.L., Lewis, S.J., Gottlier, S.S., Bernstein, V., McEwan, P., Jacobson, K., Brown, E.J., Kukin, M.L., Kantrowitz, N.E., Pfefeer, M.A., Sex differences in the management of coronary artery disease, *N. Eng. J. Med.*, 325, 226, 1991.
12. Eaker, E.D., Packard, B., Thom, T.J., Epidemiology and risk factors for coronary heart disease in women, *Cardiovasc. Clin.*, 19, 129, 1989.
13. Nagata, C., Ecological study of the association between soy product intake and mortality and heart disease in Japan, *Int. J. Epidemiol.*, 29, 832, 2000.
14. Bittner, V., Olson, M., Kelsey, S.F., Rogers, W.J., Merz, N.B., Armstrong, K., Reis, S.E., Boyette, A. and Sopko, G.: for the WISE Investigators, *Am. J. Cardiol.*, 85, 1083, 2000.
15. Smith, S.C., Clinical treatment of dyslipidemia: Practice patterns and missed opportunities, *Am. J. Cardiol.*, 86S, 62L, 2000.
16. Sueta, C.A., Chowdhury, M., Boccuzi, S.J., Smith, S.C., Alexander, C.M., Londhe, A., Lulla, A. and Simpson, R.J., Analysis of the degree of undertreatment of hyperlipidemia and congestive heart failure secondary to coronary artery disease, *Am. J. Cardiol.*, 83, 1303, 1999.
17. Danias, P.G., O'Mahony, S., Radford, M.J., Korman, L. and Silverman, D.I., Serum cholesterol levels are underevaluated and undertreated, *Am. J. Cardiol.*, 8, 1353, 1998.

18. Samuel, R.S., Hausdorff, J.M. and Wei, J.Y., Congestive heart failure with preserved systolic function: Is it a woman's disease?, *Women's Hlth. Issues*, 9, 219, 1999.

19. Calvert Finn, S., All's fair but not in diabetes: Women's unique vulnerability: Part I, *J. Women's Hlth.*, 7, 167, 1998.

20. Murray, J.C., O'Farrell, P. and Huston, P., The Experience of women with heart disease: What are their needs?, *Can. J. Public Health*, 91, 98, 2000.

21. Coronary Heart Disease In Women, A Summary of Proceedings, National Heart, Lung and Blood Institute, National Institutes of Health, Bethesda, MD, 1986.

22. National Cholesterol Education Program "Adult Treatment Panel III," National Institute of Public Health. NIH pub. No. 02-5215, Sept. 2002.

23. Kuller, L.H., Meilahn, E., Bunker, C., Yong, C., Sutton-Tyrrel, K. and Matthews, K., Development of risk factors for cardiovascular disease among women from adolescence to older ages, *Am. J. Med. Sc.*, 310S, 91, 1995.

24. Roger, V.V.L., Jacobson, S.J., Weston, S.A. and Gabriel, S.E., Sex differences and outcomes of heart disease: Population-based trends, *Lupus*, 8, 346, 1999.

25. Eaker, E.D. and Castelli, W.P., Coronary heart disease and its risk factors among women in the Framingham Study, in *Coronary Heart Disease in Women*, Eaker E.D., Packard, B., Wenger N.K., Clarkson TB and Tyroler HA, Eds., Haymarket Doyma Inc., New York, 1987, 122.

26. Burke, G.L., Arnold, A.M., Bild, D.E., Cushman, M., Fried, L.P., Neuman, A., Nunn, C., Robbins, J. for the C.H.S. Collaborative Research Group, *J. Am. Geriatr. Soc.*, 49, 254, 2001.

27. Kahn, H.S., Williamson, D.F., Stevens, F.A., Race and weight change in U.S. women: The roles of socioeconomic and marital status, *Am. J. Pub. Hlth.*, 81, 319, 1991.

28. Barrett-Connor, E. and Bush, T.L., Estrogen and coronary heart disease in women, *J. Am. Diet. Assoc.*, 265, 1861, 1991.

29. Wolk, A., Manson, J.E., Stampfer, M.J., Colditz, G.A., Hu, F.B., Speizer, F.E., Hennekens, C.H. and Willet, W.C., Long-term intake of dietary fiber and decreased risk of coronary heart disease among women, *JAMA*, 281, 1998, 1999.

30. Sundstrom, J., Lind, L., Vessby, B. Andren, B., Aro, A. and Lithell, H.O., Dyslipidemia and an unfavorable fatty acid profile predict left ventricular hypertrophy 20 years later, *Circulation*, 103, 836, 2001.

31. Mayer, E., Jacobsen, D.W. and Robinson, K., Homocysteine and coronary atherosclerosis, *J. Am. Coll. Cardiol.*, 27, 517, 1996.

32. Sklavounou, E., Economou-Petersen, E., Karadima, G., Panas, M., Avramopoulos, D., Varsou, A., Vassilopoulos, D. and Petersen, M.B., Apolipoprotein E polymorphism in Greek population, *Clin. Genet.*, 52, 216, 1997.

33. Superko, H.R., Did grandma give you heart disease? The new battle against coronary artery disease, *Am. J. Cardiol.*, 82, 34Q, 1998.

34. Schaefer, E.J., Lamon-Fava, S., Johnson, S., Ordovas, J.M., Schaefer, M.M., Castelli, W.P. and Wilson, P.W.F., Effects of gender and menopausal status on the association of apolipoprotein E phenotype with plasma lipoprotein levels: Results from the Framingham offspring study, *Arterioscler. Thromb.*, 14, 1105, 1994.

35. Colditz, G., Stampfer, M., Willett, W., A prospective study of parental history of myocardial infarction and coronary artery disease in women, *Am. J. Epidemiol.*, 123, 48, 1986.

36. Macera, C.A., Lane, M.J., Mustafa, T., Giles, W.H., Blanton, C.J., Croft, J.B. and Wheeler, F.C., Trends in mortality and health behaviors: Status of white and African-American women, *J. S.C. Med. Assoc.*, 92, 421, 1996.

37. Gandhi, S.K., Gainer, J., King, D. and Brown, N.J., Gender affects renal vasoconstrictor response to Ang I and Ang II, *Hypertension*, 31, 90, 1998.

38. Nanchahal, K., Ashton, W.D. and Wood, D.A., Association between blood pressure, the treatment of hypertension and cardiovascular risk factors in women, *J. Hypertens.*, 18, 833, 2000.

39. Reckelhoff, J.F., Gender differences in regulation of blood pressure, *Hypertension*, 37, 1199, 2001.

40. Adlercreutz, H. and Mazur, W., Phyto-oestrogens and Western diseases, *Ann. Med.*, 29, 95, 1997.

41. Cassidy, A. and Griffin, B., Phytoestrogens: A potential role in the prevention of CVD?, *Proc. Nutr. Soc.*, 58, 193, 1999.

42. Slater, C.C., Shoupe, D., Mack, W.J., Stanczyk, F.Z. and Hodis, H.N., Evaluation of baseline carotid artery intima-thickness and its progression over two years in postmenopausal women with and without intact ovaries, *Philad. Cent. Rel. Sci. Abstracts*, 75, 16S, 2001.

43. Bazzano, L.A., He, J., Ogden, L.G., Loria, C., Vupputuri, S., Myers, L. and Whelton, P.K., Dietary potassium intake and risk of stroke in U.S. men and women: National Health and Nutrition Examination Survey I – epidemiological follow-up study, *Stroke*, 32, 1473, 2001.

44. Knopp, R.H., Zhu, X. and Bonet, B., Effects of estrogens on lipoprotein metabolism and cardiovascular disease in women, *Atherosclerosis*, 110, 83S, 1994.

45. Bjorkelund, C., Lissner, L., Devine, C., Lindroos, A.K., Palm, L. and Westerstahl, A., Long-term effects of a primary health care intervention program for women: Lower blood pressure and stable weight, *Fam. Med.*, 32, 246, 2000.

46. Lipid Research Clinic Program, The lipid clinics coronary primary prevention trials results. I. Reduction in incidence of coronary heart disease, *JAMA*, 251, 351, 1984.

47. Wenger, N.K., Hypertension and other cardiovascular risk factors in women, *Am. J. Hypertension*, 8, 94S, 1995.

48. Tunstall-Pedoe, H., Woodward, M., Tavendale, R., Brook, R.A. and McCluskey, M.K., Comparison of the prediction by 27 different factors of coronary heart disease and death in men and women of the Scottish heart health study: Cohort study, *Br. Med. J.*, 315, 722, 1997.

49. Tuttle, K.R., Short, R.A. and Johnson, R.J., Sex differences in uric acid and risk factors for coronary artery disease, *Am. J. Cardiol.*, 87, 1411, 2001.

50. Thurau, R., Perceived gender bias in the treatment of cardiovascular disease, *J. Vasc. Nurs.*, 15, 124, 1997.

51. Higgins, M., Keller, J.B., Ostrander, L.D., Risk factors for coronary heart disease n women: Tecumseh community health study, 1959 to 1980, in *Coronary Heart Disease in Women*, Eaker E.D., Packard, B., Wenger N.K., Clarkson TB and Tyroler HA, Eds., Haymarket Doyma Inc., New York, 1987, 83.

52. Bush, T.L., Criqui, M.H., Cowan, L.D., Barrett-Conner, E., Wallace, R.B., Tyroler, H.A., Suchindran, C.M., Cohn, R. and Rifkind, B.M., Cardiovascular disease mortality in women, results from the Lipid Research Clinics follow-up, in *Coronary Heart Disease in Women*, Eaker E.D., Packard, B., Wenger N.K., Clarkson TB and Tyroler HA, Eds., Haymarket Doyma Inc., New York, 1987, 106.

53. Wingard, D.L. and Cohn, B.A., Coronary heart disease mortality among women in Alameda County, 1965 to 1973, in *Coronary Heart Disease in Women*, Eaker E.D., Packard, B., Wenger N.K., Clarkson TB and Tyroler HA, Eds., Haymarket Doyma Inc., New York, 99, 1987.

54. Stampfer, M.J., Colditz, G.A., Willett, W.C., Rosner, B., Speizer, F.E. and Hennekens, C.H., Coronary heart disease risk factors in women: the Nurses' Health Study experience, in *Coronary Heart Disease in Women*, Eaker E.D., Packard, B., Wenger N.K., Clarkson TB and Tyroler HA, Eds., Haymarket Doyma Inc., New York, 112, 1987.
55. Barrett-Connor, E.L., Obesity, atherosclerosis and coronary artery disease, *Ann. Intern. Med.*, 103, 1010, 1985.
56. Hubert, H.B., Feinleib, M., McNamara, P.M. and Castelli, W.P., Obesity as an independent risk factor for cardiovascular disease; A 26-year follow-up of participants in the Framingham heart study, *Circulation*, 678, 968, 1983.
57. Manson, J.E., Stampfer, M.J., Hennekens, C.H. and Willett, W.C., Body weight and longevity: A reassessment, *JAMA*, 257, 353, 1987.
58. Ballor, D.L. and Poehlman, E.T., Resting metabolic rate and coronary heart-disease risk factors in aerobically and resistance trained women, *Am. J. Clin. Nutr.*, 56, 968, 1992.
59. Kissebah, A.H., Vydelingum, N., Murray, R., Evans, D., Hartz, A., Kalkhoff, R. and Adams, P., Relation of body fat distribution to metabolic complications of obesity, *J. Clin. Endocrinol. Metab.*, 54, 254, 1982.
60. The special cholesterol concerns for women, The Johns Hopkins Medical Letter: Health after 50, 12, 4, 2000.
61. Powell, L.H., Shaker, L.A., Jones, B.A., Vaccarino, L.V., Thoresen, C.E. and Pattillo, J.R., Psychosocial predictors of mortality in 83 women with premature acute myocardial infarction, *Psychosom. Med.*, 55, 420, 1993.
62. Haynes, S.G. and Feinleib, M., The relationship of psychosocial factors to coronary heart disease in the Framingham heart study. III Eight-year incidence of coronary heart disease, *Am. J. Epidemiol.*, 111, 37, 1980.
63. Haynes, S.G. and Feinleib, M., Women, work and coronary heart disease: prospective findings from the Framingham heart study, *Am. J. Public Health*, 70, 133, 1980.
64. Matthews, K.A., Owens, J.F., Kuller, L.H., Suton-Tyrrell, K., Lassila, H.C. and Wolfson, S.K., Stress-induced pulse pressure change predicts women's carotid atherosclerosis, *Stroke*, 29, 1525, 1998.
65. Eaker, E.D., Pinsky, J. and Castelli, W.P., Myocardial infarction and coronary death among women: Psychosocial predictors from a 20-year follow-up of women in the Framingham study, *Am. J. Epidemiol.*, 135, 854, 1992.
66. Clarkson, T.B., Adams, M.R., Kaplan, J.R., Shively, C.A., Pathophysiology of coronary artery atherosclerosis: animal studies of gender differences, in *Heart Disease in Women*, Douglas P.S., Ed., F.A. Davis, Philadelphia, 1989.
67. Berkman, L.F. and Breslow, L., *Health and Ways of Living. The Alameda County Study*, Oxford University Press, New York, 1983.
68. Cottington, E.M., Matthews, K.A., Talbott, E. and Kuller, L.H., Environmental events preceding sudden death in women, *Psychosom. Med.*, 42, 567, 1980.
69. Talbott, E., Kuller, L.H., Perper, J. and Murphy, P.A., Sudden unexpected death in women — Biologic and psychosocial origins, *Am. J. Epidemiol.*, 114, 671, 1981.
70. Matthews, K.A., Kelsey, S.F., Meilahn, E.N., Kuller, L.H. and Wing, R.P., Educational attainment and behavioral and biologic risk factors for coronary heart disease in middle-aged women, *Am. J. Epidemiol.*, 129, 1132, 1989.
71. Conference on Women, Behavior and Cardiovascular disease: Task force on psychosocial factors in cardiovascular disease treatment, recovery and rehabilitation in women, National Heart, Lung and Blood Institute, Chevy Chase, MD, September, 1991.

72. Ness, R.B., Harris. T., Cobb. J., Flegal, K.M., Kelsey, J.L., Balanger, A., Stunkard, A.J. and D'Agostino, R.B., Number of pregnancies and the subsequent risk of cardiovascular disease, *N. Engl. J. Med.*, 328, 1528, 1993.

73. Chesney, M.A., Social isolation, depression and heart disease: Research on women broadens the agenda, *Psychosom. Med.*, 55, 429, 1993.

74. Kirtz-Silverstein, D., Wingard, D.L. and Barrett-Connor, E., Employment status and heart disease risk factors in middle aged women: The Rancho Bernardo study, *Am. J. Public Health*, 82, 315, 1992.

75. Winkleby, M.A., Jatulis, D.E., Frank, E. and Pertmann, S.P., Socioeconomic status and health: How education, income and occupation contribute to risk factors for cardiovascular disease, *Am. J. Public Health*, 82, 816, 1992.

76. Pitsavos, C.E., Panagiotakos, D.B., Chrysochoou, C.A., Skoumas, J., Stefanadis, C. and Toutouzas, P.K., Education and acute coronary syndromes: Results from the CARDIO2000 epidemiological study, *Bull.WHO*, 80, 371, 2002.

77. McElduff, P. and Dobson, A.J., Trends in coronary heart disease — Has the socioeconomic differential changed?, *Aust. N.Z. J. Pub. Hlth.*, 24, 465, 2000.

78. Lipid Research Clinic Program, The lipid clinics coronary primary prevention trials results. II. The relationship of reduction in incidence of coronary heart disease to cholesterol lowering, *JAMA*, 251, 365, 1984.

79. Ridker, P.M., Hennekens, C.H., Bring, J.E. and Rifai, N., C-reactive protein and other markers of inflammation in the prediction of cardiovascular disease in women, *N. Engl. J. Med.*, 342, 836, 2000.

80. La Rosa, J.C., Lipids and cardiovascular disease do the finding and therapy apply equally to men and women?, *Women's Hlth. Issues*, 20, 102, 1992.

81. Gordon, D.J., Probstfield, J.L., Garrison, R.J., Neaton, J.D., Castelli, W.P., Knoke, J.D., Jacobs, D.R., Bangdiwala, S. and Tyroler, H.A., High-density lipoprotein cholesterol and cardiovascular disease: Four prospective studies, *Circulation*, 79, 8, 1989.

82. Eaker, E.D. and Castelli, W.P., Coronary heart disease and its risk factors among women in the Framingham study, in *Coronary Heart Disease in Women*, Eaker E.D., Packard, B., Wenger N.K., Clarkson TB and Tyroler HA, Eds., Haymarket Doyma Inc., New York, 1987, 122.

83. Brunner, E.J., Marmot, M.G., White, I.R., O'Brien, J.R., Etherington, M.D., Slavin, B.M., Kearney, E.M. and Davey Smith, G., Gender and employment grade differences in blood cholesterol, apolipoproteins and hemostatic factors in the Whitehall II study, *Atherosclerosis*, 102, 195, 1993.

84. Stevenson, J.C., Crook, D. and Godsland, I.F., Influence of age and menopause on serumlipids and lipoproteins in healthy women, *Atherosclerosis*, 98, 3, 1993.

85. Seed, M., Sex hormones, lipoprotein and cardiovascular risk, *Atherosclerosis*, 90, 1, 1991.

86. Higgins, M. and Keller, J., Cholesterol, coronary heart disease and total mortality in middle-aged and elderly men and women in Tecumseh, *Ann. Epidemiol.*, 2, 69, 1992.

87. Kannel, W.B., Castelli, W.P., Gordon, T., Cholesterol in the prediction of atherosclerotic disease, *Ann. Intern. Med.*, 90, 85, 1979.

88. Bush, T.L., Barrett-Connor, E., Cowan, L.D., Criqui, M.H., Wallace, R.B., Suchindran, C.M., Tyroler, H.A. and Rifkind, B.M., Cardiovascular mortality and noncontraceptive use of estrogen in women: Results from the Lipid Research Clinics' program follow-up study, *Circulation*, 75, 1102, 1987.

89. Kannel, W.B., Castelli, W.P., Gordon, T. and Mcnamara, P.M., Serum cholesterol, lipoproteins and the risk of coronary heart disease, *Ann. Intern. Med.*, 74, 1, 1971.

90. Gordon, T., Kannel, W.B., Castelli, W.P. and Dawber, T.R., Lipoproteins, cardiovascular disease and death, *Arch. Intern. Med.*, 141, 1128, 1981.
91. Utermann, G., Menzel, H.J., Kraft, H.G., Duba, N.C., Kemmler, H.G. and Seitz, C., Lp(a)- lipoprotein concentrations in plasma, *Hum. Genet.*, 78, 47, 1988.
92. Clarkson, T.B., Soy, soy phytoestrogens and cardiovascular disease, *J. Nutr.*, 132, 566S, 2002.
93. Blankenhorn, R.H. and Hodis, H.N., Arterial imaging and atherosclerosis reversal, *J. Arterioscl. Thromb.*, 14, 177, 1994.
94. Gaziano, J.M., Hennekens, C.H., O'Donnel, C.J., Breslow, J.L. and Buring, J.E., Fasting triglycerides, high-density lipoprotein and risk of myocardial infarction, *Circulation*, 96, 2520, 1997.
95. Criqui, M.H., Heiss, G., Cohn, R., Cowan, L.D., Suchindran, C.M., Bangdiwala, S., Kritchevsky, S., Jacobs, D., O'Grady, H.K. and Davis, C.E., Plasma triglyceride level and mortality from coronary heart disease, *N. Engl. J. Med.*, 328, 1220, 1993.
96. Morena, M., Cristol, J-P., Dantione, T., Carbonneau, M-A., Descomps, B. and Canaud, B., Protective effects of high-density lipoprotein against oxidative stress are impaired in haemodialysis patients, *Nephrol. Dial. Transplant.*, 15, 389, 2000.
97. Sierksma, A., van der Gaag, M.S., Schaafsma, G., Kluft, C., Bakker, M. and Hendriks, H.F.J., Moderate alcohol consumption and fibrinolytic factors of pre- and postmenopausal women, *Nutr. Res.*, 21, 171, 2001.
98. National Center for Health Statistics, Dietary intake and cardiovascular risk factors, II. Serum urate, serum cholesterol and correlates: U.S., 1971–75, Vital and health statistics, Series 11, No 227, Department of Health and Human Services Publ. No (P.H.S.) 83–1677, Public Health Service
99. Despres, J-P., Lemieux, I., Dagenais, G-R., Cantin, B. and Lamarche, B., HDL-Cholesterol as a marker of coronary heart disease risk: The Quebec cardiovascular study, *Atherosclerosis*, 153, 263, 2000.
100. Kissebath, A.H., Freedman, D.S. and Peiris, A.N., Risks of obesity, *Med. Clin. North Am.*, 73, 111, 1989.
101. Elmstahl, S., Holmovist, O., Gullberg, B., Johansson, U. and Berglund, G., Dietary patterns in high and low consumers of meat in a Swedish cohort study, *Appetite*, 32, 191, 1999.
102. Kimm, S.Y.S., Barton, B.A., Obarzanek, E., McMahon, R.P., Sabry, Z.I., Waclawiw, M.A., Schreiber, G.B., Morrison, J.A., Similo, S. and Daniels, S.R., Racial divergence in adiposity during adolescence: The N.H.L.B.I. Growth and Health Study, *Pediatrics*, 107, 34, 2001.
103. Glueck, C.J., Taylor, H.L., Jacobs, D., Morrison, J.A., Beaglehole, R. and Williams, O.D., Plasma high-density lipoprotein cholesterol: Association with measurements of body mass. The Lipid Research Clinics Program Prevalence Study, *Circulation*, 62, 62, 1980.
104. Kesaniemi, Y.A. and Grundy, S.M., Increased low density lipoprotein production associated with obesity, *Atherosclerosis*, 3, 170, 1983.
105. Katan, M.B., Diet and HDL-C, in *Clinical and Metabolic Aspects of High-Density Lipoprotein*, Miller, N.E. and Miller, G.J., Eds., Elsevier, Amsterdam, 1984, 103.
106. Ebert, S.N., Liu, X-K. and Woosley, R.L., Female Gender as a risk factor for drug-induced cardiac arrhythmias: Evaluation of clinical and experimental evidence, *J. Womens Hlth.*, 7, 547, 1998.
107. The WISEWOMAN Workgroup, Cardiovascular disease prevention for women attending breast and cervical cancer screening programs: The WISEWOMAN Projects, *Prev. Med.*, 28, 496, 1999.

108. Larsson, B., Svardsudd, K., Welin, L., Wilhelmsen, L., Bjorntorp, P. and Tibblin, G., Abdominal adipose tissue distribution, obesity, the risk of cardiovascular disease and death: 13-year follow up of participants in the study of men born in 1913, *Br. Med. J.*, 288, 1401, 1984.

109. Anderson, A.L., Sobocinski, K.A., Freedman, D.S., Barborial, J.J., Rimm, A.A. and Gruchow, H.W., Body fat distribution, plasma lipids and lipoproteins, *Arteriosclerosis*, 8, 88, 1988.

110. Stern, M.P. and Haffner, S.M., Body fat distribution and hyperinsulinemia as risk factors for diabetes and cardiovascular disease, *Arteriosclerosis*, 6, 123, 1986.

111. Hartz, A.J., Rupley, D.C., Kalkhoff, R.D., Rimm, A.A., Relationship of obesity to diabetes: Influence of obesity level and body fat distribution, *Prev. Med.*, 12, 351, 1983.

112. Freedman, F., Jacobsen, J., Brboriak, J., Sobocinski, K. Anderson, A., Kissebah, A., Sasse, E. and Gruchow, H., Body fat distribution and male/female differences in lipids and lipoproteins, *Circulation*, 81, 1498, 1980.

113. Ryan, A., Nicklas, B., Berman, D. and Dennis, K., Dietary restriction and walking reduce fat deposition in the midthigh in obese older women, *Am. J. Clin. Nutr.*, 72, 708, 2000.

114. Hu, F.B., Stampfer, M.J., Manson, J.E., Grodstein, F., Colditz, G.A., Speizer, F.E. and Willett, W.C., Trends in incidence of coronary heart disease and changes in diet and lifestyle in women, *N. Engl. J. Med.*, 343, 530, 2000.

115. Siervogel, R.M., Wisemandle, W., Maynard, M., Guo, S., Roche, A.F., Chumlea, W.C. and Towne, B., Serial changes in body composition throughout adulthood and their relationship to changes in lipid and lipoprotein levels: The Fels Longitudinal Study, *Arterioscler. Thromb. Vasc. Biol.*, 18, 1759, 1998.

116. Meilahn, E.N., Becker, R.C. and Corrao, J.M., Primary prevention of coronary heart disease in women, *Cardiology*, 86, 286, 1995.

117. Legato, M.J., Coronary Artery Disease in Women, *Int. J. Fertil.*, 41, 94, 1996.

118. Kralikova, E., Ceska, R. and Rames, J., Diet, smoking and blood lipids in patients with combined familial hyperlipidemia, *Cent. Eur. J. Publ. Hlth*, 7, 19, 1999.

119. Lovejoy, J.C., The influence of sex hormones on obesity across the female life span, *J. Womens Hlth.*, 7, 1247, 1998.

120. Legato, M.J., Dyslipidemia, Gender and the role of high-density lipoprotein cholesterol: Implications for therapy, *Am. J. Cardiol.*, 86S, 15L, 2000.

121. Blazer, D.G., Moody-Ayers, S., Craft-Morgan, J. and Burchett, B., Depression in diabetes and obesity: Racial/ethnic/gender issues in older adults, *J. Psychosom. Res.*, 53, 913, 2002.

122. Reardon, M.F., Nestel, P.J., Craig, I.H. and Harper, R.W., Lipoprotein predictors of the severity of coronary artery disease in men and women, *Circulation*, 71, 881, 1985.

123. Liu, S., Willett, W.C., Stampfer, M.J., Hu, F.B., Franz, M., Sampson, L., Hennekens, C.H. and Manson, J.E., A prospective study of dietary glycemic load, carbohydrate intake and risk of coronary heart disease in U.S. women, *Am. J. Clin. Nutr.*, 71, 1455, 2000.

124. Liu, S., Manson, J.E., Stampfer, M.J., Holmes, M.D., Hu, F.B., Hankinson, S.E. and Willett, W.C., Dietary glycemic load assessed by food-frequency questionnaire in relation to plasma high-density lipoprotein cholesterol and fasting plasma triacylglycerols in postmenopausal women, *Am. J. Clin. Nutr.*, 73, 560, 2001.

125. Fagot-Campagna, A., Narayan, V.K.M., Hanson, R.L., Imperatore, G., Howard, B.V., Nelson, R.G., Pettitt, D.J. and Knowler, W.C., Plasma lipoproteins and incidence of non-insulin dependent diabetes mellitus in Pima Indians: protective effect of HDL-Cholesterol in women, *Atherosclerosis*, 128, 113, 1997.

126. Steinberg, H.O., Paradisi, G., Cronin, J., Crowde, K., Hempfling, A., Hook, G. and Baron, A.D., Type II diabetes abrogates sex differences in endothelial function in premenopausal women, *Circulation*, 101, 2040, 2000.

127. Falkner, B., Kushner, H., Tulenko, T., Summer, A.E. and Marsh, J.B., Insulin sensitivity, lipids and blood pressure in young American blacks, *Arterioscler. Thromb. Vasc. Biol.*, 15, 1798, 1995.

128. Giles, W.H., Croft, J.B., Greenlund, K.J., Ford, E.S. and Kitter, S.J., Total homocysteine concentration and the likelihood of nonfatal stroke: Results from the Third National Health and Nutrition Examination Survey: 1988–1994, *Stroke*, 29, 2473, 1998.

129. De Kniff, P. and Havekes, L.M., Apolipoprotein E as a risk factor for coronary heart disease: A genetic and molecular biology approach, *Curr. Opin. Lipidol.*, 7, 59, 1996.

130. Hak, A.E., Polderman, K.H., Westendrop, I.C.D., Jakobs, C., Hofman, A., Witteman, J.C.M., Stehouwer, C.D.A., Increased plasma homocysteine after menopause, *Atherosclerosis*, 149, 163, 2000.

131. Ridker, P.M., Manson, J.E., Buring, J.E., Shih, J., Matias, M. and Hennekens, C.H., Homocysteine and risk of cardiovascular disease among postmenopausal women, *JAMA*, 281, 817, 1999.

132. Bazzano, L.A., He, J., Ogden, L.G., Loria, C., Vupputuri, S., Myers, L. and Whelton, P.K., Dietary intake of folate and risk of stroke in U.S. men and women: N.H.A.N.E.S. I, epidemiologic follow-up study. National Health and Nutrition Examination Survey, *Stroke*, 33, 1183, 2002.

133. Pace-Asciak, C.R., Hahn, S., Diamandis, E.P., Soleas, G. and Goldberg, D.M., The red wine phenolics trans-resveratrol and quercetin block human platelet aggregation and eicosanoid synthesis: Implications for protection against coronary heart disease, *Clinica Chimica Acta*, 235, 207, 1995.

134. Grubben, M., Boers, G.H., Blom, H.J., Broekhuizen, R., de Jong, R., van Rijt, L., de Ruijter, E., Swinkels, D.W., Nagengast, F.M. and Katan, M.B., Unfiltered coffee increases plasma homocysteine concentrations in healthy volunteers: A randomized trial, *Am. J. Clin. Nutr.*, 71, 480, 2000.

135. Mattson, M.P., Kruman, I.I. and Duan, W., Folic acid and homocysteine in age-related disease, *Age. Res. Rev.*, 1, 95, 2002.

136. Olthof, M.R., Hollman, P.C., Zock, P.L. and Katan, M.B., Consumption of high doses of chlorogenic acid, present in coffee, or of black tea increases plasma total homocysteine concentrations in humans, *Am. J. Clin. Nutr.*, 73, 532, 2001.

137. Ueland, P.M., Refsum, H., Beresford, S.A.A. and Vollset, S.E., The controversy over homocysteine and cardiovascular risk, *Am. J. Clin. Nutr.*, 72, 324, 2000

138. Magnoni, A.A. and Jackson, S.H.D., Homocysteine and cardiovascular disease: Current Evidence and future prospects, *Am. J. Med.*, 112, 556, 2002.

139. Brattstrom, L., Wilcken, D.E.L., Homocysteine and cardiovascular disease: Cause or effect, *Am. J. Clin. Nutr.*, 72, 315, 2000.

140. Liu, S., Manson, J.E., Cole, S.R., Hennekens, C.H., Willett, W.C. and Buring, J.E., Fruit and vegetable intake and risk of cardiovascular disease: The Women's Health Study, *Am. J. Clin. Nutr.*, 72, 92, 2000.

141. Diaz, M.N., Frei, B., Vita, J.A. and Keaney, J.F., Antioxidants and Atherosclerotic heart disease, *N. Engl. J. Med.*, 337, 408, 1997.

142. Jialal, I., Devaraj, S. and Yusuf, S., Vitamin E supplementation and cardiovascular events in high-risk patients, *N. Engl. J. Med.*, 342, 1917, 2000.

143. Stamler, J., Stamler, R., Neaton, J.D., Wentworth, D., Daviglus, M.L., Garside, D., Dyer, A.R., Liu, K. and Greenland, P., Low risk-factor profile and long-term cardiovascular and noncardiovascular mortality and life expectancy, *JAMA*, 282, 2012, 1999.

144. Ridker, P.M., Manson, J.E., Buring, J.E., Shih, J., Matias, M. and Hennekens, C.H., Homocysteine and risk of cardiovascular disease among postmenopausal women, *JAMA*, 281, 1817, 1999.

145. Rissanen, T., Voutilainen, S., Nyyssonen, K., Salonen, R. and Salonen, J.T., Low plasma lycopene concentration is associated with increased intima-media thickness of the carotid artery wall, *Arterioscler. Thromb. Vasc. Biol.*, 20, 2677, 2000.

146. Mottram, P., Shige, H. and Nestel, P., Vitamin E improves arterial compliance in middle-aged men and women, *Atherosclerosis*, 145, 399, 1999.

147. Stampfer, M.J., Hennekens, C.H., Manson, J.E., Colditz, G.A., Rosner, B. and Willett, W.C., Vitamin E consumption and the risk of coronary heart disease in women, *N. Engl. J. Med.*, 328, 1444, 1993.

148. Yochum, L.A., Folsom, A.R. and Kushi, L.H., Intake of antioxidant vitamins and risk of death from stroke in postmenopausal women, *Am. J. Clin. Nutr.*, 72, 476, 2000.

149. Kushi, L.H., Folsom, A.R., Prineas, R.J., Mink, P.J., Wu, Y. and Bostick, R.M., Dietary antioxidant vitamins and death from coronary heart disease in postmenopausal women, *N. Engl. J. Med.*, 334, 1156, 1996.

150. Matthews, K.A., Kuller, L.H., Sutton-Tyrrell, K. and Chang, Y-F., Changes in cardiovascular risk factors during the perimenopause and postmenopause and carotod artery atherosclerosis in healthy women, *Stroke*, 32, 1104, 2001.

151. Cambien, F., Insight into the genetic epidemiology of coronary heart disease, *Ann. Med.*, 28, 465, 1996.

152. Klevay, L.M., Cardiovascular disease from copper deficiency — A history, *J. Nutr.*, 130, 489S, 2000.

153. Burch, G.E. and Giles, T.D., The importance of magnesium deficiency in cardiovascular disease, *Am. Heart J.*, 94, 649, 1977.

154. De Bacquer, D., De Henauw, S., De Backer, G. and Kornitzer, M., Epidemiological evidence for an association between serum calcium and serum lipids, *Atherosclerosis*, 108, 193, 1994.

155. Berge, L.N., Bonaa, K.H. and Nordoy, A., Serum ferritin, sex hormones and cardiovascular risk factors in healthy women, *Arterioscler. Thromb.*, 14, 857, 1994.

156. Iribarren, C., Sempos, C.T., Eckfeldt, J.H. and Folsom, A.R., Lack of association between ferritin level and measures of LDL oxidation: The A.R.I.C. study. Atherosclerosis Risk in Communities, *Atherosclerosis*, 139, 189, 1998.

157. Corti, M.C., Guralnik, J.M., Salive, M.E., Ferrucci, L., Pahor, M., Wallace, R.B. and Hennekens, C.H., Serum iron level, coronary artery disease and all-cause mortality in older men and women, *Am. J. Cardiol.*, 79, 120, 1997.

158. Sempos, C., Looker, A., Gillum, R., McGee, D., Vuong, C. and Johnson, C., Serum ferritin and death from all causes and cardiovascular disease: The N.H.A.N.E.S. II Mortality Study, *Ann. Epidemiol.*, 10, 441, 2000.

159. Kiechl, S., Willeit, J., Egger, G., Poewe, W., Oberhollenzer, F., for the Bruneck Study Group, Body Iron Stores and the Risk of Carotid Atherosclerosis, *Circulation*, 96, 3300, 1997.

160. Roest, M., van der Schouw, Y., de Yalk, B., Marz, J., Tempelman, M., de Groot, P., Sixma, J. and Banga, J.D., Heterozygosity for a hereditary hemochromatosis gene is associated with cardiovascular death in women, *Circulation*, 100, 1268, 1999.

161. Barrett-Connor, E., Cox, D.A. and Anderson, P.W., The potential role of SERMS for reducing the risk of coronary heart disease, *Trends Endocrinol. Metab.*, 10, 320, 1999.

162. Liu, S., Manson, J.E., Stampfer, M.J., Rexrode, K.M., Hu, F.B., Rimm, E.B. and Willet, W.C., Whole grain consumption and risk of ischemic stroke in women: A prospective study, *JAMA*, 284, 1534, 2000.

163. Liu, S., Stampfer, M.J., Hu, F.B., Giovanucci, E., Rimm, E., Manson, J.E., Hennekens, C.H. and Willett, W.C., Whole grain consumption and risk of coronary heart disease: Results from the Nurses' Health Study, *Am. J. Clin. Nutr.*, 70, 412, 1999.

164. Kant, A.K., Schatzkin, A., Graubard, B.I. and Schairer, C., A prospective study of diet quality and mortality in women, *JAMA*, 283, 2109, 2000.

165. Murphy, S.P., Rose, D., Hudes, M. and Viteri, F.E., Demographic and economic factors associated with dietary quality for adults in the 1987–88 Nationalwide Food Consumption Survey, *J. Am. Diet. Assoc.*, 92, 1352, 1992.

166. Kris-Etherton, K. and Krummel, D., Role of nutrition in the prevention and treatment of coronary heart disease in women, *J. Am. Diet. Assoc.*, 93, 987, 1993.

167. American Diabetes Association. Diabetes: 1996 Vital Statistics. Alexandria, VA, 1996.

168. Rimm, E.B., Willett, W.C., Hu, F.B., Sampson, L., Colditz, G.A., Manson, J.E., Hennekens, C. and Stampfer, M.J., Folate and vitamin B_6 from diet and supplements in relation to risk for coronary heart disease among women, *JAMA*, 279, 359, 1998.

169. Appleby, P.N., Thorogood, M., Mann, J.I. and Key, T.J.A., The Oxford Vegetarian Study: an overview, *Am. J. Clin. Nutr.*, 70, 525S, 1999.

170. Cobb, M.M., Teitlebaum, H., Risch, N., Jekel, J. and Ostfield, A., Influence of dietary fat, apolipoprotein E phenotype and sex in plasma lipoprotein levels, *Circulation*, 86, 849, 1992.

171. Shekelle, R.B. and Stamler, J., Dietary cholesterol and ischemic heart disease, *Lancet*, 1, 1177, 1989.

172. Grundy, S.M., Nix, D., Whelen, M.F. and Franklin, L., Comparison of three cholesterol lowering diets in normolipidemic men, *JAMA*, 256, 2351, 1986.

173. Jones, D.Y., Judd, J.T., Taylor, P.R., Cambell, W.S. and Nair, P.P., Influence of caloric contribution and saturation of dietary fat on plasma lipids in premenopausal women, *Am. J. Clin. Nutr.*, 45, 1451, 1987.

174. Brussard, J.H., Dallinga-Thie G., Groot, P.H.E. and Katan, M.B., Effects of amount and type of dietary fat on serum lipids, lipoproteins and apolipoproteins in man, *Atherosclerosis*, 36, 515, 1980.

175. Coulston, A.M., Liu, G.C. and Reaven, G.M., Plasma glucose, insulin and lipid responses to high-carbohydrate, low-fat diets in normal humans, *Metabolism*, 32, 52, 1983.

176. Kohlmeier, M., Strickler, G. and Schlierf, G., Influences of "normal" and "prudent" diets on biliary and serum lipids in healthy women, *Am. J. Clin. Nutr.*, 42, 1201, 1985.

177. Report of the expert panel of detection, evaluation and treatment of high blood cholesterol in adults, in National Institutes of Health Publication, National Heart, Lung and Blood Institute, Bethesda, MD, 1988, 2925.

178. Keys, A., Anderson, J.T. and Grande, F., Serum cholesterol response to changes in the diet. IV. Particular saturated fatty acids in the diet, *Metabolism*, 14, 776, 1965.

179. Boyd, N.F., Cousins, N., Beaton, M., Kriukov, V., Lockwood, G. and Tritchler, D., Quantitative changes in dietary fat intake and serum cholesterol in women: Results from a randomized controlled trial, *Am. J. Clin. Nutr.*, 52, 470, 1990.

180. Katan, M.B., van Gastel, A.C., de Rover, C.M., van Montfort, M.A.J. and Knuiman, J.T., Differences in individual responsiveness of serum cholesterol to fat-modified diets in man, *Eur. J. Clin. Invest.*, 18, 644, 1988.

181. Mensink, R.P. and Katan, M.B., Effect of monounsaturated fatty acids vs. complex carbohydrates on high-density lipoprotein in healthy men and women, *Lancet,* 1, 122, 1987.

182. Clifton, P., Kestin, M., Abbey, M., Drysdale, M. and Nestel, P., Relationship between sensitivity to dietary fat and dietary cholesterol, *Arteriosclerosis,* 10, 394, 1990.

183. Barnard, R.J., Effects of lifestyle modification on serum lipids, *Arch. Intern. Med.,* 151, 1389, 1991.

184. Mata, P., Garrido, J.A., Ordovas, J.M., Blasquez, E., Alvarez-Sala, L.A., Rubio, M.J., Alonso, R. and de Oya, M., Effect of dietary monounsaturated fatty acids on plasma lipoprotein and apolipoproteins in women, *Am. J. Clin. Nutr.,* 56, 77, 1992.

185. Nig, T.K.W., Hayes, K.C., DeWitt, G.F., Jegathesan, M., Satgunasigam, N., Ong, A.S.H. and Tan, D., Dietary palmitic and oleic acids exert similar effects on serum cholesterol and lipoprotein profiles on normocholesterolemic men and women, *J. Am. Coll. Nutr.,* 11, 383, 1992.

186. Hu, F.B., Stampfer, M.J., Manson, J.E., Rimm, E., Colditz, G.A., Rosner, B.A., Hennekens, C.H. and Willett, W.C., Dietary fat intake and the risk of coronary heart disease in women, *N. Engl. J. Med.,* 337, 1491, 1997.

187. Mata, P., Alvarez-Sala, L.A., Rubio, M.J., Nuno, J. and De Oya, M., Effects of long-term monounsaturated vs. polyunsaturated-enriched diets on lipoproteins in healthy men and women, *Am. J. Clin. Nutr.,* 55, 846, 1992.

188. Wood, P.D., Stefanik, M.L., Williams, P.T. and Haskell, W.I., The effects on plasma lipoproteins of a prudent weight-reducing diet, with or without exercise, in overweight men and women, *N. Engl. J. Med.,* 325, 461, 1991.

189. Kesteloot, H., Geboers, J. and Joossens, J.V., On the within-population relationship between nutrition and serum lipids: the BIRNH study, *Eur. Heart J.,* 10, 196, 1989.

190. Kesteloot, H., Oviasu, V.O., Obashoham, A.O., Cobbaert, C. and Lissens, W., Serum lipid and apolipoprotein levels in a Nigerian population sample, *Atherosclerosis,* 78, 33, 1989.

191. Kesteloot, H. and Sasaki, S., On the relationship between nutrition, sex hormones and high-density lipoproteins in women, *Acta Cardiol.,* 4, 355, 1993.

192. Krummel, D., Mashaly, M. and Kris-Etherton, P., Prediction of plasma lipids in a cross-sectional sample of young women, *J. Am. Diet. Assoc.,* 92, 942, 1992.

193. Van Horn, L., Ballew, C., Liu, K., Ruth, K., McDonald, A., Hilner, J., Burke, G., Savage, P., Braag, C., Caan, B., Jacobs, D., Slattery, M. and Sidney, S., Diet, body size and plasma lipids-lipoproteins in young adults: Differences by race and sex. The coronary artery risk development in young adults (CARDIA) Study, *Am. J. Epidemiol.,* 133, 9, 1991.

194. Knuiman, J.J., West, C.E., Katan, M.B. and Hautvast, J.G., Total cholesterol and high-density lipoprotein cholesterol levels in populations differing in fat and carbohydrate intake, *Arteriosclerosis,* 7, 612, 1987.

195. Baggio, G., Fellin, T., Baiocchi, M.R., Martini, S., Baldo, G., Manzato, E. and Crepaldi, G., Relationship between triglyceride-rich lipoprotein (chylomicrons and VLDL) and HDL-2 and HDL-3 in the postprandial phase in humans, *Atherosclerosis,* 37, 271, 1980.

196. Clifton, P.M. and Nestel, P.J., Influence of gender, body mass index and age on response of plasma lipids to dietary fat plus cholesterol, *Arterioscler. Thromb.,* 12, 955, 1992.

197. Denke, M., Individual responsiveness to a cholesterol-lowering diet in postmenopausal women with moderate hypercholesterolemia, *Arch. Intern. Med.,* 154, 1977, 1994.

198. Kesteloot, H., Changing trends in mortality, in *New Horizons in Preventing Cardio-vascular Diseases,* Yamori, Y. and Strasser, T., Eds. Elsevier, New York, 1989, 101.

199. Heber, D., Ashley, J.M., Leaf, D.A. and Barnard, R.J., Reduction of serum estradiol in postmenopausal women given free access to low fat high carbohydrate diet, *Nutrition,* 7, 137, 1991.

200. Ernst, N., Fisher, M., Smith, W., Gordon, T., Rifkind, B.M., Little, J.A., Mischkel, M.A. and Williams, O.D., The association of plasma high-density lipoprotein cholesterol with dietary intake and alcohol consumption. The Lipid Research Clinics program prevalence study, *Circulation,* 62, 41, 1980.

201. Gordon, T., Fischer, M., Ernst, N. and Rifkind, B.M., Relation of diet to LDL cholesterol, VLDL cholesterol and plasma total cholesterol and triglycerides in white adults, The Lipid Research Clinics program prevalence study, *Arteriosclerosis,* 2, 502, 1982.

202. Ernst, N., Fisher, M., Bowen, P., Schaefer, E.J. and Levy, R.I., Changes in plasma lipids and lipoproteins after a modified fat diet, *Lancet,* 2, 111, 1980.

203. Jones, D.Y., Judd, J.T., Taylor, P.R., Campbell, W.S. and Nair, P.P., Influence of caloric contribution and saturation of dietary fat on plasma lipids in premenopausal women, *Am. J. Nutr.,* 45, 1451, 1987.

204. Brussard, J.H., Katan, M.B., Groot, P.H., Havekes, L.M. and Hautvast, J.G., Serum lipoproteins of heathy persons fed a low-fat diet or a polyunsaturated fat diet for three months, *Atherosclerosis,* 42, 205, 1982.

205. Weisweiler, P., Janetschek, P. and Schwandt, P., Influence of polyunsaturated fats and fat restriction on serum lipoproteins in humans, *Metabolism,* 34, 83, 1985.

206. Masarei, J.R.L., Rouse, I.L., Lynch, W.J., Robertson, K., Vandongen, R. and Beilin, L.J., Effects of a lacto-ovo vegetarian diet on serum concentrations of cholesterol, triglyceride, HDL-C, HDL2-C, HDL3-C, apolipoprotein B and Lp(a), *Am. J. Clin. Nutr.,* 40, 468, 1984.

207. Cole, T., Bowen, P., Schmeisser, D., Prewitt, E., Aye, P., Langenberg, P., Dolecek, T., Brace, L. and Kamath, S., Differential reduction of plasma cholesterol by the American Heart Association phase 3 diet in moderately hypercholesterolemic, pre-menopausal women with different body mass indexes, *Am. J. Clin. Nutr.,* 40, 468, 1984.

208. Ginsberg, H.N., Kris-Etherton, P., Dennis, B., Elmer, P.J., Ershow, A., Lefevre, M., Pearson, T., Roheim, P., Ramakrishnan, R., Reed, R., Stewart, K., Stewart, P., Phillips, K. and Anderson, N., for the delta Research Group, Effects of reducing dietary saturated fatty acids on plasma lipids and lipoproteins in healthy subjects, *Arterioscler. Thromb. Vasc. Biol.,* 18, 441, 1998.

209. Mensink, R.P. and Katan, M.B., Effects of a diet enriched in monounsaturated or polyunsaturated fatty acids on levels of low-density and high-density lipoprotein cholesterol in healthy women and men, *N. Eng. J. Med.,* 321, 436, 1989.

210. Ascherio, A., Katan, M.B., Zock, P.L., Stampfer, M.J. and Willet, W.C., Trans fatty acids and coronary heart disease, *N. Engl. J. Med.,* 340, 1994, 1999.

211. Walden, C.E., Retzlaff, B.M., Buck, B.L., Wallick, S. and McCann, B.S., Differential effect of National Cholesterol Education Program (NCEP) Step II diet on HDL Cholesterol, its subfractions and Apolipoprotein A-I levels in hypercholesterolemic women and men after 1 year: The beFIT study, *Arterioscler. Thromb. Vasc. Biol.,* 20, 1580, 2000.

212. Iso, H., Stampfer, M.J., Manson, J.E., Rexrode, K., Hu, F., Hennekens, C.H., Colditz, G.A., Speizer, F.E. and Willett, W.C., Prospective study of fat and protein intake and risk of intraparenchymal hemorrhage in women, *Circulation,* 103, 784, 2001.

213. Bulliyya, G., Fish intake and blood lipids in fish eating *vs* non-fish eating communities of coastal South India, *Clin. Nutr.*, 19, 165, 2000.

214. Cleopas, T. and van der Meulen, J., Relationship of dietary folate and vitamin B6 with coronary heart disease in women, *JAMA*, 280, 417, 1998.

215. Suzukawa, M., Abbey, M., Howe, P.R., Nestel, P.J., Effects of fish oil fatty acids on low density lipoprotein size, oxidizability and uptake of macrophages, *J. Lipid Res.*, 36, 473, 1995.

216. Higdon, J.V., Liu, J., Du, S.H., Morrow, J.D., Ames, B.N. and Wander, R., Supplementation of postmenopausal women with fish oil rich in EPA and DHA is not associated with greater *in vivo* lipid peroxidation compared with oils rich in oleate and linoleate as assessed by plasma malondialdehyde and F2-isoprostanes, *Am. J. Clin. Nutr.*, 72, 714, 2000.

217. Frishman, W.H., Biologic markers as predictors of cardiovascular disease, *Am. J. Med.*, 104, 18S, 1998.

218. Stark, K.D., Park, E.J., Maines, V.A. and Holub, B.J., Effect of a fish-oil concentrate on serum lipids in postmenopausal women receiving and not receiving hormone replacement therapy in a placebo-controlled, double-blind trial, *Am. J. Clin. Nutr.*, 72, 389, 2000.

219. Brownell, K.D. and Stunkard, A.J., Differential changes in plasma high-density lipoprotein-cholesterol levels in obese men and women during weight reduction, *Arch. Intern. Med.*, 141, 1142, 1981.

220. North American Menopause Society, The role of isoflavones in menopausal health: Consensus opinion of the North American Menopause Society, *Menopause*, 7, 215, 2000.

221. Miller, V.T., Lipids, lipoproteins, women and cardiovascular disease, *Atherosclerosis*, 108, S73, 1994.

222. Lichtenstein, A.H., Got soy? *Am. J. Clin. Nutr.*, 73, 667, 2001.

223. Tonstad, S., Smerud, K. and Hoie, L., A comparison of the effects of two doses of soy protein or casein on serum lipids, serum lipoproteins and plasma total homocysteine in hypercholesterolemic subjects, *Am. J. Clin. Nutr.*, 76, 78, 2002.

224. Gardner, C.D., Newell, K.A., Cherin, R. and Haskell, W.L., The effect of soy protein with or without isoflavones relative to milk protein on plasma lipids in hypercholesterolemic postmenopausal women, *Am. J. Clin. Nutr.*, 73, 728, 2001.

225. Adams, M.R., Golden, D.L., Anthony, M.S., Register, T.C. and Williams, J.K., The inhibitory effect of soy protein isolate on atherosclerosis in mice does not require the presence of LDL receptors or alteration of plasma lipoproteins, *J. Nutr.*, 132, 43, 2002.

226. Teede, H., Dalais, F.S., Kotsopoulos, D., Liang, Y-L., Davis, S. and McGrath, B.P., Dietary soy has both beneficial and potentially adverse cardiovascular effects: A placebo-controlled study in men and postmenopausal women, *J. Clin. Endocrinol. Metab.*, 86, 3053, 2001.

227. Clarkson, T.B., Soy, Soy phytoestrogens and cardiovascular disease, *J. Nutr.*, 132, 566S, 2002.

228. Swain, J., Alekel, D.L., Dent, S.B., Peterson, C., Reddy, M.B., Iron indexes and total antioxidant status in response to soy protein intake in perimenopausal women, *Am. J. Clin. Nutr.*, 76, 165, 2002.

229. Stevenson, J.C., Flather, M., Collins, P. and Bassan, M., Comment on: Coronary artery disease in women, *N. Engl. J. Med.*, 343, 1891, 2000.

230. Herrington, D.M., Reboussin, D.M., Brosnihan, K.B., Sharp, P.C., Shumaker, S.A., Snyder, T.E., Furberg, C.D., Kowalchuk, G.J., Stuckey, T.D., Rogers, W.J., Givens, D.H. and Waters, D., Effects of estrogen replacement on the progression of coronary-artery atherosclerosis, *N. Engl. J. Med.*, 343, 522, 2000.

231. Tanis, B.C., van der Bosch, M.A.A.J., Kemmeren, J.M., Manger, V., Helmerhorst, F.M., Algra, A., van der Graaf, Y. and Rosendaal, F.R., Oral contraceptives and the risk of myocardial infarction, *N. Engl. J. Med.,* 345, 1787, 2001.

232. Vandenbrouke, J.P. and Kahlenborn, C., Oral contraceptives and the risk of myocardial infarction, *N. Engl. J. Med.*, 346, 1826, 2002.

233. Heinemann, L.A.J., Emerging evidence on oral contraceptives and arterial disease, *Contraception*, 62, 29S, 2000.

234. Heinemann, L.A.J., Lewis, M.A., Thorogood, M., Spitzer, M.O., Guggenmoos-Holz-mann, I. and Bruppacher, R., Case-control study of oral contraceptives and risk of thromboembolic stroke: Results from international study on oral contraceptives and health of young women, *Br. Med. J.*, 315, 1502, 1997.

235. Higdon, J.V., Du, S.H., Lee, Y.S., Wu, T. and Wander, R.C., Supplementation of postmenopausal women with fish oil does not increase overall oxidation to LDL*ex vivo* compared with dietary oils rich in oleate and linoleate, *J. Lipid. Res.*, 42, 407, 2001.

236. Herrington, D.M. and Potvin Klein, K., Effects of SERMS on important indicators of cardiovascular health: lipoproteins, hemostatic factors and endothelial function, *Women's Hlth. Issues*, 11, 98, 2001.

237. Eden, J., Phytoestrogens and the menopause, *Bail. Clin. Endocrinol. Metabol.*, 12, 581, 1998.

238. Tham, D.M., Gardner, C.D. and Haskell, W.L., Potential health benefits of dietary phytoestrogens: A review of the clinical, epidemiological and mechanistic evidence, *J. Clin. Endocrinol. Metab.*, 83, 2223, 1998.

239. Lucas, E.A., Wild, R.D., Hammond, L.J., Khalil, D.A., Juma, S., Daggy, B.P., Sto-ecker, B.J. and Arjmandi, B.H., Flaxseed improves lipid profile without altering biomarkers of bone metabolism in postmenopausal women, *J. Clin. Endocrinol. Metab.*, 87, 1527, 2002.

240. Nestel, P.J., Yamasita, T., Sasahara, T., Pomeroy, S., Dart, A., Komesaroff, P., Owen, A. and Abbey, M., Soy isoflavones improve systemic arterial compliance but not plasma lipids in menopausal and perimenopausal women, *Arterioscler. Thromb. Vasc. Biol.*, 17, 3392, 1997.

241. Feroz, F. and Morales, S., Cholesterol management: A review of literature and national cholesterol education program guidelines, *Prim. Care Update Ob./Gyns.*, 6, 186, 1999.

242. Goodman-Gruen, D. and Kritz-Silverstein, D., Usual dietary isoflavone intake is associated with cardiovascular disease risk factors in postmenopausal women, *J. Nutr.*, 131, 1202, 2001.

243. Chiechi, L.M., Secreto, G., Vimercati, A., Greco, P., Venturlli, E., Pansini, F., Fanelli, M., Loizzi, P. and Selvaggi, L., The effects of soy rich diet on serum lipids: The Menfis randomized trial, *Maturitas*, 41,97, 2002.

244. Wangen, K.E., Duncan, A.M., Xu, X. and Kurzer, M.S., Soy isoflavones improve plasma lipids in normocholesterolemic and mildly hypercholesterolemic postmeno-pausal women, *Am. J. Clin. Nutr.*, 73, 225, 2001.

245. Dewell, A., Hollenbeck, C.B. and Bruce, B., The effects of soy-derived phytoestro-gens on serum lipids and lipoproteins in moderately hypercholesterolemic postmeno-pausal women, *J. Clin. Endocrinol. Metab.*, 87, 118, 2002.

246. Min, J.Y., Liao, H., Wang, J.F., Sullivan, M.F., Ito, T. and Morgan, J.P., Genistein attenuates postischemic depressed myocardial function by increasing myofilament Ca^{2+} sensitivity in rat myocardium, *Exp. Biol. Med.*, 227, 632, 2002.

247. Wiseman, H., O'Reilly, J.D., Adlercreutz, H., Mallet, A.I., Bowey, E.A., Rowland, I.R., Sanders, T., Isoflavone phytoestrogens consumed in soy decrease F2-isoprostane concentrations and increase resistance of low-density lipoprotein to oxidation in humans, *Am. J. Clin. Nutr.*, 72, 395, 2000.

248. Tikkanen, M.J. and Adlercreutz, H., Dietary soy-derived isoflavone phytoesterogens: Could they have a role in coronary heart disease prevention?, *Biochem. Pharmacol.*, 60, 1, 2000.

249. Mukhtar, H. and Ahmad, N., Tea polyphenols: Prevention of cancer and optimizing health, *Am. J. Clin. Nutr.*, 71, 1698S, 2000.

250. Yannakoulia, M. and Vassilakou, T., Alcoholic Beverages In: *The Mediterranean Diet: Constituents and Health Promotion*, Matalas, A-L., Zampelas, A., Stavrinos, V., Wolinsky, I., Eds. CRC Press, 2001, Ch 8.

251. Serafini, M., Maiani, G., Ferro-Luzzi, A., Alcohol-free red wine enhances plasma antioxidant capacity in humans, *J. Nutr.*, 128, 1003, 1998.

252. Wahlqvist, M., Kouris-Blazos, A. and Polychronopoulos, E., The wisdom of the Greek cuisine and way of life, *Age Nutr.*, 2, 163, 1991.

253. Baer, D.J., Judd, J.T., Clevidence, B.A., Muesing, R.A., Cambell, W.S., Brown, E.D. and Taylor, P.R., Moderate alcohol consumption lowers risk factors for cardiovascular disease in postmenopausal women fed a controlled diet, *Am. J. Clin. Nutr.*, 75, 593, 2002.

254. Rumpler, W.V., Clevidence, B.A., Muesing, R.A. and Rhodes, D.G., Changes in women's plasma lipid and lipoprotein concentrations due to moderate consumption of alcohol are affected by dietary fat level, *J. Nutr.*, 129, 1713, 1999.

255. Fernandez-Sola, J., Estruch, R., Nicolas, J-M., Pare, J-C., Sacanella, E., Antunez, E. and Urbano-Marquez, A., Comparison of alcoholic cardiomyopathy in women versus men, *Am. J. Cardiol.*, 80, 481, 1997.

256. Sillanaukee, P., Koivula, T., Jokela, H., Pitkajarvi, T. and Seppa, K., Alcohol consumption and its relation to lipid-based cardiovascular risk factors among middle aged women: The role of HDL-3 cholesterol, *Atherosclerosis*, 152, 503, 2000.

257. Nakamura, Y., Amamoto, K., Tamaki, S., Okamura, T., Tsujita, Y., Ueno, Y., Kita, Y., Kinoshita, M. and Ueshima, H., Genetic variation in aldehyde dehydrogenase 2 and the effect of alcohol consumption on cholesterol levels, *Atherosclerosis*, 164, 171, 2002.

258. Dixon, J.B., Dixon, M.E. and O'Brien, P.E., Reduced plasma homocysteine in obese red wine consumers: A potential contributor to reduced cardiovascular risk status, *Eur. J. Clin. Nutr.*, 56, 608, 2002.

259. Caccetta, R.A., Burke, V., Mori, T.A., Beilin, L.J., Puddey, I.B. and Croft, K.D., Red wine polyphenols, in the absence of alcohol, reduce lipid peroxidative stress in smoking subjects, *Free Rad. Biol. and Med.*, 30, 636, 2001.

260. Serafini, M., Laranjinha, J.A.N., Almeida, L.M. and Maiani, G., Inhibition of human LDL lipid peroxidation by phenol rich beverages and their impact on plasma total antioxidant capacity in humans, *J. Nutr. Biochem.*, 11, 585, 2000.

261. Nigdikar, S.V., Williams, N.R., Griffin, B.A. and Howard, A.N., Consumption of red wine polyphenols reduces the susceptibility of low-density lipoproteins to oxidation *in vivo*, *Am. J. Clin. Nutr.*, 68, 258, 1998.

262. Van Golde, P., Sloots, L.M., Vermeulen, W.P., Wieldees, J.P.M., Hart, H.C., Bouma, B.N. and van de Wiel, A., The role of alcohol in the anti low density lipoprotein oxidation activity of red wine, *Atherosclerosis*, 147, 365, 1999.
263. Kerry, N. and Abbey, M., Red wine and fractionated phenolic compounds prepared from red wine inhibit low density lipoprotein oxidation *in vitro*, *Atherosclerosis*, 135, 93, 1997.
264. Auger, C., Caporiccio, B., Landrault, N., Teissedre, P.L., Laurent, C., Cros, G., Besancon, P., Rouanet, J-M., Red wine phenolic compounds reduce plasma lipids and apolipoprotein B and prevent early aortic atherosclerosis in hypercholesterolemic golden Syrian hamsters (Mesocricetus auratus), *J. Nutr.*, 132, 1207, 2002.
265. Van der Gaag, M.S., Van Tol, A., Vermunt, S.H.F., Scheek, L.M., Schaafsma, G. and Hendriks, H.F.J., Alcohol consumption stimulates early steps in reverse cholesterol transport, *J. Lipid Res.*, 42, 2077, 2001.
266. Schlienger, J.L., Alcohol et système cardiovasculaire:Mecanisme des effets protecteurs, *Pathol. Biol.*, 49, 764, 2001.
267. Fuhrman, B., Lavy, A. and Aviram, M., Consumption of red wine with meals reduces the susceptibility of human plasma and low-density lipoprotein to lipid peroxidation, *Am. J. Clin. Nutr.*, 61, 549, 1995.
268. Hodgson, J.M., Croft, K.D., Mori, T.A., Burke, V., Beilin, L.J. and Puddey, I.B., Regular ingestion of tea does not inhibit *in vivo* lipid peroxidation in humans, *J. Nutr.*, 132, 55, 2002.
269. Sasazuki, S., Kodama, H., Yoshimasu, K., Liu, Y., Washio, M., Tanaka, K., Tokunaga, S., Kono, S., Arai, H., Doi, Y., Kawano, T., Nakagaki, O., Takada, K., Koyanagi, S., Hiyamuta, K., Nii, T., Shirai, K., Ideishi, M., Arakawa, K., Mohri, M. and Takeshita, A., Relation between green tea consumption and the severity of coronary atherosclerosis among Japanese men and women, *Ann. Epidemiol.*, 10, 401, 2000.
270. Hodgson, J.M., Puddey, I.B., Croft, K.D., Burke, V., Mori, T.A., Caccetta, R.A., Beilin, L.J., Acute effects of ingestion of black and green tea on lipoprotein oxidation, *Am. J. Clin. Nutr.*, 71, 1103, 2000.
271. Sabate, J., Nut Consumption, vegetarian diets, ischemic heart disease risk and all-cause mortality: Evidence from epidemiologic studies, *Am. J. Clin. Nutr.*, 70, 500S, 1999.
272. Anderson, K.J., Teuber, S.S., Gobeille, A., Cremin, P., Waterhouse, A.L., Steinberg, F.M., Walnut polyphenolics inhibit *in vitro* human plasma and LDL oxidation, *J. Nutr.*, 131, 2837, 2001.
273. Jakovljevic, D., Sart, C., Sivenius, J., Torppa, J., Mahonen, M., Immonen-Raiha, P., Kaarsalo, E., Alhainen, K., Kuulasmaa, K., Tuomilehto, J., Puska, P. and Salomaa, V., Socioeconomic status and ischemic stroke, The FITMONICA Stroke Register, *Stroke*, 32, 1492, 2001.
274. McCullough, M.L., Feskanich, D., Stampfer, M.J., Rosner, B.A., Hu, F.B., Hunter, D.J., Variyam, J.N., Colditz, G.A. and Willett, W.C., Adherence to the Dietary Guidelines for Americans and risk of major chronic disease in women, *Am. J. Clin. Nutr.*, 72, 1214, 2000.
275. Pickering, T.G., Obesity and Hypertension: What should we do?, *Ann. Inter. Med.*, 134, 72, 2001.
276. Dowse, G.K., Gareeboo, H., Alberti, K.G.M.M., Zimmet, P., Tuomilehto, J., Purran, A., Fareed, D., Chitson, P., Collins, V.R. and Hemraj, F., Changes in population cholesterol concentrations and other cardiovascular risk factor levels after five years of the non-communicable disease intervention program in Mauritius, *Br. Med. J.*, 311, 1255, 1995.

277. Shimakawa, T., Nieto, F.J., Malinow, R., Chambless, L., Schreiner, P.J. and Szklo, M., Vitamin Intake: A possible determinant of plasma homocysteine among middle-aged adults, *Ann. Epidemiol.*, 7, 285, 1997.

278. Bramlet, D.A., King, H., Young, L., Witt, J.R., Stoukides, C.A. and Kaul, A.F., Management of hypercholesterolemia: Practice patterns for primary care providers and cardiologists, *Am. J. Cardiol.*, 80, 39H, 1997.

279. Bouchard, C., Genetic factors in obesity, *Med. Clin. North Am.*, 73, 67, 1989.

280. Bronner, L.L., Kanter, D.S. and Manson, J.E., Primary prevention of stroke, *N. Engl. J. Med.*, 333, 1392, 1995.

281. Young, L.R. and Nestle, M., The contribution of expanding portion sizes to the U.S. obesity epidemic, *Am. J. Publ. Hlth.*, 92, 246, 2002.

282. Bertone, E.R., Rosner, B.A., Hunter, D.J., Stampfer, M.J., Speizer, F.E., Colditz, G.A., Willett, W.C. and Hankinson, S.E., Dietary fat intake and ovarian cancer in a cohort of U.S. Women, *Am. J. Epidemiol.*, 156, 22, 2002.

283. McGowan, J.A. and Pottern, L., Commentary on women's health initiative, *Maturitas*, 34, 109, 2000.

284. Shapiro, J.S., Primary prevention of coronary heart disease in women through diet and lifestyle, *N. Engl. J. Med.*, 343, 1814, 2000.

285. Rich-Edwards, J.W., Manson, J.E., Hennekens, C.H. and Buring, J.E., The primary prevention of coronary heart disease in women, *N. Engl. J. Med.*, 332, 1758, 1995.

286. Stampfer, M.J., Hu, F.B., Manson, J.E., Rimm, E.B. and Willett, W.C., Primary prevention of coronary heart disease in women through diet and lifestyle, *N. Engl. J. Med.*, 343, 16, 2000.

287. Zanni, E.E., Annis, V.I., Blum, C.B., Herbert, P.N. and Breslow, J.L., Effect of egg cholesterol and dietary fats on plasma lipids, lipoproteins and apoproteins of normal women consuming natural diets, *J. Lipid Res.*, 28, 518, 1987.

288. Shepard, J., Packard, C.J., Patsch, J.R., Botto, A.M. and Taunton, O.D., Effects of dietary polyunsaturated and saturated fat on the properties and the metabolism of apolipoprotein A-I, *J. Clin. Invest.*, 61, 1582, 1978.

289. Thomas, J.L. and Brauss, P.A., Coronary artery disease in women: A historical perspective, *Arch. Intern. Med.*, 158, 333, 1998.

290. Oldroyd, J.C., Unwin, N.C., White, M., Imrie, K., Mathers, J.C. and Alberti, K.G.M.M., Randomized controlled trial evaluating the effectiveness of behavioral interventions to modify cardiovascular risk factors in men and women with impaired glucose tolerance: outcomes at 6 months, *Diab. Res. Clin. Pract.*, 52, 29, 2001.

291. Gureitz, O., Jonas, M., Boyoko, V., Rabinowitz, B. and Reicher-Reiss, H., Clinical profile and long term prognosis of women 50 years of age referred for coronary angiography for evaluation of chest pain, *Am. J. Cardiol.*, 85, 806, 2000.

292. Vinson, J.A., Teufel, K. and Wu, N., Red wine, dealcoholized red wine and especially grape juice, inhibit atherosclerosis in a hamster model, *Atherosclerosis*, 156, 67, 2001.

293. Van de Wiel, A., Hypothesis: Alcohol and insulin sensitivity, *Neth. J. Med.*, 52, 91, 1998.

294. Clevidence, B.A., Judd, J.T., Schaefer, E.J., Jenner, J.L., Lichtenstein, A.H., Muesing, R.A., Wittes, J. and Sunkin, M.E., Plasma lipoprotein (a) levels in men and women consuming diets enriched in Saturated, cis-, or trans- monounsaturated fatty acids, *Arterioscler. Thromb. Vasc. Biol.*, 17, 1657, 1997.

295. Conlin, P.R., The dietary approaches to stop hypertension (DASH) clinical trial: Implications for lifestyle modifications in the treatment of hypertensive patients, *Cardiol. Rev.*, 7, 284, 1999.

296. Brochu, M., Starling, R.D., Tchernof, A., Matthews, D.E., Garcia-Rubi, E. and Poe-hlman, E.T., Visceral adipose tissue is an independent correlate of glucose disposal in older obese postmenopausal women, *J. Clin. Endocrinol. Metab.*, 85, 2378, 2000.

297. Hu, F.B., Stampfer, M.J., Manson, J.E., Ascherio, A., Colditz, G.A., Speizer, F.E., Hennekens, C.H. and Willet, W.C., Dietary saturated fats and their food sources in relation to the risk of coronary heart disease in women, *Am. J. Clin. Nutr.*, 70, 1001, 1999.

298. Gill, J.M.R. and Hardman, A.E., Postprandial lipemia: Effects of exercise and restriction of energy intake compared, *Am. J. Clin. Nutr.*, 71, 465, 2000.

299. Williams, P.T., High-density lipoprotein cholesterol and other risk factors for coronary heart disease in female runners, *N. Engl. J. Med.*, 334, 1298, 1996.

300. Rosenberg, I.H., Is it time to standardize and to measure blood homocysteine levels in patients with heart disease?, *Am. J. Med.*, 112, 582, 2002.

14 Diabetes: A Woman's Disease?

Carolyn D. Berdanier

CONTENTS

I. INTRODUCTION

Diabetes mellitus is not a single disease. Rather, it is a collection of diseases having in common a deranged glucose-insulin relationship. It is the largest group of genetic diseases that afflict Americans. In many instances, the phenotypic expression of the diabetes genotype is dependent on lifestyle choices and environmental factors. Environmental factors include diet as well as environmental contaminants and pathogens. It has been estimated that there are probably twice as many people with a diabetes genotype than with a diabetes phenotype. In population surveys, more women than men are found with diabetes and these women with diabetes have a higher risk for developing heart disease. This chapter reviews the various forms of the disease and provides documentation on the prevalence of diabetes in the U.S. population. Gender differences in metabolism as well as reasons why there are gender differences in the disease pattern will be explored.

II. DIABETES MELLITUS: THE DISEASE

A. DIAGNOSIS

The common clinical feature of diabetes mellitus is that of deranged glucose metabolism as assessed by the glucose tolerance test. This test consists of blood sampling before and after an oral glucose challenge. There are several variations in this test

0-8493-1337-6/03/$0.00+$1.50
© 2004 by CRC Press LLC

295

but basically the test assesses how well the body uses glucose. For screening purposes, the patient may have a single blood sample drawn either after an overnight fast or 2 hours after a meal. If the glucose level is higher than normal, the patient is then given the glucose tolerance test. The NHANES III (National Health and Nutrition Examination Survey III) survey, for example, screened for diabetes using a fasting blood glucose level of greater than 140 mg/dl or a 2-hour post glucose challenge value of greater than 200 mg/dl as its cutoff point.[1]

The American Diabetes Association periodically publishes criteria for the diagnosis of diabetes. These are updated as new information becomes available. The latest report[2] provides the following criteria for the diagnosis of the disease:

- Symptoms of diabetes (excessive thirst, excessive urination, fatigue, perhaps ketones in blood and urine, unexplained and rapid weight loss) plus a casual plasma glucose level of more than 200 mg/dl (11.1 mmol/l). (In this definition, casual means a blood sample assessed without regard to the time of the last meal.)
- Fasting (at least 8 hours without food) blood glucose of more than 126 mg/dl (7.0 mmol/l).
- A 2-hour post glucose challenge blood value of more than 200 mg/dl (11.1 mmol/l). In this challenge, the glucose load should be the equivalent of 75 g of anhydrous glucose dissolved in water.

There may be people with intermediate glucose levels that do not fully meet the criteria outlined above. These people may have fasting blood glucose levels greater than 110 mg/dl but less than 126 mg/dl. These individuals should be evaluated on a continuing basis. They may develop further signs of diabetes or these results may be a "one time abnormality." People who may be ill could have this kind of result because the stress of illness can alter glucose metabolism. As these persons recover, their glucose metabolism will return to normal and no further symptoms will develop. On the other hand, some of these people with borderline glucose levels may be those in whom the stress of illness may precipitate the more serious diabetes sequellae.

The NHANES III study also used the fasting blood glucose level of greater than 126 mg/dl as the cut-off for diabetes diagnosis.[1] When they used the more time consuming and rigorous criteria (the 2 hour glucose tolerance screening test), they reported a prevalence of 14.26% of individuals with diabetes between the ages of 40–74 whereas, when they used the second criteria (the single fasting blood glucose value), they reported a prevalence of 12.27%. The difference in prevalence is significant but can be explained by the difference in the rigor of the testing. Using the less rigorous fasting blood glucose level without a follow-up glucose challenge misses those people with diabetes who have target tissue disease. These people will likely have normal fasting blood glucose levels but, because they are not able to normally metabolize glucose in the peripheral tissue, their post-glucose challenge values will be higher than normal. These higher than normal values would not be detected using only fasting blood glucose values as the diagnostic criterion.

B. Classification of Diabetes Mellitus

Typically, people with diabetes are divided into two groups based on the management of their clinical state. Those who require insulin replacement from the time of diagnosis are type 1 patients, while those whose clinical condition can be managed with diet and exercise are type 2 patients. Type 2 patients may use oral hypoglycemic agents to help manage glucose homeostasis or may require daily insulin supplements later in the time course of their disease. Those with type 1 disease are about 10% of the total population with diabetes and probably have one or more mutations in the genes that encode components of the immune system. Patients with type 1 disease usually are those with autoimmune disease, although there are instances where certain viruses can either trigger the autoimmunity that in turn causes the destruction of the insulin-producing islet cells or directly cause the destruction of these cells. [3-10] Autoimmune diabetes or viral diabetes can strike at any age, but children seem to be the most vulnerable. In the north-central parts of the country (North Dakota, Wisconsin, Colorado) more boys than girls have this disease whereas, in areas with a significant black or Hispanic population, more girls than boys are affected. [11] The onset of type 1 disease is rapid and the symptoms of excessive thirst, polyuria, hyperglycemia, sudden weight loss and elevated blood and urine ketones are observed. If not diagnosed quickly and insulin replacement administered, the individual could die. Because type 2 patients can progress to insulin dependence, it is difficult to segregate type 1 adult patients from type 2 patients in surveys of adult populations. Thus, estimates of the number of type 1 adults are not as good as those for type 1 children.

In contrast, type 2 diabetes usually appears in the adult and may be associated with increasing fat stores. Over the last 20 years, the age of onset has been declining. Recently, adolescents have been reported to have type 2 disease. As this population group is becoming increasingly obese, it is not surprising that they are also becoming diabetic. The appearance of type 2 disease is gradual and may go undiagnosed for many years until another medical emergency develops or unless the person is routinely screened for diabetes as part of a yearly physical. In many, the diabetes is preceded by the accumulation of excess fat stores; in others, obesity and diabetes co-develop. There is a strong genetic contribution to the development of both diseases. Equally as strong are lifestyle choices, including food intake (type and amount of food) and physical activity. In this respect, one might suggest that diabetes, particularly type 2, is the result of a nutrient–gene interaction that can be modified by physical activity. A number of genes for type 2 diabetes have been identified and some of these are also associated with obesity. [12-19] Mutations in the insulin gene, the gene that encodes the enzyme that splits proinsulin into the active insulin, the genes for the insulin receptor at the adipocyte or muscle cell, the gene for the insulin receptor substrate and genes that encode proteins in the downstream signaling of insulin binding and glucose use have all been found to associate with the type 2 diabetes phenotype. [20-35]

That diabetes is a genetic trait has been shown by studies of twins. In identical twins in North America, concordance for type 1 diabetes was reported as 33%. [36] That is, in 33% of all the identical twin pairs studied, both members of the pair were afflicted with type 1 diabetes. In the remaining pairs, only one twin had the disease.

In type 2 diabetes, close to 100% concordance has been reported. In these twin pairs, if one became diabetic, in almost all cases the other did also.

In addition to these general categories of patients, there are four other groups of people who are susceptible to diabetes. The first of these are women who develop diabetes while they are pregnant. These patients have gestational diabetes. They may lose the diabetic trait after delivery or they may progress to the chronic diabetic state. Gestational diabetes complicates about 4% of all pregnancies in the U.S., resulting in approximately 135,000 cases annually.[37] The prevalence may range from 1–14% depending on the population studied. Women with gestational diabetes are at greater risk with respect to fetal malformation, to having very large babies, for complications of pregnancy — especially hypertension — and their babies may be at greater risk for neonatal difficulties.[38] Maternal or neonatal death is greater in gestational diabetes than in normal pregnancy. Physicians monitor women with gestational diabetes very carefully, using ultrasound to monitor the growth of the fetus. Other tests as well are used to assess the status of the woman and her child. Some women with gestational diabetes will need daily insulin supplementation, while others can be managed with careful attention to diet, weight gain and daily exercise. Many physicians will induce labor or schedule cesarean deliveries if the baby appears to be of excessive size, which, in turn, indicates that delivery will not be normal. Reports of babies in the 12–15-lb (about 4–6 kg) range have appeared in the medical literature and the mothers of these babies were found to be gestationally diabetic. Newborns of gestationally diabetic mothers (as well as newborns of either type 1 or 2 diabetics) need to be monitored with respect to hypoglycemia. These babies may have produced compensatory amounts of insulin during gestation and this hyperinsulinemia may continue after birth. Excessive insulin release after birth would then result in hypoglycemia that, if not quickly diagnosed and treated, could result in the death of the newborn.

The second group of people with diabetes are those having a mutation in the mitochondrial genome.[39] While people with types 1 and 2 diabetes have the disease as a result of one or more mutations in the nuclear genome, people with mitochondrial diabetes have one or more mutations in the mitochondrial genome. Typically, these people are thin yet have a fatty liver. With time, their insulin producing islet cells become depleted of insulin and hormone replacement is needed. People with this form of diabetes frequently have sensory losses (partial or complete deafness, blindness,) and may have neuromuscular losses as well. Sometimes, this form of diabetes is secondary to more devastating neuromuscular and central nervous system diseases such as epilepsy. Estimates of the prevalence of people with these disorders are not very good and range from 0.1 to 9% of the population with diabetes. The reason these figures are poor is that people with devastating mitochondrial disease in which diabetes is a secondary feature are not reported as people with diabetes. In addition, people with these diseases are short lived. Their numbers within the total population are affected by their early deaths. In contrast to the inheritance patterns of diabetes due to nuclear mutation (autosomal dominent or recessive), mitochondrial diabetes is inherited from the mother, not the father. Both males and females phenotype with the disease but only females can pass it to their progeny.

The third group of people are those with maturity-onset diabetes of the young, abbreviated MODY.[40–48] People with MODY have insulin secretory defects that ultimately require hormone replacement because the islet cell is unable to appropriately recognize the glucose signal for insulin release. The number of people with this defect is very small, probably accounting for ~0.1% of the population with diabetes. Mutations in the genes for glucokinase (the glucose sensor in the islet cell) and in hepatocyte nuclear transcription factors 1∀ and 4∀ have been identified as the causative factors for this group of diabetes diseases. The MODY trait is inherited as an autosomal dominant trait and many different mutations in these three genes have been found.

The fourth special category of people includes those with impaired glucose tolerance. They may have glucose intolerance secondary to some other endocrine disease, or secondary to one or more prescribed drugs or may have glucose intolerance due to malnutrition. Some people fall into none of these categories. Indeed, their glucose intolerance may progress into type 2 diabetes mellitus requiring diet and exercise management and perhaps oral hypoglycemic drugs or daily insulin therapy. This special category of people is quite diverse and difficult to generalize with respect to management and outcome. However, many of the people with this condition normalize once their primary condition is resolved. The primary endocrine disorder is normalized or the drug that affected glucose tolerance is discontinued or the malnourished individual is rehabilitated.

The distribution of these classes in the population with diabetes is shown in Figure 14.1. Not shown, because the condition may exist but may not be recognized, are people with unrecognized type 2 diabetes. The American Diabetes Association estimates that one person in 14 either has the disease or will develop it during his or her lifetime.

Diabetic Population

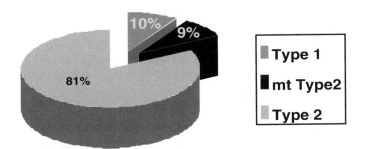

FIGURE 14.1 Distribution of people with type 1, type 2 or mitochondrial diabetes in the population with this disease. Not shown are those with gestational diabetes or those whose diabetes is secondary to some other disorder. Also not shown or included in the total population with diabetes are those who have impaired glucose tolerance. Because the population with MODY is so small (about 0.1%) it is not shown as a separate entity in this pie chart.

As screening efforts are increased, it is hoped that more Americans having diabetes will be identified and the number of people with unrecognized diabetes will decrease.

C. PREVALENCE

Diabetes mellitus is widespread and of concern to health professionals not just because of their interest in the disease per se, but because diabetes may precipitate a number of health problems including heart disease, renal disease, blindness and loss of circulation in the lower limbs necessitating amputation. The cost to society for diabetes with respect to lost productivity and health care expense is tremendous. The American Diabetes Association estimates that the health care costs exceed $44 billion per year. When this cost is added to the cost of lost productivity the figure could easily exceed $100 billion per year.

The National Centers for Chronic Disease Prevention and Health (the CDC) reported in 1999 that there has been a rise in the number of people in the U.S. with diabetes.[49] In 1980 there were 5.8 million people with diabetes. In 1996 (the last year for which there are reliable figures) there were 8.4 million. This is a 45% increase in diabetes prevalence. However, if these figures are age adjusted, the rise is not as great. A rate of 25/1000 was reported in 1980, whereas 30/1000 was reported for 1996. This is an increase of 20% rather than 45%. Age adjustment allows for the fact that, as people age, they are more likely to develop diabetes. Thus, in an aging population such as that in the U.S., an adjustment for increasing age is important for disease prevalence figures. One of the more interesting aspects of these surveillance figures is the difference in age-standardized prevalence between blacks, Hispanics and nonHispanic whites. Gender differences in prevalence have also been noted. These are illustrated in Figure 14.2.

The prevalence of diabetes in whites has been stable over the reporting period (1980–96), whereas the prevalence of diabetes in black males and females is higher. In the 1980–1996 period, the prevalence of diabetes in the white population was about 22/1000. In the black male population in 1980 it was about 37/1000 and by 1996 it had risen to about 45/1000. The black female population had a prevalence of about 45/1000 in 1980 and by 1996, this prevalence had risen to about 55/1000. When segregated further into specific age-race-gender groups, the difference between the races is more striking. In the groups that were less than 44 years of age, the rates were not different (about 10/1000). In the 45–60 years of age group, white males and females had similar rates (about 50/1000) but the black males had rates of about 130/1000 and the black females had rates close to 150/1000. After the age of 65 there were further age, gender and race differences in prevalence. Between the age of 65 and 75, white males had a rate of about 125/1000. White females had a rate of 80/1000; black males 170/1000 and black females had a prevalence of just over 200/1000. After the age of 75, the prevalence of diabetes in white males and females fell slightly but the rate rose again in the black males to about 185/1000, while the prevalence in black females fell slightly to about 190/1000. When the population figures are further divided so as to identify Hispanic people, the prevalence in these specific groups is striking.

Prevalence of diabetes in adults

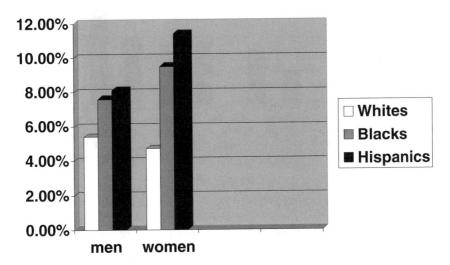

FIGURE 14.2 Estimated age-adjusted prevalence of physician-diagnosed diabetes in adults 20+ years of age segregated by gender and race. Data are from NHANES II and III studies.[1]

There are geographical differences in prevalence as well. High (49–59/1000) age-standardized prevalence rates were reported in Maryland, Virginia, Michigan, Indiana, Illinois, Alabama, Mississippi, Louisiana, Texas, New Mexico and California while low age-standardized prevalence rates were reported in Maine, Minnesota, North Dakota, South Dakota, Montana, Wyoming, Colorado, Idaho, Kansas, Oklahoma, Arizona and Washington state.

In some instances, these geographical differences may simply be due to poor surveillance and reporting due to the sparse population in some areas of these states. Particularly surprising was the reported low prevalence in Arizona, since this is the home state of the southwest Indian tribes (the Pimas and others) that have been studied so intensively. In these tribes, the prevalence of type 2 diabetes is quite high. More than half of all adults 35 years of age and older have type 2 diabetes mellitus.[50–53] Excess body fat and alcoholism also characterize these Native American groups. There may be a group of genes in these peoples that can account for these characteristics.

As mentioned above, obesity may precipitate type 2 diabetes or may co-develop with it. Obesity is rising in America just as diabetes is. Shown in Figure 14.3 are the time trends in the percent of adolescents, men and women who are overweight. In part, this trend toward excessive body fat stems from a lack of physical activity coupled with an increase in food intake and an interaction of these factors with a genetically determined predisposition to store excess fat. Excess fat stored in the adipocyte has effects on glucose utilization. As the fat cell size increases, it is less responsive to the glucose lowering effect of insulin. Insulin receptors are less abundant and the binding of insulin less active. A reduction in physical activity also

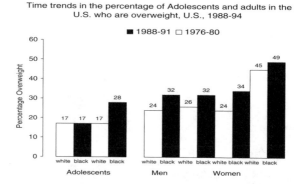

FIGURE 14.3 Time trends in the percentage of adolescents, men and women who are overweight in the United States. Data are from the NHANES II and III studies.[1]

has effects on glucose metabolism. The active exercising muscle uses glucose in a non-insulin dependent manner. The resting muscle requires insulin for glucose use. Hence, those people who are physically active require less overall insulin to maintain glucose homeostasis. In addition, muscle mass is less in the sedentary person. In active individuals with a normal muscle mass, this tissue can account for up to 40% of the non-insulin dependent glucose use. As people become more and more sedentary, the proportion of glucose used by the active muscle decreases and these people become more dependent on insulin to facilitate glucose use. The increased fat cell size and number plus the decreased muscle activity, in turn requires that the insulin producing cells of the pancreas release more insulin. Eventually, the pancreas is no longer able to meet these demands and diabetes develops. In overweight people, insulin resistance is a typical characteristic. Insulin resistance is just that. The muscle and fat cells are resistant to the action of insulin in promoting the entry and use of glucose. If individuals with this problem were able to lose some of the excess fat stores and increase their physical activity this insulin resistance would be mitigated.

Note in Figure 14.3 that black teenagers are becoming fatter than are white teenagers. Note too that almost half the black female population is overweight. Among men, the trend toward overweight is about the same. Both the black and white male groups are 32% overweight. The white female adult group was fatter in 1988–91 NHANES III survey than they were in the 1976–80 NHANES II survey but not as fat as the black female population.[1] More recent but smaller surveys have reported that the population that is considered obese is rising. Childhood obesity is becoming more prevalent and these children are at high risk for type 2 diabetes.[54] Generally, a population is first considered overweight when the body mass index (a weight/height ratio) exceeds 25. When it approaches 30, the person is considered obese. Obesity is a significant health risk with respect to not only diabetes but also to heart disease and other health problems. A recent survey by Mokdad et al.[55] reported that in Mississippi 24.3% of the adult population was obese, and 11.1% of the African-American population in this state had diagnosed diabetes. If this state is like other states, there is probably an equal number of African-Americans who have diabetes but do not know it.

D. GENDER DIFFERENCES IN OBESITY AND DIABETES

Gender dimorphism in size, shape and body composition of teenagers has been reported by Katch et al. [56] These investigators reported that 12-year-old females were generally fatter than males of the same age. This gender difference might be due to differences in the age of onset of puberty. Females generally mature faster than males. In addition, as males mature, they tend to increase their muscle mass rather than fat mass, thus influencing their overall body composition. As males mature, they tend to deposit fat in the abdomen even as they are gaining fat stores in other areas as well. This increase in visceral fat is associated with an increase in risk for a number of degenerative conditions such as heart disease and diabetes. In adults, there are gender differences in visceral fat. Females have less visceral fat than males when corrections are made for total body fat stores.[57] Women who accumulate excess visceral fat are at greater risk for developing diabetes than men with similar amounts of similar visceral fat.[58,59]

The reasons that there are gender differences in body fatness and distribution may relate to the influence of the sex hormones on metabolism. These hormones influence insulin release and action. Both males and females produce and release testosterone but in different amounts. Testosterone influences fat mass as well as glucose homeostasis. Haffner[60] has reported that females who produce excess androgens also become fatter than normal and show insulin resistance. The androgen is produced by the ovaries and is bound by a protein called the sex hormone binding protein (SHBP).[60] Insulin inhibits the release of this binding protein but, in those individuals producing excess androgen, SHBP production is also increased and this in turn appears to interfere with the action of insulin. Some investigators have suggested that the gender difference in severity of diabetes complications might be due to this same phenomenon.[61–63] That is, complications of diabetes are more frequent and more severe in men than in premenopausal women and that this difference is due to the testosterone production (and associated SHBP) in males. Postmenopausal women also have more severe complications than premenopausal women and again the difference could be due to testosterone production and SHBP.

These gender differences are seen in the impact of coexistent diabetes on the survival of patients with coronary heart disease.[61] Diabetes confers a substantially higher risk of mortality in women than in men when it occurs in the presence of coronary heart disease.[62,63] In part, this gender difference in heart disease-diabetes mortality may be due to a gender related difference in peroxidized lipids.[63] Females have higher levels of these lipids than males and it has been proposed that peroxidized lipids, particularly in the vascular system, play an important role in the pathophysiology of coronary vessel disease.

Gender effects on metabolism apart from diabetes have shown that insulin secretion is influenced by estrogen. Females release significantly more insulin in response to glucose than do males.[64] Indeed, cyclic variations in glucose tolerance that reflect the menstrual cycle have been found in women.[65] Estrogen effects on fat cell insulin receptors have also been reported.[66] When estrogen levels are high, there is more insulin resistance than when estrogen levels are low. In postmenopausal women given hormone replacement therapy there seems to be some question as to whether there could be an estrogen effect on glucose homeostasis. Thus, there may be a variety of factors at work that determine whether a woman is fatter than a man and whether she will develop diabetes and its complications. Perhaps the gender difference in obesity is due to gender differences in physical activity. Perhaps men are more active and thus use more glucose in an insulin independent manner. Studies of physical activity (including work) in men and women with and without diabetes are needed.

Given that there are gender differences in metabolism, there is also a need to demonstrate whether these gender differences carry over to the gender differences in diabetes mellitus and indeed whether the sexes differ in their response to dietary manipulation. Studies of males and females with and without diabetes are needed to determine whether diet and exercise elicit the same responses with respect to glucose homeostasis.

III. SUMMARY AND CONCLUSIONS

Population studies have shown that women are more at risk for developing diabetes than men in certain subsets of the population. The explanations for this sexual dimorphism probably involve the differences in hormonal status but also may be due to differences in physical activity and differences in food selection and intake. Gender differences in fat stores as well as gender differences in diabetes prevalence suggest that the woman should limit her body fatness if she wishes to avoid developing diabetes and the complications diabetes offers. There are, however, certain inherited defects associated with diabetes that may not be amenable to dietary intervention. These defects may not be associated with obesity and as described in the text may be related to type 1 diabetes, MODY or to mitochondrial diabetes, rather than to the diabetes that is linked to excessive fat stores.

REFERENCES

1. NHANES http://www.cdc.gov/nchs (accessed 10/04/01).
2. Report of the Expert Committee on the diagnosis and classification of diabetes mellitus. *Diabetes Care* 2002 25: S5–20.
3. Atkinson, M.A., Maclaren, N.K. The pathogenesis of insulin dependent diabetes. *N. Engl. J. Med.* 331, 1428–1436, 1994.
4. Atkinson, M.A., Maclaren, N.K. Islet cell autoantigens in IDDM. *Diabetes Rev.* 1, 191–203, 1993.
5. Faustman, D. Mechanisms of autoimmunity in type 1 diabetes. *J. Clin. Immunol.* 13,1–7, 1993.
6. Lan, M.S., Wasserfall, C., Maclaren, N.K., Notkins, A.L. IA-2, a transmembrane protein of the protein tyrosine phosphatase family is a major autoantigen in insulin-dependent diabetes mellitus. *Proc. Natl. Acad. Sci.* (U.S.A) 93, 2307–2311, 1996.

7. Huang, W., Conner, E., DelaRosa, T., Muir, A., Schatz, D., Silverstein, J., Crockett, S., She, J.X., Maclaren, N.K. Although DR3-DQB1* may be associated with multiple component diseases of the autoimmune polyglandular syndromes, the human leukocyte antigen DR4-DQB110302 haplotype is implicated only in ∃ cell autoimmunity. *J. Clin. Endocrinol Metab.* 81, 1–5, 1996.

8. Vreugdenhil, G.R., Geluk, A., Ottenhoff, T.H.M., Melchers, W.J.G., Roep, B.O., Galama, J.M.D. Molecular mimicry in diabetes mellitus: The homologous domain in coxsackie B virus protein 2C and islet autoantigen GAD$_{65}$ is highly conserved in the coxsackie B-like enteroviruses and binds to the diabetes associated HLA-DR3 molecule. *Diabetologia* 41: 40–46, 1998.

9. Foulis, A.K., McGill, M., Farquharson, M.A., Hilton, D.A. A search for evidence of viral infection in pancreases of newly diagnosed patients with IDDM. *Diabetologia* 40, 53–61, 1997.

10. Szopa, T.M., Ward, T., Dronfield, D.M., Portwood, N.D., Taylor, K.W. Coxsackie B4 viruses with the potential to damage ∃ cells of the islets are present in clinical isolates. *Diabetologia* 33, 325-328, 1990.

11. Karvonen, M., Pitkaniemi, M., Pitkaniemi, J., Kohtamaki, K., Tajima, N., Tuomilehto, J. Sex differences in the incidence of insulin dependent diabetes mellitus: An analysis of recent epidemiological data. *Diabetes Metab. Rev.* 13, 275-291, 1997.

12. Golay, A., Munger, R., Felber, J-P Obesity and Type 2 diabetes: The retrograde regulation concept *Diabetes Rev.* 5, 69-82, 1997.

13. Leibel, R. Single gene obesities in rodents: Possible relevance to human obesity. *J. Nutr.* 127,1908S-1015S, 1997.

14. Bouchard, C. (Ed.) *The Genetics of Obesity.* CRC Press, Boca Raton, 1–247,1994.

15. Lundgren, H., Bengtsson, C., Blohme, G., Lapidus, L., Sjostrom, L. Adiposity and adipose tissue distribution in relation to incidence of diabetes in women: Results from a prospective population study in Gothenburg Sweden. *Int. J. Obesity* 13, 413–423, 1988.

16. Forsen, T., Eriksson, J., Tuomilehto, J., Reunanen, A., Osmond, C., Barker, D. The fetal and childhood growth of persons who develop type 2 diabetes. *Ann. Intern. Med.* 133, 176–182, 2000.

17. Young, T.K., Dean, H.J., Flett, B., Wood-Steiman, P. Childhood obesity in a population at high risk for type 2 diabetes. *J. Pediat.* 136, 365–369, 2000.

18. Goldberg, A.P., Coon, P.J. Non-insulin dependent diabetes mellitus in the elderly. Influence of obesity and physical inactivity. *Endocrinol. Aging* 16, 843–865, 1987.

19. Leiter, E.H., Herberg, L. The polygenetics of diabesity in mice. *Diabetes Rev.* 5, 131–148, 1997.

20. Hanis, C.L., Boerwinkle, E., Chakaraborty, R., Ellsworth, E.L., Concannon, P., Stirling, B., Morrison, V.A., Wapelhorst, B., Speilman, R.S., Gogolin-Ewens, K.J., Shepard, J.M., Williams, S.R., Risch, N., Hinds, D., Iwasaki, N., Ogata, M., Omori, Y., Petzold, C., Rietzsch, H., Schroder, H.E., Schulze, J., Cox, N.J., Menzel, S., Boriraj, V.V., Chen,X., Lim, L.R., Lindner, T., Mereu, L.E., Wang, Y-Q., Xiang, K., Yamagata, K., Yang, Y., Bell, G.I. A genome wide search for human non-insulin-dependent (type 2) diabetes genes reveals a major susceptibility locus on chromosome 2. *Nature Genet.* 13, 161–174, 1996.

21. Stern, M.P., Mitchell, B.D., Blangero, J., Reinhart, L., Kammerer, C.M., Harrison, C.R., Shipman, P.A., O'Connell, P.O., Frazier, M.L., MacCluer, J.W. Evidence for a major gene for type II diabetes and linkage analysis with selected candidate genes in Mexican Americans. *Diabetes* 45, 563–568, 1996.

22. Elbein, S.C., Bragg, K.L., Hoffman, M.D., Mayorga, R.A., Leppert, M.F. Linkage studies of Type 2 diabetes with 23 chromosome 11 markers in a sample of whites of northern European descent. *Diabetes* 45, 370–375, 1996.

23. Elbein, S.C., Chiu, K.C., Hoffman, M.D., Mayorga, R.A., Bragg, K.L., Leppert, M.F. Linkage analysis of 19 candidate regions for insulin resistance in familial Type 2 diabetes. *Diabetes* 44, 1259–1265, 1995.

24. Hani, E.H. Boutin, P., Durand, E., Inoue, H., Permutt, M.A., Velho, G., Froguel, P. Missense mutations in the pancreatic islet beta cell inwardly rectifying K⁺ channel gene (K1R6.2/BIR): a meta analysis suggests a role in the polygenic basis of type II diabetes mellitus in Caucasians. *Diabetologia* 41, 1511–1515, 1998.

25. Ghosh, S., Schork, N.J. Genetic analysis of Type 2 diabetes. The study of quantitative traits. *Diabetes* 45, 1–14, 1996.

26. Lev-Ran, L. Thrifty genotype: How applicable is it to obesity and type 2 diabetes? *Diabetes Rev.* 7, 1–22, 1999.

27. Rich, S.S. Mapping genes in diabetes. Genetic epidemiological perspective. *Diabetes* 39, 1315–1319, 1990.

28. Velho, G., Froguel, P.H. Genetic determinants of non-insulin-dependent diabetes mellitus: Strategies and recent results. *Diabetes Metab.* 23, 7–17, 1997.

29. Bell, G.I. Molecular defects in diabetes mellitus. *Diabetes* 40, 413–422, 1991.

30. Rich, S.S. Positional cloning works! Identification of genes that cause IDDM. *Diabetes* 44, 139–140, 1995.

31. Bell, G.I., Cox, N.J., Lindner, T., Concannon, P., Speilman, R.S., Boerwinkle, E., Hanis, C.L. Genetics of Type 2 diabetes in the Mexican Americans of Starr County Texas: An update. *Diabetes Rev.* 5, 277–283, 1997.

32. Weir, G.C., Sharma, A., Zangen, D.H., Bonner-Weir, S. Transcription factor abnormalities as a cause of beta cell dysfunction in diabetes: A hypothesis. *Acta diabetol.* 34, 177–184, 1997.

33. Yamagata, K., Takeda, J., Menzel, S., Chen, X., Eng, S., Lim, L.R., Concannon, P., Hanis, C.L., Speilman, R.S., Cox, N.J., Bell, G.I. Searching for Type 2 diabetes susceptibility genes: Studies of genes with triplet repeats expressed in skeletal muscle. *Diabetologia* 39:725–730, 1996.

34. Vionnet, N., Hani, E.H., Lesage, S., Philippi, A., Hager, J., Varret, M., Stoffel, M., Tanizawa, Y., Chin, K.C., Glasser, B., Permutt, M.A., Passa, P., Demenais, F., Froguel, P. Genetics of Type 2 diabetes in France. Studies with 19 candidate genes in affected sib pairs. *Diabetes* 46, 1062–1068, 1997.

35. DeFronzo, R.A. Pathogenesis of type 2 diabetes: Metabolic and molecular implications for identifying diabetes genes. *Diabetes Rev.* 5, 177–269, 1997.

36. Kumar, D., Gemayel, N.S., Deapen, D., Kapadia, D., Yamashita, P.H., Lee, M.L., Dwyer, J.H., Roy-Burman, P., Bray, G.A., Mack, T.M. North American twins with Type 2 diabetes. Genetic, etiological and clinical significance of disease concordance according to age, zygosity and the interval after diagnosis in the first twin. *Diabetes* 42, 1351–1363, 1993.

37. Engelgau, M.M., Heerman, W.H., Smith, P.J., German, R.R., Aubert, R.E. The epidemiology of diabetes and pregnancy in the U.S. in 1988. *Diabetes Care* 18, 1029–1033, 1995.

38. Ratner, R.E. Gestational diabetes mellitus In:*Diabetes Mellitus. A Fundamental and Clinical Text* (LeRoith, D., Taylor, S.I., Olefsky, J.M., Eds.) Lippincott-Raven, Philadelphia. 710–718, 1996.

39. Mathews, C.E., Berdanier, C.D. Non insulin dependent diabetes mellitus as a mitochondrial genomic disease. *Proc. Soc. Exp. Biol. & Med.* 219, 97–108, 1998.

40. Froguel, P. Vaxillaire, M., Velho, G. Genetic and metabolic heterogeneity of maturity-onset diabetes of the young. *Diabetes Rev.* 5, 123–130, 1997.

41. Fajans, S.S., Bell, G.I., Bowden, D.W., Halter, J.B., Polonsky, K.S. Maturity-onset diabetes of the young. *Life Sci.* 55, 413–422, 1994.

42. Gragboli, C., Lindner, T., Cockburn, B.N., Kaisaki, P.J., Gragnoli, F., Marozzi, G., Bell, G.I. Maturity-onset diabetes of the young due to a mutation in the hepatocyte nuclear facto 4∀ binding site in the promoter of the hepatocyte nuclear factor 1∀ gene. *Diabetes* 46, 1648–1651, 1997.

43. Lesage, S., Hani, ElH., Philippi, A., Vaxillaire, M., Hager, J., Passa, P., Demenais, F., Froguel, P., Vionnet, N. Linkage analyses of the MODY 3 locus on chromosome 12q with late-onset Type 2 diabetes. *Diabetes* 44, 1243–1247, 1995.

44. Vaxillaire, M., Rouard, M., Yamagata, K., Oda, N., Kaisaki, P.J., Boriraj, V.V., Chevre, J-C., Boccio, V., Cox, R.D., Lathrop, G.M., Dussoix, P., Philippe, J., Timsit, J., Charpentier, G., Velho, G., Bell, G.I., Froguel, P. Identification of nine novel mutations in the hepatocyte nuclear factor 1 ∀ gene associated with maturity-onset diabetes of the young (MODY 3). *Hum. Mol. Genet.* 6, 583–586, 1997.

45. Yamagata, K., Oda, N., Kaisaki, P.J., Menzel, S., Furuta, H., Vaxillaire, M., Southam, L., Cox, R.D., Lathrop, G.M., Boriraj, V.V., Chen, X., Cox, N.J., Oda, Y., Yano, H., Le Beau, M.M., Yamada, S., Nishigori, H., Takeda, J., Fajans, S.S., Hattersley, A.T., Iwasaki, N., Hansen, T., Pedersen, O., Polonsky, K.S., Turner, R.C., Velho, G., Chevre, J-C., Froguel, P., Bell, G.I. Mutations in the hepatocyte nuclear factor-1 ∀ gene in maturity-onset diabetes of the young (MODY3). *Nature* 384, 455–458, 1997.

46. Vaxillaire, M., Vionnet, N., Vigouroux, C., Sun, F., Espinoza, R., Lebeau, M.M., Stoffel, M., Lehto, M., Beckmann, J.S., Detheux, M., Passa, P., Cohen, D.,Van Schaftingen, E., Velho, G., Bell, G.I., Froguel, P. Search for a third susceptibility gene for maturity-onset diabetes of the young. Studies with eleven candidate genes. *Diabetes* 43, 389–395, 1994.

47. Glucksmann, M.A., Lehto, M., Tayber, O., Scotti, S., Berkemeir, L., Puliddo, J.C., Wu, Y. Nir, W-J., Fang, L., Markel, P., Munnelly, K.D., Goranson, J., Orho, M., Young, B.M., Whitacre, J.L., McMenimen, C., Wantman, M., Tuomi, T., Warram, J., Forsblom, C.M., Carlsson, M., Rosenzweig, J., Kennedy, G., Duyk, G.M., Krolewski, A.S., Groop, L.C., Thomas, J.D. Novel mutations and a mutational hotspot in the MODY 3 gene. *Diabetes* 46, 10811–1086, 1997.

48. Furuta, H., Iwasaki, N., Oda, N., Hinokio, Y., Horikawa, Y., Yamagata, K., Yano, N., Sugahiro, J., Ogata, M., Ohgawara, H., Omori, Y., Iwamoto, Y., Bell, G.I. Organization and partial sequence of the hepatocyte nuclear factor-4 "/MODY1 gene and identification of a missense mutation, R127W in a Japanese family with MODY *Diabetes* 46, 1652–657, 1997.

49. http://www.cdc.gov/diabetes/statistics/surv199/chap2/(accessed 10/04/01)

50. Knowler, W.C., Williams, R.C., Pettitt, D.J., Steinberg, A.G. Gm3; 5,13,14 and type 2 diabetes mellitus: An association in American Indians with genetic admixture. *Am. J. Hum. Genet.* 43, 520–526, 1988.

51. Knowler, W.C., Pettitt, D.J., Saad, M. F., Bennett, P.H., Diabetes mellitus in the Pima Indians: Incidence, risk factors and pathogenesis. *Diabetes Metab. Rev.* 6, 1–27, 1990.

52. Sakul, H., Pratley, R., Cardon, L., Rauvissin, E., Mott, D., Bogardus, C., Familiality of physical and metabolic characteristics that predict the development of non-insulin dependent diabetes mellitus in Pima Indians. *Am. J. Hum. Genet.* 60, 651–656, 1997.

53. Bogardus, C., Lillioja, S. Pima Indians as a model to study the genetics of Type 2 diabetes. *J. Cell. Biochem.* 48, 337–343, 1992.

54. Young, T.K., Dean, H.J., Flett, B., Wood-Steiman, P. Childhood obesity in a population at high risk for type 2 diabetes. *J. Pediat.* 136, 365–369, 2000.

55. Mokdad, A.H., Bowman, B.A., Ford, E.S., Vinicor, F., Marks, J.S., Koplan, J.P. The continuing epidemics of obesity and diabetes in the United States. *J. Am. Med. Assoc.* 280, 1195–1200, 2001.

56. Katch, V., Becque, M.D., Marks, C., Moorhead, C., Rocchini, A. Gender dimorphism in size, shape and body composition of child-onset obese and non-obese adolescents. *Int. J. Obesity* 15, 267–282, 1990.

57. Lemieux, S., Prud'homme, D., Bouchard, C., Tremblay, A., Despres, J-P. Sex difference in the relation of visceral adipose tissue accumulation total body fatness. *Am. J. Clin. Nutr.* 58, 463–467, 1993.

58. Haffner, S., Mitchell, B.D., Hazuda, H.P., Stern, M.P. Greater influence of central distribution of adipose tissue on the incidence of non-insulin dependent diabetes in women than in men. *Am. J. Clin. Nutr.* 53, 1312–1317, 1991.

59. Lundgren, H., Bengtsson, C., Blohme, G., Lapidus, L., Sjostrom, L., Adiposity and adipose tissue distribution in relation to incidence of diabetes in women: Results from a prospective population study in Gothenburg, Sweden. *Int. J. Obesity* 13, 413–423, 1989.

60. Haffner, S.M. Sex hormone-binding protein, hyperinsulinemia, insulin resistance and non-insulin-dependent diabetes. *Hormone Res.* 45, 233–237, 1996.

61. Liao, Y., Lansky, D., Cooper, R.S., Cao, G, Ghali, J.K., Lee, J. Sex differences in the impact of coexistent diabetes on survival in patients with coronary heart disease. *Diabetes Care* 16, 708–713, 1993.

62. Gordon, T, Castelli, W.P., Hjortland, M.M., Kannel, W.B., Dawber, T.R. Diabetes, blood lipids and the role of obesity in coronary heart disease risk for women. *Ann. Internal Med.* 87, 393–397, 1977.

63. Evans, R.W., Orchard, T.J. Oxidized lipids in insulin-dependent diabetes mellitus: a sex-diabetes interaction? *Metabolism* 43, 1196-1200, 1994.

64. Ruhe, R.C., Curry, D.L., Herrmann, S., McDonald, R.B. Age and gender effects on insulin secretion and glucose sensitivity of the pancreas. *Am. J. Physiol.* 262, R671–R676, 1992.

65. Macdonald, I., Crossley, J.N. Glucose tolerance during the menstrual cycle. Diabetes 19, 450-452, 1970.

66. Sharp, S.C., Diamond, M.P. Sex steroids and diabetes. *Diabetes Rev.* 1, 318–342, 1993.

15 Nutritional Issues in Arthritis and Rheumatic Disease

Tammy O. Utset

CONTENTS

I. INTRODUCTION

Arthritis and musculoskeletal disorders are among the most common medical disorders. While it has been estimated that 15% of Americans (40 million) had some sort of arthritis in 1995, this is expected to increase to 18.2% (59.4 million) by 2020. Most types of arthritis have a predilection for women. The most common form, osteoarthritis, affects 29.6% in women versus 17% of men over 60 years of age.[1] In addition to direct disability from arthritis, musculoskeletal pain among older women, mostly ascribable to osteoarthritis, has been shown to increase the risk for falling,[2] and thus contributes to the morbidity and mortality from bone fractures among elderly women.

Among young people, the most common form of chronic arthritis is rheumatoid arthritis, which occurs in 1% of the general population, but affects women two to three times as often as men.[1] In one study assessing the impact of various diseases on self-perceived health, the diagnosis of rheumatoid arthritis was more strongly associated with self-perceived ill health than cancer or diabetes mellitus among middle-aged women and was second only to renal disease in its association with self-perceived ill health among women older than 65. When prevalence of disease was also considered, rheumatoid arthritis was second only to cardiovascular disease as an attributable cause of self-perceived ill health among women 65 and older, while among men, the presence of diseases such as cancer, cardiovascular disease and neurological disease predominantly explained self-reported ill health.[3] Thus, arthritis and musculoskeletal disease have an exceptionally prominent role in the health of women.

Globally, most arthritis can be divided into degenerative arthritis (osteoarthritis), metabolic arthritis (prototypically gout) and inflammatory arthritis due to autoimmune disorders. In the autoimmune disease rheumatoid arthritis, joints are the major sites of inflammation in most patients. In other autoimmune diseases such as systemic lupus or scleroderma, the joints or various internal organs may be affected. Because issues differ greatly among these conditions, they will be discussed separately.

II. OSTEOARTHRITIS

Osteoarthritis (OA), or degenerative arthritis, is by far the most common form of arthritis and is a near-universal part of aging. Prior to menopause, the frequency of osteoarthritis is equal between the sexes. After menopause, the frequency of osteoarthritis in women markedly rises for unknown reasons.[4] Radiographic evidence of moderate to severe hand OA is present in 1% of women under 45, but increases to 5% in ages 45–54 and to 21–37% in women over 55.[5] This, combined with the increased life expectancy of women, results in a disproportionate burden of osteoarthritis among elderly women. Limitations in activity due to arthritis contribute, not only to disability, but also to obesity and obesity-related disease such as diabetes mellitus and coronary artery disease, discussed elsewhere in this volume.

Age is the greatest known risk factor for osteoarthritis. With aging, the cartilage, which lines and cushions joints, loses elasticity and water content. This results in brittleness, which predisposes to cracking in the setting of mechanical stressors. Traumatic injury to cartilage is more likely to occur from normal activity due to these changes. Such microtrauma then triggers the release of inflammatory factors such as interleukin-1β and tumor necrosis factor. These inflammatory factors trigger the synthesis of proteolytic enzymes that may further damage cartilage.[6]

Despite its relative acellularity, cartilage is always in a state of turnover, being constantly dissolved and rebuilt by the body. The maintenance of normal cartilage is dependent on the balance between anabolic and catabolic forces. While catabolic factors such as the matrix metalloproteinases attempt to destroy cartilage, inhibitors of matrix metalloproteinases and growth factors such as transforming growth factor-β and insulin-like growth factor-1 try to rebuild cartilage. As cartilage ages, it may become less responsive to anabolic factors and thus the balance may be shifted toward catabolism and cartilage thinning.[7]

Underlying articular bone depends on healthy cartilage to shield it from trauma. As cartilage thins, the underlying bone is injured. In an attempt to heal itself, the bone develops sclerosis, or scarring, and grows bone spurs at the margins of joints. This loss of joint space, sclerosis and spurring are the pathognomonic changes of osteoarthritis.

Obesity is highly associated with the development of osteoarthritis.[4] Because obesity increases the mechanical forces on weight-bearing joints, this association is not surprising. Of interest, obese women are prone not only toward OA of weight-bearing joints such as knees, but also toward OA of the hands. This association is not understood, but may represent a derangement in the balance of growth factors affecting articular structures in the setting of obesity.

While aging is inevitable, obesity is not. Weight control represents a very important site for intervention to prevent and minimize OA. A significant protective effect of weight loss on incident knee OA was demonstrated in the large population study, the Framingham Knee Osteoarthritis Study.[8] Relatively modest weight losses in the range of 12 lbs (5 kg) resulted in a more than 50% reduction in risk of incident knee OA at 10-year follow-up. Educating obese patients about the impact of weight loss on future disability can be helpful in motivating patients to pursue a weight loss program.

Indirect epidemiological associations suggest that a relative deficiency in micro-nutrients may predispose to OA. The Framingham Knee Osteoarthritis Study found that progression of established knee OA was increased threefold in those individuals in the lowest tertile of vitamin C intake relative to the individuals in the middle and highest tertiles of vitamin C consumption.[9] A similar protective effect was seen in individuals in the middle and highest tertiles of vitamin D intake.[10] Beta-carotene intake was not as strongly associated with OA risk. High vitamin E intake was protective among men but not women.[9] There is no evidence to suggest that supra-physiological doses of vitamins provide any further protection than standard doses. Although this data represents a simple epidemiological association, it seems reasonable to support the use of a simple daily vitamin with the standard recommended daily allowances of vitamin C, D and E in patients with established OA and in those individuals at high risk of OA.

The role of estrogen replacement in prevention or treatment of OA is controversial. Because OA becomes much more common after menopause, a protective effect of estrogen on cartilage health has been postulated. However, observational studies have shown mixed results, most likely related to confounding health practices among women who chose to take hormone replacement therapy.[4] While it is possible that estrogen replacement might decrease the risk of OA, the magnitude of any such benefit is not known. Recommendations to take estrogen primarily to benefit OA cannot be made at this time.

The use of nonprescription nutritional supplements has become extremely popular for self-treatment of OA. The most well-studied of these supplements are glucosamine sulfate and chondroitin sulfate. Glucosamine is a hexosamine sugar, which is a substrate for synthesis of cartilage by chondrocytes, while chondroitin is a compound naturally present in articular cartilage. Both are orally absorbed in the sulfate form. Countless studies of these nutritional supplements in OA suggest that they do have utility in reducing symptoms related to OA.[11] However, due to limitations in the methodologies of these studies, it is difficult to estimate the degree of benefit gained. One study has found decreased disease progression in patients on long-term supplementation with glucosamine, but, to estimate joint space, used radiological techniques that have been criticized as inaccurate.[12] Further studies with modified radiological techniques will be needed to clarify any potential disease-modifying role of glucosamine sulfate in OA.

Other nutritional supplements purported to help OA pain include methylsulfo-
nylmethane (MSM) and S-adenosyl-methionine (SAMe). MSM, also called
DMSO2, is found in plants and animal tissue. Its physiological roles are not known.
Unlike its cousin dimethyl sulfoxide (DMSO), no reports of toxic side effects from
MSM have been made. SAMe is a substrate for synthesis of neurotransmitters and
other compounds. No peer-reviewed trials with MSM have been reported in the
medical literature, while there has been one small controlled trial of SAMe in OA.[13]
This study suggested reduction in some parameters of OA symptomatology, but
reported severe gastrointestinal side effects in significant numbers of participants.
Currently, the data on SAMe and MSM is inadequate to recommend the use of either
compound for symptomatic OA.

Because products like the glucosamine and chondroitin sulfate, MSM and SAMe
are classified as nutritional supplements, they are not monitored by any U.S. regulatory agencies for quality and accuracy of content. An independent consumer group
(www.consumerlab.com) has found that substantial numbers of products do not
contain the labeled quantities of supplements. Patients need to be made aware of
this problem with quality control and make personal decisions about whether to buy
these supplements. If glucosamine and chondroitin can be clearly demonstrated to
affect the natural progression of OA in future studies, one can hope that the Federal
Drug Administration will consider making this a regulated drug and thus enforce
quality control on prescription versions of these products.

In summary, the most important nutritional issue in OA is obesity. Even relatively
modest weight losses can markedly decrease the risk of OA. Although the data
associating vitamins C, D and E with OA is indirect and may be confounded by
other protective health practices, a standard multivitamin supplement could be considered as a simple intervention that might impact the risk for OA and its progression.
While glucosamine and chondroitin sulfate may alleviate the symptoms of OA in
some individuals, it is not yet known if the long-term ingestion of these supplements
affects disease progression in individuals with established OA. Other popular supplements such as MSM and SAMe cannot be recommended as they have not been
adequately studied.

III. GOUT

Classically considered a "man's disease," gouty arthritis is thought to be increasingly
prevalent in women due to the aging of the population. In the 1960s, clinical gout
occurred in 0.72% of men and 0.48% of women over the age of 20. The frequency
of gout has doubled since that time, with an overall self-reported prevalence of
0.84% across all ages and sexes. Over age 65, 4.4% of men and 1.8% of women
report having gout.[1] Increases in the prevalence of obesity has also been cited as a
causative factor in this increased prevalence of gout.[14]

Gout occurs due to excessive build-up of uric acid in the blood, with secondary
precipitation of uric acid crystals in joints. These crystals can trigger a dramatic
inflammatory response that causes exquisite joint pain and swelling. At least initially,
attacks of gout are self-limited and subside over a few weeks. Although classically
involving the great toe, almost any joint can be affected.[15]

Premenopausally, women have lower levels of uric acid than men and thus are at lower risk for gouty arthritis. After menopause, the serum levels of uric acid increase in women. The widespread use of thiazide diuretics in treatment of hypertension in the elderly have further accelerated the frequency of gout in women, as these drugs result in increased serum uric acid concentrations.[16]

Uric acid is a byproduct of purine metabolism. The body endogenously produces the majority of its purines. Only about 1 mg/dl of serum uric acid is ascribable to dietary purine intake in individuals with normal renal function. In patients with impaired renal function, dietary intake may play a greater role.[17]

Some dietary practices can have significant impact on gouty arthropathy. Among these factors, alcohol ingestion is the most prominent. Excessive ethanol ingestion is associated with both hyperuricemia and gout. The mechanisms of hyperuricemia with ethanol ingestion are complex and include decreased urinary excretion of urate, the purine content of alcohol, effects on turnover of purine substrates and dehydration.[15,18]

Obesity is clearly associated with hyperuricemia and gout. Population studies reveal that approximately 3% of individuals in the lowest 20% of weight have hyperuricemia, while 11% of individuals in the highest 20% of weight are hyperuricemic.[19] Weight loss correlates with lower uric acid levels and a decreased frequency of gouty attacks.[20] Obesity and hyperuricemia may be part of "syndrome X," a constellation of insulin resistance, hyperlipidemia, hypertension, gout and coronary artery disease observed in some individuals. The presence of gout should suggest the possibility of these associated disorders and screening should be considered for hypertension, diabetes mellitus, hyperlipidemia and coronary artery disease.[19]

General dietary recommendations to gout patients thus include abstention or strict limitation of alcohol intake and weight loss if obese. A generous water intake will decrease the risk of nephrolithiasis and avoid dehydration, which may acutely elevate uric acid level. The purine content of foods varies, but strict avoidance of purines is not feasible as they are widespread in food groups. The highest levels of purines will be found in organ meats, meat extracts, scallops and canned small fish such as anchovies, herring and mackerel. Intermediate are protein sources such as red meat, poultry and other shellfish. The vegetables asparagus, cauliflower, legumes, spinach, mushrooms, peas, wheat germ and bran are also intermediate in purine content. Lowest in purines are non-whole-grain breads and cereals, dairy products, fish roe, fruits, nuts, gelatins and other vegetables. Limitation of the intake of high-purine foods, reduction of the amount of meat protein and dependence more heavily on dairy products for protein intake are reasonable dietary adjustments for patients with gouty arthropathy.[21]

In addition to these dietary changes, it is prudent for the physician to specifically review the patient's medications for drugs that might incite gout. Along with thiazide diuretics, loop diuretics such as furosemide will exacerbate hyperuricemia. Pyrazinamide, ethambutol and nicotinic acid will elevate serum uric acid levels and the transplant drugs cyclosporin and tacrolimus often cause a very severe gouty arthropathy. While high-dose salicylates lower uric acid levels, low-dose salicylates, as used for prevention of cardiovascular disease, elevate uric acid levels.[15]

Because dietary effects on uric acid levels are modest, patients with recurring episodes of gout will often require pharmacological therapy. Tophaceous gout or urate nephrolithiasis are clear indications for urate-lowering medications. Acute gouty episodes are managed with nonsteroidal anti-inflammatory medications, colchicine or corticosteroids. Chronic preventive therapy may include colchicine, allopurinol, or uricosuric agents such as probenecid.[22]

IV. RHEUMATOID ARTHRITIS

Rheumatoid Arthritis (RA) is an inflammatory arthritis usually involving the wrists and small joints of the hands, in addition to other joints. In RA, inflammatory cells and synovial cells proliferate around involved joints, causing pain, swelling, limitations in movement and eventually may result in joint destruction and consequent disability. While the inflammatory mediators are actually similar to that seen in OA (interleukin 1-β and tumor necrosis factor-α), the levels of these cytokines are much higher. RA is a systemic disease not limited to the joints, and elevations in these cytokines may be detectable in the blood. Patients with highly active RA typically have severe fatigue and may have weight loss and low-grade fevers. Inflammation from RA may occur in nonarticular structures such as the lungs, nerves, pericardium and skin in addition to the joints.[22]

Rheumatoid arthritis occurs in approximately 1% of the population, but is twice as common in women as in men.[1] Average age of onset is during the 50s, but the range of onset is wide. Rheumatoid arthritis may start in very young adult life or in the extremely aged. Disability from the arthritis is frequent and often individuals with RA will become unable to work after years of arthritis activity.[23] The frequency of disability from RA may soon decrease due to recent advances in the treatment of RA by tumor necrosis factor inhibitors.

Several environmental factors have been recognized as increasing the risk of developing RA. Smoking cigarettes increases the risk of RA.[24,25] Low serum levels of antioxidants, including beta-carotene, alpha-tocopherol and selenium are risk factors for developing RA.[26,27] A high-fish diet has been associated with decreased risk for RA in a case-control study.[28] A high intake of decaffeinated but not conventional coffee is associated with a higher risk of RA, while tea-drinking appears to be protective.[29]

Many lay sources claim the effectiveness of dietary changes in controlling RA. Studies of fasting support a transient improvement in RA, most likely due to the global immunosuppression associated with the fasting state. Obviously, this is not a viable long-term strategy for the control of a chronic disease. Other diets eliminating foods such as red meats, wheat, corn, dairy products, citrus and tomatoes or a strict vegan diet have been touted as useful, but the studies are contradictory and do not show effectiveness in the majority of patients.[30,31] Individual patients may occasionally find foods they feel strongly exacerbate their arthritis, but there is no uniform food list that is likely to exacerbate disease activity in the average patient.

The best data in the area of dietary supplements in RA is the use of fish oils for RA.[32–35] Fish oils from cold-water fish contain eicosapentaemoic acid and docosahexaenoic acids, which are known to decrease production of interleukin-1, tumor necrosis factor-α and arachidonic acid. Several studies have demonstrated modest improvement in disease activity in RA with the use of these supplements. These studies primarily used very high doses of fish oil (18 gm of fish oil concentrate daily, or fish oil containing 60% (n-3) fatty acids at 40 mg/kg/day) and the effectiveness of lower doses as often used by the lay population is not known. Vitamin E can prevent oxidation of encapsulated fish oil both during storage and with ingestion and it is recommended that vitamin E α-tocopherol, 3 mg per gram of fish oil, be included in fish oil supplements.[36] The best results of fish oil supplementation have been found in individuals who markedly decrease (n-6) saturated fats along with increasing fish oil intake in order to improve the n-3 to n-6 fatty acid ratios. While this dietary change may have multiple health benefits, including a decrease in risk of cardiovascular disease and some cancers, it may be hard for patients to sustain long-term.

Based on animal models of RA, vitamin E may play an important role in preventing bony destruction by downregulating interleukin-1,[37] although joint inflammation itself is not affected by vitamin E. Human RA studies of vitamin E supplementation in the prevention of joint damage have not yet been done.

It has long been observed that RA patients die younger than predicted, with mortality occurring 10 years earlier than in non-RA populations.[38] While cardiovascular disease is especially increased, the increased mortality is ascribed to a wide variety of illnesses and seems to indicate a general frailty of these patients. While the excess mortality is likely multifactorial, poor reserves in body cell mass (BCM), or "RA cachexia," may be a significant contributor. Loss of BCM is highly correlated with death in a variety of chronic medical conditions. A 40% reduction in BCM strongly predicts death regardless of clinical setting. Anthromorphometric studies demonstrate that the majority of RA patients have cachexia, or a decrease in BCM.[39,40] The BCM is reduced an average 13% in RA patients, which is one third of the dispensable BCM.[41] Thus, when illness strikes RA patients, they have less physical reserve than other individuals.

This cachexia is highly associated with the RA-associated cytokine tumor necrosis factor-α and to a lesser degree with interleukin 1-β.[41] Animal models demonstrate weight loss in the setting of high tumor necrosis factor levels even with controlled feeding conditions.[42] Tumor necrosis factor is known to affect insulin sensitivity while interleukin 1-β affects central appetite factors.[43]

Metabolic studies of humans with RA demonstrate an increased metabolic rate with superimposed relative anorexia — that is, the appetite is not increased as much as the metabolic rate.[41] Nutritional supplementation has not been shown to be effective in RA cachexia, yet, in frail patients with poor intake, the use of general nutritional supplements seems reasonable. Progressive resistance exercise programs may improve protein catabolism in these patients. However, the most effective treatment for RA cachexia is likely to be effective disease control, with concomitant decreases in tumor necrosis factor production.[44] Consistent with the importance of disease control in decreasing mortality, aggressive disease control with the immunosuppressive drug methotrexate has been shown to improve survival in RA patients.[45] With the new generation of drugs that directly inhibit tumor necrosis factor, perhaps RA cachexia will be reversed and mortality improved in the future.

Rheumatoid arthritis patients are predisposed to osteoporosis, even if they are not maintained on corticosteroid therapy.[46] Thus, close attention to bone health is appropriate in this population. All RA patients should maintain a calcium intake of 1500 mg per day along with vitamin D in the range of 400–800 IU per day.[47] A baseline measurement of bone density is reasonable in many RA patients to determine if there is a further need for prophylactic or therapeutic doses of osteoporosis medications, particularly in RA patients on chronic low-dose corticosteroids, in peri- or postmenopausal females or in patients who have any other risk factors for osteoporosis. Hormone replacement therapy is not thought to impact RA disease activity adversely and could be considered along with selective estrogen receptor modulators and bisphosphonates for osteoporosis therapy in RA patients.[48,49]

V. SYSTEMIC LUPUS ERYTHEMATOSUS

Systemic lupus erythematosus (SLE), or lupus, is a systemic autoimmune disease most often affecting women in their 30s and 40s. It occurs in approximately 1 in 1000 people, with greater than 90% of affected individuals being women. It can have a very wide variety of manifestations, including skin rashes, arthritis, inflammation of the lining tissues of the lungs and heart, blood abnormalities, kidney or brain involvement.[22] Because patients with SLE often have to take prolonged courses of oral corticosteroids, most nutritional issues in SLE involve side effects from corticosteroid therapy.

High-dose corticosteroid therapy has well-established side effects that include weight gain, induction of diabetes mellitus, hypertension, hypercholesterolemia and osteoporosis.[50] Weight gain in corticosteroid-treated patients is caused by a variety of factors including increase in appetite, decrease in metabolic rate and increase in the body's resistance to insulin. The increase in appetite that occurs with high-dose corticosteroids makes dietary self-discipline very problematic. It is best for patients to limit the availability of fattening foods — that is, not to keep such foods in the house. When children or other household members expect to have fatty food available, purchasing foods that the patient doesn't like may be a helpful strategy for some patients. Because of the complexity and potential severity of SLE, the use of pharmacological appetite suppressants is not prudent. Despite the increase in fatty tissue, high-dose corticosteroids cause atrophy of muscle and thus dieting must be undertaken with caution to not further waste muscle mass. Although no diet is formally tested for use in these patients, it may be beneficial to be referred to a trained dietitian. If renal function is normal, a high-protein modified diet and strength training may be considered to minimize weight gain and muscle mass loss, particularly in lupus patients who are already obese prior to initiation of corticosteroid therapy. Further studies in dietary, behavioral and pharmacological interventions to minimize weight gain and other steroid morbidities during prolonged corticosteroid therapy in lupus are obviously needed.

Lupus patients are prone to atherosclerotic heart disease,[51] so treating modifiable risk factors for heart disease such as hypercholesterolemia and hypertension should be a high priority. Corticosteroid-induced hypertension is common and is dose- and duration-dependent.[50] Dietary adjustments to minimize weight gain and salt intake may have some beneficial effect, but pharmacological treatment is often needed.[50] Patients with hypercholesterolemia should decrease the saturated fat intake in their diet, but may require pharmacological agents to lower cholesterol.[52] Lupus patients with kidney involvement and heavy protein losses in the urine, or nephrotic syndrome, are most prone to hypercholesterolemia and nearly all such patients should be treated with lipid-lowering medications until their renal disorder improves.[53]

Obesity at baseline may be a risk factor for the development of steroid-induced diabetes mellitus.[54,55] In addition, a high current dose and the total cumulative dose of exogenous corticosteroids administered are associated with diabetes risk.[54] The effect of glucocorticoids on blood sugar is dose-dependent and diabetes may subside after steroids are lowered.[50,55] Because obesity increases the body's resistance to insulin, minimizing weight gain during steroid therapy may make it more likely that diabetes will abate when steroid doses are lowered. A prudent diet avoiding concentrated sweets and simple carbohydrates may minimize glucose intolerance in individuals on high-dose corticosteroids. Empiric diabetes medications such as metformin, or lifestyle modifications including strict dietary control and exercise have been shown to lower the incidence of diabetes mellitus in normal individuals at high risk for diabetes.[56] However, the role of such interventions in preventing the onset of diabetes mellitus in patients initiating corticosteroid therapy has not been studied.

Osteoporosis is a more insidious complication in lupus, occurring gradually over years of corticosteroid use.[57] While corticosteroids have direct effects on bone, promoting osteoporosis, there may be other contributing factors.[58] The active form of vitamin D is often decreased in lupus patients and these decreases are associated with the use of the common lupus medication hydroxychloroquine.[59] However, hydroxychloroquine use is protective against osteoporosis in other studies.[60] Based on this protective effect, the inhibition of vitamin D conversion by hydroxychloroquine is likely not clinically significant or is overridden by the steroid-sparing effects of this drug. Exogenous corticosteroid therapy also suppresses sex hormone production, including both estrogens and androgens; thus the protective effect of these hormones on bone is decreased. Intestinal absorption of calcium is impaired by corticosteroids.[58] Simple supplementation of the diet to ensure the intake of 1500 mg of calcium and 400-800 IU of vitamin D is taken daily has been shown to be useful to inhibit bone loss in many patients on low doses of corticosteroids (less than 10 mg per day of prednisone) and may be adequate if patients are premenopausal and without other risk factors for osteoporosis.[61] However, baseline bone density measurement is reasonable in patients initiating 7.5 mg or more of prednisone daily for an expected 3-month or greater duration. If baseline measurement indicates osteopenia or osteoporosis, or if repeated bone density at 6–12 months indicates a significant decline in bone density, then addition of pharmacological agents for bone protection is indicated. If high-dose steroids are initiated with the expectation of long-term therapy, simple calcium and vitamin D supplementation alone is unlikely to be adequate to prevent significant bone loss. The active form of vitamin D, calcitriol, is somewhat more potent in bone protection in this setting but can result in significant hypercalcemia and requires careful monitoring. In most patients on high-dose corticosteroids,

baseline bone density measurement can again give guidance on the need for
pharmacological prevention of bone loss. If bone density is normal and only
calcium/vitamin D is used, repeat densitometry at 6 months is indicated to follow
the degree of bone loss on therapy.[47,58] Further discussion of osteoporosis can be
found elsewhere in this volume.

Dihydroepiandrosterone (DHEA), which is available over the counter as a nutritional supplement, has been used in lupus as a steroid-sparing agent in clinical
trials.[62] DHEA is usually produced in the adrenal glands along with natural glucocorticoids in response to adrenocorticotropin (ACTH) secretion by the pituitary
gland. When exogenous steroids are given, ACTH is inhibited and thus DHEA
secretion drops. DHEA is a weak androgen and has anabolic effects on muscle and
bone that may partially offset toxicities of exogenous corticosteroid administration.[63]
Bone density is relatively preserved in SLE patients on corticosteroids when DHEA
supplements are used.[64] The usual dose in SLE is 50–200 milligrams per day. Side
effects of DHEA supplementation include possible mild hirsutism and irregularity
of menses. Because DHEA is currently an unregulated nutritional supplement, the
acceptance of DHEA by the mainstream medical community has been limited by
concern about quality control. Lupus researchers are attempting to develop a pre-
scription-only form of DHEA to ensure product quality regulation for the medical
treatment of lupus.[65]

VI. SCLERODERMA

Scleroderma is a rare autoimmune disease that typically causes Raynaud's phenomenon (abnormal sensitivity of blood vessels to cold exposure) and fibrosis of
vascular endothelium, skin and other organs. It has a predilection for women, with
a mean age of onset around 50.[66] Disability often arises from contractures in the
hands due to thickened skin and ulceration of the fingertips. Variably, it may cause
scar tissue deposition in respiratory, cardiac, gastrointestinal or renal organ systems,
with potentially serious health consequences.[22]

The dominating nutritional issue in scleroderma is weight loss.[67] Weight loss is
most often due to sclerodermatous involvement of the gastrointestinal system. The
most common site of involvement is the esophagus.[68,69] Both deposition of scar tissue
and neuronal dysfunction in the esophagus interfere with normal contractility of the
esophageal muscles. Reflux esophagitis, dilation of the esophagus or esophageal
strictures may result. Patients adapt best to this by the use of small meal portions
and may unintentionally decrease their food intake while trying to minimize gastrointestinal discomfort. Pharmacological treatment of reflux esophagitis with proton
pump inhibitors can be extremely helpful in these patients, although high doses of
these agents are often necessary.[70]

Scleroderma may also directly affect the bowels, causing disorders in bowel
motility and direct difficulties in nutrient malabsorption. Slow motility may result
in either constipation or diarrhea. Constipation occurs due to impaired bowel motility
and may be so severe that a pseudo-obstruction may develop in some patients.[69,70]
The use of fiber supplements has been associated with the provocation of pseudo-
obstruction in scleroderma[69]and such supplements, if used, should be started at low

doses and very cautiously increased. While osmotic agents such as lactulose are sometimes used in these patients, no clinical trials have been performed to document the safety of osmotic agents for constipation in scleroderma patients.

Alternatively, diarrhea may ensue in scleroderma patients when slow motility allows overgrowth of bacteria in the bowel. These bacteria deconjugate bile salts, secondarily causing fat malabsorption-associated diarrhea. Twenty-four-hour stool fat measurements are often elevated in scleroderma patients, even in the absence of diarrhea. Vitamin deficiencies may occur due to competition for nutrients with overgrown enteric bacteria in the atonic bowel.[70] Cyclical use of antibiotics to control bacterial overgrowth is the most helpful strategy for these types of scleroderma bowel disease.[69]

Rarely clinically apparent, scleroderma can also affect pancreatobiliary function, resulting in steatorrhea and fat malabsorption.[71] This should also be considered in scleroderma patients with weight loss and refractory gastrointestinal disorder despite treatment for bacterial overgrowth.[70]

In the most severe cases, refractory vomiting or pseudo-obstruction may make central venous hyperalimentation necessary. Studies on the utility of long-term hyperalimentation in scleroderma are mixed, with some showing very high mortality rates and others showing substantial benefits.[69,70,72]

While there have been small uncontrolled studies implicating nutritional factors in the onset of scleroderma, there is no established role of micronutrients or nutritional supplements for the treatment of scleroderma.[67,73] The major focus of nutritional care for these patients relates to vigilance to progressive weight loss and prompt action on treatable causes such as reflux esophagitis or bacterial overgrowth syndromes.

VII. SUMMARY

Arthritis and musculoskeletal disease are particularly common in women and have a major impact on women's health. Significant epidemiological evidence supports the importance of weight loss in the management of OA and gouty arthropathy. Inadequate vitamin intake (particularly vitamins C and D) may contribute to the development and progression of OA. Nutritional supplements such as glucosamine sulfate and chondroitin sulfate may ameliorate symptoms but have not yet been shown to impact the long-term progression of this disease. Amongst gouty patients, weight loss and avoidance of alcohol are the most reasonable targets for intervention. In RA, a variety of environmental factors may be risk factors for the development of RA, but their impact on established RA is not known. Fish oil supplementation is mildly effective in the treatment of RA and may be a useful adjunct to standard therapy. RA patients appear excessively frail due to loss of body cell mass. This cachexia appears to be related to excessive tumor necrosis factor production in this condition. In lupus, the major nutritional issues are in the management of morbidities of chronic corticosteroid therapy, while in scleroderma, nutritional issues generally involve prevention and treatment of weight loss due to gastrointestinal dysfunction.

REFERENCES

1. Lawrence, R.V., Helmick, C.G., Arnett, F.C., Deyo, R.A., Felson, D.T., Giannini, E.H., Heyse, S.P., Hirsh, R., Hochberg, M.C., Hunder, G.G., Liang, M.H., Pillemer, S.R., Steen, V.D., Wolfe, F. Estimates of the prevalence of arthritis and selected musculoskeletal disorders in the United States, *Arthritis Rheum.*, 41:778, 1998.

2. Leveille, S.G., Bean, J., Bandeen-Roche, K., Jones, R., Hochberg, M.C., Guralnik, J.M. Musculoskeletal Pain and the risk of falls in older disabled women living in the community, *J. Am. Geriatr. Soc.*, 50:671, 2002.

3. Molarius, A., Janson, J. Self-rated health, chronic diseases and symptoms among middle-aged and elderly men and women, *J. Clin. Epidemiol.*, 55:364, 2002.

4. Felson, D.T., Lawrence, R.C., Dieppe, P.A., Hirsh, R., Helmick, C.J., Jordan, J.M., Kington, R.S., Lane, N.E., Nevitt, M.C., Zhang, Y., Sowers, M., McAlindon, T., Spector, T.D., Poole, A.R. Osteoarthritis: New insights. Part 1: The disease and its risk factors, *An. Intern. Med.*,133:635, 2000.

5. Lawrence, R.C., Hochberg, M.C., Kelsey, J.L., McDuffie, F.C., Medsger, T.A. Jr., Felts, W.R., Shulman, L.E. Estimates of the prevalence of selected arthritis and musculoskeletal diseases in the United States. *J. Rheumatol.* 16:427, 1989.

6. Pelletier, J.P., Martel-Pelletier, J., Abramson, S.B. Osteoarthritis, an inflammatory disease: potential implication selection of new therapeutic targets, *Arthritis Rheum.*, 44:1237, 2001.

7. Van der Kraan, P.M., van den Berg, W.B. Anabolic and destructive mediators in OA, *Curr. Opin. Clin. Nut. Metab. Care*, 3:205, 2000.

8. Felson, D.T., Zhang, Y., Anthony, J.M., Naimark, A., Anderson, J.J. Weight loss reduces the risk for symptomatic knee OA in women, *Ann. Int. Med.*, 116:535, 1992.

9. McAlindon, T.E., Jacques, P., Zhang, Y., Hannan, M.T., Aliabadi, P., Weissman, B., Rush, D., Levy, D., Felson, D.T. Do antioxidant micronutrients protect against the development and progression of knee OA? *Arthritis Rheum.*, 39:648, 1996.

10. McAlindon, T.E., Felson, D.T., Zhang, Y., Hannan, M.T., Aliabadi, P., Weissman, B., Rush, D.,Wilson, P.W.F., Jacques, P., Relation of dietary intake and serum levels of vitamin D to progression of OA of the knee among participants in the Framingham Study, *Ann. Intern. Med.*, 125:353, 1996.

11. McAlindon, T.E., LaValley, M.P., Gulin, J.P., Felson, D.T., Glucosamine and chondroitin for treatment of OA, *J. Amer. Med. Assoc.*, 283:1469, 2000.

12. Reginster, J.Y., Deroisy, R., Rovati, L.C., Lee, R.L., Lejeune, E., Bruyere, O., Giacovelli, G., Henrotin, Y., Dacre, J.E., Gossett, C., Long-term effects of glucosamine sulphate on OA progression: A randomized, placebo-controlled clinical trial, *Lancet*, 357:251, 2001.

13. Montrone, F., Fumagalli, M., Sarzi Puttini, P., Boccassini, L., Santandrea, S., Volpato, R., Locati, M., Caruso, I., Letter: Double-blinded study of s-adenosyl-methionine versus placebo in hip and knee arthrosis. *Clin. Rheumatol.*, 4:484, 1985.

14. Harris, C.M., Lloyd, D.C.E.F., Lewis, J. The prevalence and prophylaxis of gout in England. *J. Clin. Epidemiol.*, 48:1153–1158, 1995.

15. Becker, M.A. *Arthritis and Allied Conditions,* 14th ed., Lippincott Williams and Wilkins. Philadelphia, 2001, Ch. 114.

16. Puig, J.G., Michan A.D., Jimenez, M.L., Perez de Ayala, C., Mateos, F.A., Capitan, C.F., de Miguel, E., Gijon, J.B., Female gout. Clinical spectrum and uric acid metabolism. *Arch. Intern. Med.*, 151:726, 1991.

17. Rall, C.L. and Roubenoff, R., *Encyclopedia of Human Nutrition*, Academic Press, San Diego, CA, 1999, 978.

18. Faller, J. and Fox, I.H., Ethanol-induced hyperuricemia: Evidence for increased urate production by activation of adenine nucleotide turnover, *New Eng. J. Med.*, 307:1598, 1982.

19. McGill, N.W., Gout and other crystal-associated arthropathies, *Bailliere's Best Prac. Res.*, 14:445, 2000.

20. Dessein, P.H., Shipton, E.A., Stanwix, A.E., Joffe, B.I., Ramokgadi, J., Beneficial effects of weight loss associated with moderate calorie/carbohydrate restriction and increased proportional intake of protein and unsaturated fat on serum urate and lipoprotein levels in gout: A pilot study, *Annals Rheum. Disease*, 59:539, 2000.

21. Pennington, J.A.T. *Bowes & Church's Food Values of Portions Commonly Used.* 17th ed., Lippincott, Philadelphia, 1998, p 391.

22. Klippel, J.H., Dieppe, P.A., Eds., *Rheumatology*, 2nd ed., Mosby, London, 1998.

23. Young, A., Dixey, J., Kulinskaya, E., Cox, N., Davies, P., Devlin, J., Emery, P., Gough, A., James, D., Prouse, P., Williams, P., Winfield, J. Which patients stop working because of rheumatoid arthritis? Results of five years' follow up in 732 patients from the Early RA Study (ERAS), *Ann. Rheum. Dis.*, 61:335, 2002.

24. Criswell, L.A., Merlino, L.A., Cerhan, J.R., Mikuls, T.R., Mudano, A.S., Burma, M., Folsom, A.R., Saag, K.G., Cigarette smoking and the risk of rheumatoid arthritis among postmenopausal women: Results from the Iowa Women's Health Study. *Am. J. Med.*, 112:465, 2002.

25. Albano, S.A., Santana-Sahagun, E., Weisman, M.H., Cigarette smoking and rheumatoid arthritis, *Semin. Arthritis Rheum.*, 31:146, 2001.

26. Knekt, P., Heliovaara, M., Aho, K., Alfthan, G., Marniemi, J., Aromaa, A., Serum selenium, serum alpha-tocopherol and the risk of rheumatoid arthritis, *Epidemiology*, 11:402, 2000.

27. Heliovaara, M., Knekt, P., Aaran., R-K., Alfthan, G., Aromaas, A., Serum antioxidants and the risk of rheumatoid arthritis, *Ann. Rheum. Dis.*, 53:51, 1996.

28. Shapiro, J.A., Koepsell, T.D., Voigt, L.F., Dagowson, C.E., Kestin, M., Nelson, J.I., Diet and rheumatoid arthritis in women: A possible protective effect of fish oil consumption, *Epidemiology*, 7:256, 1996.

29. Mikuls, T.R., Cerhan, J.R., Criswell, L.A., Merlino, L., Mudano, A.S., Burma, M., Folsom, A.R., Saag, K.G., Coffee, tea and caffeine consumption and risk of rheumatoid arthritis: Results from the Iowa Women's Health Study, *Arthritis Rheum.*, 46:83, 2002.

30. Mangge, H., Hermann, J., Schauenstein, K., Diet and rheumatoid arthritis — a review, *Scand. J. Rheumatol.*, 28:201, 1999.

31. Haugen, M., Fraser, D., Forre, O., Diet therapy for the patient with rheumatoid arthritis? *Rheumatology (Oxford)*, 38:1036, 1999.

32. Volker, D., Fitzgerald, P., Major, G., Garg, M., Efficacy of fish oil concentrate in the treatment of rheumatoid arthritis, *J. Rheumatol.*, 27:2343, 2000.

33. Ariza-Ariza, R., Mestanza-Peralta, M., Cardiel, M.H., Omega-3 fatty acids in rheumatoid arthritis: An overview, *Semin. Arthritis Rheum.*, 27:366, 1998.

34. Kremer, J.M., Lawrence, D.A., Petrillo, G.F., Litts, L.L., Mullaly, P.M., Rynes, R.I., Stocker, R.P., Parhami, N., Greenstein, N.S., Fuchs, B.R. et al. Effects of high-dose fish oil on rheumatoid arthritis after stopping nonsteroidal anti-inflammatory drugs. Clinical and immune correlates, *Arthritis Rheum.*, 38:1107, 1995.

35. Geusens, P., Wouters, C., Nijs, J., Jiang, Y., Dequeker, J., Long-term effect of omega-3 fatty acid supplementation in active rheumatoid arthritis. A 12-month, double-blind, controlled study, *Arthritis Rheum.*, 27:824, 1994.

36. Darlington, L.G., Stone, T.W., Antioxidants and fatty acids in the amelioration of rheumatoid arthritis and related disorders, *Br. J. Nutr.*, 85:251, 2001.
37. De Bandt, M., Grossin M., Driss., F., Pincemail, J., Babin-Chevaye, C., Pasquier, C., Vitamin E uncouples joint destruction and clinical inflammation in a transgenic mouse model of rheumatoid arthritis, *Arthritis Rheum.*, 46:522, 2002.
38. Guedes, C., Dumont-Fischer, D., Leichter-Nakache, S., Boissier, M.C. Mortality in rheumatoid arthritis, *Rev. Rheum. Engl Ed.*, 66:492, 1999.
39. Roubenoff, R., Roubenoff, R.A., Ward, L.M., Holland, S.M., Hellmann, D.B., Rheumatoid cachexia: Depletion of lean body mass in rheumatoid arthritis. Possible association with tumor necrosis factor, *J. Rheumatol.*, 19:1505, 1992.
40. Hernandez-Beriain, J.A., Segura-Garcia C., Rodriguez-Lozano B., Bustabad S., Gantes M., Gonzalez T., Undernutrition in rheumatoid arthritis patients with disability, *Scand. J. Rheumatol.*, 25:383, 1996.
41. Roubenoff, R., Roubenoff, R.A., Cannon, J.G., Kehayias, J.J., Zhuang, H., Dawson-Hughes, B., Dinarello, C.A., Rosenberg, I.H. Rheumatoid cachexia: Cytokine-driven hypermetabolism accompanying reduced body cell mass in chronic inflammation, *J. Clin. Invest.*, 93:2379, 1994.
42. Roubenoff, R., Freeman, L.M., Smith, D.E., Abad, L.W., Dinarello, C.A., Kehayias, J.J. Adjuvant arthritis as a model of inflammatory cachexia, *Arthritis Rheum.*, 40: 534, 1997.
43. Argiles, J.M and Lopez-Soriano, F.J. Catabolic proinflammatory cytokines, *Metab. Care*, 1: 245, 1998.
44. Rall, L.C., Rosen, C.J., Dolnikowski, G., Hartman, W.J., Lundgren, N., Abad, L.W., Dinarello, C.A., Roubenoff, R. Protein metabolism in rheumatoid arthritis and aging. Effects of muscle strength training and tumor necrosis factor α, *Arthritis Rheum.*, 39:1115, 1996.
45. Choi, HK, Hernan, M.A., Seeger, J.D., Robins, J.M., Wolfe, F., Methotrexate and mortality in patients with rheumatoid arthritis: A prospective study, *Lancet*, 359:1173, 2002.
46. Haugeberg, G., Uhlig, T., Falch, J.A., Halse, J.I., Kvien, T.K., Bone mineral density and frequency of osteoporosis in female patients with rheumatoid arthritis: Results from 394 patients in the Oslo County Rheumatoid Arthritis register, *Arthritis Rheum*, 43:522, 2000.
47. ACR ad hoc committee on glucocorticoid-induced osteoporosis. Recommendations for the prevention and treatment of glucocorticoid-induced osteoporosis, *Arthritis Rheum.*, 44:1496, 2001.
48. Yilmaz, L., Ozoran, K., Gunduz, O.H., Ucan, H., Yucel, M. Alendronate in rheumatoid arthritis patients treated with methotrexate and glucocorticoids. *Rheumatol. Int.*, 20:65, 2001
49. Julkunen, H. Hormone replacement therapy in women with rheumatic diseases. *Scand. J. Rheumatol.*, 29:146,2000.
50. Ginzler, E.M., Aranow, C., Prevention and treatment of adverse effects of corticosteroids in systemic lupus erythematosus, *Baillieres Clin. Rheumatol.*, 12:495, 1998.
51. Karrar, A., Sequeira, W., Block, J.A., Coronary artery disease in systemic lupus erythematosus: A review of the literature, *Semin. Arthritis Rheum.*, 30:436, 2001.
52. Hearth-Holmes, M., Baethge, B.A., Broadwell, L., Wolf, R.E. Dietary treatment of hyperlipidemia in patients with systemic lupus erythematosus, *J. Rheumatol.*, 22:450, 1995.
53. Austin, H.A., Antonovych, T.T., MacKay, K., Boumpas, D.T., Balow, J.E. NIH conference. Membranous nephropathy. *Ann. Intern. Med.*, 116:672, 1992.

54. Raul Ariza-Andraca, C., Barile-Fabris, L.A., Frati-Munari, A.C., Baltazar-Montufar, P. Risk factors for steroid diabetes in rheumatic patients. *Arch. Med. Res.*, 29:259,1998.

55. Hoogwerf, B., Danese, R.D. Drug Selection and the management of corticosteroid-related diabetes mellitus. *Rheum. Dis. Clin. North Am.*, 25:489, 1999.

56. Diabetes Prevention Program Research Group, Reduction in the incidence of type 2 diabetes with lifestyle intervention or metformin, *New Eng. J. Med.*, 346:393, 2002.

57. Cunnane, G., Lane, N.E., Steroid-induced osteoporosis in systemic lupus erythematosus, *Rheum. Dis. Clin. N. Am.*, 26:311, 2000.

58. Adachi, J.D., Olszynski, W.P., Hanley, D.A., Hodsman, A.B., Kendler, D.L., Siminoski, K.G., Brown, J., Cowden, E.A., Goltzman, D., Ioannidis, G., Josse, R.G., Ste-Marie, L.-G., Tenenhouse, A.M., Davison, K.S., Blocka, K.L.N., Pollock, A.P., Sibley, J., Management of corticosteroid-induced osteoporosis, *Semin. Arthritis Rheum.*, 29:228, 2000.

59. Huisman, A.M., White, K.P., Algra, A., Harth, M., Vieth, R., Jacobs, J.W.G., Bijlsma, J.W.J., Bell, D.A., Vitamin D levels in women with systemic lupus erythematosus and fibromyalgia, *J. Rheumatol.*, 28:2535, 2001.

60. Lakshminarayanan, S., Walsh, S., Mohanraj, M., Rothfield, N., Factors associated with low bone mineral density in female patients with systemic lupus erythematosus, *J. Rheumatol.*, 28:102, 2001.

61. Amin, S., LaValley, M.P., Simms, R.W., Felson, D.T. The role of vitamin D in corticosteroid-induced osteoporosis. *Arthritis Rheum.*, 42:1740, 1999.

62. Van Vollenhoven, R.F., Dehydroepiandrosterone in systemic lupus erythematosus, *Rheum. Dis. Clinics N. Am.*, 26:349, 2000.

63. Straub, R.H., Scholmerich, J., Zietz, B., Replacement therapy with DHEA plus corticosteroids in patients with chronic inflammatory diseases — substitutes of adrenal and sex hormones, *Z. Rheumatol.*, 59, suppl. 2, 108, 2000.

64. Van Vollenhaven, R.F., Park, J.L., Genovese, M.C., West, J.P., McGuire, J.L., A double-blind, placebo-controlled, clinical trial of dehydrepiandrosterone in severe systemic lupus erythematosus, *Lupus*, 8:181, 1999.

65. Norman, P., GL-701 Genelabs, *Curr. Opin. Investig. Drugs*, 2:231, 2001.

66. Silman, A.J. Scleroderma — demographics and survival. *J. Rheumatol., Suppl.*, 48:58, 1997.

67. Lundberg, A.C., Akesson, A., Akesson, B., Dietary intake and nutritional status in patients with systemic sclerosis, *Ann. Rheum. Dis.*, 51:143, 1992.

68. Poirier, T.J., Rankin, G.B., Gastrointestinal manifestations of Progressive systemic scleroderma based on a review of 364 cases, *Am. J. Gastroenterol.*, 58: 30, 1972.

69. Rose, S., Young, M.A., Reynolds, J.C. Gastrointestinal manifestations of scleroderma, *Gastroenterol. Clin. N. Am.*, 27:563, 1998.

70. Sjogren, R.W., Review: Gastrointestinal motility disorders in scleroderma, *Arthritis Rheum.*, 37: 1265, 1994.

71. Hendel, L., Worning, H. Exocrine pancreatic function in patients with progressive systemic sclerosis. *Scan. J. Gatroenterol.*, 24:461, 1989.

72. Ng, S.C, Clements, P.J., Berquist, W.E., Furst, D.E., Paulus, H.E., Home central venous hyperalimentation in fifteen patients with severe scleroderma bowel disease, *Arthritis Rheum.*, 32:212, 1989.

73. Werbach, M.R.., *Textbook of Nutritional Medicine*, Third Line Press, Inc., Tarzana, CA, 1999.

16 Thyroid Hormones in Health and Disease

Carolyn D. Berdanier

CONTENTS

I. INTRODUCTION

The thyroid hormones are important regulators of intermediary metabolism. They function at the whole organism level, at the cellular level and at the gene level. The active hormone, triiodothyronine, is a universal metabolic regulator, yet disorders of thyroid function are found more frequently in females rather than males. Overactive and underactive thyroid hormone production can have serious effects on metabolism. In addition, thyroid hormone metabolism and its deviations may have a role in the development of obesity. This chapter reviews the anatomy and physiology of the thyroid gland, showing how thyroid hormone is synthesized and released and how it functions. The nutritional aspects of thyroid metabolism will be indicated where relevant.

II. THYROID GLAND ANATOMY AND PHYSIOLOGY

The thyroid gland is a shield-like structure located at the base of the neck (Figure 16.1). It can be palpated by gently moving the fingers over the windpipe between the hyoid bone and the sternal notch. The patient should sit relaxed with the head in the normal position (not elevated or with chin lifted) and be asked to swallow. In

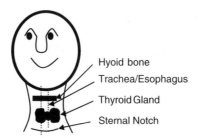

Hyoid bone
Trachea/Esophagus
Thyroid Gland
Sternal Notch

FIGURE 16.1 Location of the thyroid gland.

healthy individuals the gland will feel like a soft palpable mass around the trachea/esophagus above the sternal notch. Goiter, characterized by gland enlargement, is a typical feature of iodine deficiency. In people with goiter the gland will be larger and firmer. In advanced cases of goiter, the gland can be seen without palpation. Some of these goiters will regress spontaneously if the diet is supplemented with iodine or if the primary reason (excess dietary iodine or an iodine-rich drug) for the enlargement is removed. Other goiters will advance and enlarge. The reasons that the gland enlarges are various: It can be due to dietary iodine deficiency or excess, due to the consumption of goitrogens (compounds that inhibit the production of hormone), it may be congenital or it may be due to some other reason.

Goiter used to be endemic in the areas far removed from the sea. Seafood is an excellent source of this essential mineral. However, with the discovery of the importance of iodine in the diet and its role in the synthesis of thyroid hormone, the incidence of goiter has dramatically fallen. A prevalence of less than 5% in the U.S. has been reported.[1]

III. GENDER DIFFERENCES IN THYROID DISEASES

Most of the cases of nontoxic goiter are female.[2] Table 16.1 provides some information on the female:male ratio in a variety of thyroid diseases. There is practically no difference between the sexes in thyroid cancers but almost all other diseases of the thyroid have a female predominance. The ratio of female:male varies with the disease. For example, the ratio is 2:1 in coast goiter. This is an enlargement of the thyroid gland due to excess consumption of iodine. It was described in a Japanese coastal community where the consumption of seaweed and fish was high.[3] When these people reduced their iodine intake through elimination of the high-iodine-containing foods, the goiters regressed.[4] In most instances, it took about 6 months for the enlargements to disappear. In iodine-induced thyrotoxicosis the female:male ratio varies from 6:1 to 10:1.[5] As with the coast goiter, this condition is due to excess iodine intake.

There is also a drug-induced thyrotoxicosis due to the use of iodine-rich drugs. This condition is uncommon. Nontoxic goiter, usually due to an inadequate iodine intake, has a female:male ratio of 4:1.[6] If diagnosed early and treated with a dietary iodine supplement, the enlargement regresses. Hashimoto's thyroiditis, an inflammation of the thyroid gland due to autoimmune disease, is characterized by elevated

TABLE 16.1
Female to Male Ratio in Various Thyroid Diseases

Disease	Female:Male Ratio
Coast Goiter (excess I Intake)[3,4]	2:1
Iodine-Induced Thyrotoxicosis[5]	6:1 to 10:1
Drug Induced Thyrotoxicosis[6]	1:1
Goiter, Non-Toxic (Iodine deficiency)[6]	4:1
Hashimoto's Thyroiditis (autoimmune disease)[7]	2:1
Substernal Goiter (late onset)[8]	1:6:1-3.2:1
Thyroid Cancer	1:1
Graves Disease (severe hyperthyroidism)	5:1
Postpartum Thyroiditis[9]	1:0
Subacute Granulomatus Thyroiditis	F>M (not enough cases to give good ratio)
Hypothyroidism	10:1

levels of thyroid stimulating hormone (TSH). It is more common in middle-aged persons and more common in females than in males.[7]

Late-onset substernal goiter has a female:male ratio of 1.6:1 to 3.2:1.[8] This goiter is sometimes hard to diagnose and occurs primarily in the elderly. Cancer of the thyroid gland occurs equally in males and females, whereas Graves disease has a 5:1 female:male ratio. Graves disease is a severe form of hyperthyroidism. It can be treated by administration of propylthiouracil (PTU) or through ablation of some of the thyroid gland. PTU inhibits thyroid hormone synthesis as well as the conversion of thyroxine to triiodothyronine. Administration of PTU to women who then become pregnant results in neonatal hypothyroidism.[9]After birth, the maternal PTU effect disappears and, within 3 days, the infant normalizes. Whether there are long-lasting effects of maternal PTU on the infant has not been determined. The ablation of some of the thyroid hormone producing cells using the short-lived isotope I^{131} is also used. With the isotope treatment, the woman must be careful to avoid pregnancy for at least 6 months after treatment.

Pregnancy induces an increase in thyroid hormone production as the woman's body supports the growth and development of the unborn child. Sometimes, after birth, the thyroid gland continues to be stimulated to produce high amounts of hormone and hyperthyroidism can occur. Sometimes this resolves itself but sometimes medical intervention is required. Either PTU or gland ablation as described above can be used. Hyperthyroidism can also occur at other critical states in the female's reproductive life. Menarche and menopause each seem to precipitate changes in thyroid gland activity, and hyperthyroidism may develop at these stages. Again, sometimes this condition resolves itself but in other instances medical intervention is needed. Regardless of the cause, hyperthyroidism can have serious long-term effects on the health of women. For example, hyperthyroidism and thyrotoxicosis reduce bone mineral and muscle mass.[10] As well, intestinal calcium absorption is lower in women with hyperthyroidism than in normal women.[11] These two results of hyperthyroidism are a concern for women, who develop osteoporosis more frequently than do men.

Finally, hypothyroidism or under-production of thyroid hormones has a 10:1 female:male ratio. In adults, the condition is known as myxedema; in children, it is cretinism. Regardless of whether there is excess or deficient gland activity, females seem to predominate in these disorders.

Since thyroid hormone is so important in the regulation of metabolism, it is no surprise to find that the features of hyperthyroidism (excess thyroid hormone production and release) and hypothyroidism (inadequate thyroid hormone production and release) are manifested as changes in metabolism. Listed in Table 16.2 are the features of each.

Increased oxygen consumption and basal metabolic rate are key diagnostic features of hyperthyroidism, while the reverse (below normal oxygen consumption and basal metabolic rate) characterizes hypothyroidism.[12–18] The other characteristics are more subjective and difficult to measure. However, taken all together, the characteristics are related to the metabolism of the tissue or organ involved. In hyperthyroidism, the patient is heat intolerant; there is excess sweating, nervousness, anxiety, insomnia, perhaps depression, a rapid heart beat, weight loss, diarrhea, hair loss and a number of skin-related symptoms. In hypothyroidism, there is cold intolerance. Patients frequently complain of being cold all the time no matter the temperature of the environment. Mental activity is affected, with memory loss being a critical characteristic. If hypothyroidism occurs in an infant or young child, the memory problem may be permanent if not caught early. Mental retardation (cretinism), somnolence, depression, weight gain, constipation, dry coarse skin, coarse hair, fatigue and peripheral pain are among the characteristics of hypothyroidism.

IV. NUTRITIONAL ASPECTS OF THYROID GLAND FUNCTION

The disappearance of the once-common condition goiter can be attributed to a variety of factors. The mandated iodination of table salt plus the development of the technology to distribute seafood throughout the nation has ensured that the diet of the average American is adequately supplied with this essential nutrient. Other food sources include milk and bread. As farmers realized that iodine was essential to farm animals, they fed dairy cows iodine-supplemented feed. This iodine passes to their milk. Iodates are also used as dough conditioners in the making of bread, so this foodstuff is also a source for this essential nutrient.

Normal thyroid iodine economy can be maintained on an intake of 50–70 µg iodine/day. Iodine (I_2), an essential mineral and a member of the halogen family of elements, is found in fish, shellfish, milk, bread and sea products (seaweed and its derivatives). It is consumed as either a salt or as the element. Iodine in excess is excreted in the urine and urinary iodine reflects intake fairly accurately. Urinary iodine excretion varies from 45–700 µg/day, whereas in goiter it may be as low as 3 µg/day. The average intake in the U.S. is estimated at 350–450 µg/day. Elemental iodine or inorganic iodide salts are reduced to iodide once ingested. Iodide is then available for use in the synthesis of the thyroid hormones. This is its sole function.

In addition to the essentiality of iodine intake, the status of other nutrients may affect thyroid status. Protein malnutrition in children is one of these. Thyroid

TABLE 16.2
Features of Disordered Thyroid Function

Hyperthyroidism	Hypothyroidism
Heat intolerance	Cold intolerance
Nervousness, agitation	Memory loss
Anxiety	Somnolence
Depression	Depression
Insomnia	Periorbital edema
Eye Grittiness, tearing	Hoarseness
Rapid heart beat	Chest pain
Dyspnea	Peripheral edema
Increased appetite	Decreased appetite
Weight loss	Weight gain
Diarrhea	Constipation
Increased sweating	Decreased sweating
Hair loss	Dry coarse skin
Pruritis	Coarse hair
Polyurea	Hair loss
Ammenorrhea	Menorrhagia
Decreased libido	Decreased libido
Fatigue, muscle weakness	Fatigue
Tremor	Arthralgias, myalgias
Increased oxygen consumption	Decreased oxygen consumption
Increased BMR	Decreased BMR

hormone production is decreased in these children, who are characterized by a reduced basal metabolic rate, reduced iodine uptake by the thyroid gland and growth failure.[19]

The thyroid hormone (see next section) is synthesized from the amino acid tyrosine. In protein-malnourished individuals, tyrosine is in short supply, hence less is available for thyroid hormone synthesis. In addition, the protein hormones that regulate thyroid hormone synthesis and release are also synthesized in reduced quantities because of the reduced supply of the amino acids needed for their synthesis. Altogether, protein malnutrition has devastating effects on the health of the child with respect to thyroid hormone status.

Another nutritional condition is selenium deficiency. In rats, severe selenium deficiency has been shown to result in decreased activity of the 5′ deiodinase, an enzyme essential to the conversion of thyroxine to triiodothyronine, the active thyroid hormone (see next section). However, in humans, this enzyme is very protected; it is very unlikely to be decreased in activity in selenium-deficient people.[20]

A. THYROID HORMONE SYNTHESIS

Thyroid hormone synthesis occurs in the thyroid gland. The synthesis begins with the movement of iodide from the blood into thyroid cells. TSH stimulates the removal of iodide from the blood capillary network that supplies the thyroid gland. Iodide ions move to the apex of the thyroid cell, where the iodination of the amino acid tyrosine occurs. This is the so-called organification of the iodide ion. The iodination of tyrosine requires a heme-containing peroxidase enzyme. The regulation of this enzyme is but one of the factors important to the regulation of thyroid hormone synthesis. If there is a sudden increase in iodide, there is down regulation of the peroxidase enzyme. This occurs through a reduction in the amount of peroxide(H_2O_2) needed for the iodination reaction. Down regulation of the peroxidase enzyme helps to protect against iodine toxicity. Should there be a congenital deficiency of peroxidase, goiter and cretinism with an associated loss in mental function may result. This is a very rare condition.

The tyrosine that is used for iodination is actually part of the thyroglobulin molecule. This tyrosine-rich protein is rather large (660,000 Da). It has 110 tyrosine residues, of which 8–10 can be used for thyroid hormone synthesis. Mutations have been reported in the gene for thyroglobulin, however, these are very rare. The iodination of tyrosine involves the substitution of an iodide for the hydrogen on the tyrosyl ring. This occurs in a step-wise fashion, as illustrated in Figure 16.2. The first substitution produces monoiodotyrosine, the second, diiodotyrosine. These two substituted tyrosines are then joined together (coupled) to form triiodothyronine (T_3) or tetraiodothyronine, thyroxine (T_4). The newly formed hormone remains a part of thyroglobulin. The coupling occurs at the phenol end of the tyrosine, where one ring is donated to the other to form T_4. This leaves a residual dehydroalanine at the donor site in the thyroglobulin molecule. All of these steps are under the control of TSH, the thyroid stimulating hormone produced by the pituitary. Once the T_4 is formed as part of thyroglobulin, it is packaged and stored in the Golgi apparatus until a signal for its release into the circulation occurs. The thyroglobulin is gathered into a colloid space at the center of the thyroid cell. It is inaccessible to the circulation at this point. Slowly it is released. Estimated release rates are about 1% per day and this small percent is replaced. If there is constant TSH stimulation, more hormones are secreted and less colloid is stored. This occurs in hyperthyroidism.

Approximately 90 µg of T_4 and 30 µg of T_3 are released daily in normal individuals. Turnover is carefully regulated such that serum levels of 8 µg T_4/dL and 140 ng T_3/dL are maintained. Less than 1% of each of these is active. 99% is bound to a transport protein called thyroid-binding globulin. This is a glycoprotein that binds about 75% of the circulating hormone; the other 24% is bound by other blood proteins including albumin (10%) and prealbumin (14%). The binding of the hormone by these proteins can be influenced by a number of clinical situations: excess estrogen, pregnancy, oral contraceptives, hepatitis, porphyria (excess porphyrins in the blood) and heredity. All of these factors increase the binding of the thyroid hormones by the blood proteins and in turn, this can cause an increase in TSH production with its effects on hormone synthesis and release. In addition to the above, there are factors that can have the opposite effect.

Decreased binding can occur with the androgens, in cirrhosis, nephrosis and again heredity. Note the gender difference in these factors. Female hormones in general increase binding and TSH production while male hormones decrease binding. Here may be another factor in the female prevalence in thyroid diseases.

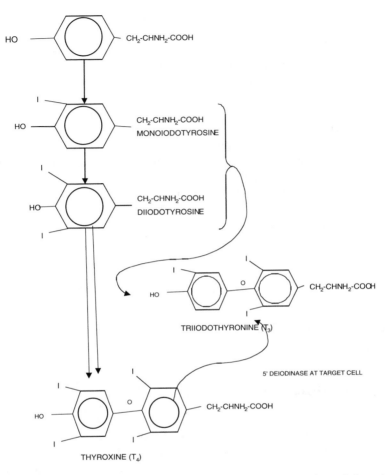

FIGURE 16.2 Thyroid hormone synthesis from tyrosine and conversion of thyroxine to triiodothyronine at the target cell.

Once at the target cell, T_4 is deiodinated to T_3. Most cell types have this deiodination ability, however, the liver, kidney and pituitary are the most important. In the pituitary, the deiodination step is essential to the regulation of the thyroid axis. Deiodination is stepwise and is catalyzed by the enzyme 5′deiodinase. There are three types of deiodinases. All are dependent on the availability of sulfhydryl compounds. This deiodination accounts for 85% of the production of active T_3 each day. Sometimes, this conversion is not very active and the condition known as "euthyroid ill" develops. It is a situation where there is little deiodinase activity. There is ample T_4, but little T_3 is produced. Conditions such as starvation, glucocorticoid therapy, use of beta blockers, thionamides and chronic or acute illness can affect thyroid hormone status. There is some suggestion that the lack of diet- or cold-induced thermogenesis in the obese may be due to an aberrant deiodinase activity.[21,22] Diet- or cold-induced thermogenesis is an important element in energy balance. Himms-Hagen et al.[21,22] have studied this phenomenon extensively. Genetically obese rodents have an impaired capacity to increase deiodinase activity when cold exposed. Cold exposure normally stimulates an increase in norepinephrine release that in turn stimulates both thermogenesis by brown fat cells and deiodinase activity. The deiodinase has been found to be defective in the obese mouse and may account for some of the obesity problem. Where energy wasting through thermogenesis does not occur normally, there can be excess energy storage as fat. In animals made hyperlipogenic through starvation–refeeding, 5'deiodinase activity adjusted to accommodate the dietary change. However, in genetically obese animals, such adjustments did not occur.[23] Again, this may contribute to their obesity development. In addition, obese Zucker rats provided with thyroid hormone supplements reduced their food intake and lost body fat.[24] As mentioned in the section on hypothyroidism, thyroid hormone deficiency exhibits reduced appetite as a feature of the condition. In the obese female rat, hyperphagia, not hypophagia, is a feature. Clearly, the role of the thyroid hormone in these genetically obese rats with respect to appetite control is different from that in the human.

Selenium is an essential component of Type I 5'deiodinase and secondary thyroid hormone deficiency in rats can occur where selenium deficiency occurs.[25,26] Types II and III deiodinases do not contain selenium, however, their activity is linked to that of the Type I. Should there be a less active Type I because of selenium deficiency, all three deiodinases will be less active. Restoration of selenium to the deficient diet fed to rats reverses the impaired thyroid state. Analogous studies in humans have not been conducted nor have there been any studies showing a gender difference in response to selenium deficiency.

B. Thyroid Hormone Regulation

As mentioned above, thyroid hormone status is closely regulated (Figure 16.3). Neurotransmitters from the brain signal the hypothalamus to release thyrotropin releasing hormone (TRH). The neuropeptides responsible for this signaling are poorly understood. Both adrenergic and peptinergic signals may be involved.[27]

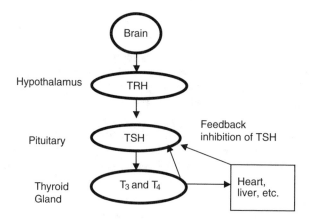

FIGURE 16.3 Thyroid hormone regulation. TRH, thyrotropic hormone; TSH, thyroid stimulating hormone; T_3, triiodothyronine; T_4, thyroxine.

The release of TRH then stimulates the pituitary to release TSH and, as described above, this hormone stimulates the synthesis as well as release of the thyroid hormones T_4 and T_3. As the levels of these compounds rise in the blood, there is a feedback to the pituitary such that TSH release is inhibited. As T_4 and T_3 exert their effects and disappear from the circulation, the blood levels fall and this inhibition is released, thus completing the regulatory circuit.

C. THYROID HORMONE FUNCTION

The function of the thyroid hormones is a regulatory one in metabolism. It affects both anabolic and catabolic reactions and truly is one of the central regulators of energy balance. At the core of this function is its effect on the expression of those genes that encode the key regulatory steps in intermediary metabolism.

Shown in Table 16.3 is an effect of thyroid hormone on mitochondrial oxygen consumption as well as thermogenesis. With thyroid hormone administration there is no increase in ATP synthesis.[14,17,28] That is, mitochondrial respiration can be increased but, unless coupled with an increase in ATP production, the energy generated by the respiratory chain is released as heat — hence, the observation of an increase in heat production in the hyperthyroid individual. Coupled with the increase in mitochondrial respiration is an increase in both the α-glycerol phosphate shuttle and the malate-aspartate shuttle.[28,29] Both of these must increase to support an increase in respiration. These two shuttles are responsible for the indirect transfer (via substrate conversions on each side of the mitochondrial membrane) of reducing equivalents into the mitochondrial compartment.

TABLE 16.3
Metabolic Activity Induced by Thyroid Hormone Administration

Enzyme	Activity Change[*]
Malic enzyme	
FAD linked Glycerol-3-phosphate dehydrogenase	increased
α Glycerol phosphate shuttle	increased
Malate-aspartate shuttle	increased
Glycolysis	increased
Gluconeogenesis	increased
Glycogen synthesis and degradation	increased
Lipolysis	increased
Thermogenesis	increased
Mitochondrial oxygen consumption	increased
Membrane fluidity	increased
Citric acid cycle enzymes	increased
Proteolysis	increased

[*]Compared with euthyroid animals or humans

The first is dependent on the activity of the FAD linked α glycerol phosphate dehydrogenase in the mitochondria. Its activity is unregulated by thyroid hormone via an effect on the expression of the gene that encodes the FAD α glycerol phosphate dehydrogenase.[30]

The second shuttle, the malate-aspartate shuttle, is essential to respiration and indeed is the major transporter of reducing equivalents into the mitochondrial compartment. The activity of this shuttle is dependent on the phosphorylation state of the cytosol. As mentioned, although thyroid hormone increases respiration, it has little effect on ATP synthesis. Hence, there is an abundant supply of ADP to drive the malate-aspartate shuttle forward.

Glycolysis is, in part, rate-controlled by the α glycerol phosphate shuttle because it generates, in the cytosol, the NAD needed by this pathway. Similarly, gluconeogenesis is, in part, dependent on the activity of the malate aspartate shuttle and, as noted, this shuttle is up regulated by thyroid hormone.[31] The citric acid cycle, located in the mitochondrial compartment, is responsive to all of these metabolic changes and it too is more active so as to accommodate the use of the end product of glycolysis (pyruvate) as well as to produce the necessary entry points for mitochondrial respiration.

As thyroid hormone also stimulates lipolysis,[32,33] it is surprising to find that mitochondrial membranes are more fluid in a hyperthyroid animal.[34–36] An increase in lipolysis means that more of the stored fatty acids are released for use and are in circulation. It suggests that the unsaturated fatty acids are preferentially incorporated into the mitochondrial membrane and so explain the increase in fluidity. Finally, the thyroid-treated animal has an increased rate of amino acid oxidation and protein turnover.[37] One assumes that these amino acids are mobilized from the muscle and thus explain the loss in body protein that occurs in the hyperthyroid individual.[10] It also ties in to the increase in gluconeogenesis because this process uses nonglucose metabolites to produce glucose; in this instance, it uses the carbon chains of some of the amino acids released from the proteolysis. Altogether, thyroid hormone in excess seems to induce some futile cycling of metabolites and, with this futile cycling, there is an increase in heat production.

D. ROLE IN GENE EXPRESSION

Thyroid hormone has these effects because of its effect on gene expression in both the nucleus and the mitochondria.[38–46] In the cytosol, T_3 is bound to a specific thyroid hormone binding protein. It is then transferred into the nucleus or into the mitochondria. Upon transfer into either of these compartments, it is bound to another protein, the thyroid receptor protein. This protein binds to DNA at specific base sequences in the promoter region for specific genes. Figure 16.4 illustrates this process. The receptor utilizes zinc fingers for its binding to DNA. The receptor has two transacting domains: one at the NH_3 end of the protein and one at the COOH end of the protein. The latter can dimerize to other receptors, such as the RXR receptor, such that together, the hormone and the vitamin (retinoic acid, the gene active form of vitamin A), can have additive effects on gene expression. The thyroid receptor can also dimerize to the estrogen receptor and, as mentioned earlier in this chapter, estrogen plus the thyroid hormone can be especially active. Without the

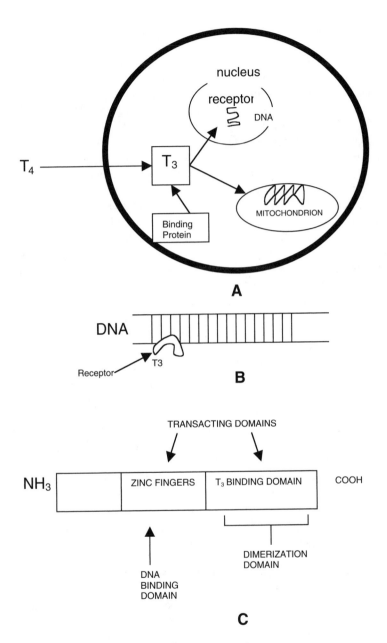

FIGURE 16.4 Thyroid hormone action in gene expression.

estrogen and its receptor binding to DNA to stimulate gene expression, the effects of the thyroid hormone are minimal. Here is another explanation for the predominance of females with thyroid disease.

A number of genes have promoter regions with thyroid binding elements, as suggested by the large number of reactions that can be modified with the addition of thyroid hormone or its removal. In general, nuclear genes each have their own promoter regions. However, with the mitochondrial genome, there is only one promoter region — the D-loop (the displacement loop) — and this promoter regulates the expression of all of the 13 structural genes found in this genome.[47] Thyroid hormone, bound to its receptor, increases the expression of all of these genes.[47] These genes encode components of the mitochondrial respiratory chain and two units of the ATP synthesizing enzyme complex, the F_1F_0ATPase.[48] Although thyroid hormone addition can up regulate the expression of the mitochondrial genome, it cannot induce an increase in oxidative phosphorylation efficiency. This is because this genome encodes only a small percentage of the total number of proteins in the oxidative phosphorylation system. All units must simultaneously be expressed to allow an increase in both the respiratory chain and ATP synthesis. Thus, thyroid hormone, if it is to have an effect on this process, must have effects on the nuclear genes as well. If any one is not up regulated, a simultaneous increase in respiration and ATP synthesis will not occur. This has been reported. For example, the ATPase b unit gene is unresponsive to thyroid hormone treatment.[46] As described earlier, ATP production is not increased in hyperthyroidism. In addition, rats with a mutation in the ATPase 6 gene of the mitochondrial genome did not increase their respiratory chain activity when treated with thyroid hormone.[49] These rats have less efficient mitochondria than normal rats and thyroid treatment did not improve their mitochondrial efficiency.

A number of mutations have been reported that affect the responsiveness of cells to thyroid hormone action.[50] One of these is a mutation of the thyroid receptor in the nucleus.

Thyroid hormone receptor mutant cells have been prepared that mimic humans with hormone resistance.[51] The mutations in the receptor appear to occur in the portion that is in the dimerization domain. Mutations in the ligand-binding region of the receptor have been reported in humans with an autosomal dominant syndrome of generalized thyroid hormone resistance. These people have elevated free thyroid hormone levels, inappropriate TSH levels and resistance to thyroid hormone by target cells. The clinical features are a mixture of those of hypothyroidism and hyperthyroidism. There are tachycardia, abnormal growth (short stature, poor muscle development), attention deficit disorder and alterations in metabolism. It would appear that these mutations affect the ability of the thyroid hormone receptor to dimerize with other DNA binding proteins. In turn, this can explain the features of this inherited disorder.[50,51]

It also provides insight into the mechanism of action of the thyroid hormone receptor with respect to gene expression. Other mutations in genes that encode other elements of the regulation of thyroid hormone status have likewise provided information on how the thyroid axis works.

V. SUMMARY

Diseases of the thyroid gland are found primarily in females rather than in males. The reason for this gender difference has little to do with nutrition, but has much to do with the interacting effects of the estrogens with the expression of thyroid-sensitive genes. As well, this female bias has to do with the effects of estrogen and other female hormones on the regulation of the thyroid axis.

REFERENCES

1. Matovinovic, J. Endemic goiter and cretinism at the dawn of the third millennium. *Ann. Rev. Nutr.* 3:341, 1983.
2. Davis, P.J., Davis, F.B. Nontoxic goiter, In: *Principles and Practice of Endocrinology and Metabolism* (K.L. Becker, Ed.) J.B. Lippincott, Philadelphia, 1990, 306–318.
3. Suzuki, H., Higuchi, T., Sawa K. Endemic coast goiter in Hokkaido, Japan, *Acta Endocrinol.* (Copenhagen) 50:141, 1965.
4. Wolff, J. Iodide goiter and the pharmacologic effects of excess iodide. *Am. J. Med.* 47:101, 1969.
5. Ermans, A.M., Camus, M. Modification of thyroid function induced by chronic administration of iodide in the presence of autonomous thyroid tissue. *Acta Endocrinol.* (Copenhagen) 70:463, 1972.
6. Vander, J.B., Gaston, E.A., Dawber, T.R. The significance of nontoxic thyroid nodules. *Ann. Internal Med.* 69:537.
7. Brown, J., Soloman, D.H., Beall, G.N. Autoimmune thyroid disease — Graves disease and Hashimoto's. *Ann. Internal Med.* 88:379, 1978.
8. Katlic, M.R., Wang, C.A., Grillo, H.C. Substernal goiter. *Ann. Thorac. Surg.* 39:391, 1985.
9. Cheron, R.G., Kaplan, M.M., Larsen, P.R., Selenkow, H.A., Crigler, J.F. Neonatal thyroid function after propylthiouracil therapy for maternal Grave's disease. *New Eng. J. Med.* 304:525, 1981.
10. Bayley, T.A., Harrison, J.E., McNeill, K.G., Mernagh, J.R. Effect of thyrotoxicosis and its treatment on bone mineral and muscle mass. *J. Clin. Endocrinol. Metab.* 50:916, 1980.
11. Haldimann, B., Kaptein, E.M., Singer, F.R., Nicoloff, J.T., Massry, S.G. Intestinal calcium absorption in patients with hyperthyroidism. *J. Clin. Endocrinol. Metab.* 51:995, 1980.
12. Nolte, J., Pette, D., Bachmair, B., Kiefhaber, P., Schneider, H., Scriba, P.C. Enzyme response to thyrotoxicosis and hypothyroidism in human liver and muscle: Comparative aspects. *Eur. J. Clin. Invest.* 2:141, 1972.
13. De Nayer, P. Thyroid hormone action at the cellular level. *Hormone Res.* 26:48, 1987.
14. Gregory, R.B., Berry, M.N. On the thyroid hormone-induced increase in respiratory capacity of isollated rat hepatocytes. *Biochem. Biophs. Acta* 1098:61, 1991.
15. Luvisetto, S., Schmehl, I., Intravaia, E., Conti, E., Azzone, G.F. Mechanism of loss of thermodynamic control in mitochondria due to hyperthyroidism and temperature. *J. Biol. Chem.* 267:15348, 1992.
16. Soboll, S., Horst, C., Hummerich, H., Schumacher, J.P., Seitz, H.J. Mitochondrial metabolism in different thyroid states. *Biochem. J.* 281:171, 1992.
17. Soboll, S. Thyroid hormone action on mitochondrial energy transfer. *Biochem. Biophys. Acta* 1144:1, 1993.
18. Harper, M-E., Brand, M.D. Use of top-down elasticity analysis to identify sites of thyroid hormone induced thermogenesis. *Proc. Soc. Exp. Biol. Med.* 208:228, 1995.
19. Monckeberg, F., Beas, F., Horwitz, I., Dabancens, A., Gonzalez, M. Oxygen consumption in infant malnutrition. *Pediatrics* 33: 554, 1964
20. Rayman, M.P. The importance of selenium to human health. *Lancet* 356:233, 2000.

21. Kates, A.-L., Himms-Hagen, J. Defective regulation of thyroxine 5'-deiodinase in brown adipose tissue of ob/ob mice. *Am. J. Physiol.* 258:E7, 1990.

22. Kates, A.-L., Himms-Hagen, J. Adrenergic effects on thyroxine 5' deiodinase in brown adipose tissue of lean and ob/ob mice. *Am. J. Physiol.* 258: R430, 1990.

23. McIntosh, M.K., Berdanier, C.D., Kates, A-L. Studies of 5'deiodinase in rats differing in hepatic lipogenic activity. *FASEB J.* 3:1734, 1989.

24. Parente, J.A., Berdanier, C.D. Hyperthyroidism reduces food intake by obese female Zucker rats. *Biochem Arch.* 13: 277, 1997.

25. Arthur, J.R., Nicol, F., Beckett, G.J. Selenium deficiency, thyroid hormone metabolism and thyroid hormone deiodinases. *Am. J. Clin. Nutr.* 57:236S, 1993.

26. Ahren, B. Thyroid neuroendocrinology: Neural regulation of thyroid hormone secretion. *Endocrinol. Rev.* 7:149, 1986.

27. Harper, M-E, Ballantyne, J.S., Leach, M., Brand, M.D. Effects of thyroid hormone on oxidative phosphorylation. *Biochem. Soc. Trans.* 21:785, 1993.

28. Tobin, B.B., Berdanier, C.D., Eckland, R.E., DeVore, V., Canton, C. Mitochondrial shuttle activities in hyperthyroid and normal rats and guinea pigs. *J. Environ. Path. Toxicol.* 3:289, 1980.

29. Tobin, R.B., Berdanier, C.D., Eckland, R.E. Effect of thyroidectomy upon the activity of three mitochondrial shuttles in rats. *J. Environ. Path. Toxicol.* 3:307, 1980.

30. Muller, S., Seitz, H.J. Cloning of a cDNA for the FAD-linked glycerol-3-phosphate dehydrogenase from rat liver and its regulation by thyroid hormones. *Proc. Natl. Acad. Sci. USA* 91:10581, 1994.

31. Berdanier, C.D. Effects of thyroid hormone on the gluconeogenic capacity of lipemic BHE rats. *Proc. Soc. Exp. Biol. Med.* 172:187, 1983.

32. Jung, R.T., Shetty, P.S., James, W.P.T. Nutritional effects of thyroid and catecholamine metabolism. *Clin. Sci.* 58:183, 1980.

33. Pou, M-A., Torresani, J. Coordinated stimulation by triiodothyronine of fatty acid synthesis and isoproterenol-sensitive fatty acid release in two preadipocyte cell lines of lean and genetically obese mice. *Horm. Metab. Res.* 21:468, 1989.

34. Berdanier, C.D. Interaction of dietary fat type and thyroxine on the hepatic phospholipid fatty acids of BHE rats. *Nutrition* 4:293, 1988.

35. Hoch, F.L., Subramanian, C., Dhopeshwarkar, G.A., Mead, J.F. Thyroid control over biomembranes: VI. Lipids in liver mitochondria and microsomes of hypothyroid rats. *Lipids* 16:328, 1981

36. Hoch, F.L., Depierre, J.W., Ernster, L. Thyroid control over biomembranes. Liver-microsomal cytochrome b_3 in hypothyroidism. *Eur. J. Biochem.* 109:301, 1980.

37. Kim, M.J.C., Berdanier, C.D. Nutrient–gene interactions determine mitochondrial function. *FASEB J.* 12:243, 1998.

38. Tsalikian, E., Lim, V.S. L-triiodothyronine at a slightly over physiologic dose increases leucine flux, which suggests an increase in protein degradation in normal subjects. *J. Lab. Clin. Med.* 114:171, 1989

39. Zilz, N.D., Murray, M.B., Towle, H.C. Identification of multiple thyroid hormone response elements located far upstream from the S14 promoter. *J. Biol. Chem.* 265:8136, 1990.

40. McNabb, F.M.A. Thyroid hormones, their activation, degradation and effects on metabolism. *J. Nutr.* 125:1773S, 1995.

41. Pillar, T.M., Seitz, H.J. Thyroid hormone and gene expression in the regulation of mitochondrial respiratory function. *Eur. J. Endocrinol.* 136:231, 1997.

42. Hoppner, W., Rasmussen, U.B., Abuerreish, G., Wohlrab, H., Seitz, H.J. Thyroid hormone effect on gene expression of the adenine nucleotide translocase in different rat tissues. *Mol. Endocrinol.* 2:1127, 1988.

43. Shupnik, M.A., Chin, W.W., Habener, J.F., Ridgway, E.C. Transcriptional regulation of the thyrotropin subunit genes by thyroid hormone. *J. Biol. Chem.* 260:2900, 1985.

44. Sterling, K. Thyroid hormone action at the cell level. *New Eng. J. Med.* 300:117, 1979.

45. Jump, D.B. Rapid induction of rat liver S_{14} gene transcription by thyroid hormone. *J. Biol. Chem.* 259:2789, 1989.

46. Martin, I., Villena, J.A., Giralt, M., Iglesias, R., Mampel, T., Vinas, O., Villarroya, F. Influence of thyroid hormones on the human ATP synthase β-subunit gene promoter. *Mol. Cell. Biochem.* 154:107, 1996.

47. Berdanier, C.D., Everts, H.B., Hermoyian, C., Mathews, C.E. Role of vitamin A in mitochondrial gene expression. *Diab. Res. Clin. Prac.* 54:511, 2001.

48. Anderson, S., Bankier, A.T., Barrell, B.G., Bruijn. M. H. L., Coulsen, A.R., Drouin, J., Epperon, I.C., Nielich, D.P., Roe, B.A., Sannger, F., Schreier, P.H., Smith, A.J.H., Staden,R., Young, I.G. Sequence and organization of the human mitochondrial genome. *Nature* (London) 290:457, 1981.

49. Berdanier, C.D., Kim, M-J. C., Hyperthyroidism in BHE/Cdb rats does not induce an increase in mitochondrial respiration. *J. Nutr. Biochem.* 4:10, 1993.

50. Kopp, P., Kitajima, K., Jameson, J.L., Syndrome of resistance to thyroid hormone: Insights into thyroid hormone action. *Proc. Soc. Exp. Biol. Med.* 211:49, 1996.

51. Nagaya, T., Madison, L.D., Jameson, J.L., Thyroid hormone receptor mutants that resistance to thyroid hormone. *J. Biol. Chem.* 267:13014, 1992.

17 Nutritional Factors in Women's Cancers: Breast, Cervical, Endometrial and Ovarian

Barbara C. Pence

CONTENTS

I. INTRODUCTION

Many investigators have examined the impact of diet and nutrition on both total cancer incidence and mortality. Their results are based on evaluating the relationship between dietary factors and the observed cancer risk, migrant studies in which there are definite shifts in site-specific cancer rates among those peoples migrating to the U.S., supportive evidence from animal studies, as well as the biological relevance of diet to a particular type of cancer.[1] In 1981, Doll and Peto[2] estimated that 35% of all cancer mortality in the United States was related to diet; previously, Wynder and Gori[3] estimated that nearly 40% of cancers among women are related to diet. Although it is not possible to quantify the contribution of diet to cancer risk for a particular site, it is sufficient to say that — excluding colon cancer, which is not specific to women — there appears to be a significant role for diet and nutrition in the etiology and prevention of women's cancers. In this chapter, the role of nutrition in the potential prevention or causation of those cancers specific to women will be discussed, by site (breast, cervical, endometrial and ovarian) and by nutrient class.

II. BREAST CANCER

Breast cancer is the second most common cancer diagnosis in American women, as well as the most common cause of cancer mortality. It is second only to lung cancer, which is not considered to be a nutritionally related cancer. Cancer at this site is associated with hormonal activity, but diet has long been suspected as a major cause.[4] Many descriptive epidemiologic studies of migrants have demonstrated an association between life-style factors and risk for breast cancer. Diet has been implicated extensively in the etiology of this disease, especially dietary fat, but results are still inconclusive to date and have been the subject of much controversy in recent years.

Several types of studies will be discussed that provide evidence supporting the importance of dietary factors in breast cancer: descriptive epidemiological studies, correlation studies, evaluation of nutritionally mediated risk factors, case control, cohort studies and meta-analyses. This review will focus solely on human studies, with animal data mentioned only where it might add pertinent support.

A. DESCRIPTIVE EPIDEMIOLOGICAL STUDIES

The evidence from descriptive epidemiological studies suggests that cultural factors or life-style, especially diet, are important etiological factors in the development of breast cancer. Kolonel[5] reported that Japanese migrant women living in Hawaii have a higher incidence of this disease than Japanese women living in Japan. Migrant studies have shown that the incidence of breast cancer among premenopausal Japanese-American women living in California is now almost as high as that for Caucasian women, whereas the incidence of cancer among them was similar to the low rate in Japan when they first migrated.[6] Other descriptive studies[7] have shown that changes in cancer incidence for certain populations can be related to changes in life-style of successive birth cohorts.

B. CORRELATION STUDIES

A second type of evidence for dietary factors in breast cancer has been provided by studies correlating breast cancer incidence and mortality with per capita intake of total fat and other nutrients in different countries[8] and the U.S. Early correlation studies[9] with various dietary constituents have shown a correlation between dietary fat and mortality from breast cancer in a number of countries. Gaskill et al.[10] found a direct correlation between cancer mortality and intake of milk, table fats, beef, calories, protein and fat and an inverse correlation with intake of eggs.

C. NUTRITIONALLY MEDIATED FACTORS

Factors that are considered nutritionally related, but are not nutrients themselves, have been analyzed with respect to breast cancer risk. These include weight, height, body mass (which is dependent on weight and height), body mass index (BMI) and age at menarche. Women who experience menarche at an early age, especially before age 12, are at higher risk.[4, 11] Evidence that body weight and food intake are related to early onset of estrus in rats[12] supports the hypothesis that the rat's body must contain a minimum amount of fat for estrus to occur. This also appears to be essential for menarche in women, [13] although not all studies have confirmed these findings.[14] To confuse the results further, an evaluation of the effects of per capita intake of total fat and animal protein on the international incidence and mortality rates for breast cancer found a significant effect of these variables, even after controlling for height, weight and age at menarche.[15] Most studies examining weight and breast cancer risk support an association of weight with increased breast cancer risk.[16] In the Nurses' Health Study, a significant positive association was seen between weight and breast cancer risk in postmenopausal women.[17] As an additional variable, the BMI (weight/height^2) has been studied, suggesting an interaction between BMI, breast cancer and menopausal status.[18]

Out of 13 case-control studies of BMI and breast cancer risk, 11 show a greater relative risk for postmenopausal women in the highest BMI category, [16] but this is an inverse association in premenopausal women. In the Nurses' Health Study, a similar inverse association was seen between weight at age 18 and risk of breast cancer in premenopausal women.[17] A recent analysis of the association between anthropomorphic indices and the risk of breast cancer used pooled data from seven prospective cohort studies, with a combined total of 337, 819 women and 4385 incident breast cancer cases.[19] These authors concluded that height was an independent risk factor for postmenopausal breast cancer, but for premenopausal women, this relationship was inconsistent. The relationship of BMI to breast cancer varied by menopausal status. Their final comment was that weight control may reduce the risk of breast cancer among postmenopausal women.[19]

Exercise appears to be an independent risk determinant for cancers in general and breast cancer specifically. A recent review of the association between physical activity and cancer prevention[20] not only describes methodological limitations in the previous studies, but also gives detailed recommendations for future research in the field. For the role of physical activity in breast cancer, Friedenreich had concluded that 24 of 26 studies[20] demonstrated a consistency of evidence for risk reduction with increased physical activity levels, with an average risk reduction for breast cancer of 30–40%. Friedenreich concluded that, for breast cancer, the overall level of scientific evidence for the role of physical activity in breast cancer prevention was "convincing."[20] The relationship between BMI, physical activity and breast cancer risk has also been reviewed in women from several racial and ethnic backgrounds.[21] Seven studies were included in the review and integrated women from Asian-, African- and Mexican-American backgrounds.[21] McTiernan has concluded that obesity and a sedentary lifestyle may be important modifiable risk factors for breast cancer, especially in women from multiethnic backgrounds. However, the cultural acceptance of weight loss and physical activity may vary by ethnicity and therefore, further research is needed in this area.[21]

D. Case-Control or Cohort Studies

Case-control or cohort studies should provide the most conclusive evidence we have on dietary factors and breast cancer risk. In 1975, an early case-control study reported five categories of foods that were associated with breast cancer: fried foods, fried potatoes, hard fat used for frying, dairy products except milk and white bread, with the relative risks ranging from 1.6 to 2.6.[22] In another early case-control study[23] the strongest association for dietary factors and breast cancer risk was seen for total fat consumption in both premenopausal and postmenopausal women, although the relative risks were low and there was no dose-response. Yet another study[24] reported that the relative risk of breast cancer increased significantly with more frequent consumption of beef and other red meat, pork and sweet desserts. More recent studies have not supported the connection between dietary fat and breast cancer. Graham et al.[25] compared the fat intake of 2024 breast cancer cases with 1463 controls and found that both animal fat and total fat intake were nearly identical in the two groups. A number of smaller case-control studies have been summarized in a meta-analysis by Howe et al.[26] Only 4 of 12 studies showed positive associations between fat intake and breast cancer risk. However, when all the data were pooled, a significant but weak association was observed for both total and saturated fat in postmenopausal women. Also supporting the same hypothesis, Kushi et al.[27] reported a modest positive association of total fat intake with risk of breast cancer in a study of 34, 388 postmenopausal women from Iowa. Another prospective population-based study of dietary fat, calories and the risk of breast cancer demonstrated that women who developed breast cancer had significantly higher age-adjusted intake of all fats with a stepwise increase in risk across tertiles of intake.[28] However, in the largest prospective cohort study, [29] the Nurses' Health Study, 89, 494 women were followed for 8 years and the relative risk for developing breast cancer for the highest quintile of dietary fat intake was only 0.90, indicating no effect of this dietary factor on the risk of developing breast cancer.

E. Meta-Analyses

The role of meta-analyses in nutritional epidemiology has become widespread, although it remains controversial.[30] Usually, data are combined from a number of studies that have met specific criteria. The value of meta-analyses goes beyond a summary measure of association[31] and also allows possible explanation for the causes of heterogeneity among studies.[31] A commonly used alternative to meta-analysis is the pooling of data, allowing an analysis to be made on the combined primary data from a number of studies, where the data meet specified criteria.[30] In pooled analyses, it is possible to evaluate associations across a wider range than may be available within individual studies and Willett has stated that "the advantages of pooled analyses in nutritional epidemiology are so substantial that this should become common practice for important issues."[30] Indeed, this methodology has become an extremely common one in the recent literature on nutrition and cancer. To better achieve this understanding of how diet and cancer are related, the Pooling Project of Prospective Studies of Diet and Cancer was established and a standardized approach adopted for use of the primary data from combined studies.[32]

F. ANTIOXIDANT VITAMINS (A, C, AND E)

Vitamin A consists of both preformed vitamin A as retinol and retinyl esters, as well as the carotenoids found primarily in fruits and vegetables. A number of case-control studies have examined the role of vitamin A intake and all have found a protective association.[16] Howe et al.[26] reported a significant protective association between total vitamin A and breast cancer in a meta-analysis of nine case-control studies with data on dietary intake of vitamin A. The data are more supportive of carotenoid vitamin A than for the preformed type. In the Nurses' Health Study, Hunter et al.[33] prospectively studied the cohort of 89,494 women and assessed their intake of vitamins A, C and E from foods and supplements at baseline and in 1984. They found a significant inverse association of vitamin A intake with the risk of breast cancer. They also found that large intakes of vitamin C or vitamin E did not protect the women in this study from breast cancer. In a previous study of postmenopausal women in New York, Graham et al.[25] reported no increase in risk related to the ingested amount of calories, vitamins A, C, or E, dietary fiber, or fat. In a case-control study on women in Buffalo, Potischman et al.[34] reported no overall association between plasma retinol and breast cancer, but a positive relationship was observed between retinol and breast cancer in the subgroup with low plasma beta-carotene values, suggesting that low plasma carotene may be a risk factor for breast cancer. There have been few published studies linking vitamin E and breast cancer. Three case-control studies have reported protective associations, whereas another two report no effect or a direct effect.[16] In the only prospective study published, as mentioned previously,[33] no protective effect was seen for vitamin E. Howe et al.[26] in their meta-analysis observed a significant inverse association for ascorbic acid and breast cancer risk. Hunter et al.,[33] again in the only prospective study on the antioxidant vitamins, reported a weak positive association.

G. FRUITS AND VEGETABLES

A number of recent epidemiologic studies of diet and breast cancer have suggested that increased fruit and vegetable consumption is associated with a decreased risk. Smith-Warner and Giovanucci's review contained few cohort studies, however.[35] Using the Pooling Project and Food frequency questionnaires,[32] fruit and vegetable intake was assessed from 351,825 women with 7377 incident cases of invasive breast cancer. These authors concluded that fruit and vegetable consumption during adult-hood is not significantly associated with breast cancer risk.[32] This result is consistent with a previous analysis combining five prospective studies of comparative mortality between vegetarians vs. nonvegetarians that found no significant difference with regard to breast cancer.[36] However, another meta-analysis examined the relationship between breast cancer, fruit and vegetable consumption and the intake of beta-carotene and vitamin C.[37] This analysis of 26 studies supports the association between breast cancer and intake of vegetables and, to a lesser extent, fruits (relative risk (RR = 0.75 for vegetables and 0.94 for fruits)). The authors conclude that increasing vegetable consumption may be protective.

H. SELENIUM

Ecologic studies have demonstrated strong inverse associations between selenium exposure and breast cancer.[38–40] In addition, although the nutrition and cancer liter-ature is represented extensively with animal studies of selenium and its protective effect on mammary carcinogenesis, a substantial body of evidence appears to indicate a lack of any appreciable effect of selenium intake on breast cancer risk, at least within the range of human diets.[41] In a recent case-control study in Sweden, [42] plasma selenium and glutathione peroxidase in erythrocytes were analyzed. In individuals without supplemental selenium intake, a preventive effect for breast cancer was found, increasing with plasma selenium level.[42] This was significant for women over 50 years of age and a nonsignificant effect was seen in women under 50. In a prospective study in the Nurses' Health Study, Hunter et al.[43] collected toenail clippings and determined selenium concentration. The relative risk for selenium concentration from highest to lowest quintile was not different. The authors con-cluded that selenium intake later in life is not likely to be an important factor in the etiology of breast cancer.[43] More recent studies have also drawn the conclusion that selenium is not an important etiological factor in breast cancer.

I. VITAMIN D

Although dietary vitamin D deficiency may be a risk factor for mammary carcino-genesis in rodents[44] and the vitamin in its active form has demonstrated protective effects in experimental models, [45] the only reported study investigating the hypothesis of vitamin D deficiency and cancer of the breast showed no differences between cases and controls in their mean daily intake of the vitamin.[46] Therefore, there is no evidence at this time that vitamin D has any role in the etiology of human breast cancer. However, patients with vitamin D receptor-positive tumors had longer dis-ease-free survival than those with receptor-negative tumors[45] and vitamin D receptor status has potential as a prognostic indicator.[47]

J. ALCOHOL CONSUMPTION

In recent years, a substantial body of evidence has accumulated to support a positive association between alcohol consumption and breast cancer.[16] Longnecker et al.[48]

performed a meta-analysis on 12 case-control studies and concluded that there is an increased relative risk of about 1.4 for each two drinks of alcohol per day. Reichman et al.[49] have reported that in a controlled diet study, alcohol consumption was associated with statistically significant increases in levels of several estrogenic hormones and that this could be a possible explanation for the positive association seen between alcohol consumption and breast cancer. In a Polish case-control study of breast cancer, smoking and vodka drinking, Pawlega[50] reported that the habit of drinking vodka 20 years earlier significantly increased breast cancer risk in women under 50 years old. In a Canadian study of 56,837 women, Friedenreich et al.[51] reported only a small association of alcohol consumption with breast cancer risk (RR of 1.11) and no association at all for postmenopausal women. An Italian case-control study of alcohol and breast cancer risk also reported a moderate increase in risk for the highest quintile of alcohol consumption.[52] Also in a case-control study in Moscow (Russia), Zaridze et al.[53] reported an odds ratio for risk of breast cancer in postmenopausal women of 3.39, thus supporting a hypothetical role of alcohol as an etiologic factor in breast cancer. The most recent study on alcohol and breast cancer[54] is another pooled analysis of six prospective studies from the Pooling Project, described previously.[32] This review included the alcohol intake of 322,647 women from Canada, the United States and northern Europe.[54] The authors concluded that alcohol consumption was associated with a linear increase in breast cancer risk, with RR = 1.09 for 10g/day or less and RR = 1.41 for intakes between 30 and 60 g/day.[54] There did not appear to be additional risk for consumption of more than 60 g/day. For women who consume alcohol, it is recommended that reduction in intake may decrease breast cancer risk.

K. OTHER DIETARY FACTORS

Caffeine consumption has been examined as a risk factor for breast cancer since elimination of caffeine from the diet has been proposed as a treatment for benign breast disease.[55] However, most case-control studies show no positive association with the disease. In contrast, Hunter et al.[56] observed a weak, but significant inverse association between caffeine consumption and breast cancer risk. The dietary intake of fiber has also been investigated as a potential risk factor for human breast cancer. Van't Veer et al., [57] in a Netherlands study of the association between dietary fiber, beta-carotene and breast cancer, reported a statistically significant lower intake of dietary fiber observed in breast cancer cases than in controls. The corresponding odds ratio (OR) for intake of dietary fiber was 0.55, but was nonsignificant. The authors suggest that a high intake of cereal products, especially those rich in fiber, may be inversely related to breast cancer risk. Another potential etiological dietary component might be fish. Lund and Bonaa[58] reported reduced breast cancer mortality among fishermen's wives in Norway by comparing death rates and husbands' occupations (fishermen vs. unskilled workers). The authors state that their study supports the hypothesis that fish consumption may be associated with lower breast cancer mortality.[58]

Phytoestrogens are another dietary component that may be associated with a protective effect against breast cancer risk. It has been suggested that dietary phytoestrogens, which are present in legumes and grains, provide potential prevention of estrogen-dependent cancers such as breast cancer. Most of the data so far have come from cell culture and animal studies and few human studies have been reported.[59] However, a recent study by Adlercreutz et al.[60] demonstrated that these compounds in the diet (lignans, plant heterocyclic phenols similar in structure to estrogens, and isoflavonoids) may affect uptake and metabolism of sex hormones in postmenopausal women and thus may inhibit cancer cell growth by competing for estrogen binding sites. Heterocyclic amines generated from the high-temperature cooking of meats have also been hypothesized to be associated with increased risk of breast cancer, but no firm conclusions can be drawn.[61] Recently, the findings of a new case-control study in California did not support a role for heterocyclic amines from meat in the etiology of breast cancer.[62]

L. PESTICIDES

Recent attention has been drawn to the issue of organochlorine residues and breast cancer. Although this is not specifically a dietary exposure route, Wolff et al.[63] reported that blood levels of organochlorines such as DDT insecticide and PCBs used as fluid insulators of electrical components were higher for breast cancer patients than for controls. These findings suggest that environmental chemical contamination with organochlorine residues may be an important etiologic factor in breast cancer. Given the widespread dissemination of organochlorine insecticides in the environment and the food chain, the implications are that this could be a dietary etiological agent for human breast cancer. However, a recent review of case-control and nested case-control studies have not supported this association between breast cancer risk and blood levels of DDT and DDE.[64]

M. SUMMARY

Nutritional factors in the etiology of breast cancer are summarized in Table 17.1. The data implicating dietary fat in the etiology of breast cancer appear to be weak at best. Hormonal factors such as age at menarche, which is only partially related to diet, seem to be more important than body weight or size. However, the emerging importance of controlling obesity and the role of physical activity are prominent. The data on the antioxidant vitamins seem to demonstrate a reasonably consistent protective effect for vitamin A and a weakly positive protective effect for vitamin C, with not enough data for evaluating vitamin E. Recent data suggest that the increased consumption of fruits and vegetables does not appear to play a significant role. The role of selenium as a breast cancer inhibitory agent is inconclusive at this time. Alcohol seems to be gaining momentum as a culprit in the etiology of breast cancer, [48–54] although the increased risk is not substantial. Any other dietary factors do not appear to have enough evidence at this time to draw any conclusions as to their role in breast cancer. The World Cancer Research Fund/American Institute for Cancer Research in their massive 1997 review Food, Nutrition and the Prevention of Cancer: a Global Perspective, concluded there is probable evidence for the role of fruits and vegetables in decreasing risk of breast cancer and a possible role for carotenoids and fiber.[65]

TABLE 17.1
Studies of Nutrients and Breast Cancer Risk

Nutrient	Type of Study/Factor Studied	Reference
Dietary fat	Descriptive	5–7
	Correlation	8–10
	Nutritionally mediated factors, exercise	11–15, 17–21
	Case-control, cohort	16, 22–29
	Meta-analyses	30, 32
Vitamin A	Dietary	16, 25, 26, 33, 34
Vitamin C	Dietary	16, 26, 33, 34
Vitamin E	Dietary	16, 33
Fruits and Vegetables	Meta-analyses	35–37
Selenium	Ecologic	38–40
	Dietary	41
	Serologic	42
	Toenails	43
Vitamin D	Dietary	46
	Receptors	45, 47
Alcohol	Consumption	16, 48, 53, 54
Other Factors	Caffeine ingestion	55, 56
	Fiber intake	57
	Fish consumption	58
	Phytoestrogens	59, 60
	Heterocyclic amines	61, 62
	Pesticide exposure	63, 64

The most recent American Cancer Society Guidelines on Nutrition and Physical Activity for Cancer Prevention (2002) have recommended that to reduce the risk of breast cancer one must:

- Engage in vigorous physical activity at least four hours per week
- Avoid or limit intake of alcoholic beverages to one drink per day
- Minimize lifetime weight gain through calorie reduction and exercise.[66]

No mention is made of specific foods that may reduce breast cancer risk.

III. CERVICAL CANCER

Although the cervical cancer incidence rates have decreased in the U.S. in the past 40 years, this cancer site remains a significant problem in the lower socioeconomic strata, as well as in other parts of the world.[67] Nutritional influences on the development of cervical cancer have long been of interest. Many nutrients have been studied for a possible relationship to cervical neoplasia, as well as other nondietary factors in this disease. These etiological factors include a number of sexual and reproductive factors, as well as oral-contraceptive use and smoking, none of which will be discussed in this review.

A. VITAMIN A AND CAROTENOIDS

The majority of reports have found no association between the dietary intake of preformed vitamin A and risk of cervical dysplasia, *in situ* cancer, or invasive disease (for an excellent review, see Potischman[67]). Most of the serologic studies agree with the dietary intake studies[67] in concluding that there is no relation between vitamin A and cervical neoplasia. Results from analysis of carotenoid intakes and cervical cancer were mixed, which is not surprising, since this was a very heterogeneous group of studies (Table 17.2). A recent case-control study conducted in Latin America showed no trend with extent of disease, although stage IV cases had lower carotene values than other cases.[68]

In analyses of carotenoid intakes, seven studies[69-75] found that the cases consumed lower intakes than controls, four[69, 76-78] found no difference and one[79] reported intakes higher for cases than controls. Serologic studies of carotenoid levels were slightly more consistent, with lower levels of carotenoids among cases than controls in eight[70, 75, 80-85] out of 12 studies.[80, 86-88] To summarize, although there was some indication that carotenoids may be protective, the studies were not consistent.

TABLE 17.2
Case-Control Studies of Nutrients and Cervical Cancer

Nutrient/Type of Study	Association w/Risk	Reference
Carotenoids		
Dietary	No difference	69, 76–78
	Inverse	69–75
	Positive	79
Serologic	No difference	80, 86–88
	Inverse	70, 75, 80–85
Vitamin C		
Dietary	No difference	76–78
	Inverse	70, 72, 73, 75, 79, 89
Serologic	No difference	86
	Inverse	83, 90
Vitamin E		
Dietary	No difference	77
	Inverse	72
Serologic	No difference	84, 88
Folate	Inverse	80, 91, 92
Dietary	No difference	70, 72, 73, 76, 78
	Inverse	93, 94
Serologic	No difference	96
	Inverse	83, 94, 95

Adapted from Potischman, N., *J. Nutr.*, 123, 424, 1993

B. Vitamin C

Most studies[70–73, 75, 79, 83, 89, 90] of vitamin C (both dietary and serologic) seemed to be associated with a reduction in risk for cervical neoplasia. Two studies found a protective effect only among smokers.[77, 78] However, this is not inconsistent, since smoking is a risk factor for this disease and is also related to vitamin C status. Two serologic studies have also suggested that vitamin C may play a protective role in cervical cancer.[83, 90]

C. Vitamin E

Vitamin E has not been studied extensively in terms of cervical neoplasia, [72, 77, 82, 84, 88, 91, 92] however, two serologic studies of cervical dysplasia demonstrated lower levels of vitamin E to be associated with a higher-grade lesion and even lower concentrations in those with invasive cancers.[82, 91] Overall, studies with vitamin E and cervical cancer risk showed mixed results, with no clear-cut conclusion that could be drawn.

D. Folate

The case for folate in the etiology of cervical cancer is probably stronger than for any other nutrient studied.[93–96] Since 1977, several reports have indicated an increased incidence of cervical cancer among oral contraceptive users.[97–100] An early study reported morphologic similarities between megaloblastic anemia and those features present in the cervical cells of oral contraceptive users.[101] Supplementation with folate improved the cervical dysplasia associated with oral contraceptive use.[102] There is also an association of human papilloma virus (HPV) type 16 prevalence and lowered folate status, which may suggest that folate status might be linked with HPV infection and not with dysplastic progression.[103] In a clinical intervention trial, the data did not confirm the hypothesis that oral folate supplements would improve cervical dysplasia.[103] There were no statistically different rates of normal biopsies between the folate-treated subjects and those receiving placebo. However, as in the case-control study, there was a higher incidence of HPV-16 positives among those cases with low red blood cell folate initially, leading the authors to conclude that folate deficiency may exert a cocarcinogenic effect in the presence of HPV-16 exposure.[104]

E. Other

In a study of the associations between cervical cancer and serological markers of nutritional status in Latin America, an inverse trend for cholesterol and triglyceride concentrations was observed with stage of disease, suggesting a clinical effect of cervical cancer on blood lipids.[68] A single study has associated pork intake and HPV-related disease. Schneider et al.[105] reported that international correlations suggest that pork intake is positively associated with incidence of cervical cancer, a disease also related to HPV. Pork meat or dietary factors associated with pork meat consumption may be involved in the development of HPV-related diseases.[105] Nutrition scientists continue to study the role of fruits and vegetables in cancer prevention, and an intervention has been conducted in women with cervical intraepithelial neoplasia.[106] However, no conclusions for the cervical neoplasia were available, only that dietary counseling can effectively promote increased fruit and vegetable intake in premenopausal women.[106]

F. SUMMARY

The relation between nutrients and cervical neoplasia appears to be predominantly limited to the effects of folate. Preformed vitamin A did not appear to be related to risk of any preinvasive or invasive cervical lesions, whereas vitamin C has been associated with a reduced risk for dysplasia, *in situ* cancer and invasive disease, especially among smokers. There was some evidence of reduced risks associated with various carotenoids and vitamin E at all stages of the disease, but the overall results were inconsistent. Folate was the only nutrient that appeared to be protective for dysplastic lesions, but not related to the risk of *in situ* or invasive disease. Red blood cell folate was the best predictor of dysplasia, better than serum or dietary folate. It has also been suggested that more research is needed into the interactions between nutrients and other risk factors for this disease, such as smoking and HPV infection. The World Cancer Research Fund/American Institute for Cancer Research 1997 report concluded there was no convincing evidence that any dietary factors modify the risk of cervical cancer, nor evidence of any probable causal relationships with diet.[65] They further concluded there was possibly no relationship at all with either folate or retinol and cervical cancer.[65] The American Cancer Society (ACS) 2002 nutrition and cancer recommendations do not even mention any dietary associations for cervical cancer.[66]

IV. ENDOMETRIAL CANCER

Endometrial cancer has been correlated with cancers of the breast, ovary, colon and rectum.[11] It tends to be more common in the U.S. than in other parts of the world and to be more frequent in Caucasian women of higher socioeconomic status. The only established etiologic cause for this cancer appears to be the use of exogenous estrogens at the high doses commonly prescribed years ago.[1] Obesity has been cited as a risk factor in a number of studies[107-111] and a hormonal mechanism has been postulated for this association. There also appears to be an association between endometrial cancer risk and body fat distribution, with certain studies demonstrating that women with upper body fat have an increased risk of endometrial cancer.[112] A longitudinal population study[113] of 1462 women in Sweden examined adipose tissue distribution and the occurrence of endometrial cancer. Abdominally localized adipose tissue was associated with irregular ovulation and menstruation, as well as an increased risk of endometrial cancer.[113] Additionally, in a case-control study in China, [114] obesity proved to be a strong risk factor for endometrial cancer, even in a country where supplemental estrogen use is uncommon. However, another study has shown no association between obesity and endometrial cancer. A case-control study of endometrial adenocarcinoma in Greece investigated the epidemiology of this cancer in a low-risk setting.[115] No relationship was found between weight and endometrial cancer. A population-based case-control study done on Hawaiian women examined the association between diet, body size, physical activity and the risk for endometrial cancer.[116] These authors found a strong dose-response effect of increased body size on risk for endometrial cancer, even after adjusting for energy intake.[116]

In terms of specific dietary factors and endometrial cancer, one of the first studies, in which a case-control study collected data on the frequency of consumption of selected dietary items, was performed in Italy.[109] The cases with endometrial cancer reported a greater fat intake and a less frequent intake of fruits, vegetables and grains. A subsequent study by the same investigator[117] examined Italian regional diets and their correlation to breast, ovarian and endometrial cancer rates. Diets high in fat, protein and calories increased the incidence rates of all three cancers and diets high in green vegetable and fresh fruit consumption had a protective effect. The relation between diet and endometrial cancer was more recently examined in China.[118] Women in the highest quartile of total caloric intake had a 2.1-fold increased risk of endometrial cancer and that risk varied according to the source of calories, with the highest risk attributable to caloric intake from fat and protein confined to foods of animal origin. Following adjustment for total calories, no significant association of risk was found with intake of vegetables, dark green/yellow vegetables, or esti-mated carotene intake, although fruit and allium vegetables were associated with some reduction in risk. These results suggest that animal fat and protein may play a role in the etiology of endometrial cancer. In the Hawaiian study, [116] the authors' dietary analyses concluded that consumption of vegetables and fruits, particularly those high in lutein, were inversely associated with endometrial cancer risk.[116] In another Hawaiian study by the same authors, [117] high consumption of soy products and other legumes was associated with a decreased risk of endometrial cancer with an OR of 0.46, and similar reductions in risk were seen for increased consumption of whole grains, vegetables, fruits and seaweeds. These results may explain the lower incidence of endometrial cancer in Asian countries compared with the United States.[119] Another recent study in the United States mainland examined the associ-ations of dietary fat, as well as selected plant foods, with endometrial cancer and concluded that consumption of fruits or vegetables was inversely associated with endometrial cancer risk (OR = 0.65).[120]

In a case-control study of diet and endometrial cancer conducted in Birmingham, Alabama, [121] a high intake of certain micronutrients was found to be associated with a decreased risk of endometrial cancer for those in the upper tertile of carotene and nitrate intake. There was also an inverse association between endometrial cancer and protein consumption, as well as a direct association with cholesterol intake. More frequent consumption of several vegetables and certain dairy products was associated with a statistically significant decreased risk of endometrial cancer, sug-gesting that diet plays an important role in this cancer. An Italian case-control study[122] examined the association between intake of certain micronutrients and the risk of endometrial carcinoma. They reported the following RR's: 0.5 for beta-carotene, 0.6 for ascorbic acid and 0.7 for folate, suggesting that some micronutrients may have a protective effect against endometrial carcinoma.[122] Although the focus of this review of nutrition and women's cancers does not emphasize all of the experimental studies, a recent rodent study of endometrial cancer is worthy of mention. The study[123] was conducted to examine the possible inhibiting effect of indole-3-carbinol, a constituent of cruciferous vegetables, on the spontaneous occurrence of endometrial adenocarcinoma in female Donryu rats. The high incidence of endometrial cancer in this rat strain is thought to be related to increased estrogen/progesterone ratio with aging. Dietary indole-3-carbinol significantly decreased the frequency of endometrial carcinoma, preneoplastic lesions and mammary fibroadenoma, while it increased the 2-hydroxylation of estradiol. These results suggest that cruciferous vegetables may be protective against the development of endometrial cancer.

Physical activity has been linked to cancer risk reduction at a number of sites.[66] Littman et al. investigated the association between recreational physical activity and endometrial cancer risk.[124] They reported an OR of 0.62 for regular exercise compared with no exercise in a population-based case-control study in Washington state.[124] Another nondietary factor that has recently been studied in terms of association with endometrial cancer is persistent environmental pollutants such as organochlorines.[125] In a population-based case-control study in Sweden, the authors determined that the serum concentrations of a number of chlorinated pesticides did not increase the risk for endometrial cancer (OR of 1.2).[125]

A. SUMMARY

In summary, endometrial cancer is primarily associated with excess estrogenic stimulation, and obesity may contribute significantly to this risk. Other potential dietary factors have not been established with any certainty, although there appears to be a growing body of evidence linking high-fat diets, especially animal fats, to this risk and consumption of vegetables and fruits with protection. The World Cancer Research Fund/American Institute for Cancer Research review concluded that the evidence that high BMI increases risk is convincing, and that diets high in fruits and vegetables may possibly reduce risk.[65] The ACS 2002 Guidelines recommend that to reduce risk, a woman should maintain a healthful weight through diet and regular physical activity and eat at least five servings of fruits and vegetables daily.[66]

V. OVARIAN CANCER

Similar to endometrial cancer, ovarian cancer is more common in the U.S. and other western countries than in Asia and is also correlated with cancers of the breast, colon and endometrium. There is a greater-than-expected risk of second primary cancers of the corpus uteri, colon and breast in patients with ovarian cancer.[126] This supports the hypothesis that there are common etiological factors for these cancer sites. Ovarian cancer also tends to occur more frequently in women in the higher socioeconomic groups and less frequently in women who use oral contraceptives.[127–130] In one case-control study, Annegers et al.[131] observed that obesity is not a risk factor for ovarian cancer and in another there was no effect of height or weight.[132] In terms of dietary influences, Cramer et al.[133] found that ovarian cancer cases consumed significantly greater amounts of animal fat and considerably less vegetable fat than did controls. In contrast, Byers et al.[134] found no such association. Most studies of weight and height did not find an association with ovarian cancer risk.[1] Two studies[135, 136] have reported an association between coffee drinking and an increased risk of ovarian cancer and another one[134] did not. Therefore, coffee's role as an etiologic agent in ovarian cancer is not conclusive. A study of mortality trends of breast, colorectal, ovarian and prostate cancer in Spain, Italy, Greece, Yugoslavia, England and Wales implicated consumption of fat-containing foods in the increase in cancer at these sites in Mediterranean countries, [137] whereas in England and Wales a decrease in ovarian and colorectal cancer among women was observed.[137] More recent studies of ovarian cancer risk and diet have reported an inverse association with total and green leafy vegetable intake in the Iowa Women's Health Study[138] and an OR of 1.5 for the association of red meat intake and ovarian cancer in an Italian case-control study.[139] Interestingly, in the Nurses' Health Study, [140] no association was observed between ovarian cancer risk and antioxidant vitamin consumption from foods, or foods plus supplements; the authors concluded that their data do not support a role for fruits and vegetables in protection against cancer of the ovary. In contrast, Italian epidemiologists have concluded that vegetable consumption appears to be inversely related to risk.[141]

A. SUMMARY

Although the risk for ovarian cancer has been linked inversely to extended oral contraceptive use, no clear-cut dietary associations have been discerned for this cancer site. The World Cancer Research Fund/American Institute for Cancer Research review reported the conclusions that there is as yet no convincing evidence that any dietary factors modify risk of ovarian cancer, nor any probable causal relationships with diet, although they note that diets high in fruits and vegetables may possibly reduce risk.[65] The ACS 2002 Guidelines state that there are no established nutritional risk factors and that consumption of fruits and vegetables may lower risk.[66] Since screening and early detection are not available for this cancer, more research is needed.

VI. SUMMARY AND CONCLUSIONS

The overwhelming message that emerges from all of the data on nutrition and women's cancers is that few nutrients demonstrate a compelling role in the development of these cancers. The role of dietary fat in breast cancer is far from resolved and the role of alcohol is just beginning to surface. Vitamin A intake and, to a lesser extent, vitamin C, appear to be protective, but that does not mean their role is causative in nature. The role of fruits and vegetables in lowering risk appears to be less compelling for breast than for other cancers. More work needs to be undertaken into the mechanisms of the antioxidant vitamins in protection against human breast cancer. As more research into the genetics of breast cancer emerges, it becomes more important to understand the nutritional factors in this disease in the context of the genetic risk factors. This should become a focus for future research efforts.

In terms of nutritional factors in cervical cancer, folate is the only dietary component that appears to demonstrate any consistent protective effect that can be readily assessed and this has recently been questioned. There is also some promise for a protective role for vitamin C, but this is not compelling. The overwhelming risk factors for cervical cancer appear to be smoking and HPV infection and we should begin to direct research efforts to the effects of nutritional variables interacting with these risk factors.

Endometrial cancer is primarily associated with excess estrogenic stimulation, but obesity may contribute to this risk. Any future research efforts should perhaps investigate how dietary components actually influence this risk. Ovarian cancer does not appear to have any major dietary factor associated with its etiology, although animal fats may play an obscure role. Ovarian cancer is an enigma in terms of early diagnosis and possible causation, so clearly more research into this cancer is needed.

In conclusion, the implications for women and their risks for cancers unique to women, in terms of what types of diets would potentially protect them, are limited to the same dietary recommendations that have been promoted by all health groups in recent years: maintain ideal body weight, eat plenty of fruits and vegetables, decrease fat and fatty meat consumption and limit alcohol consumption to modest intakes. However, the prominent role of physical activity cannot be underestimated in a cancer prevention regimen for most women's cancers and it is this one that may show the most promise in reducing circulating levels of estrogen, which appear to be the common denominator for all women's cancers.

REFERENCES

1. Committee on Diet and Health, Food and Nutrition Board, Commission on Life Sciences, National Research Council, *Diet and Health, Implications for Reducing Chronic Disease Risk,* National Academy Press, Washington, D.C., 1989, ch. 22.
2. Doll, R. and Peto, R., The causes of cancer: Quantitative estimates of avoidable risks in the United States today, *J. Natl. Cancer Inst.,* 66, 1191, 1981.
3. Wynder, E.L. and Gori, G.B., Contribution of the environment to cancer incidence: An epidemiological exercise, *J. Natl. Cancer Inst.,* 58, 825, 1977.
4. MacMahon, B., Cole, P. and Brown, J., Etiology of human breast cancer: A review, *J. Natl. Cancer Inst.,* 50, 21, 1973.
5. Kolonel, L.N., Cancer patterns of four ethnic groups in Hawaii, *J. Natl. Cancer Inst.,* 65, 1127, 1980.
6. Dunn, J.E., Jr., Breast cancer among American Japanese in the San Francisco Bay area, *Natl. Cancer Inst. Monog.,* 47, 157, 1977.
7. Moolgavkar, S.H., Day, N.E. and Stevens, R.G., Two-stage model for carcinogenesis: Epidemiology of breast cancer in females, *J. Natl. Cancer Inst.,* 65, 559, 1980.
8. Committee on Diet, Nutrition and Cancer, Assembly of Life Sciences, National Research Council, *Diet, Nutrition and Cancer,* National Academy Press, Washington, D.C., 1982, ch. 17.
9. Carroll, K.K. and Khor, H.T., Dietary fat in relation to tumorigenesis, *Prog. Biochem. Pharmacol.,* 10, 308, 1975.
10. Gaskill, S.P., McGuire, W.L., Osborne, C.K. and Stern, M.P., Breast cancer mortality and diet in the United States, *Cancer Res.,* 39, 3628, 1979.
11. Miller, A.B., An overview of hormone-associated cancers, *Cancer Res.,* 38, 3985, 1978.

12. Frisch, R.E., Hegsted, D.M. and Yoshinaga, K., Body weight and food intake at early estrus of rats on a high-fat diet, *Proc. Natl. Acad. Sci. USA*, 72, 4172, 1975.

13. Frisch, R.E. and McArthur, J.W., Menstrual cycles: Fatness as a determinant of minimum weight for height necessary for their maintenance or onset, *Science*, 185, 949, 1974.

14. Miller, A.B., Epidemiology of gastrointestinal cancer, *Compr. Ther.*, 7, 53, 1981.

15. Gray, G.E., Pike, M.C. and Henderson, B.E., Breast cancer incidence and mortality rates in different countries in relation to known risk factors and dietary practice, *Br. J. Cancer*, 39, 1, 1979.

16. Willett, W., Diet and breast cancer, *Contemp. Nutr.*, 18, 1, 1993.

17. London, S.J., Colditz, G.A., Stampfer, M.J., Willett, W.C., Rosner, B., Speizer, F.E., Prospective study of relative weight and breast cancer, *JAMA*, 262, 2853, 1989.

18. Hunter, D.J. and Willett, W.C., Diet, body size and breast cancer, *Epidemiol. Rev.*, 15, 110, 1993.

19. van den Brandt, P.A., Spiegelman, D., Yaun, S.S., Adami, H.O., Beeson, L., Folsom, A.R., Fraser, G., Goldbohm, R.A., Graham, S., Kushi, L., Marshall, J.R., Miller, A.B., Rohan, T., Smith-Warner, S.A., Speizer, F.E., Willett, W.C., Wolk, A. Hunter, D.J., Pooled analysis of prospective cohort studies on height, weight and breast cancer risk, *Amer. J. Epidemiol.*, 152, 514, 2000.

20. Friedenreich, C.M., Physical activity and cancer prevention: From observational to intervention research, *Cancer Epidemiol. Biomarkers Control*, 10, 287, 2001.

21. McTiernan, A., Associations between energy balance and body mass index and risk of breast carcinoma in women from diverse racial and ethnic backgrounds in the U.S., *Cancer*, 88, 1248, 2000.

22. Phillips, R.L., Role of life-style and dietary habits in risk of cancer among Seventh-Day Adventists, *Cancer Res.*, 35, 3513, 1975.

23. Miller, A.B., Kelly, A., Choi, N.W., Matthews, V., Morgan, R.W., Munan, L., Burch, J.D., Feather, J., Howe, G.R, Jain, M., A study of diet and breast cancer, *Am. J. Epidemiol.*, 107, 499, 1978.

24. Lubin, J.H., Blot, W.J. and Burns, P.E., Breast cancer following high dietary fat and protein consumption, *Am. J. Epidemiol.*, 114, 422, 1981.

25. Graham, S., Marshall, J., Mettlin, C., Rzepka, T., Nemoto, T., Byers, T., Diet in the epidemiology of breast cancer, *Am. J. Epidemiol.*, 116, 68, 1982.

26. Howe, G. R., Hirohata, T., Hislop, T.G., Iscovich, J.M., Yuan, J.M., Katsouyanni, K., Lubin, F., Marubini, E., Modan, B., Rohan, T., Dietary factors and risk of breast cancer: Combined analysis of 12 case-control studies, *J. Natl. Cancer Inst.*, 82, 561, 1990.

27. Kushi, L.H., Sellers, T.A., Potter, J.D., Nelson, C.L., Mumger, R.G., Kaye, S.A., Folsom, A.R, Dietary fat and postmenopausal breast cancer, *J. Natl. Cancer Inst.*, 84, 1092, 1992.

28. Barrett-Connor, E. and Friedlander, N.J., Dietary fat, calories and the risk of breast cancer in postmenopausal women: A prospective population-based study, *J. Am. Coll. Nutr.*, 12, 390, 1993.

29. Willett, W.C., Hunter, D.J., Stampfer, M.J., Colditz, G., Manson, J.E., Spiegelman, D., Rosner, B., Hennekens, C.H., Speizer, F.E., Dietary fat and fiber in relation to risk of breast cancer, *JAMA*, 268, 2037, 1992.

30. Willett, W.C., *Nutritional Epidemiology*, 2nd ed., Oxford University Press, New York, 1998, 340.

31. Greenland, S., A meta-analysis of coffee, myocardial infarction and coronary death, *Epidemiology*, 4, 366, 1993.

32. Smith-Warner, S.A., Spiegelman, D., Yaun, S.S., Adami, H.O., Beeson, W.L., van den Brandt, P.A., Folsom, A.R., Fraser, G.E., Freudenheim, J.L., Goldbohm, R.A., Graham, S., Miller, A.B., Potter, J.D., Rohan, T.E., Speizer, F.E., Toniolo, P., Willett, W.C., Wolk, A., Zeleniuch-Jacquotte, A., Hunter, D.J., Intake of fruits and vegetables and risk of breast cancer: A pooled analysis of cohort studies, *JAMA,* 285, 769, 2001.

33. Hunter, D.J., Stampfer, M.J., Colditz, G.A., Manson, J., Rosner, B., Hennekens, C.H., Speizer, F.E., Willett, W.C., A prospective study of consumption of vitamins A, C and E and breast cancer risk, *Am. J. Epidemiol.,* 134, 715, 1991.

34. Potischman, N., McCulloch, C.E., Byers, T., Nemoto, T., Stubbe, N., Milch, R., Parker, R., Rasmussen, K.M., Root, M., Graham, S., Breast cancer and dietary and plasma concentrations of carotenoids and vitamin A, *Am. J. Clin. Nutr.,* 52, 909, 1990.

35. Smith-Warner, S.A and Giovanucci, E., Fruit and vegetable intake and cancer, In: Heber, D., Blackburn, G.L., Go, V.L.W., Eds., *Nutritional Oncology,* Boston, Mass: Academic Press, 1999, p. 153.

36. Key, T.J., Fraser, G.E., Thorogood, M., Appleby, P.N., Beral, V., Reeves, G., Burr, M.L., Chang-Claude, J., Frentzel-Beyme, R., Kuzma, J.W., Mann, J., McPherson, K., Mortality in vegetarians and non-vegetarians: Detailed findings from a collaborative analysis of five prospective studies, *Am. J. Clin. Nutr.,* 70(suppl), 516S, 1999.

37. Gandini, S., Merzenich, H., Robertson, C., Boyle, P., Meta-analysis of studies on breast cancer risk and diet: The role of fruit and vegetable consumption and the intake of associated micronutrients, *Eur. J. Cancer,* 36, 636, 2000.

38. Shamberger, R.J., Tytko, S.A and Willis, C.E., Antioxidants and cancer. VI. Selenium and age-adjusted human cancer mortality, *Arch. Environ. Hlth.,* 31, 231, 1976.

39. Clark, L.E., The epidemiology of selenium and cancer, *Fed. Proc.,* 44, 2584, 1985.

40. Schrauzer, G.D., White, D.A. and Schneider, C., Cancer mortality correlation studies. III. Statistical associations with dietary selenium intake, *Bioinorg. Chem.,* 7, 23, 1977.

41. Garland, M., Willett, W.E., Manson, J.E., Hunter, D.J., Antioxidant micronutrients and breast cancer, *J. Am. Coll. Nutr.,* 12, 400, 1993.

42. Hardell, L., Danell, M., Angqvist, C.A., Marklund, S.L., Fredriksson, M., Zakari, A.L., Kjellgren, A., Levels of selenium in plasma and glutathione peroxidase in erythrocytes and the risk of breast cancer: A case-control study, *Biol. Trace Elem. Res.,* 36, 99, 1993.

43. Hunter, D.J., Morris, J.S., Stampfer, M.J., Colditz, G.A., Speizer, F.E., Willett, W.C., A prospective study of selenium status and breast cancer risk, *JAMA,* 264, 1128, 1990.

44. Jacobson, E.A., James, K.A., Newmark, H.L., Carroll, K.K., Effects of dietary fat, calcium and vitamin D on growth and mammary tumorigenesis induced by 7, 12-dimethylbenz(a)anthracene in female Sprague-Dawley rats, *Cancer Res.,* 49, 6300, 1989.

45. Colston, K.W., Berger, U. and Coombes, R.C., Possible role for vitamin D in controlling breast cancer cell proliferation, *Lancet,* 28, 188, 1989.

46. Simard, A., Vobecky, J. and Vobecky, J.S., Vitamin D deficiency and cancer of the breast: An unprovocative ecological hypothesis, *Can. J. Public Health,* 82, 300, 1991.

47. Berger, U., McClelland, R.A., Wilson, P., Greene, G.L., Haussler, M.R, Pike, J.W., Colston, K., Easton, D., Coombes, R.C., Immunocytochemical determination of estrogen receptor, progesterone receptor and 1, 2-dihydroxyvitamin D3 receptor in breast cancer and relationship to prognosis, *Cancer Res.,* 51, 239, 1991.

48. Longnecker, M., Berlin, J.A., Orza, M.J., Chalmers, T.C., A meta-analysis of alcohol consumption in relation to risk of breast cancer, *JAMA,* 260, 652, 1988.

49. Reichman, M. E., Judd, J.T., Longcope, C., Schatzkin, A., Clevidence, B.A., Nair, P.P., Campbell, W.S., Taylor, P.R, Effects of alcohol consumption on plasma and urinary hormone concentrations in premenopausal women, *J. Natl. Cancer Inst.*, 85, 722, 1993.
50. Pawlega, J., Breast cancer and smoking, vodka drinking and dietary habits: A case-control study, *Acta. Oncol.*, 31, 387, 1992.
51. Friedenreich, C.M., Howe, G.R, Miller, A.B., Jain, M.G., A cohort study of alcohol consumption and risk of breast cancer, *Am. J. Epidemiol.*, 137, 512, 1993.
52. Ferraroni, M., Decarli, A., Willett, W.C., Marubini, E., Alcohol and breast cancer risk: A case-control study from northern Italy, *Int. J. Epidemiol.*, 20, 859, 1991.
53. Zaridze, D., Lifanova, Y, Maximovitch, D., Day, N.E., Duffy, S.W., Diet, alcohol consumption and reproductive factors in a case-control study of breast cancer in Moscow, *Int. J. Cancer,* 48, 493, 1991.
54. Smith-Warner, S.A., Spiegelman, D., Yaun, S.S., van den Brandt, P.A., Folsom, A.R, Goldbohm, RA., Graham, S., Holmberg, L., Howe, G.R, Marshall, J.R, Miller, A.B., Potter, J.D., Speizer, F.E., Willett, W.C., Wolk, A., Hunter, D.J., Alcohol and breast cancer in women: A pooled analysis of cohort studies, *JAMA,* 279, 535, 1998.
55. Minton, J.P., Foecking, M.K., Webster, D.J., Matthews, R.H., Response of fibrocystic disease to caffeine withdrawal and correlation of cyclic nucleotides with breast disease, *Am. J. Obstet. Gynecol.*, 135, 157, 1979.
56. Hunter, D.J., Manson. J.E., Stampfer, M.J., Colditz, G.A., Rosner, B., Hennekens, C.H., Speizer, F.E., Willett, W.E., A prospective study of caffeine, coffee, tea and breast cancer, *Am. J. Epidemiol.*, 136, 1000, 1992.
57. Van't Veer, P., Kolb, C.M., Verhoef, P., Kok, F., Schouten, E.G., Hermus, R.J.J., Sturmans, F., Dietary fiber, beta-carotene and breast cancer: Results from a case-control study, *Int. J. Cancer,* 45, 825, 1990.
58. Lund, E. and Bonaa, K.R., Reduced breast cancer mortality among fishermen's wives in Norway, *Cancer Causes Control,* 4, 283, 1993.
59. Kurzer, M.S., Diet, estrogen and cancer, *Contemp. Nutr.,* 17, 1, 1992.
60. Adlerkreutz, R., Mousavi, Y., Clark, J., Rokerstedt, K., Hamalainen, E., Wahala, K., Makela, T., Hase, T., Dietary phytoestrogens and cancer: *In vitro* and *in vivo* studies, *J. Steroid Biochem. Mol. Biol.*, 41, 331, 1992.
61. Pence, B.C. and Dunn, D.M., *Nutrition and Women's Cancers,* CRC Press, Boca Raton, FL, 1998, p. 40.
62. Delfino, R.J., Sinha, R., Smith, C., West, J., White, E., Lin, R.J., Liao, S.Y., Gim, J.S., Ma, R.L., Butler, J., Anton-Culver, R., Breast cancer, heterocyclic aromatic amines from meat and N-acetyltransferase 2 genotype, *Carcinogenesis,* 21, 607, 2000.
63. Wolff, M.S., Toniolo, P.G., Lee, E.W., Rivera, M., Dubin, N., Blood levels of organochlorine residues and risk of breast cancer, *J. Natl. Cancer Inst.,* 85, 648, 1993.
64. Snedeker, S.M., Pesticides and breast cancer risk: A review of DDT, DDE and dieldrin, *Environ. Hlth. Perspec.,* 109(Suppl), 35, 2001.
65. World Cancer Research Fund in association with American Institute for Cancer Research, Food, Nutrition and the Prevention of Cancer: a Global Perspective, World Cancer Research Fund, Washington, D.C., 1997.
66. Byers, T., Nestle, M., McTiernan, A., Doyle, C., Currie-Williams, A., Gansler, T., Thun, M. and the American Cancer Society 2001 Nutrition and Physical Activity Guidelines Advisory Committee, American Cancer Society Guidelines on Nutrition and Physical Activity for Cancer Prevention (2002), *CA Cancer J. Clin.,* 52, 92, 2002.
67. Potischman, N., Nutritional epidemiology of cervical neoplasia, *J. Nutr.,* 123, 424, 1993.

68. Potischman, N., Hoover, R.N., Brinton, L.A., Swanson, C.A., Herrero, R., Tenorio, F., de Britton, R.C., Gaitan, E., Reeves, W.C., The relations between cervical cancer and serological markers of nutritional status, *Nutr. Cancer,* 21, 193, 1994.

69. La Vecchia, C., Decarli, A., Fasoli, M., Parazzini, F., Franceschi, S., Gentile, A., Negri, E., Dietary vitamin A and the risk of intra epithelial and invasive cervical neoplasia, *Gynecol. Oncol.,* 30, 187, 1988.

70. Brock, K.E., Berry, G., Mock, P.A, MacLennan, R., Truswell, A.S., Brinton, L.A., Nutrients in diet and plasma and risk of *in situ* cervical cancer, *J. Natl. Cancer Inst.,* 80, 580, 1988.

71. Marshall, J.R., Graham, S., Byers, T., Swanson, M., Brasure, J., Diet and smoking in the epidemiology of cancer of the cervix, *J. Natl. Cancer Inst.,* 70, 847, 1983.

72. Verreault, R., Chu, J., Mandelson, M., Shy, K., A case-control study of diet and invasive cervical cancer, *Int. J. Cancer,* 43, 1050, 1989.

73. Herrero, R., Potischman, N., Brinton, L.A., Reeves, W.C., Brenes, M.M. Tenorio, F., de Britton, R.C., Gaitan, E., A case-control study of nutrient status and invasive cervical cancer. I.Dietary indicators, *Am. J. Epidemiol.,* 134, 1335, 1991.

74. Wylie-Rosett, J.A., Romney, S.L., Slagle, N.S., Wassertheil-Smollen, S., Miller, G.L., Palan, P.R., Lucido, D.J., Duttagupta, C., Influence of vitamin A on cervical dysplasia and carcinoma *in situ,* *Nutr. Cancer,* 6, 49, 1984.

75. Van Eenwyk, J., Davis, F.G. and Bowen, P.E., Dietary and serum carotenoids and cervical intraepithelial neoplasia, *Int. J. Cancer,* 48, 34, 1991.

76. Ziegler, R.G., Jones, C.J., Brinton, L.A., Norman, S.A., Mallin, K., Levine, R.S., Lehman, H.F., Hamman, R.F., Trumble, A.C., Rosenthal, J.F., Diet and the risk of *in situ* cervical cancer among white women in the United States, *Cancer Causes Control,* 2, 17, 1991.

77. Slattery, M.L., Abbott, T.M., Overall, J.C. Jr., Robison, L.M. French, T.K., Jolles, C., Gardner, J.W., West, D.W., Dietary vitamins A, C and E and selenium as risk factors for cervical cancer, *Epidemiology,* 1, 8, 1990.

78. Ziegler, R.G., Brinton, L.A., Hamman, R.F., Lehman, H.F., Levine, R.S., Norman, S.A., Mallin, K., Rosenthal, J.F., Trumble, A.C., Hoover, R.N., Diet and the risk of invasive cervical cancer among white women in the United States, *Am. J. Epidemiol.,* 132, 432, 1990.

79. de Vet, H.C., Knipschild, P.G., Grol, M.E., Schouten, H.J., Sturmans, F., The role of beta carotene and other dietary factors in the aetiology of cervical dysplasia: Results of a case-control study, *Int. J. Epidemiol.,* 20, 603, 1991.

80. Harris, R.W., Forman, D., Doll, R, Vessey, M.P., Wald, N.J., Cancer of the cervix uteri and vitamin A, *Br. J. Cancer,* 53, 653, 1986.

81. Palan, P.R., Romney, S.L, Mikhail, M., Basu, J., Vermund, S.H., Decreased plasma beta-carotene levels in women with uterine cervical dysplasias and cancer, *J. Natl. Cancer Inst.,* 80, 454, 1988.

82. Palan, P.R, Mikhail, M.S., Basu, J., Romney, S.L, Plasma levels of antioxidant beta-carotene and alpha-tocopherol in uterine cervix dysplasias and cancer, *Nutr. Cancer,* 15, 13, 1991.

83. Orr, J.W. Jr., Wilson, K., Bodiford, C., Cornwell, A., Soong, S.J., Honea, K.L, Hatch, K.D., Shingleton, H.M., Nutritional status of patients with untreated cervical cancer. II. Vitamin assessment, *Am. J. Obstet. Gynecol.,* 151, 632, 1985.

84. Potischman, N., Herrero, R., Brinton, L.A., Reeves, W.C., Stacewicz- Sapuntzakis, M., Jones, C.J., Brenes, M.M., Tenorio, F., de Britton, R.C., Gaitan, E., A case-control study of nutrient status and invasive cervical cancer. II. Serologic indicators, *Am. J. Epidemiol.,* 134, 1347, 1991.

85. Smith, A.H. and Waller, K.D., Serum beta-carotene in persons with cancer and their immediate families, *Am. J. Epidemiol.*, 133, 661, 1991.

86. Basu, J., Palan, P.R, Vermund, S.H., Goldberg, G.L, Burk, RD., Romney, S.L, Plasma ascorbic acid and beta-carotene levels in women evaluated for HPV infection, smoking and cervix dysplasia, *Cancer Detect. Prevent.*, 15, 165, 1991.

87. Lambert, B., Brisson, G. and Bielman, P., Plasma vitamin A and precancerous lesions of cervix uteri: A preliminary report, *Gynecol. Oncol.*, 11, 136, 1981.

88. Heinonen, P.K., Kuoppala, T., Koskinen, T., Punnonen, R., Serum vitamins A and E and carotene in patients with gynecologic cancer, *Arch. Gynecol. Obstet.*, 241, 151, 1987.

89. Wassertheil-Smoller, S., Romney, S.L., Wylie-Rosett, J., Slagle, S., Miller, G., Lucido, D., Duttagupta, C., Palan, P.R., Dietary vitamin C and uterine cervical dysplasia, *Am. J. Epidemiol.*, 114, 714, 1981.

90. Romney, S.L., Duttagupta, C., Basu, J., Palan, P.R., Karp, S., Slagle, N.S., Dwyer, A., Wassertheil-Smoller, S., Wylie-Rosett, J., Plasma vitamin C and uterine cervical dysplasia, *Am. J. Obstet. Gynecol.*, 151, 976, 1985.

91. Cuzick, J., De Stavola, B.L., Russell, M.J., Thomas, B.S., Vitamin A, vitamin E and the risk of cervical intraepithelial neoplasia, *Br. J. Cancer*, 62, 651, 1990.

92. Knekt, P., Serum vitamin E levels and risk of female cancers, *Int. J. Epidemiol.*, 17, 281, 1988.

93. McPherson, R.S., Nutritional factors and the risk of cervical dysplasia, *Am. J. Epidemiol.*, 130, 830, 1989.

94. Van Eenwyk, J., Davis, F.G. and Colman, N., Folate, vitamin C and cervical intraepithelial neoplasia, *Cancer Epidemiol. Biomarkers Prevent.*, 1, 119, 1992.

95. Butterworth, C.E., Jr., Hatch, K.D., Macaluso, M., Cole, P., Sauberlich, H.E., Soong, S.J., Borst, M., Baker, V.V., Folate deficiency and cervical dysplasia, *JAMA*, 267, 528, 1992.

96. Potischman, N., Brinton, L.A., Laiming, V.A., Reeves, W.C., Brenes, M.M., Herrero, R., Tenorio, F., de Britton, R.C., Gaitan, E., A case-control study of serum folate levels and invasive cervical cancer, *Cancer Res.*, 51, 47785, 1991.

97. Peritz, E., Ramcharan, S., Frank, J., Brown, W.L., Huang, S., Ray, R., The incidence of cervical cancer and duration of oral contraceptive use, *Am. J. Epidemiol.*, 106, 462, 1977.

98. Stem, E., Steroid contraceptive use and cervical dysplasia: Increased risk of progression, *Science*, 196, 1460, 1977.

99. Swan, S.H. and Brown, W.L., Oral contraceptive use, sexual activity and cervical carcinoma, *Am. J. Obstet. Gynecol.*, 139, 52, 1981.

100. Vessey, M.P., Lawless, M., McPherson, K., Yeates, D., Neoplasia of the cervix uteri and contraception: A possible adverse effect of the pill, *Lancet*, 2, 930, 1983.

101. Whitehead, N., Reyner, F. and Lindenbaum, J., Megaloblastic changes in the cervical epithelium. Association with oral contraceptive therapy and reversal with folic acid, *JAMA*, 226, 1421, 1973.

102. Butterworth, C.E., Jr., Hatch, K.D., Gore, H., Mueller, H., Krumdieck, C.L., Improvement in cervical dysplasia associated with folic acid therapy in users of oral contraceptives, *Am. J. Clin. Nutr.*, 35, 73, 1982.

103. Butterworth, C.E., Jr., Hatch, K.D., Soong, S.J., Cole, P., Tamura, T., Sauberlich, H.E., Borst, M., Macaluso, M., Baker, V., Oral folic acid supplementation for cervical dysplasia: A clinical intervention trial, *Am. J. Obstet. Gynecol.*, 166, 803, 1992.

104. Borst, M., Butterworth, C.E. Jr., Baker, V., Kuykendall, K., Gore, H., Soong, S.J., Hatch, K.D., Human papillomavirus screening for women with atypical papanicolaou smears, *J. Reprod. Med.,* 36, 95, 1991.

105. Schneider, A., Morabia, A., Papendick, U., Kirchmayr, R., Pork intake and human papillomavirus-related disease, *Nutr. Cancer,* 13, 209, 1990.

106. Rock, C.L., Moskowitz, A., Huizar, B., Saenz, C.C., Clark, J.T., Daly, T.L., Chin, H., Behling, C., Ruffin, M.T., IV, High vegetable and fruit diet in premenopausal women with cervical intraepithelial neoplasia, *J. Am. Diet. Assoc.,* 101, 1167, 2001.

107. Elwood, J.M., Cole, P., Rothman, K.J., Kaplan, S.D., Epidemiology of endometrial cancer, *J. Natl. Cancer Inst.,* 59, 1055, 1977.

108. Henderson, B.E., Casagrande, J.T., Pike, M.C., Mack, T., Rosario, I., Duke, A., The epidemiology of endometrial cancer in young women, *Br. J. Cancer,* 47, 749, 1983.

109. La Vecchia, C.A., Decarli, A., Fasoli, M., Gentile, A., Nutrition and diet in the etiology of endometrial cancer, *Cancer,* 57, 1248, 1986.

110. Lew, E.A. and Garfinkel, L., Variations in mortality by weight among 750,000 men and women, *J. Chronic Dis.,* 32, 563, 1979.

111. Wynder, E.L., Escher, G.C. and Mantel, N., An epidemiological investigation of cancer of the endometrium, *Cancer,* 19, 489, 1966.

112. Schapira, D.V., Nutrition and cancer prevention, *Prim. Care,* 19, 481, 1992.

113. Lapidus, L., Helgesson, O., Merck, C., Bjorntorp, P., Adipose tissue distribution and female carcinomas. A 12-year follow-up of participants in the population study of women in Göteborg, Sweden, *Int. J. Obesity,* 12, 361, 1988.

114. Shu, X.O., Brinton, L.A., Zheng, W., Gao, Y.T., Fan, J., Fraumeni, J.F., Jr., A population-based case-control study of endometrial cancer in Shanghai, China, *Int. J. Cancer,* 49, 38, 1991.

115. Koumantaki, Y., Tzonou, A., Koumantakis, E., Kaklamani, E., Aravantinos, D., Trichopoulos, D., A case-control study of cancer of the endometrium in Athens, *Int. J. Cancer,* 43, 795, 1989.

116. Goodman, M.T., Hankin, J.H., Wilkens, LR., Lyu, LC., McDuffie, K., Liu, LQ., Kolonel, L.N., Diet, body size, physical activity and the risk of endometrial cancer, *Cancer Res.,* 57, 5077, 1997.

117. LaVecchia, C., Nutritional factors and cancers of the breast, endometrium and ovary, *Eur. J. Cancer Clin. Oncol.,* 25, 1945, 1989.

118. Shu, X.O., Zheng, W., Potischman, N., Brinton, L.A., Hatch, M.C., Gao, Y.T., Fraumeni, J.F., Jr., A population-based case-control study of dietary factors and endometrial cancer in Shanghai, People's Republic of China, *Am. J. Epidemiol.,* 137, 155, 1993.

119. Goodman, M.T., Wilkens, L.R., Hankin, J.H., Lyu, L.C., Wu, A.H., Kolonel, LN., Association of soy and fiber consumption with the risk of endometrial cancer, *Am. J. Epidemiol.,* 15, 146, 1997.

120. Littman, A.J., Beresford, S.A. and White, E., The association of dietary fat and plant foods with endometrial cancer (United States), *Cancer Causes Control,* 12, 691, 2001.

121. Barbone, F., Austin, H. and Partridge, E.E., Diet and endometrial cancer: A case-control study, *Am. J. Epidemiol.,* 137, 393, 1993.

122. Negri, E., LaVecchia, C., Franceschi, S., Levi, F., Parazzini, F., Intake of selected micronutrients and the risk of endometrial carcinoma, *Cancer,* 77, 917, 1996.

123. Kojima, T., Tanaka, T. and Mori, H., Chemoprevention of spontaneous endometrial cancer in female Donryu rats by dietary indole-3-carbinol, *Cancer Res.,* 54, 1446, 1994.

124. Littman, A.J., Voigt, L.F., Beresford, S.A, Weiss, N.S., Recreational physical activity and endometrial cancer risk, *Am. J. Epidemiol.,* 15; 154, 2001.

125. Weiderpass, E., Adami, H.O., Baron, J.A, Wicklund-Glynn, A, Aune, M., Atuma, S., Persson, I., Organochlorines and endometrial cancer risk, *Cancer Epidemiol. Biomarkers Prev.,* 9, 487, 2000.

126. Reimer, R.R, Hoover, R., Fraumeni, J.F., Jr., Young, R.C., Second primary neoplasma following ovarian cancer, *J. Natl. Cancer Inst.,* 61, 1195, 1978.

127. Casagrande, J.T., Louie, E.W., Pike, M.C., Roy, S., Ross, RK., Henderson, R.E., "Incessant ovulation" and ovarian cancer, *Lancet,* 2, 170, 1979.

128. Cramer, D.W., Hutchinson, G.B., Welch, W.R., Scully, R.E., Knapp, R.C., Factors affecting the association of oral contraceptives and ovarian cancer, *New Engl. J. Med.,* 307, 1047, 1982.

129. Nasca, P.C., Greenwald, P., Chorost, S., Richart, R., Caputo, T., An epidemiologic case-control study of ovarian cancer and reproductive factors, *Am. J. Epidemiol.,* 119, 705, 1984.

130. Weiss, N.S., Lyon, J.L., Liff, J.M., Vollmer, W.M., Daling, J.R., Incidence of ovarian cancer in relation to the use of oral contraceptives, *Int. J. Cancer,* 28, 669, 1981.

131. Annegers, J.F., Strom, H., Decker, D.G., Dockerty, M.B., O'Fallon, W.M., Ovarian cancer: Incidence and case-control study, *Cancer,* 43, 723, 1979.

132. Hildreth, N.G., Kelsey, J.L., Li Volsi, V.A., Fischer, D.B., Holford, T.R., Mostov, E.D., Schwartz, P.E., White, C., An epidemiologic study of epithelial carcinoma of the ovary, *Am. J. Epidemiol.,* 114, 398, 1981.

133. Cramer, D.W., Welch, W.R., Hutchison, G.B., Willett, W., Scully, R.E., Dietary animal fat in relation to ovarian cancer risk, *Obstet. Gynecol.,* 63, 833, 1984.

134. Byers, T., Marshall, J., Graham, S., Mettlin, C., Swanson, M., A case-control study of dietary and nondietary factors in ovarian cancer, *J. Natl. Cancer Inst.,* 71, 681, 1983.

135. La Vecchia, C., Franceschi, S., Decarli, A., Gentile, P., Liati, M., Regallo, M., Tognoni, G. Coffee drinking and risk of epithelial ovarian cancer, *Int. J. Cancer,* 33, 559, 1984.

136. Trichopoulos, D., Papapostolou, M. and Polychronopoulou, A., Coffee and ovarian cancer, *Int. J. Cancer,* 28, 691, 1981.

137. Serra-Majem, L., La Vecchia, C., Ribas-Barba, L., Prieto-Ramos, F., Lucchini, F., Ramon, J.M., Salleras, L., Changes in diet and mortality from selected cancers in southern Mediterranean countries, *Eur. J. Clin. Nutr.,* 47, S25, 1993.

138. Kushi, LH., Mink, P.J., Folsom, A.R., Anderson, K.E., Zheng, W., Lazovich, D., Sellers, T.A., Prospective study of diet and ovarian cancer, *Am. J. Epidemiol.,* 149, 21, 1999.

139. Tavani, A., La Vecchia, C., Gallus, S., Lagiou, P., Trichopoulos, D., Levi, F., Negri, E., Red meat intake and cancer risk: A study in Italy, *Int. J. Cancer,* 86, 425, 2000.

140. Fairfield, K.M., Hankinson, E.E., Rosner, B.A., Hunter, D.l., Golditz, G.A., Willett, W.C., Risk of ovarian carcinoma and consumption of vitamins A, C and E and specific carotenoids: A prospective analysis, *Cancer,* 92, 2318, 2001.

141. La Vecchia, C., Epidemiology of ovarian cancer: A summary review, *Eur. J. Cancer Prev.,* 10, 125, 2001.

18 Women and Weight: A Model-Based Perspective

Ellen S. Parham and Adrienne A. White

CONTENTS

I. INTRODUCTION

Fatness is a matter of intense concern for our time. From health care professionals to the media to consumers, avoiding fatness is a major issue. Although men, women and children are all affected by this issue, it seems to have special urgency for women. In this chapter, weight issues will be explored with primary focus on the concerns of women. The definitions and meanings or interpretation of fatness will be examined. Factors contributing to the accumulation of fat will be considered and the safety and effectiveness of various weight management interventions will be evaluated. In gathering and interpreting information, the authors have tried to maintain a perspective of recognizing human diversity.

0-8493-1337-6/03/$0.00+$1.50
© 2004 by CRC Press LLC

Overweight, fat, heavy, obese — are all terms describing a condition of having excessive body fat. How much fat is too much is a topic of considerable debate.[1] The focus of the debate is on the appropriate criteria to apply, and the criteria are dependent on the meaning or model of fatness being considered.

II. MODELS OF OBESITY

Attitudes and behaviors related to weight are the products of how our culture views fatness. The meanings, interpretations and conceptualizations of weight are guided by a number of models existing simultaneously in the Western culture (Figure 18.1). Some of these models are ancient, whereas others are unique to the last 50–60 years. Their influence is subtle, but so powerful that we may come to think that one model or a combination of several represent the whole truth about weight. All models seem to encompass some truths about fatness, but also seem to distort or greatly magnify some attitudes. For example, almost everyone would recognize the beauty in a woman's trim and well-toned body, but does that mean that no physical beauty exists except in slenderness?

Traditional cultures nearly universally viewed fatness as evidence of power, strength and well-being.[2] Although that model probably existed among indigenous Americans, it has largely, if not totally, disappeared in the Western world today. We are, however, still very much influenced by two early models: the moral model and the aesthetic model. The moral model defines fatness as sin, gluttony and sloth. The sin may be viewed as a religious issue or as a violation of being a good "world citizen," an ecological fault. The Judeo-Christian concept of the body as a temple is an illustration of this model. We hear our contemporaries refer to themselves as "bad" or "guilty" because they have violated their diets, clear evidence of the continued influence of the moral model.

The aesthetic model is a powerful force in our contemporary culture. Media bombard us with messages that good things go only to attractive people and that only slender people can be attractive. Women are especially targeted with these messages but men and children do not escape them. Comparison of the pin-up girls of several decades ago with today's media stars clearly illustrates the fact that the body size and shape considered beautiful is a fickle judgment. Such relativity is totally lost, however, in our contemporary message that it is impossible to be too thin.

In both the moral and aesthetic models, the individual who deviates from the narrowly defined range of acceptable fatness is blamed. Therefore, the evolution of a medical model that viewed fatness as a disease was somewhat of a relief. Although obesity had long been considered unhealthy, it was only in the middle of the last century that it began to receive serious medical attention.[2] The medical model views a heavy person as someone who needs to be cured. This model is supported by a vast body of literature demonstrating an array of health risks associated with obesity.[3]

The triple influences of the moral, aesthetic and medical interpretations of obesity have created extraordinary pressures for slenderness. The three models interact as illustrated in this quote from a young woman entering a weight-loss program: "I owe it to my husband and children to lose this fat so that I can be the healthy, attractive wife and mother they deserve. I have been bad in allowing myself

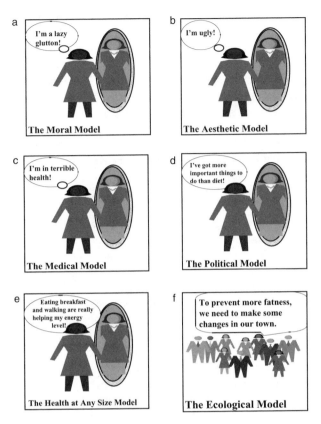

FIGURE 18.1 Models of obesity. Each model interprets the meaning of obesity in a different manner. All of these models exist in our culture simultaneously, exerting subtle, but powerful, influences on our understanding of obesity.

to get this way and now I just have to suffer to lose it."[4] Another outcome of the interaction of these models is the fact that slenderness has come to represent not only beauty but also being in control of one's life, being powerful. This view has great salience for both women and men. In a recent Australian study, women revealed that they considered themselves overweight at levels of fatness well within the range considered healthy by medical definitions.[5]

Stigmatization of obese persons supports the huge weight loss industry that, in turn, generates an increased demand for its goods and services by encouraging further fat phobia. With sales estimated at $35 billion annually, the weight loss industry has capitalized on women's desire for thinness.[6] Advertising designed to encourage body dissatisfaction will ensure profit-making in the diet industry.[7] Use of weight loss centers, meal replacements and appetite suppressants is increasing.[8] Medical interpretations of weight may actually legitimize weight stigmatization and support unnecessary dieting practices.[9] Moore implied that the economic opportunity extends to physicians and researchers who study obesity.[10]

In the 1970s, some women began to observe how much time and energy they and other women devoted to trying to be thin. They asked themselves what they might accomplish if they could harness these resources for other goals. They came to view emphasis on a small slender body as a means to weaken women. Striving for thinness was seen as disempowering. The title of Suzy Orbach's 1978 book *Fat is a Feminist Issue* summarizes this political model.[11]

The political model opened the door for people to begin to question the precepts of the moral, aesthetic and medical models: Were heavy people guilty of gluttony and laziness? Did not restricting the definition of beauty only to those of a narrowly prescribed size and shape deny the diversity of the human species? Were all heavy people at risking their health? If diets do not work, why should we pressure ourselves and others to diet? A new model began to emerge, characterized by some as a militant call to disavow dieting and to accept one's body regardless of its level of fatness. Because it denies what is presented as truth by the more traditional models,[12] this model is quite threatening to those who view it as a refusal to face facts and as a matter of "giving up."[13] A more constructive model has grown out of the earlier absolutes — the health-at-any-size paradigm focuses on health and well-being, not weight.

Advocates of the health-at-any-size model do not view "thinness" as synonymous with being "healthy," but instead, promote health rather than weight loss.[14] Inherent in the model is "size acceptance," which means seeing oneself as a person of value and putting body size into perspective in terms of one's total persona.[15] Diversity in body size is accepted as one of many other physical attributes that differ among people, such as the colors of skin, hair and eyes.

The basic tenets of the model have been delineated by Ikeda:[16]

- Human beings come in a variety of sizes and shapes. There is no ideal body size, shape or weight that every individual should strive to achieve.
- Self esteem and body image are strongly linked. Helping people feel good about their bodies and about who they are can motivate and maintain healthy behaviors.
- Appearance stereotyping is inherently unfair to the individual because it is based on superficial factors over which the individual has little or no control.
- Good health is not defined by body size; it is a state of physical, mental and social well-being.
- People of all sizes and shapes can reduce their risk of poor health by adopting a healthy lifestyle.

The model is predicated on a holistic approach to health with the importance placed on balancing eating according to hunger and satiety signals, participating in regular enjoyable physical activity, maintaining a strong network for social support, positive emotional health and spiritual well-being.[17,18]

The authors of this chapter, believing that the health-at-any-size model is honest and constructive, have framed this chapter around it. How such a paradigm can be implemented is discussed more fully toward the end of the chapter. As we review concepts associated with earlier models, we attempt to provide perspective so that the reader can sort truths from distortions.

Very recently, leaders in the field of weight management have begun to call for an additional model, one that recognizes the impact of environmental factors in the development and maintenance of obesity.[19] All earlier models have viewed obesity as a concern of the individual. In fact, as is discussed below, major environmental factors influence the likelihood of large numbers of persons developing obesity. These factors, such as the ready access of high calorie foods and the need to rely on automobiles for personal transportation are, in large part, beyond the control of the individual. They are characteristics of the community and are determined by formal and informal policies and practices of the community as a whole. For that reason, some advocate the name public health model[19] for this paradigm. The term *public health* has disease connotations, however, and may be viewed as a mere extension of the medical model. Possibly a better label is ecological model. Ecology is defined as the relations and interactions between organisms and their environment. Those who have dealt with efforts to prevent obesity have found that prevention involves changes beyond the capacity of individuals. For that reason, the ecological model has great relevance to prevention.

III. STANDARDS OF FATNESS

The models of obesity influence terms used to describe fatness, methods to assess and definitions of severity. For example, "cellulite," a term used to describe dimpled subcutaneous fat, is the focus of much concern to those influenced by the aesthetic model, whereas it goes without recognition in the medical model. Although we could point out terms and measures associated with the various models, the assessment approaches and definitions of the medical model are clearly the "gold standard" today. Dozens of highly technical means of determining fatness are currently available but the most commonly used are based on simple measures of weight, height and body circumference. The most popular of these is body mass index (BMI). BMI is the ratio of body weight expressed in kilograms divided by the square of the height in meters. The value produced is equally applicable to adult males and females. The most usual definitions of a healthy BMI are supposedly based on the range of minimal risk to physical health. The World Health Organization (WHO) defines this healthy range as a BMI of 18.5–24.9.[20] We think that it is rarely useful to apply categories to fatness and prefer to use the terms overweight, fatness, obesity and heaviness in a qualitative way, rather than a means to distinguish between levels of adiposity. We recommend that the use of the classifications of overweight (BMI 25.0–29.9) and obesity (BMI>30) be reserved for those rare situations requiring a more precise definition. There is considerable concern that there is inadequate evidence to classify persons with BMIs of 25.0–29.9 as being at increased risk for degenerative disease.[21]

As will be shown below, BMI alone does not adequately explain health risks. The location of the fat is a major factor contributing to risk. Females are prone to depositing fat in the buttocks, thighs and lower abdomen, sites much deplored by aesthetic interpretations of fatness but actually relatively benign as far as physical health is concerned. On the other hand, fat in the waist area, particularly visceral fat that is inside the abdominal cavity is especially dangerous. WHO recommends that waist circumferences above 800.01 mm (31.5 in.) for women be considered indicative of the likelihood of metabolic complications and that circumferences above 881.38 mm (34.7 in.) be considered to represent substantial risk.[20] Waist circumferences cannot, however, distinguish subcutaneous and visceral fat. More sophisticated, but not readily available scanning techniques can show the location.[22] A more viable alternative may be to measure blood triglyceride levels, high levels being associated with increased visceral fat.[23] Routine physical examinations often include measurement of serum triglyceride levels.

Proponents of the health-at-any-size model advocate an entirely different definition of healthy weight. Being sensitive to individual differences in genetically determined body sizes and shapes and aware of the limitations of lasting change in weight, advocates of this model have suggested a working definition of healthy weight as the weight that an adult can sustain by eating a healthy diet and engaging in appropriate amounts of regular exercise.[24,25] Some might modify this definition to stipulate that the individual be free of risk factors like hypertension or impaired glucose tolerance .[26]

IV. ARE WE EXPERIENCING AN OBESITY EPIDEMIC?

During the last quarter of the 20th century, dramatic increases in the prevalence of obesity were observed. Relatively mild obesity (BMI 25–29.9) showed very little increase, but the incidence of extreme fatness (BMI>30) almost doubled from 1960 to 1994.[27] Although there were some differences associated with age, gender and race or ethnicity, no group escaped the trend. Consequently, at the close of the century, more than half of American women (50.7%) had BMIs beyond the recommended level. In a longitudinal study of young adults from the mid-1980s to mid-1990s, almost all groups gained weight over the observation period.[28] Most successful in maintaining their weights were normal-weight white women. The weight gains were most dramatic in African-American women, among whom the prevalence of normal weight decreased from 52% initially to 28.4% finally. This trend of increasing fatness continued during the last decade of the century with greatest increases found among 18 to 29 year olds, those with some college education and those of Hispanic ethnicity.[29] Given the fact that numerous researchers have found a severe and widespread increase in childhood obesity,[30] it would seem that the obesity epidemic can be expected to continue for some time into the future.

Given the stigma of obesity and the seeming rewards of being slender, how is it that Americans continue to fatten? Changes in body weight are a function of the balance between energy intake and expenditure. The increase in fatness is clear evidence that in recent decades this balance has been positive, intake exceeding expenditure. Although, as discussed below, numerous factors affect this balance, practically speaking one must look to quantities of food eaten and levels of physical activity for explanation of the obesity epidemic.

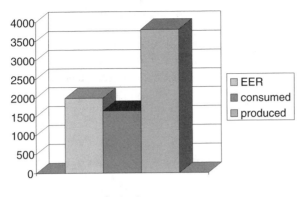

Daily Calories

FIGURE 18.2 Dramatic differences exist between the estimated energy requirement (EER) for adult women (30 years of age, sedentary and with BMI of 24.99), reported intakes (consumed) and the energy content of food produced per person daily in this country.

Although, compared with energy intake earlier in the last century, American women were eating less, in the 1990s, there were more-recent upturns in intake. In the 1977–78 surveys, American women were eating food providing 1534 kcal daily; in 1994–96 this amount had increased to 1646 kcal[31] (Figure 18.2). A positive energy balance of 112 kcal continued day after day would be expected to lead to significant weight gains. However, before concluding that women should eat less, one should consider that, depending on their size and activity level, women 30 years of age are recommended to consume approximately 2000 kcal daily.[32] When energy intake drops below these levels, it becomes extremely difficult to meet nutrient needs.

Recent decades have also been marked by changes in the American food supply, creating what some refer to as a food environment toxic to weight control.[19] The food industry produces 3800 kcal per day for every person in the United States, up from 3300 kcal daily in the 1970s.[31] Much of this food is high sugar and high fat, as well as highly available. Food served away from home is dished up in huge portions[33] and most people eat all they are served most of the time.[34] Usually "up-sized" portions provide much more food for the money, enticing customers to choose this option, an option that is more profitable for the producer. The staggering amounts of food intended for American consumers are marketed at a cost of $30 billion annually.[31]

Food marketing creates a tremendous pressure to consume. Nevertheless, Americans keep trying to control their weight by dieting. Typically, more than half of American women report having dieted in the last year.[35] Women are almost twice as likely than men to diet, but similar percentages of men and women say they are "watching what I eat."[35]

In a recent Gallup poll, persons 50 and older were most likely to attribute obesity to overeating whereas younger adults were more likely to blame lack of exercise.[36] When attempting to explain the obesity epidemic, experts tend to agree with the younger adults that lack of physical activity is the primary problem.[19,37] Recent decades have seen expansion of the sedentary quality of American life. More than 60% of Americans do not participate in regular physical activity and 25% report no activity at all.[19] More insidious is the ever-increasing utilization of labor-saving devices, with the result that one's working hours often involve little movement beyond the hands. For an active person, physical activity can account for a large portion of energy expenditure, but for sedentary persons activity represents only 20–30% of total expenditure. If activity drops, one can gain weight without eating more.

V. SYSTEMS FOR REGULATING ENERGY BALANCE

Humans have several mechanisms that allow us to adjust to irregularities in our energy intake. These mechanisms are designed to protect us from both under and over supplies of energy, but they are more powerful in the direction of prevention of starvation.[38] The very traits that served our hungry ancestors well contribute to our difficulty in living in a world of abundant food without getting fat. These adaptive mechanisms include the ability to store energy and remove it from storage, primarily in the form of fat. This storage capacity provides us with the ability to tolerate days of eating very little, as well as days of excessive consumption.

Other systems for regulating our energy balance include adjustment in the rate at which we use energy and control of our food intake. For sedentary persons, the majority of energy used is devoted to doing the internal work of the body. This work goes on 24 hours a day every day. Our bodies can adjust the efficiency of this work so as to squander energy when there is a positive energy balance or to conserve energy when resources are scarce. Once again, the capacity to slow weight loss is greater than the ability to use metabolic adjustments to prevent weight gain.[38]

Our intake controls include the experience of hunger and satiety and our voluntary decisions to act on those experiences. Hunger and satiety are produced in response to deprivation and eating through an extremely complex system of many components that monitor our body's energy status and inform our brains of our need to eat or cease eating. These components vary from immediate responses to the presence of food in the stomach to feedback responses to the post-absorptive changes in the blood to monitoring the state of energy stores. The recently discovered hormone leptin is just one component of the system, but it coordinates a variety of responses in adjusting energy balance.[39] Leptin is formed in fat cells in amounts proportional to the fat content of the cell. So, when the fat levels of the body are elevated as in obesity, or after several days of positive energy balance, high levels of leptin are found in the bloodstream. Generally, high circulating leptin levels lead to a reduction of food intake.

How can it be that, guarded by this finely tuned and integrated system of controls, we still fail to balance food intake with our needs? Sometimes the system fails to produce the usual effect. For example, obese people, in spite of the presence of high leptin levels, do not experience the brain responses that should lead to reduction in eating. This lack of responsiveness may be due to a failure in brain uptake of leptin.[39] Probably even more important than failures in the physiological systems are the urges to eat or not eat that come from our thoughts and feelings, as well as pressures from the environment.

As observed above, the food environment in 21st century America is one of almost constant exposure to an abundance of rich and tempting foods. We are bombarded with cues to eat from this environment. Although our responsiveness to environmental cues is enhanced by hunger, we are often lured into eating in the absence of hunger. Most people have "comfort" foods to which they turn in times of stress. Ideally, we would rely exclusively on our physiological cues to guide our eating, but in the complex modern world this is rarely possible.

VI. THE ROLE PLAYED BY GENETICS

In spite of all the factors contributing to the likelihood of accumulation of excessive fat, some people stay thin. Familial patterns of thinness suggest that there are genetic factors that make it possible for some people to avoid obesity even in a fat-toxic environment. Do fatness and thinness run in families because family members share genetic material, a common environment, or both? By observing the body composition of monozygotic and dizygotic twins reared together or apart by their biologic or adopted parents, scientists have been able to observe genetic influences apart from the influence of an environment shared with one's parents. Genes seem responsible for up to two thirds of the variation in fatness among adults .[40] Their influence is exerted by affecting energy intake, energy expenditure, or the molecular forms in which energy is stored in the body.[41]

Except for a few rare conditions, the genetic contribution to obesity is accomplished not by a single gene, but by non-Mendelian inheritance involving multiple genes, interactions between genes and interactions with environmental factors. It has been estimated that more than 250 genetic loci are associated with fat disposition.[42] Some of these genes are responsible for male/female differences in patterns of fat location and others contribute to racial differences in fatness, as well as many other factors affecting fat accumulation.

There has been a great deal of interest recently in the *ob* gene, which controls the production of the hormone leptin. Only rarely have mutations in this gene been found among humans.[43] As important as leptin appears to be in energy metabolism, it explains only a small portion of the genetically mediated variation in human fatness.

No genetic influences can make it possible to get fat in the absence of a positive calorie balance, but they can influence the extent of response to energy in excess of need. Bouchard[44] elegantly demonstrated this fact in a series of studies by manipulating the energy intake of monozygotic twins. When consuming 1000 kcal daily beyond their energy needs, all twins gained weight. There was close correlation in weight gain between the two twins within each pair, but differences in gain between pairs varied from less than 4.05 kg. (9 lb.) to almost 13.05 kg. (29 lb.). Similar findings resulted when energy intake was reduced below needs.

In light of the interaction between genetic makeup and environmental factors, the question as to whether genes or environment are responsible for the current obesity epidemic becomes moot. In the face of differing environmental conditions, various genes and gene interactions become more or less influential. In recent decades, the environment in this country has promoted over-consumption of food and discouraged physical activity.

The moral and medical models of obesity interpret genetic influences as "guilt-free" explanations of obesity. On the other hand, environmental factors are "guilt-laden," possibly because they are viewed as being under voluntary control. There is no evidence that guilt is productive in combating obesity.[13]

VII. HEALTH RISKS ASSOCIATED WITH LEVEL OF FATNESS

The medical model of obesity is most clear in the documentation of the association of fatness and health risks. There is strong evidence that human bodies function best when the amount of body fat is low to moderate. Both too much and too little body fat has been shown to be related to disease risk and life expectancy.

Most dramatic is the increased likelihood among heavy people of developing one or more of a cluster of diseases — diabetes, hypertension and cardiovascular disease (CVD) — that form a group of related diseases having in common high levels of blood triglycerides.[23] Insulin is also high, but, because the body is resistant to the insulin's action, the body is actually insulin poor.[23] This cluster of symptoms and risks is called syndrome x or the metabolic syndrome. Figure 18.3 shows an example of the distribution of the diseases of this syndrome among persons of varying sizes.

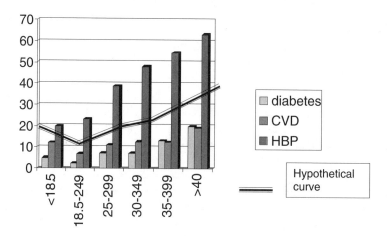

FIGURE 18.3 Typical association of body fatness with prevalence ratios for diabetes, cardiovascular disease (CVD) and hypertension (HBP). Based on 7689 women in the Third National Health and Nutrition Examination Survey, these data show the usual J-shaped curve wherein the lowest prevalence is found among individuals of normal weight. The exception is HBP, for which the lowest prevalence is among women considered underweight.

Type 2 diabetes (formerly called noninsulin-dependent diabetes) is the most common form of the disease and 60–90% of people with type 2 diabetes are overweight.[45] One third of all obese people have hypertension.[46] CVD, the number one cause of death among most adult groups in the United States, becomes more likely as weight increases. In the Nurses' Health Study, a study of more than a 100,000 female nurses followed for 14 years, even women in the higher ranges of "normal" weight suffered more coronary heart disease than did lean women.[47] Although obesity may increase other health risks including osteoarthritis, gout, gallbladder disease and certain types of cancer, it is the diseases of the metabolic syndrome that constitute the major risks.[46]

Generally, graphs of life expectancy at various levels of fatness show a J-shaped curve, with some increased mortality among persons with very low fat, minimum mortality among those with low to moderate levels and a steep increase in mortality among those who are quite fat.[48] When considered from an epidemiological perspective, the association is quite clear. On the other hand, when considering individuals, a remarkable heterogeneity in the health of heavy persons exists. Some follow the statistical pattern quite predictably but others, equally fat, seem to escape the foretold consequences. Age is one differentiating factor; although the likelihood of being fat increases with age, the health risks of extreme fatness are much more pronounced among younger adults.[49] On the other hand, age appears to be an independent risk factor, the prevalence of numerous risk factors increasing with age, regardless of adiposity. Gender is another factor: In the longitudinal Alameda County Study of more than 6000 adults, there was a higher relative risk of mortality for underweight women than underweight men but lower relative risk for moderately to extremely obese women than men in the same weight category.[21] Differences in risk between the sexes may be related to differences in the amount of visceral fat. Although women may acquire large quantities of visceral fat, men are more likely to do so.

Postmenopausal women experience an increased risk of CVD.[50] The postmenopausal period is associated with an increase in visceral fat, a factor contributing to insulin insensitivity and to increased vulnerability to CVD.[51] Although research findings are not completely consistent, there is some evidence that hormone replacement therapy is associated with lessened accumulation of visceral fat.[52]

Blair and his colleagues have shown that cardiorespiratory fitness, rather than fatness, best predicted mortality among 9925 women observed over an average of 11.4 years.[53] Not unexpectedly, the number of fit and heavy women was relatively low, but even at BMI levels exceeding 37.1, there were almost 21% who met the criteria of having moderate or high fitness levels. Blake et al.[54] found further evidence that heavy women can improve their fitness when they compared the performance of slender and heavy women in a 14-week exercise program. The investigators found no significant differences in the effort (attendance and time in exercise) or in fitness outcomes. Both groups improved in aerobic fitness, muscular strength, muscular endurance and flexibility; neither group lost weight.

Given that some heavy women seem to enjoy excellent health, it is disappointing that the medical community has seen fit to concentrate only on the unhealthy. It would seem advantageous to know more clearly why some people seem to escape the health risks of obesity. Raising such questions is not popular, often being interpreted by zealous advocates of the medical model of obesity as irresponsibly encouraging obesity.[12,37,55]

VIII. EFFECTS OF WEIGHT LOSS ON PHYSICAL HEALTH

Although removal of the stigma of obesity associated with the moral, aesthetic and medical models requires the achievement of slenderness, significant improvements in medical status have been repeatedly demonstrated with losses of 5–20% of body weight.[56] Blood pressure lowers, serum lipids decline, insulin resistance improves and general well-being increases with losses of 5–10% of initial weight.[56] In contrast to the more stable fat stores in the thighs and buttocks, abdominal fat responds quickly and preferentially to a negative energy balance;[51] a 10% loss of body weight can mean a 30% reduction in dangerous visceral fat.[23]

Given the dramatic improvement with modest weight losses, one would expect to find strong evidence of a long-term effect of weight loss on morbidity and mortality. This evidence is not present.[57,58] Even when data are limited to intentional weight loss, either a neutral or slight positive effect on longevity exists.[59] In the Nurses' Health Study, weight gains after age 18 were associated with increased mortality, but weight losses did not have a comparable benefit.[47] Many explanations have been offered for this failure to find expected benefits:

- Longitudinal studies are difficult and may involve self-reported data or losses of large numbers of subjects.
- It is not always possible to distinguish between voluntary and spontaneous weight losses.
- In the long run, weight loss efforts may in themselves be risky, outweighing the benefits of the accompanying loss.
- Over time, there may be unidentified changes in nature and location of body fat without significant changes in weight.

In this chapter, only risks of fatness to physical health have been reviewed. This perspective is limited, since the risks to emotional and social well-being are substantial.[60] The moral and aesthetic models are associated with the stigmatization of obesity that contributes to these risks. For many women, this stigma is probably more pressing than the risks to physical health and may be responsible for their high levels of dieting.

IX. SHIFTING THE FOCUS FROM WEIGHT LOSS TO WEIGHT MANAGEMENT

Figure 18.4 shows the typical cyclic pattern that characterizes weight loss attempts. Rather than making a single weight loss attempt that produces lasting slenderness, most individuals make repeated efforts that bring them back to obesity.[61]

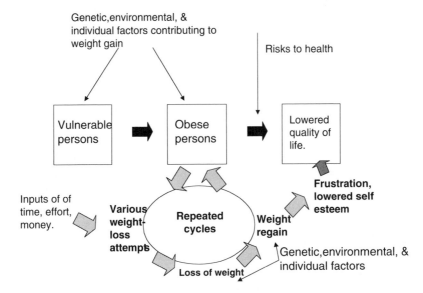

FIGURE 18.4 Most heavy individuals repeatedly try to lose weight only to regain their losses. These repeated futile cycles sustain the obesity and lead to negative emotional and social consequences, contributing to the lowered state of well-being associated with obesity.

Some years ago, the Institute of Medicine[62] recommended the term "weight management" rather than weight-control or weight-loss programs in an effort to refocus attention on overall health. The primary purpose of weight management was to achieve and maintain good health through a stable weight.[63] The focus was still on "healthy *weight* goals" and achieving and maintaining small weight losses.[64,65] At a time when weight gain and weight cycling are commonplace, the goals of weight management, which include stopping weight gain, stabilizing weight or reducing health risks, seem prudent. The authors of the American Dietetic Association's 1997 position paper on weight management admitted the challenge of dietitians to teach clients the concept of health without both food restriction or deprivation and the good food–bad food connotations.[63]

Parham[15] added the challenge of replacing the "normative discontent" of American women[66] with "body size acceptance." Accepting body size is critical for the many heavy women who will not attain culturally defined slenderness, but who quite possibly can improve their physical, emotional and social health. They are more likely to remain heavy even as they reduce health risks through such measures as lowering blood pressure and maintaining appropriate serum lipid levels.[67] Even those women who do achieve slenderness often find it hard to accept their bodies and continue to torment themselves about the threat of fatness.

To become a promoter of size acceptance, one must come to terms with one's own belief about how size acceptance fits into weight management. Clients and other health care professionals must also recognize that size acceptance is not blind acceptance of being heavy, but rather a way to provide alternatives to a lifestyle of diet restrictions, frantic exercise and hating oneself.[68] Advocates of size acceptance may need to gain credibility by substantiating claims with scientific evidence[68,69] and establishing a climate that allows for questions and sharing of personal experiences.

Miller[70] identified four components necessary for a program to have the greatest potential for successful weight maintenance:

1. Preevaluation to determine medical and behavioral history, identification of determinants of success[71] and setting realistic goals and objectives
2. Integrating an enjoyable, individualized exercise and activity program
3. Using a client-designed behavioral plan[72]
4. Having a client-designed maintenance plan that includes constant monitoring of diet and exercise behaviors[73,74] and client commitment to develop internal direction for monitoring new behaviors[61,69,75]

In 2002, the American Dietetic Association adopted a position that a lifelong commitment to enjoyable and sustainable healthful behaviors emphasizing eating practices and daily physical activity can help in successful weight management and overall health.[76] Goals for weight management were identified to include the following:[76]

• Prevention of weight gain or stopping weight gain in individuals who have been seeing a steady increase in their weight[77]
• Varying degrees of improvement in physical and emotional health[78]
• Small maintainable weight losses or more extensive weight losses achieved through sensible and tolerable eating and exercise behaviors[79]
• Improvements in eating, exercise and other behaviors apart from any weight loss

X. EVALUATION OF CURRENT PROGRAMS AND PLANS FOR WEIGHT MANAGEMENT

Planning a personal weight management effort should start with identification of one's individual weight management goals. Bearing these goals in mind, one can then consider the array of currently available weight management treatments and strategies. Through a thorough personal and professional assessment, underlying contributors to obesity as well as a person's expectations, readiness to change and lifestyle factors can be determined.[63] Underlying contributors to obesity may include sedentary living and responses to the ubiquitous availability of tempting high-calorie food, as well as psychological problems,[80] binge eating disorders and other disordered eating patterns[81] or weight cycling.[82] In any weight management plan there should be components to consider and address the contributing factors.

A. FOOD AND MACRONUTRIENT RESTRICTIONS

Daily intakes of ≤800 kcal are termed very low-calorie diets (VLCDs); these usually involve a commercially prepared formula. Wadden[83] reported that an average 12- to

16-week program resulted in a 20 kg. body weight loss, with regains of 35–50% of body weight after a 1-year follow-up. Drop-out rates as high as 80%[65] and gradual body weight regain indicate low long term success for such programs.[84] Acting as a protein sparing modified fast, VLCDs are composed of liquid or animal protein with vitamin and mineral supplements. In spite of its weight loss maintenance limitations, the diet has been used with quite heavy persons who have been unsuccessful with other approaches.[76] VLCDs should be closely supervised by medical professionals to avoid serious complications such as dehydration, ketosis, hyperuricaemia, hypokalemia, hypoglycemia, loss of body protein and psychological disorders.[85,86] Weight loss maintenance has been difficult after transition to a mixed diet. In fact, a mixed diet of equal calorie content has been found to be as effective in producing weight loss as the VLCD.[87,88]

Compared with the VLCD, following a low-calorie diet (LCD) (1200 kcal) for a longer time (20 weeks) can result in less than half of the amount of body weight loss (8.5 kg) (83). Following an LCD for 6–12 months can result in an 8–10% body weight loss. To achieve weight loss, reduction of total kcal, fat kcal to less than 30% of kcal[89] saturated fats reduction and portion control help to ensure an energy deficit of 500–1000 kcal per day.[76] While there may be body weight loss maintenance of 66% after 1 year, little long-term success has been noted.[83,90,91] Results of a meta-analysis by Miller et al.[92] of both VLCD and LCD programs were that average body weight loss was 11 kg. during a 15-week program, with 35% regained after 1 year. Miller[70] concluded that weight loss was ample when using energy-restricting diets, but gradual regain followed.

Another way to control kcal is the meal replacement method, in which premeasured frozen meals or liquids containing around 200 kcal per serving replace a meal.[76] The macronutrient composition of the meal is 50–60% carbohydrate, 30% protein and 10% fat. Flechtner-Mors et al.[93] found small, sustained weight losses ranging from 3.2–8.4% over 4 years. The benefits of meal replacements are that portion control is predetermined and sensory stimulus is minimized.[76]

Low-fat diets, diets containing 1200–1700 kcal, of which 10–15% are fat kcal, do not appear to result in substantial weight loss.[94] To lose weight, the balance must be manipulated between the food quotient (fat intake) and the respiratory quotient (fat oxidation).[95,96] A low-fat diet does help to shift the balance between fat intake and oxidation toward fat oxidation.[70]

High-protein diets are composed of low carbohydrate and may be high-fat (as much as 50–75% fat kcal) or low-fat (30% fat kcal). When protein and fat are high in the diet, muscle catabolism is avoided and ketosis contributes to appetite suppression. It is the low dietary carbohydrate content that contributes to rapid body weight loss due to glycogen depletion and diuresis. However, associated health risks of low-carbohydrate diets include nausea, hyperuricemia, elevated blood pressure, gout and kidney stones, which lead to increased risks for heart disease, cancer and osteoporosis.[76,97] Carbohydrate additions to the diet are accompanied by body weight regain.[76,97] Skov et al.[98] reported body weight losses of 8.9 kg in overweight individuals who followed a 25:45:30 protein-to-carbohydrate-to fat ratio. While health risks are reduced with this nutrient ratio, no documentation of long-term success is available.

B. Pharmacotherapy

Pharmacotherapy may be recommended for a BMI >30 or BMI > 27–29 with one or more obesity-related disorders.[76] For treatment of obesity, the Food and Drug Administration has approved Sibutramine, a centrally acting serotonin and adrenergic reuptake inhibitor (modifying internal signals for satiety and hunger), and Orlistat, a pancreatic lipase inhibitor, causing malabsorption of up to 30% of dietary fat. These pharmacologic agents have been effective in producing a 7–10% initial weight loss over the first 4 to 6 months of use, followed by a slowing and then stopping of weight loss.[99–101] Pharmacotherapy should be combined with dietary intervention, physical activity and behavior therapy.[76,102] The benefits of pharmacotherapy are that maintenance of weight loss is facilitated and that less time and effort are required by both patient and health professional.[103] Sibutramine is associated with hypertension and increased heart rate. Orlistat complications include steatorrhea, bloating and distension, anal linkage and possible deficiencies of fat-soluble vitamins.[76]

C. Surgery

When other methods for long-term weight management have been unsuccessful, surgery to restrict food intake and decrease absorption is an acceptable intervention for persons with either a BMI > 40 or BMI 35–39 with one or more obesity-related disorders.[76] Food intake is restricted with the use of a gastric band so only a small amount of food enters the stomach (gastric banding) or by banding and stapling to make a small pouch (vertical banded gastroplasty).[76] Bypassing parts of the small intestine, including the duodenum, contributes to malabsorption. The benefit of this method has been the high success rate of more than 90% of patients losing >20–25% body weight and between 50–80% maintaining loss for over 5 years.[104] Although the operation results in a low mortality rate of 1–2%, there are common troublesome side effects including nutritional complications and the need for additional surgery.[105] Long-term close monitoring by health professionals and high commitment to lifestyle changes by patients are necessary to maintain weight loss and avoid postoperative complications.[76,89]

D. Exercise

Results of the meta-analysis by Miller et al.[92] were that the amount of weekly body weight lost through exercise was only 0.2±0.04 kg. However, Miller and co-workers, as well as others,[106–112] have identified that exercise is of major importance in maintaining body weight loss following treatment. Miller[70] asserted that body weight-loss maintenance is almost guaranteed with exercise. In his review of literature, he found that the diet macronutrient composition following exercise can influence exercise effectiveness. When high-fat diets followed exercise, energy intakes increased, while *ad libitum* low-fat diets resulted in short-term negative energy balance .[113,114] When exercise was combined with VLCD body weight-loss programs, reductions in metabolism commonly seen in low-calorie diets were eliminated.

The most noteworthy benefits of exercise are related to health rather than directly to weight. Improvements have been seen in blood pressure, glucose and lipid levels, psychological well-being and overall cardiorespiratory fitness.[67,115–117] Exercise during weight loss preserves lean body mass, an important influence on resting metabolic rate[118,119] and reduces visceral abdominal fat, an independent risk factor for the development of type 2 diabetes, coronary heart disease, hypertension and some cancers.[120]

Exercise can be divided into either programmed or lifestyle activities.[121,122] Programmed activities are regularly planned events such as aerobics, running, swimming, or cycling.[103] Life-style activities are day-to-day activities such as walking rather than driving and taking the stairs rather than the elevator. Both types of exercise are encouraged.[123] Anderson et al.[124] encouraged walking for obese individuals because it can be both a programmed and life-style activity. As a programmed activity, the recommendation has been to walk two to three times per week for 15–20 minutes each time, gradually increasing times and amount to four to five times per week for 40–45 minutes per day at 60–80% of target heart rate.[103,124] For lifestyle activities, the recommendation is to expend an additional 100 kcal/day by such things as using fewer energy-saving devices.

XI. LIMITED SUCCESS OF WEIGHT LOSS EFFORTS

Losing weight and, more importantly, maintaining lost weight are challenging and frustrating tasks.[103] No quick solutions exist and even when women commit to weight-loss programs, success means only a 5–15% decrease in initial weight. For maintenance, women must acknowledged the chronic nature of obesity and accept a lifelong focus on weight management. As well as their own commitment, most women will require the long-term support of health care professionals, including weight management personnel. Since eating is an unavoidable behavior, the challenges to maintain changes are unique and difficult.[125] Eating occasions throughout the day and the "powerful biological reward of satiety" compete with the need for moderation.[125] In addition, the regulation of an obese state may be a condition of body energy regulation at an elevated set-point.[126] Discrimination and prejudice toward the obese discourage women from seeking needed health care and contribute to the psychological burden placed on those living in a culture that glorifies thinness.[75] Overweight patients have been described by physicians as being indulgent, emotionally disturbed, weak-willed and ugly.[127,128]

Goodrick et al.[129] found that individuals overestimated the overall success rate of programs and blamed themselves for failures. Treatment goals may be set that are overly ambitious relative to the limited number of contacts that occur typically between health professionals and clients. Such ambitious goals may exceed the individual's perceived self-efficacy.[130] Health care professionals, as well, may feel the sense of helplessness and lack of competence when therapeutic goals are not met.[80] Thus, they can become disinterested and apathetic about weight control, compounding the individual's feelings of helplessness.[103]

Exercise is important during the weight loss period and is a major key for weight loss maintenance. Yet access to fitness activities is lacking for obese women.[75,131,132] Lyons and Miller[75] cited intimidation and embarrassment, fear of hurting oneself and the cultural image of equating fitness with thinness as barriers to exercise for obese individuals. During the weight loss period, the low average weekly weight loss attributed to exercise (0.2 ± 0.04 kg.) could frustrate an individual with a high weight loss goal. Individuals who have exercised as part of their weight-loss programs have reported that the key to their lack of success in maintaining weight loss was exercise cessation.[133] Reported drop-out rates for exercise programs are as high as 50% within the first 6 months of starting a new program and about 70% after 12 months.[134]

A. A FEW PEOPLE SUCCEED. WHAT IS THEIR SECRET?

Klem et al.[135] reported on the strategies weight maintainers used for weight loss and maintenance. The maintainers (n = 629 women) enrolled in the National Weight Control Registry, had lost an average of 30 kg., maintained a minimum of 13.6 kg. loss for an average of 5.5 years. Fifty-five percent of subjects had used formal programs or professional assistance and most (89%) used both dietary and physical activity to lose weight. The dietary methods most commonly used were to limit intake of certain foods (87.6%), limit quantities of food eaten (44.2%) and to count kcal (43.75%). They reported consuming an average of 1381 ± 526 kcal per day during weight loss maintenance. Most of the meals were prepared or eaten at home. Compared with the men (n = 155), women were more likely to report that they limited quantities of food eaten and used the exchange system for diet planning. Liquid formulas were used by 20% of the sample. Dietary fat was maintained at less than 30% of total kcal. About 30% of maintainers reported ≥20% of total kcal from fat. Use of medication and surgery was minimal.

Almost all maintainers used physical activity to lose weight, 92% exercising at home, 31.3% exercising with groups and 40.3% exercising with friends. Women were more likely than men to use walking and aerobic dancing. Reported kcal used in physical activity were about 400 kcal per day, equivalent to 44.8 km. (28 miles) per week. Most of the sample weighed themselves at least once per week (75%), while over one third weighed themselves daily. Contrary to findings,[65] subjects (42%) felt that weight maintenance was less difficult than weight loss. Improvements in quality of life included level of energy, physical mobility, general mood, self confidence and physical health.

McGuire et al.[73] found that the only strategy for weight loss that differed between maintainers and regainers was that those who were successful at weight maintenance did not report membership in self-help groups such as Take Off Pounds Sensibly. Strategies used by both maintainers and regainers included losing weight on their own, using a physician-prescribed diet or a commercial program and using over-the-counter meal replacements. Maintainers incorporated more weight-controlling behaviors than the regainers, such as using more ways to lower dietary fat intake, engaging in more strenuous exercise and weighing themselves at least once per week.

Anderson et al.[136] conducted a meta-analysis to address the issue of long-term maintenance. While the low number of studies inhibited their analysis, they found that exercise appeared to be positively related to successful weight-loss maintenance and the use of very low-energy diets or weight loss $\geq$ 20 kg. was strongly related to weight maintenance.

While some women have been successful using the methods recommended for body weight loss and maintenance, a greater number of women have failed in their efforts, leading to weight fluctuations, weight gain and ultimately higher levels of obesity.[137,138] It is for these women especially that the health-at-any-size model holds promise. It may also be a liberating model for all women who struggle with size acceptance whatever their body weight may be.

XII. APPROACHES BASED ON THE HEALTH-AT-ANY-SIZE MODEL

When the health-at-any-size model is implemented, health and well-being for everyone at whatever size are promoted.[139] The premise is that health is a multifaceted condition involving the physical, mental, emotional, social and spiritual self. Being healthy means practicing behaviors that together achieve wellness, such as:

- Eating with balance and regularity
- Engaging in physical activity
- Getting sufficient rest and sleep
- Not abusing addictive substances
- Seeking ways for self development and expression
- Developing enduring, supportive relationships
- Finding peace and meaning in life

Thus, many of the signs of a healthy life-style are independent of body weight.[69] And, according to Jonas, the "lack of any one health-related personal behavioral outcome does not mean that a person is totally 'unhealthy.' In fact, if an overweight person undertakes health-promoting behaviors other than weight loss, it is indeed possible to be both overweight and healthy at the same time."[24]

While the model applies to "any size," the focal point has centered on issues of overweight and obesity. Health care professionals who advocate the health-at-any-size model see the obsession with body weight and thinness contributing to the increased prevalence of obesity and the lack of acceptance in diversity in body sizes.[1,61,75,140–143] Health-at-any-size, say Miller and Jacob, "assumes that the overweight person innately wants to eat healthy food and be active and that once diet restrictions and barriers to activity have been removed, the individual will develop healthier eating and activity patterns which lead to a genetically determined healthy body weight."[69] With this inherent nondiet approach, rather than seeking to reach a certain body weight, improved health and quality of life become the goals. The woman is able to stop dieting and exercising just to lose weight and start focusing on skills to recognize the body's wants and needs.[1,61,75,140–143]

Miller and Jacob[69] reviewed the research documenting the effectiveness of the health-at-any-size model. Although the number of studies was limited, moderate weight loss occurred during treatment and, more importantly, continued following treatment.[144–146] Polivy and Herman[147] reported that women scoring in the range of disordered eating participated in a nondiet intervention and maintained weight after 6 months. Sbrocco et al.[148] tested the health-at-any-size model with one group receiving 1800 kcal for 2 weeks with behavioral training about intuitive eating, compared with another group that followed a traditional weight-loss program of 1200 kcal for 2 weeks, with behavioral training on food restriction. At the 1-year follow-up, the health-at-any-size group maintained a stable diet and the traditional weight loss group increased consumption over time. Goodrick et al.[149] reported that women with combined obesity and binge-eating disorder increased weight slightly and decreased binge eating.

Mellin et al.[145] trained 21 women to manage their obesity using six intrapsychic developmental skills believed to regulate adaptive mind, body and life-style patterns. Termed "the solution method," the intervention was designed to be delivered by a trained registered dietitian and a licensed mental health professional. Eighteen 2-hour sessions were used to practice:

- Mind skills, such as identifying feelings, recognizing needs and having reasonable expectations
- Body skills, such as honoring and accepting the body and using health care effectively
- Lifestyle skills, such as eating in response to hunger and satiety
- Engaging in physical activity
- Receiving fulfillment

Between sessions, participants contacted other members of the group, kept journals and recorded progress in using the skills. The results for weight loss, blood pressure and exercise were positive and significant differences were noted after 2 years. While change in weight at 3 months was –4.2 kg., it was remarkable that the mean weight change was greater at each assessment, reaching –7.9 kg. at 24 months.

While a standardized treatment model using health-at-any-size is still evolving,[69] use of the model with cognitive-behavioral methods resulted in numerous improvements in overall mental health, quality of life and self-acceptance.[145,147–151] Variables measured included self esteem, depression, body image and eating psychopathology.

In their review, Miller and Jacob[69] identified the liabilities of the paradigm. Since many programs focus on emotional well-being and do not assess physiological measures, they may be perceived as ignoring physiological health risks, making it hard to convince other health professionals that the health-at-any-size model is the preferred method of treatment.[15] Women who are preoccupied with body weight and have food relationship problems may receive the greatest benefit from the approach because obesity is treated from a psychological perspective.[152] A cultural bias may be present as well, since these psychological issues may not be prevalent across cultural groups.[153] Women who have a strong genetic predisposition toward obesity may not benefit from the health-at-any-size model. The need for licensed professionals trained in cognitive behavioral therapy will inhibit widespread use of the model.[69,148] Coordination of medical and psychological services is needed to support the life-style changes necessary for long-term success.[69]

XIII. PREVENTION OF OBESITY

Given the limited effectiveness of currently available weight-loss interventions, the greatest hope in avoiding the risks associated with obesity is prevention. Prevention is usually interpreted to mean arresting the development of new cases of obesity and avoiding further weight gain among those already heavy. Laudable as these prevention goals may be, if they are limited to focus upon weight, they are not likely to prevent the full range of risks associated with obesity. As has been shown above, the risks of obesity are not limited to physical responses to a large accumulation of body fat. There are important risks and costs associated with weight stigmatization and repeated dieting. So-called prevention efforts derived from the moral, aesthetic and medical interpretations of obesity are highly likely to "blame the victim," leading to more and more frantic weight-loss efforts or to highly defended denial. The health-at-any-size approach has potential in avoiding the denial and destructive self-blaming. It has not, however, been demonstrated to produce major impacts on adiposity.

It seems clear that given the genetic, environmental and individual factors promoting weight gain, none of the models of obesity that focus on the individual are adequate to guide programs of prevention. The efforts involved exceed the capacity of most individuals. Widespread weight management requires changes in our environment so that the individual effort required is less monumental. The ecological model, with its focus on the relationship of persons with their environment provides a useful framework for community — or even culture-wide prevention efforts.

Even if we were able to mount effective changes in environmental factors influencing energy intake and expenditure, individual efforts would remain essential. Figure 18.5 shows a prevention process based on the ecological and the health-at-any-size models. The latter approach addresses body dissatisfaction, love–hate relationships with food and other social and psychological factors, empowering individuals to make positive changes in their attitudes and behaviors. Without environmental changes, however, these efforts will be limited in scope and effectiveness.

As we have already seen, the physical, economic and cultural conditions of the Western world contribute to obesity by making food too available and physical activity too unavailable. Avoidance of the risks of obesity is probably more likely to be achieved through programs that emphasize changes in life-style behaviors and give less attention to weight changes per se.[58] To increase individual self-efficacy in making life-style changes, the burden of obesity stigmatization must be lifted. Competing emotions of love and hate about food need to be discharged so that individuals can come to trust their own hunger and satiety.[14] Consumers need ready access to a wide variety of wholesome food and the knowledge to distinguish the relative nutritive values of these foods. They need to be spared the bombardment of high-pressure promotion of the most calorie-dense products. Food served away from home should present plates emphasizing vegetables rather than huge quantities of meat, fried potatoes and sugar-sweetened beverages. Work places need to offer access to both high-nutrient-dense foods and exercise opportunities. Neighborhoods should include safe and free or low-cost exercise opportunities. Residential areas should be planned with the idea that walking and bicycling will be major means of locomotion.

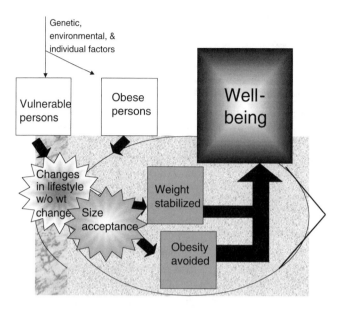

FIGURE 18.5 Obesity prevention approaches. Widespread and long-term avoidance of weight gain requires changes both in the environment and within individuals. Environmental changes will facilitate opportunities for and reduce the barriers to enjoyable, sustainable, healthy behaviors, with emphasis on eating practices and physical activity. Health-at-any-size approaches will enable individuals of any size to achieve well-being through improved health and quality of life.

How do we bring about such changes? It will take commitment from all parts of our culture. Only through a partnership of consumers, industry and trade organizations, government and the media can we really hope to bring about changes of the magnitude that widespread obesity prevention requires.[20] For example, government agencies can establish policies that change the nature of food to which consumers are exposed. These policies might include:

- Regulation of the energy density of food products or of the package or serving size so that high-calorie products are offered only in small quantities
- Controls over food advertising practices
- Limitation of sales conditions for some foods while encouraging sales of others
- Taxation of problematic foods
- Support for exercise opportunities
- Education to de-stigmatize obesity and accurately portray the realities of weight loss interventions[154]

Obviously, there will be considerable debate about the wisdom of such policies and the cost to implement them. Although similar campaigns for smoking cessation have been shown to be successful, there are no data demonstrating the effectiveness for obesity prevention.

Are there any efforts that have been successful? Most of the obesity-prevention programs to date have been limited in scope and many have focused on children. Programs limited to educational approaches have had some success in promoting the consumption of low-fat milk and high-fiber cereal and in increasing daily walking.[155] Improving the availability and relative cost of healthy food items in cafeterias and vending machines has led to some success in changing food choices.[155] Intensive intervention programs with adults have been more successful in changing multiple risk behaviors than in having a long-term impact on obesity.[20,155] Obviously we have much to learn about how to prevent obesity.

XIV. SUMMARY

Fatness is a major concern for most women in our culture. How women perceive fatness is, in large part, influenced by the model(s) of obesity they espouse. The subtle but powerful influence of six models, singularly or in combination, provides the foundation for women's and, in a larger sense, society's perspective of truth about fatness as it relates to body weight. From the perspective of the moral model, fatness is sinful and a sign of gluttony. Never being too thin is the epitome of the aesthetic model. Curing fatness is paramount in the medical model. In a militant reaction to these traditional views of fatness, the political model emerged, characterized by the desire to accept one's body whatever the level of fatness. Over the last decade, advocates of the health-at-any-size model have incorporated size acceptance into a health and well-being model. The public health model was promoted recently to show the impact of environmental factors on body weight and fatness. The ecological model, presented here, is an attempt to move away from a medical approach to illustrate the relations and interactions between women and their environment.

More than half of American women, regardless of age, race or ethnicity have BMIs beyond the recommended level. Contributing factors have included the 3800 kcal per day produced by the food industry for individual consumption, high sugar and fat content of the food supply, large food portions served away from home, lack of physical activity and ever-increasing utilization of labor-saving devices. Health risks are associated with fatness. Most dramatic is the increased likelihood among heavy people of developing one or more of a cluster of related diseases: diabetes, hypertension and cardiovascular disease. However, when comparing cardiorespiratory-fit heavy women to fit, slender women, fitness rather than fatness has been a better predictor of mortality.

With the knowledge that even small weight losses of 5–20% of body weight can result in significant improvements in immediate medical status, weight-loss programs and methods abound. Yet, success among weight-loss programs has been meager. The same limited effectiveness has been true for the two approved weight-loss medications, Sibutramine and Orlistat. Only surgery to reduce the size of the stomach and the absorptive surface of the intestine has been shown to have lasting results in the majority of patients and, unfortunately, the risks and side effects of surgery are substantial. The evidence for long-term effect of weight loss on morbidity and mortality does not exist.

The focus has shifted from weight loss to weight management in an effort to stop weight gain, stabilize weight and reduce health risks. Size acceptance is an important component of weight management. Emphasis on healthy eating practices and daily physical activity is needed. Maintenance is challenging and frustrating, requiring a lifetime of commitment by women and support of health care professionals. Access to fitness activities are lacking for obese women. Discrimination and prejudice toward the obese discourage them from seeking needed health care. Those rare women successful at weight maintenance have established demanding routines that they sustain independently through behavior change measures.

The health-at-any-size model offers a mechanism for weight management consistent with the current goal of a lifelong commitment to enjoyable, sustainable, healthy behaviors with the emphasis on eating practices and daily physical activity, not on achieving thinness or a certain body weight. At this time, the greatest potential for addressing the obesity epidemic lies in widespread prevention efforts based on the health-at-any-size and ecological interpretations of weight. The goals of prevention are avoidance of new obesity, especially among children, adolescents and young adults and limiting of further weight gain among those already heavy. Essential are changes in the environment so as to support individual efforts to making lasting changes in eating and activity behaviors. Rather than promoting guilt, effective prevention programs are designed to lessen stigmatization and promote size acceptance.

REFERENCES

1. Berg, F.M., *Women Afraid to Eat*, 2nd ed., Healthy Weight Network, Hettinger, 2001, 1–376.
2. Sobal, J., The medicalization and demedicalization of obesity, in *Eating Agendas: Food and Nutrition as Social Problems*, Sobal, J. and Maurer, D., Eds., Aldine de Gruyter, Hawthorne, 67–90, 1995.
3. National Task Force on the Prevention and Treatment of Obesity, Overweight, obesity and health risks, *Arch. Intern. Med.,* 160, 898–904, 2000.
4. Anonymous personal communication, 1994.
5. Crawford, D. and Campbell, K., Lay definitions of ideal weight and overweight, *Int. J. Obes.,* 23, 738–745, 1999.
6. Gleick, E., Get Thin Quick — an update. www.time.com/time/magazine. retrieved Aug. 2002.
7. Smith, S., The great diet deception, *USA Today.,* January, 76–78, 1995.
8. Valendi, C., Battling the bulge, http://abcnews.go.com/sections/business/The Street/diet00626.html., Retrieved June 26, 2002.
9. Germov, J. and Williams, L., The epidemic of dieting women: The need for a sociological approach to food and nutrition, *Appetite.* 27, 97–108, 1996.
10. Moore, T.J., *Lifespan: Who Lives Longer — and Why*, Simon & Schuster, New York, 1993.
11. Orbach, S., *Fat Is a Feminist Issue: The Anti-Diet Guide to Permanent Weight Loss,* Paddington Press, New York, 1978.
12. Strain, G., Response to promoting size acceptance in weight management counseling, *J. Am. Diet. Assoc.,* 99, 926–928, 1999.

13. Parham, E.S., Meanings of weight among dietitians and nutritionists, in *Weight Issues: Fatness and Thinness as Social Problems*, Sobal, J. and Maurer, D., Eds., Aldine de Gruyter, Hawthorne, 1999, 183–208.

14. Neumark-Sztainer, D., The weight dilemma: a range of philosophical perspectives, *Int. J. Obes.*, 23, S31– S37, 1999.

15. Parham, E. S., Promoting body size acceptance in weight management counseling, *JAMA*, 99, 920–925, 1999.

16. Ikeda, J., A size acceptance approach to health promotion, *Healthy Weight J.*, 14, 12–14, 2000.

17. Gingras, J.F., Body image dissatisfaction: A framework of development and recommendations for dietitians, *Can. J. Diet. Prac. Res.*, 59, 132–137, 1998.

18. American Dietetic Association., Obesity, in *Manual of Clinical Dietetics*, 6th ed., American Dietetic Association, Chicago, 2000.

19. Brownell, K.D., The environment and obesity, in *Eating Disorders and Obesity*, Fairburn, C.G. and Brownell, K.D., Eds., Guilford Press, New York, 2002, 433–438.

20. World Health Organization, Obesity: Preventing and managing the global epidemic: Report of a WHO Consultation on Obesity (WHO/NUT/NCD/98.1), WHO, Geneva, 1998.

21. Strawbridge, W.J., Wallhagen, M.I. and Shema, S.J., New NHLBI clinical guidelines for obesity and overweight: Will they promote health?, *Am. J. Pub. Hlth.*, 90, 340–343, 2000.

22. Heymsfield, B.S. and Heshka, S., Measurement of total energy stores, in *Eating Disorders and Obesity*, Fairburn, C.G. and Brownell, K.D., Eds., Guilford Press, New York, 2002, 122–125.

23. Despres, J.-P., The metabolic syndrome, in *Eating Disorders and Obesity*, Fairburn, C.G. and Brownell, K.D., Eds., Guilford Press, New York, 477–483 2002.

24. Jonas, S., A healthy approach to the "Health at Any Size" movement, *Healthy Weight J.*, 16, 45–47, 2002.

25. Hawks, S.R. and Gast, J.A., The ethics of promoting weight loss, *Healthy Weight J.*, 14, 25–26, 2000.

26. Campbell, L.A., Role of pharmacological agents in the treatment of obesity, in *Overweight and Weight Management*, Dalton, S., Ed., Gaithersberg, MD, 1997, 471–473.

27. Flegal, K.M., Carroll, M.D. and Johnson, C.L., Overweight and obesity in the United States: Prevalence and trends, 1960–1994, *Int. J. Obes.*, 22, 9–47, 1998.

28. Lewis, C.E., Jacobs, D.R. and McCreath, H., Weight gain continues in the 1990s: 10 year trends in weight and overweight from the CARDIA Study, *Am. J. Epidemi.*, 151, 1172–1181, 2000.

29. Mokdad, A.H., Seruda, M.K., Dietz, W.H., Bowman, B.A., Marks, J.S. and Koplan, J.P., The spread of the obesity epidemic in the United States, 1991–1998, *JAMA*, 282, 1519–1522, 1999.

30. James, W.P.T., A world view of the obesity problem, in *Eating Disorders and Obesity*, Fairburn, C.G. and Brownell, K.D., Eds. Guilford Press, New York, 2002, 411–416.

31. Nestle, M., *Food Politics: How the Food Industry Influences Nutrition and Health*, University of California Press, Berkeley, 2002.

32. Institute of Medicine, Dietary Reference Intakes for energy, carbohydrate, fiber, fat, fatty acids, cholesterol, protein and amino acids, *Food and Nutrition Board*, National Academy Press, Washington, D.C., 2002.

33. Young, L.R. and Nestle, M., The contribution of expanding portion sizes to the U.S. obesity epidemic, *Am. J. Pub. Health.*, 92, 246–249, 2002.

34. From wallet to waistline: The hidden costs of super sizing, Washington, D.C.: National Alliance for Nutrition and Activity, in *Eating Disorders and Obesity,* Fairburn, C.G. and Brownell, K.D., Eds., Guilford Press, New York, 2002, 442–428.

35. Hill, A.J., Prevalence and demographics of dieting, in *Eating Disorders and Obesity,* Fairburn, C. G. and Brownell, K.D., Eds. Guilford Press, New York, 2002, 80–83.

36. Wheat Food Council, Setting the Record Straight: What America Thinks About Fad Diets, Nutrition Advice and Food, Parker, 1999.

37. Koplan, J.P. and Dietz, W.H., Caloric imbalance and public health policy, *JAMA,* 282, 1579–1581, 1999.

38. Das, S.K. and Roberts, S.B., Energy metabolism, in *Present Knowledge in Nutrition,* 8th ed., Bowman, B.A. and Russell, R., Eds., International Life Sciences Institute Press, Washington, D.C., 2001, 3–12.

39. Campfield, L.A., Leptin and body weight regulation, in *Eating Disorders and Obesity,* Fairburn, C.G. and Brownell, K.D., Eds., Guilford Press, New York, 2002, 32–36.

40. Price, R.A., Genetics and common obesities: Background, current status, strategies and future prospects, in *Handbook of Obesity Treatment,* Wadden, T.A. and Stunkard, A.J., Eds., Guilford Press, New York, 2002, 73–94.

41. Leibel, R.L., The molecular genetics of body weight regulation, in *Eating Disorders and Obesity,* Fairburn, C.G. and Brownell, K.D., Eds., Guilford Press, New York, 2002, 26–31.

42. Rankinen, T., Perusse, L., Weisnagel, S.J., Snyder, E. E., Chagnon, Y.C. and Bouchard, C., The human obesity gene map: The 2001 update, *Obes. Res.,* 10, 196–243, 2002.

43. Chula, S.C. and Leibel, R.L., Bodyweight regulation: Neural, endocrine and autocrine mechanisms. In: Wadden, T.A., Stunkard A.J., Eds. *Handbook of Obesity Treatment.* New York: Guilford Press, 2002, 19–41.

44. Bouchard, C., Genetic influences on body weight, in *Eating Disorders and Obesity,* Fairburn, C.G. and Brownell, K.D., Eds., Guilford Press, New York, 2002, 16–21.

45. Wing, R. R., Treatment of obesity in patients with type 2 diabetes, in *Eating Disorders and Obesity,* Fairburn, C.G. and Brownell, K.D., Eds., Guilford Press, New York, 2002, 578–582.

46. Pi-Sunyer, F. X., Medical complications in obesity in adults, in *Eating Disorders and Obesity,* Fairburn, C.G. and Brownell, K.D., Eds., Guilford Press, New York, 2002, 467–476.

47. Willett, W.C., Manson, J.E., Stampfer, M.J., Colditz, F.A., Rosner, B., Speizer, F.E. and Hennekens, C.H., Weight, weight change and coronary heart disease in women, *JAMA,* 273, 461–465, 1995.

48. Manson, J.E., Skerrett, P.T. and Willett, W.C., Epidemiology of health risks associated with obesity, in *Eating Disorders and Obesity,* Fairburn, C.G. and Brownell, K.D., Eds., Guilford Press, New York, 2002, 422–428.

49. Must, A., Spadano, J., Coakley, E.H., Field, A.E., Colditz, G. and Dietz, W.H., The disease burden associated with overweight and obesity, *JAMA,* 282, 1523–1529, 1999.

50. Poehlman, E.T., Toth, M.J. and Gardner, A.W., Changes in energy balance and body composition at menopause: A longitudinal study, *Ann. Intern. Med.,* 123, 673–675, 1995.

51. Jebb, S.A. and Prentice, A.M., Lessons from body composition analysis, in *Present Knowledge in Nutrition, 8th ed.,* Bowman, B.A. and Russell, R., Eds., International Life Sciences Institute Press, Washington, D.C., 2001, 13–21.

52. Munoz, J., Derstine, A. and Gower, B.A., Fat distribution and insulin sensitivity in postmenopausal women: Influence of hormone replacement, *Obes. Res.,* 10, 421–431, 2002.

53. Farrell, S.W., Braun, L., Barlow, C.E., Cheng, Y.J. and Blair, S.N., The relation of body mass index, cardiorespiratory fitness and all-cause mortality in women, *Obes. Res.,* 10, 417–423, 2002.
54. Blake, A., Miller, W.C. and Brown, D.A., Adiposity does not hinder the fitness response to exercise training in obese women, *J. Sports Med. Phys. Fitness,* 40, 170–177, 2000.
55. Kirschenbaum, D.S. and Fitzgibbon, M.L., Controversy about the treatment of obesity: Criticisms or challenges, *Behav. Ther.,* 26, 43–68, 1995.
56. Blackburn, G. L., Weight loss and risk factors, in *Eating Disorders and Obesity,* Fairburn, C.G. and Brownell, K.D., Eds., Guilford Press, New York, 2002, 484–489.
57. Ernsberger, P. and Koletsky, R.J., Biomedical rationale for a wellness approach to obesity: An alternative to a focus on weight loss, *J. Social Issues.,* 55, 221–260, 1999.
58. Gaesser, G.A., Thinness and weight loss: Beneficial or detrimental to longevity, *Med. Sci. Sports Exerc.,* 3, 1118–1128, 1999.
59. Valdez, R., Gregg, E.W. and Williamson, D.F., Effects of weight loss on morbidity and mortality, in *Eating Disorders and Obesity,* Fairburn, C.G. and Brownell, K.D. Eds., Guilford Press, New York, 2002, 490–494.
60. Wadden, T.A., Womble, L.G., Stunkard, A.J. and Anderson D.A., Psychosocial consequences of obesity and weight loss, in *Handbook of Obesity Treatment,* Wadden, T.A and Stunkard, A.J., Eds., Guilford Press, New York, 2002, 144–169.
61. Miller, W.C., Fitness and fatness in relation to health: Implications for a paradigm shift, *J. Soc. Issues.,* 55, 207–219, 1999.
62. Food and Nutrition Board, Institute of Medicine, *Weighing the Options: Criteria for Evaluating Weight Management Programs.* Committee to Develop Criteria for Evaluating the Outcomes of Approaches to Prevent and Treat Obesity. Thomas, P.R., Ed., National Academy Press, Washington, D.C., 1995.
63. Position of The American Dietetic Association: Weight Management, *J. Am. Diet. Assoc.,* 97, 71–74, 1997.
64. Meisler, J.G. and St. Jeor, S., Summary and recommendations from the American Health Foundation's Expert Panel on Healthy Weight, *Am. J. Clin. Nutr.,* 63, 474S–477S, 1996.
65. NIH Technology Assessment Conference Panel, Methods for voluntary weight loss and control. *Ann. Intern. Med.,* 119, 764–770, 1993.
66. Rodin, J., Siberstein, L. and Striegel-Moore, R., Women and weight: Normative discontent, in *Nebraska Symposium of Motivation,* Sonderegger, T.B., Ed., University of Nebraska Press, Lincoln, 1984, 267–303.
67. Martin, D.A., Barnard, R.J. and Ugianskis, E.J., Role of diet and exercise in the management of hyperinsulinemia and associated atherosclerotic risk factors, *Am. J. Cardiol.,* 69, 440–444, 1992.
68. Parham, E.S., Bringing size acceptance to resistant audiences, *Healthy Weight J.,* 15, 78–80, 2001.
69. Miller, W.C. and Jacob, A.V., The health at any size paradigm for obesity treatment: The scientific evidence, *Obes. Rev.,* 2, 37–45, 2001.
70. Miller, W.C., Effective diet and exercise treatments for overweight and recommendations for interventions, *Sports Med.,* 31, 717–724, 2001.
71. Miller, W.C. and Lindeman, A.D., The role of diet and exercise in weight management, in *Overweight and Weight Management: the Health Professionals' Guide to Understanding and Practice,* Dalton, S., Ed., Gaithersburg, MD, 1997, 405–438.
72. Miller, W.C., *Negotiated Peace: How To End the War Over Weight,* Allyn & Bacon, Boston, 1998.

73. McGuire, M.T., Wing, R.R., Klem, M.L. and Hill, J.O., Behavioral strategies of individuals who have maintained long-term weight losses, *Obes. Res.*, 7, 334–341, 1999.
74. Kayman, S.M., Bruvold, W. and Stern, J.S., Maintenance and relapse after weight loss in women: Behavioral aspects, *Am. J. Clin. Nutr.*, 52, 800–807, 1990.
75. Lyons, P. and Miller, W.C., Effective health promotion and clinical care for large people, *Med. Sci. Sports Exerc.*, 31, 1141–1146, 1999.
76. Position of the American Dietetic Association: Weight Management, *J. Am. Diet. Assoc.*, 102, 1145–1155, 2002.
77. Grommet, J. Weight management: Framework for changing behavior, in *Overweight and Weight Management*. Dalton, S., Ed., Gaithersburg, MD, 1997, 332–347.
78. Van Gaal, L.F., Dietary treatment of obesity, in *Handbook of Obesity,* Bray, G.A., Bouchard, C. and James, W.P.T., Eds., Marcel Dekker, New York, 1998, 875–890.
79. McFarlane,.T, Polivy, J. and McCabe, R.E., Help, not harm: Psychologic foundation for a nondieting approach toward health. *J. Social Issues.* 55:261–276, 1999.
80. Wooley, S. and Garner, D., Obesity treatment: The high cost of false hope, *J. Am. Diet. Assoc.,* 91, 1248–1251, 1991.
81. Spitzer, R.L., Devlin, M., Walsh, B.T., Hasin, D., Wing, R., Marcus, M., Stunkard, M.M.A., Wadden, T., Yanovski, S., Agras, S., Mitchell, J. and Nonas, C., Binge eating disorder: a multi-site field trial of the diagnostic criteria, *Int. J. Eat. Disord.* 11, 191–204, 1992.
82. Robison, J.I., Hoerr, S.L., Peteismarch, K.A. and Anderson, J.V., Redefining success in obesity intervention: The new paradigm, *JAMA,*95, 422–423, 1995.
83. Wadden, T.A., Treatment of obesity by moderate and severe calorie restriction: Results of clinical research trials, *Ann. Intern. Med.,* 119, 688–693, 1993.
84. National Task Force on the Prevention and Treatment of Obesity., Very low-calorie diets, *JAMA,* 270, 967–976, 1993.
85. Berg, F.M., Health Risks Associated with Weight Loss, 3rd ed., Hettinger, *Healthy Weight J.*, 1–156, 1995.
86. Polivy, J., Psychological consequences of food restriction, *J. Am. Diet. Assoc.*,96, 589–592, 1996.
87. Wadden, T.A., Foster, G.D. and Letizia, K.A., One-year behavioral treatment of obesity: Comparison of moderate and severe caloric restriction and effects of weight maintenance therapy, *J. Consult. Clin. Psychol.,* 62, 165–171, 1994.
88. Stein, K., High-protein, low-carbohydrate diets: Do they work?, *J. Am. Diet. Assoc.,* 100, 760–761, 2000.
89. National Institutes of Health, National Heart, Lung and Blood Institute. Clinical guidelines on the identification, evaluation and treatment of overweight and obesity in adults — the evidence report, *Obes. Res.,* 6 (Suppl 2), 121–122, 1998.
90. Brownell, K.D. and Jeffery, R.W., Improving long-term weight loss: Pushing the limits of treatment, *Behav. Ther.,* 18, 353–374, 1987.
91. Kramer, J., Jeffery, R.W., Forster, J.L. and Snell, M.K., Long-term follow-up of behavioral treatment for obesity: Patterns of weight regain in men and women, *Int. J. Obes.,* 13, 123–136, 1989.
92. Miller, W.C., Koceja, D.M. and Hamilton, E.J., A meta-analysis of the past 25 years of weight loss research using diet, exercise or diet plus exercise intervention, *Int. J. Obes.,* 21, 941–947, 1997.
93. Flechtner-Mors, M., Ditschuneit, H.H., Johnson, T.D., Suchard, M.A. and Adler, G., Metabolic and weight loss effects of long-term dietary intervention in obese patients: Four year results, *Obes. Res.,* 8, 399–402, 2000.

94. National Institutes of Health, National Heart, Lung and Blood Institute., Obesity Education Initiative Expert Panel. Clinical guidelines on the identification, evaluation and treatment of overweight and obesity in adults: The evidence report, *Obes. Res,.* 6 (Suppl 2), 51–209, 1998.

95. Flatt, J.P., Ravussin, E., Acheson, K.J. and Jequier, E., Effect of dietary fat on postprandial substrate oxidation and on carbohydrate and fat balances, *J. Clin. Invest.,* 76, 1019–1024, 1985.

96. Pi-Sunyer, R.X., Metabolic efficiency of macronutrient utilization in humans. *Clin. Rev. Food Sci. Nutr.,* 33, 359–361, 1993.

97. Zeman, F., *Clinical Nutrition and Dietetics,* Macmillan Publishing Company, New York, 1991.

98. Skov, A.R., Toubro, S. and Astrup, A., Randomized trial on protein vs. carbohydrate in *ad libitum* fat reduced diet for the treatment of obesity, *Int. J. Obes.,* 23, 528–536, 1999.

99. Sjostrom, L., Rissanen, A., Anderson, T., Boldrin, M., Golay, A., Kopeschaar, H.P.F. and Krempg, M., Randomized placebo-controlled trial of Orlistat for weight loss and prevention of weight regain in obese patients, *Lancet.,* 352, 167–172, 1998.

100. Jones, S.P., Smith I.G., Kelly, F. and Gray, J.A., Long-term weight loss with sibutramine, *Int. J. Obes.,* 19 (Suppl), 41, 1995.

101. Davidson, M.H., Hampton, J., DiGirolamo, M., Foreyt, J.P., Halsted, C.H., Heber, D., Heimburger, D.C., Lucas, C.P., Robbins, D.C., Chung, J. and Heymsfield, S.B., Weight control and risk factor reduction in obese subjects for 2 years with orlistat: A randomized control trial, *JAMA,* 28, 235–242, 1999.

102. NIH and NAASO, The Practical Guide: Identification, Evaluation and Treatment of Overweight and Obesity in Adults, *National Institutes of Health.,* NIH Publication Number 00-4084, 2000, 35–38.

103. Sarwer, D.B. and Wadden, T.A., The treatment of obesity: What's new, what's recommended, *J. Women's Hlth. Gender-Based Med.,* 8, 483–493, 1999.

104. MacLean, L.D., Rhode, B.M. and Nohr, C.W., Late outcome of isolated gastric bypass, *Ann. Surg.,* 231, 524–528, 2000.

105. Latifi, R., Kellum, J.M., DeMaria, E.J. and Sugerman, H.J., Surgical treatment of obesity, in *Handbook of Obesity Treatment,* Wadden, T.A. and Stunkard, A.J., Eds., Guilford Press, New York, 2002, 339–356.

106. Cowburn, G., Hillsdon, M. and Hankey, C.R., Obesity management by lifestyle strategies, *Br. Med. Bull.,* 53, 389–408, 1997.

107. Saris, W.H.M., Fit, fat and fat-free: The metabolic aspects of weight control, *Int. J. Obes.,* 22, S15–S21, 1998.

108. Wing, R.R., Physical activity in the treatment of adulthood overweight and obesity: Current evidence and research issues, *Med. Sci. Sports Exer.,* 31 (Suppl), 547–552, 1999.

109. Westerterp, K.R., Obesity and physical activity, *Int. J. Obes.,* 23 (Suppl 1), 59–64, 1999.

110. Votruba, S.B., Horvitz, M.A. and Schoeller, D.A., The role of exercise in the treatment of obesity, *Nutrition,* 16, 179–188, 2000.

111. Harris, J.E., The role of physical activity in the management of obesity. *J. Am. Osteopath. Assoc.,* 99 (Suppl 4), 15–19, 1999.

112. Rippe, J.M. and Hess, S., The role of physical activity in the prevention and management of obesity, *JAMA,* 98 (Suppl 2), 31–33, 1998.

113. King, N.A. and Blundell, J.E., High-fat foods overcome the energy expenditure induced by high-intensity cycling or running. *Eur. J. Clin. Nutr.,* 49, 114–123, 1995.

114. Tremblay, A., Almeras, N., Boer, J., Kranenberg, E.K. and Despres, J.-P., Diet composition and postexercise energy balance, *Am. J. Clin. Nutr.,* 59, 975–979, 1994.

115. Pronk, N. and Wing, R., Physical activity and long-term maintenance of weight loss, *Obes. Res.,* 2, 587–599, 1994.

116. Grilo, C., Brownell, K.D. and Stunkard, A.J., The metabolic and psychological importance of exercise in weight control, in *Obesity: Theory and Therapy,* Stunkard, A.J. and Wadden, T.A., Eds., Raven Press, New York, 1993, 253–273.

117. Byfield, C., A lifestyle physical activity intervention for obese sedentary women: Effect on cardiovascular disease risk factors, *Am. Coll. Sports Med.,* Indianapolis, IN, 2000.

118. Ballor, D.L., Katch, V.L., Becque, M.D. and Marks, C.R., Resistance weight training during caloric restriction enhances lean body weight maintenance, *Am. J. Clin. Nutr.,* 319, 1173–1179, 1988.

119. Porcari, J., Ward, A., Morris, D., Cuneo, M.M.P., O'Hanley, S. and Reppe, J.M., Comparison of weight loss in males and females after 16 weeks of fitness walking and/or diet, *Med. Sci. Sports Exers.,* [abstract] 21, S102, 1986.

120. Mourier, A., Gautier, J.-F. and Cathelineau, G., Mobilization of visceral adipose tissue related to the improvement in insulin sensitivity in response to physical training in Type 2 diabetes: Effects of branched-chain amino acid supplements, *Diabetes Care,* 20, 385–391, 1997.

121. Brownell, K.D., *The LEARN Program for Weight Control,* American Health Publishing Company, Dallas, 1991.

122. Brownell, K.D. and Stunkard, A.J., Physical activity in the development and control of obesity, *Obesity,* Stunkard, A.J., Ed., Saunders, Philadelphia, 1980, 300–324.

123. Fox, K.R., A clinical approach to exercise in the markedly obese, in *Treatment of the Seriously Obese Patient,* Wadden, T.A. and Van Itallie, T.B., Eds., Guilford Press, New York, 1992, 354.

124. Anderson, R, E., Wadden, T.A., Bartlett, S.J., Zemel, B., Verde, T.J. and Franckowaik, S.C., Effects of lifestyle activity vs. structured aerobic exercise in obese women: A randomized trial, *JAMA,* 281, 335–340, 1999.

125. Stunkard, A.J. and Penick, S.B., Behavior modification in the treatment of obesity: The problem of maintaining weight loss, *Arch. Gen. Psychiatr.,* 36, 801–806, 1979.

126. Keesey, R.E., Set-point model of body weight regulation, in *Eating Disorders and Obesity,* Brownell, K. and Fairburn, C.G., Eds., Guilford Press, New York, 1995, 46–50.

127. Maiman, L. A., Wang, V.L., Becker, M.H., Finlay, J. and Simonson, M., Attitudes toward obesity and the obese among professionals, *J. Am. Diet. Assoc.,* 74, 331–336, 1979.

128. Maddox, G.l., Beck, K.W. and Leiderman, V.R., Overweight as social deviance and disability, *J. Hlth. Soc. Behav.,* 9, 287–298, 1968.

129. Goodrick, G.K., Raynoud, A.S. and Pace, P.W., Outcome attribution in a very low calorie weight loss program. *Int. J. Eat. Disord.* 12, 117–120, 1992.

130. Wadden, T.A., New goals of obesity treatment: A healthier weight and other ideals, *Primary Psychia.,* 5, 45–54, 1998.

131. Lyons, P. and Burgard, D., *Great Shape: The First Fitness Guide for Large Women,* Bull Publishing, Palo Alto, CA, 1990.

132. Kline, G., Exercise: Easy for you to say, *Healthy Weight J.,* 14,93–94, 2000.

133. Miller, W.C. and Eggert, K.E., Weight loss perceptions, characteristics and expectations for an overweight male and female population, *Med. Exerc. Nutr. Health.,* 1, 42–47, 1992.

134. Martin, J.E., Duppert, P.M., Katell, A.D., Thompson, J.K., Raczynski J.R., Lake, M., Smith, P.O., Webster, J.S., Sikora, T. and Cohen, R.E., Behavioral control or exercise in sedentary adults: Studies 1 through 6, *J. Consult. Clin. Psychol.*, 52, 795–811, 1984.

135. Klem, M.L., Wing, R.R., McGuire, M.T., Seagle, H.M. and Hill, J.O., A descriptive study of individuals successful at long-term weight loss, *Am. J. Clin. Nutr.*, 66, 239–246, 1997.

136. Anderson, J.W., Konz, E.C., Frederich, R.C. and Wood, C.L., Long-term weight-loss maintenance: A meta-analysis of U.S. studies, *Am. J. Clin. Nutr.*, 74, 579–584, 2001.

137. Kassirer, J.P. and Angell, M., Losing weight — an ill-fated New Year's resolution [editorial], *New Engl. J. Med.*, 338, 52–54, 1998.

138. Garner, D.M. and Wooley, S.C., Confronting the failure of behavioral and dietary treatments for obesity, *Clin. Psychol. Rev.*, 11, 729–780, 1991.

139. Berg, F.M., Breaking free: The health at any size revolution, *Healthy Weight J.*, 14, 15–16, 2000.

140. Lyons, P. and Burgard, D., *Great Shape: the First Fitness Guide for Large Women*, Bull Publishing, Palo Alto, CA, 1990.

141. Parham, E.S., Is there a new weight paradigm? *Nutr. Today.*, 31, 155–161, 1996.

142. Robison, J., Weight management: Shifting the paradigm, *J. Hlth. Educ.* 28, 28–34, 1997.

143. Gast, J. and Hawks, S.R., Weight loss education: the challenge of a new paradigm, *Hlth. Educ. Behav.* 25, 464–473, 1998.

144. Ciliska, D., Evaluation of two nondieting interventions for obese women, *West. J. Nutr. Res.*, 20, 119–135, 1998.

145. Mellin, L., Croughan-Minihane, M. and Dickey, L., The solution method: 2 year trends in weight, blood pressure, exercise, depression and functioning of adults trained in development skills, *J. Am. Diet. Assoc.*, 97, 1133–1138, 1997.

146. Tanco, S., Linden, W. and Earle, T., Well-being and morbid obesity in women: A controlled therapy evaluation, *Int. J. Eat. Disord.*, 23, 325–339, 1998.

147. Polivy, J. and Herman, C.P., Undieting: A paradigm to help people stop dieting, *Int. J. Eat. Disord.*, 11, 261–268, 1992.

148. Sbrocco, T., Nedgegaard. R.C., Stone, J.M. and Lewis, E.L., Behavioral choice treatment promotes continuing weight loss: Preliminary results of cognitive-behavioral decision-based treatment for obesity, *J. Consult. Clin. Psychol.*, 67, 260–266, 1999.

149. Goodrick, G.K., Poston, W.S.C., Kimball, K.T., Reeves, R.S. and Foreyt, J.P., Nondieting versus dieting treatment for overweight binge-eating women, *J. Consul. Clin. Psychol.*, 66, 363–368, 1998.

150. Carrier, K. M., Steinhardt, M. A. and Bowman, S., Rethinking traditional weight management programs: A 3 year follow-up evaluation of a new approach, *J. Psychol.*, 128, 517–535, 1993.

151. Roughan, P., Seddon, E. and Vernon-Robers, J., Long-term effects of a psychologically based group programme for women preoccupied with body weight and eating behavior, *Int. J. Obes.*, 14, 135–147, 1990.

152. Hawks, S.R. and Gast, J.A., Weight loss management: A path lit darkly, *Hlth. Educ. Behav.*, 25, 371–382, 1998.

153. Molley, B.I. and Herzberger, S.D., Body image and self-esteem: A comparison of African-American and Caucasian women, *Sex Roles.*, 38, 631–643, 1998.

154. Jeffery, R.W., Public health approaches to the management of obesity, in *Eating Disorders and Obesity*, Brownell, K.D. and Fairburn, C.G., Eds. Guilford Press, New York, 2002, 613–623.

155. Schmitz, K.H. and Jeffery, R.W., Prevention of obesity, in *Handbook of Obesity Treatment*, Wadden, T.A. and Stunkard, A.J., Eds., Guilford Press, New York, 2002, 556–593.

19 Nutritional Concerns of Female Recreational Athletes

Catherine G. Ratzin Jackson

CONTENTS

I. INTRODUCTION: IDENTIFYING THE FEMALE RECREATIONAL ATHLETE

A. POPULATION AND STUDY DIFFICULTIES

Accurate numbers are difficult to estimate; however, it has been reported that approximately 125 million of the over-18-year-old female population of the United States exercise or play sports regularly.[1] The activity chosen most — close to 40% or approximately 50 million women — is "exercise walking." Other activities in descending order are swimming (25%), exercising with equipment (19%), camping (17%), bicycle riding (16%) and aerobic exercise (16%).[1] This large population is rarely included in scientific studies related to nutrition and performance. Also, there are no clear definitions of recreational athletes; it is generally agreed that recreational activities involve an element of choice and the desire for a pleasurable experience or fun.[2]

The recreational athlete is frequently defined as one who does not receive coaching. Many women exercise at relatively high levels with no coach; they follow suggestions from the popular press and take tips from other exercisers. While inundated with information and misinformation in the popular press, this population must rely on extrapolated nutrition and exercise information from high-performance female athletes who make up the very small percentages of women who exercise and who themselves are rarely studied.

It is of interest that the reason sometimes given for lack of attention in research studies is that females have only "recently" begun to exercise regularly; however, the personal experiences of many women contradict this belief. There has been an explosive growth of the numbers of women in organized sport over the last 25 years; prior to that women have exercised primarily as work activities. Women have only "recently" been recognized due to their own persistent clamor for more information. It is well known that the population of convenience for many studies is the college-age male, about whom we have more information than any other group. They are chosen partially because there is a large database with which to compare results and partially because research is done at colleges and universities that they attend. Research using females includes small sample sizes, and there are few if any studies with which to compare findings, thereby making the research more difficult to interpret. It may also be necessary to include the influence of menstrual cycle on findings, thereby making comprehension even more complex. The current trend in research is to fill this gap for more than one half of the population.

B. ADDITIONAL FACTORS

When females are studied there tends to be a focus on psychological factors, as has been shown to be prevalent in the medical treatment of women for quite some time. Physiological factors are not as well understood as they are in males and are sometimes discounted due to lack of information. This bias can be found in the most fundamental areas of information dissemination, particularly in medical school texts.[3] It is often reported that females have lower relative values in performance indicators and higher values for body fat that suggest that women will not be as fast or strong but may have more endurance. The effect of sex hormones on temperament is widely accepted as an explanation for a less aggressive approach to sports and activity.[3] There is no doubt that testosterone promotes aggressiveness and that estrogen is associated with a milder temperament. "Certainly a large part of competitive sports is the aggressive spirit that drives a person to maximum effort, often at the expense of judicious restraint."[3] This quote from a text widely used in medical schools defines a stereotype for women athletes. One of the results of such a stereotype is that women recreational athletes are rarely studied and are infrequently included in studies where they are sometimes listed as "active" with no definition of the term. Women in the little studied age group between 40 and 50 find that they are treated as if they do not exist. Women are reestablished as research subjects when they become postmenopausal. Information must thus be extrapolated from studies of high-performance female athletes and from studies where the recreational athlete has not been the major focus of the research. Dietary information for recreational athletes is difficult to find.[4]

II. DIETARY ISSUES

A. ENERGY PRODUCTION

There are many misconceptions about nutrition and exercise that can be traced back to a poor understanding of energy metabolism. Not all dietary practices support all activities, as the concept of specificity of nutritional practice has been recognized for specific types of exercise.[5]

In general, short-term, highly intense activities are nonaerobic and do not depend greatly on anything besides stores of ATP available in the exercising muscle. Dietary practices have little effect on energy availability for nonaerobic work. When exercise progresses 1 to 3 min, it stresses the lactic acid system with its high reliance on carbohydrate stores for energy production. If activity progresses at least 5 min, it is characterized as aerobic metabolism and, while carbohydrate stores are necessary for the process to continue, the muscle can now use fat and protein for energy production. While the contribution of fat and carbohydrate is somewhat understood, energy delivery from protein is still not clear. It is thought that a person who exercises aerobically uses protein to a greater degree for energy production than one who exercises anaerobically.

B. OVERVIEW

Methods of dietary assessment that might include self-reporting may not produce completely accurate information, but trends for the prevention of disease can be noted.[6] The concern for ever-increasing levels of obesity and the high incidence of cardiovascular disease in the American population dictates the dissemination of much dietary information related to lowering fat and cholesterol in the diet. However, there is another concern when caloric intake is reduced without making appropriate food choices to cover the needs of the body, a practice to which women are particularly prone. The American diet in general has been changing and healthier patterns seem to be developing but data show that the majority of women 19–50 years old failed to consume recommended amounts of iron, calcium, magnesium, zinc, vitamin B_6, vitamin A and folacin.[7] This fact is particularly disturbing when it is recognized that 6 out of 10 women take supplements in addition to their normal diet. When assessed at regular intervals, fat intakes in the population seem to be decreasing, although they are not yet low enough for health, while carbohydrate intakes seem to be increasing. Dietary fiber intakes are not yet high enough to eliminate concerns about cancer.[7] The implications are clear; sound nutritional advice is still an extremely important issue for the recreational female athlete.

C. Changes in Methods of Recommendations

Recent pronouncements by the Institute of Medicine's (IOM) Food and Nutrition Board[8] have changed dietary guidelines, or RDA's, recommended since 1943. There is considerable additional terminology which, while more scientific in approach and appropriate for more accurate information, will be confusing for consumers for a while. Food labels will contain DVs (Daily Values), a dietary reference term that consists of DRVs (Daily Reference Values) and RDIs (Reference Daily Intakes). DRVs apply to fat, saturated fat, carbohydrate, fiber, protein, cholesterol, sodium and potassium; values are uppermost limits based on the number of calories consumed per day. RDIs are dietary references based on the DRIs for essential vitamins and minerals, which sometimes includes protein. RDI replaces "U.S. RDA" which has been used since 1973. Included in recent recommendations are slight increases in suggested fat intakes from 30% to 35%. Low-fat, high-carbohydrate diets have been found to lower levels of HDL cholesterol and may therefore not reduce the risk of cardiovascular diseases as was thought in the past.

One IOM recommendation was to increase daily activity to 1 hour of moderate exercise per day. Previous recommendations of 30 min per day made in the 1996 Surgeon General's Report on Physical Activity and Health,[9] the American College of Sports Medicine (ACSM),[10] the Centers for Disease Control (CDC),[11] and the National Institutes of Health (NIH),[12] were doubled by the IOM. It should be noted that the recommendation of 30 min of moderate activity done on most days of the week is still valid for the health benefits that will be derived by increased physical activity. One can increase, over time, to 60 min but should not be dissuaded from exercise by the perhaps overwhelming recommendation of an hour per day. The IOM document was primarily a nutritional recommendation that did not evaluate moderate activity for health benefit. The female recreational athlete should begin with 30 min per day on most days of the week and can increase to more time as she becomes conditioned. The cardiovascular benefits of moderate physical activity cannot be ignored.

D. Macronutrients

It is difficult to recommend general guidelines for energy intake, since individual needs should be carefully assessed, but patterns can be seen. It is known that particular groups of female athletes are at risk for diet-related health problems if they consume too few calories and make poor food choices.[13–15] While competitive athletes are known to have difficulty, it is thought that female recreational athletes fare better in dietary practices than their inactive counterparts; however, they continue to have lower than recommended intakes of iron and calcium.[16–19]

The ideal diet for an individual athlete or sport is still uncertain but recommendations are similar to those made for the general population. The National Academy of Sciences has, for the first time, set a recommended daily intake of 130 g/day for carbohydrate.[8] This will most certainly be debated for quite some time as the popular press has focused on low-carbohydrate regimens for weight loss. It was also advised that fat intakes can range from 20–35%. The first recommendations have also been set for fiber with 25 g/day for women ages 50 and younger. While there is great variation in specific intakes of these macronutrients for athletes, 10–15% protein, 30–35% fat and 50–60% carbohydrate is well accepted.[20,21] There are sport-specific recommendations[22] but, in general, recreational athletes should have a nutritional analysis done to determine their particular eating pattern and then modify it if necessary.

The macronutrient with the greatest effect for the recreational athlete is water. The greatest decrements in performance are seen when hydration is compromised. The less conditioned the individual the greater the effect of hydration state for the proper functioning of the body with respect to sweat response and maintenance of proper blood volume. In general, if individuals are thirsty, they are already dehydrated; it may take 2 days to return to a properly hydrated state. There are many sources of detailed information on this topic for the recreational athlete in general[21,23,24] and for women in particular.[25–27]

E. MICRONUTRIENTS

As previously stated, women in the United States show that they ingest levels of iron, calcium, magnesium, zinc, vitamin B_6, vitamin A and folacin below recommended levels.[7] It is recognized that intakes below recommendations do not necessarily indicate deficiency states. The Food and Nutrition Board sets allowance levels for large population groups; they are intentionally set high to meet the needs of almost everyone within a specific category of healthy people. With respect to athletes, vitamin and mineral supplements are commonly used[28] and deficiencies frequently coexist with restricted food intake.[29,30] Deficiencies seem to be specific to the groups investigated, but it is recognized that, as seen in the general population, female athletes have low intakes of calcium, iron and zinc.

Vitamin and mineral supplements are generally safe unless large doses are consumed or herbs are added; caution should be used in self-administered megadoses where the supplement may achieve pharmacological levels. Since vitamin and mineral supplements are more commonly used by females, attention should be given to safety of their use. The recently published Dietary Reference Intakes (DRIs) have now included Tolerable Upper Intake Levels[8] (UL), which are the maximum levels of daily nutrient intake unlikely to pose adverse health-effect risk for almost all individuals in a particular group. Fat-soluble vitamins are generally more toxic than water-soluble vitamins; several concerns can be noted.[31-34] High dosage problems are recognized for Vitamins A and E. Vitamin A intoxication has been reported at approximately 25,000 IU/day.[31-34] Symptoms of toxicity include abdominal pain, anorexia, blurred vision, headache, drowsiness, muscle weakness, nausea and vomiting. Vitamin E side effects appear when 300 IU/day is exceeded. Symptoms of toxicity include nausea, fatigue, headache, elevation of serum lipids and double vision; high intakes also interfere with the activity of vitamin K.[32]

Water-soluble vitamins are not as safe as previously thought. Pyridoxine (Vitamin B_6) is neuroactive; high levels can produce symptoms of sensory neuropathy. The level shown to produce symptoms has consistently been reported lower and lower; the toxicity threshold may be as low as 300–500 mg/day. Controversy over vitamin C continues; several of the widely reported effects have proven to be incorrect. Conditioned scurvy, while speculated, has not been substantiated, oxalate kidney stones have not been seen and vitamin B_{12} destruction was incorrectly reported. Other clearly substantiated effects include:

- Gastrointestinal distress (nausea, abdominal pain, diarrhea) with doses as low as 1000 mg perhaps related to acidity, not the vitamin itself.
- Tissue oxygen demand is increased and problems may occur at altitude.
- Dental enamel may be eroded if chewable tablets are used daily.
- Copper intake and absorption may be decreased.
- Some individuals develop a rash indicating delayed hypersensitivity allergy.[32]

Two minerals of concern, iron and calcium, are reviewed later in this chapter. Deficiencies of vitamin A, iron and zinc are most often seen with protein deficiency, which is common in high-performance athletes. Adequate zinc intake is a concern for athletes;[29, 35-37] toxicity levels are difficult to determine due to its association with copper, iron and phytates. One of the most toxic trace minerals is copper; its supplementation should be discouraged. Selenium in excess can cause extensive tissue damage; however, its threshold is not known. Excess manganese intakes may be a problem in individuals whose iron status is compromised.[32]

As an individual ages, there is often a change in vitamin status; deficiencies in one or more of the B vitamins may develop.[38] Vitamin B_6 has been investigated in female athletes and it has been shown that there are effects of training status and age.[22,39] It becomes clear that there should be a minimum reliance on supplementation and care should be taken that amounts do not exceed 100–150% of recommended levels. However, supplementation may be warranted for iron and calcium.[40]

F. WEIGHT CONTROL ISSUES

It is not known how to categorize the female recreational athlete for evaluation of energy intake but it is reported that approximately 26% of the female population of the United States self reports that they are 20% or more over desirable weight standards.[1] Thus, there is a belief among the females in the U.S. that they are overweight. Many recreational athletes act on this belief by dieting and overexercising with no knowledge of their eating patterns or their energy expenditure during exercise.

Conditioning changes the physiology of the body; not all is understood as to how this affects long-term weight control. The physiology of the obese individual may be altered to maintain obesity since it has been shown that fat calories may be stored preferentially in obese women who reduce their weight; this assures reacquisition of the weight lost.[41] Obese individuals tend to consume higher amounts of dietary fat and sugar than lean individuals, even when overall energy intakes are the same; fats and sugars are preferentially chosen.[42] Exercise helps metabolize the lipids in the diet if they are consumed.[43] The regional distribution of fat may also play a role in the ease with which weight can be maintained or lost; upper body obesity in females is more closely associated with abnormalities in metabolism than lower body obesity.[44] Diet composition and activity patterns seem to have a greater effect on the amount of body fat than the number of calories consumed.[42] Exercise combined with diet to the extent that energy intake reduction is matched by the same amount of energy expended through activity has been shown to be the most effective way to keep weight stable.[45] A stable adult weight is considered the most healthy.[45–47]

The recidivism rate for weight loss is very high, but is lowered when exercise practices developed during weight loss are maintained.[48] Dieting alone without an exercise component has serious consequences as there is a loss of muscle protein. Metabolic changes occur that assure that the weight loss will not be maintained for long periods of time.[49] Exercise may also change brain regulation of appetite and basal metabolic rate, which has the effect of placing the individual in energy deficit with ultimate weight loss.[50]

III. IRON

A. ACTIONS

Iron is a trace mineral recognized as an essential component of the diet present in all body cells. It directly affects many biochemical reactions where oxygen is metabolized or DNA is synthesized. Iron acts in metabolic pathways where oxygen is transported; it is vital in the synthesis of oxygen-carrying proteins such as myoglobin in muscle and hemoglobin in blood. Iron is also a component of the electron transport system, where iron-containing cytochromes are used to cycle electrons and hydrogens in the synthesis of the energy carrier molecule ATP. Therefore, iron is directly related to energy production within the body.[51] However, iron deficiency may be the most common nutritional deficiency in the world.[52]

B. RECOMMENDED INTAKE

The RDA for men and postmenopausal women is 8 mg/day.[53] The RDA for premenopausal women is 18 mg/day. It has been determined that premenopausal women have a median intake of 12 mg/day, which shows that iron deficiency is common. The UL associated with gastric distress is 45 mg/day. These intakes depend on energy intake but it is difficult to determine exactly how much iron may be consumed by an average person. To cover the iron needs of adult menstruating women, and recognizing that only about 15% of the iron consumed can be absorbed, 2.84 mg/day should be provided. Women using anovulatory drugs have lower needs, which are met by 1.89 mg/day or 12.6 mg available iron, 6.3 mg of iron for every 1000 kcal if 2000 kcals/day are consumed. Therefore, the average American diet for the woman not on anovulatory drugs should contain 9.45 mg of iron for every 1000 kcal if 2000 kcals/day are consumed,[54] while this may not represent the diet of a female recreational athlete. Calculations done by Manore et al.[55] showed that an average of 6 mg/1000 kcals was ingested by female long distance runners, who also tend toward vegetarian eating habits due to the persistent quest for carbohydrate in the diet. If this represents female recreational athletes as well, it would be difficult for them to consume enough iron if the RDA is followed. A caloric intake of 2200 is the RDA for 11–50 year olds and they would then consume 13.2 mg/day below the RDA. If caloric intake is increased to 2500, then the RDA for iron is met but the cost might be excess body fat, which creates a dilemma. The woman over 50 years will consume slightly more than the RDA with the recommended energy intake of 1900 kcals.

The estimated average requirement (EAR) is the average intake level that meets the estimated nutrient needs of half of the individuals in a group. The EAR for women 19–50 years of age is 8.1 mg/day; 51 to over 70 is 5mg/day. Vegetarians require 1.8 times the recommendations for mixed Western diets, as there is a 10% bioavailability of iron in vegetarian diets versus 18% bioavailability in normal mixed diets.

C. IRON STATUS IN WOMEN WHO EXERCISE

There is little understanding of the relationships among dietary iron intake, voluntary supplementation and performance in high-performance female athletes. There is even less known about the female recreational athlete. A lack of standardized criteria and terminology for normal and deficiency states further confuses attempts at interpretation and recommendation. Studies on female athletes tend to focus on the role of menstruation in blood loss and rarely consider other issues.[52]

Newhouse et al.[56] reported that females do not consume adequate iron in their diets. The majority of the 111 female subjects between the ages of 18–40 trained regularly three times per week at three-fourths maximal effort for at least 120 minutes; thus, over half of the randomly selected women were recreational athletes. 40% were either iron depleted or iron deficient. Iron supplementation (320 mg ferrous sulfate or 100 mg elemental iron/day taken for 12 weeks) successfully brought values to normal and did not affect serum copper, calcium, zinc or magnesium levels, a concern when iron supplementation occurs.

Female recreational athletes tend to fare better nutritionally than female high-performance endurance athletes. Pate et al.[15] observed that female recreational runners, defined as those who ran regularly but were not competitive, had diets much closer to recommendations for optimum dietary regimens given by public health officials than female competitors. They consumed more carbohydrate and less fat than their inactive counterparts, while protein intake was less. Although these dietary practices are considered healthy, iron and calcium intakes were as low as in the inactive women. The number of athletes, both competitive and recreational, representing iron deficiency is no more than the level found in the general female population.[57] Endurance performance is impaired when iron depletion results in anemia.

Symptoms of iron deficiency are vague and include fatigue, decreased appetite, headache, heartburn, shortness of breath or excessive menstrual discharge. If deficiency does occur, it is in progressive stages, the last of which is iron deficiency anemia. It has been observed that some female athletes who are initially normal develop iron deficiency during the course of a season of conditioning, suggesting that they may require more iron than an inactive woman.[57] A long-term study that followed collegiate female field hockey players over a period of 3 consecutive competitive years found that body iron stores and iron reserves tended to become progressively more depleted with consecutive seasons.[58] The reasons for the observations found in the previous studies were linked to dietary practices linked to reduced energy intake, as it has been reported that activity per se does not necessarily lead to depletion in the mineral status of iron, copper and zinc when intakes are adequate.[59]

An iron deficiency anemia can be mild but will still impair performance[60] and iron therapy is suggested (325 mg three times/day for 2 months). This level of supplementation may be successful in correcting the iron deficiency but may not necessarily improve work capacity.[61] Iron deficiency may also predispose females to impaired thermogenesis and thermoregulatory responses, thus decreasing their ability to withstand cold.[62] Women who are mildly iron deficient are less satisfied with their performance than women who are normal; treatment does not necessarily change performance or "mood."[57] The cause of iron deficiency in women is predominantly insufficient iron in the diet. Other contributing factors might be loss of iron in urine and the gastrointestinal tract,[63] menstrual losses and hemolysis during high levels of conditioning.[64] Iron is lost in sweat; however, all potential losses coupled with low dietary intake contributes to negative iron balance.[65,66]

D. Iron Absorption

Iron absorption is known to be affected by numerous dietary practices. Some inhibitors of iron absorption are phytic acids that are found in legumes, rice and grains; polyphenols found in tea, coffee and grain products; soybean proteins; and calcium. Iron absorption is enhanced when up to 100 mg of ascorbic acid are consumed with a meal; other ways to enhance absorption are through the simultaneous consumption of citric acid, lactic acid, malic acid, meat, fish and poultry. There is some evidence that excessive iron intakes increase the risk of cardiovascular disease. All evidence suggests that iron supplementation should be done after assessment of iron status and should be monitored by a physician. Self determination and excessive supplementation are discouraged.

E. Effect of Protein Intake on Iron Status

Females who exercise are often given the advice to elevate carbohydrate intake to levels that sometimes exceed 60% of caloric intake. Levels of fat and protein intake would concomitantly be reduced and, therefore, so would the nutrients supplied by these sources. Telford et al.[64] reported that iron status may have a greater association with percentage protein intake than overall energy intake than is frequently suggested. It appears that when one approaches vegetarian dietary practices, iron intake should be monitored and elevated.

IV. CALCIUM, HORMONES AND BONE DENSITY

A. GENERAL INFORMATION

A known consequence of aging is loss of bone mass that results in osteoporosis, a disorder of epidemic proportions in the United States. Osteoporosis is a major public health concern in the U.S., for an estimated 44 million individuals; it affects mostly women who are 50 and older. Many Americans attempt to lose weight by reducing caloric and cholesterol consumption with the reduction of dairy products that contain the calcium bone needs. Loss of calcium from the skeleton predisposes bone to fractures and compressions of the spine leading to deformity. Concern for reducing risk factors for cardiovascular disease through weight loss may increase the risk for osteoporosis. The integrity of bone requires a complex integration of estrogen and testosterone, diet and exercise. Manipulating a single parameter cannot ameliorate the problem.

Bone is a dynamic tissue that continuously adapts, albeit slowly, to the stresses that are either placed on or removed from the skeleton. The highest bone densities are found in male weight lifters, suggesting an interaction of muscle mass, which places stress and weight on bone that forces it to adapt by either increasing or maintaining density.[67]

Weight-bearing exercise was thought to be the best type of stimulus in the female to protect bone integrity, which is compromised by age, immobility, corticosteroid use and peri- and postmenopausal loss of estrogen. Exercises proposed and evaluated have been running and resistance training. Heinrich and co-workers[68] found that weight training or resistance training may provide a better stimulus for increasing bone mineral content due to increased muscle weight.

The interactions among exercise, hormones, diet and bone density are complex in the female. It is not certain when the greatest bone mass is achieved. It is known that bone gains density during adolescence and plateaus in the third decade, where it is somewhat stable, although decline has been observed. At approximately age 50, there is a gradual and progressive loss.[69] In females, this coincides with menopause; the loss of bone density within the first 5 years after this event is dramatic.[70] If a line were drawn for bone mass throughout a lifetime it would show progressive decline after the third decade, with the angle of decline modified by diet, exercise and hormone balance. Much attention has been focused on understanding how to slow this loss; however, 75% of the variance may be hereditary, with only 20% modifiable by activity, strength, hormone or dietary interventions.[69] Any female who develops amenorrhea while she is an active exerciser should be professionally evaluated, as the low estrogen levels associated with this syndrome may predispose her to osteoporotic bone changes.[71,72] It has been shown that diet has a strong effect on bone status, since stress fractures are more common in dancers with restrictive diets than those whose diets are more liberal.[73] A female recreational athlete who has a mother or grandmother with osteoporosis should become educated in interventions and practices that maintain bone mass, and should take an active role in preserving her bone density throughout her lifetime.

B. ESTROGEN

Bone status is probably most affected by female estrogen status. However, the effects of diet and exercise are also important. It has long been recommended that estrogen status should be maintained as long as possible, calcium intake should be high throughout the lifetime and the female should adopt a lifestyle that includes exercise — the exact type, frequency, intensity and duration of which is yet to be determined.

Controversy has erupted over hormone replacement therapy (HRT) after menopause. A study conducted by the NIH assessing the risks and benefits of estrogen and progestin treatment in more than 16,600 healthy menopausal women, half of whom were in a placebo group, was abruptly terminated in July of 2002. It was determined that the risks of the hormone therapy outweighed the benefits, as a rise was seen in the incidence of breast cancers, heart attacks, strokes and blood clots in the veins or lungs. The results did show that therapy resulted in reductions in risks for colorectal cancer and hip fractures. On November 29, 2002, the NIH released a news bulletin confirming the risk of breast cancer in those taking HRT. The risk was reported to plummet after halting treatment. Estrogen alone was not evaluated as of the time of the completion of this chapter.

HRT is used by an estimated 38% of postmenopausal women. At this point in time, there is a wait-and-see attitude in the medical community that should be monitored by the female recreational athlete. Alternative therapies have been shown to confer fewer benefits than the HRT previously used in large numbers of women. A female recreational athlete with a strong genetic predisposition to osteoporosis should become as well informed about bone health as early in life as possible and should aggressively follow the current controversy in order to make an informed decision as to her choices.

C. RECOMMENDED INTAKE OF CALCIUM AND SUPPLEMENT ISSUES

The RDIs for women aged 19–50 are 1000 mg (25 mmol)/day.[74] For ages 51–70, the recommended intake is 1200 mg (30 mmol)/day. It is known that males tend to consume about 25% more calcium per day than women, thus suggesting that supplementation is important for the female recreational athlete.

There is no biochemical assay that reflects calcium nutritional status, therefore knowledge about absorption is important. Lactose-intolerant individuals are at risk for deficiency states due to their avoidance of milk products; they need to monitor intake carefully. While previous work suggested that vegetarians were at risk for low calcium absorption due to the increased oxalate and phytates in their diets, recommendations are not different from those for omnivores. It has been shown that calcium supplementation alone has a small positive effect on bone density in post-menopausal osteoporosis.[75]

High sodium, protein and caffeine intakes are associated with a loss of urinary calcium. Calcium carbonate is preferred due to its greater absorbability and should be consumed between meals. However, calcium tends to inhibit nonheme iron absorption when both calcium and iron are consumed at the same time.

V. GENERAL CONSIDERATIONS FOR IRON, CALCIUM AND DIET

Since iron and calcium represent two major nutritional deficiencies for women in the United States today, they will also represent problems for recreational athletes. If both iron and calcium supplementation are chosen, it is important to coordinate their consumption. If consumed at the same time, the degree of absorption is unpredictable.[76]

Female recreational athletes should consume adequate energy (calories) in their diets to assure good iron and calcium availability, since the cause of deficiency is most likely low intake.[19,77,78] If iron deficiency is suspected, the athlete should have her blood tested before beginning a self prescribed program of iron supplementation. A physician who understands athletic performance should be chosen. Acidic beverages such as orange juice consumed at meals and consumption of meats, poultry and fish enhance iron absorption.[79] Inhibitors of iron absorption are known to be tea, coffee and wheat bran.[53,54] If calcium supplements are also used, both the iron and calcium in carbonate form should be taken between meals. If weight loss is also desired, the female recreational athlete should follow the recommendations of the American College of Sports Medicine[45] that suggest that caloric deficit be matched equally with dietary caloric restriction, causing weight loss to occur in a gradual manner. Recommendations for cardiovascular fitness will not necessarily result in weight loss.

VI. DISORDERED EATING AND BODY COMPOSITION ISSUES

A. DISORDERED EATING

Research on females who exercise shows that low iron status and many other indicators of poor nutrition are highly associated with low energy intake,[13,14] which can become so low that life-threatening disorders can result. The incidence of disorders in recreational female athletes is unknown, but it would be reasonable to assume that they occur in similar percentages as in the general population. While the term "eating disorders" has become quite recognizable over the last decade, clinical diagnosis remains difficult. Estimates of incidence vary widely; an approximation is 1–3% of the U.S. population.[80] Athletes in particular sports such as the triathlon may have a much higher incidence of eating disorders in both females (28%) and males (11%).[81]

Excessive physical activity is a common observation in disordered eating. The activity most chosen usually has an aerobic or endurance component. Estimates of prevalence are difficult due to varying criteria and the sport analyzed. Female dancers are frequently identified as at risk for eating disorders, but their prevalence may be no greater than that in the general population.[82] Pathogenic weight control behaviors are found in competitive adolescent female gymnasts[83] and college varsity level athletes.[84] However, it has been observed that female athletes as a group may have a lower active incidence rate than nonexercising females in their age categories.[85]

Disordered eating continues to be a problem in female exercising populations and potentially presents the risk for developing a full disorder if there is excessive concern over body image.[86] The spectrum of eating difficulties is defined on a continuum from normal concerns about body weight to diagnosable eating disorders. These disorders are largely confined to women, while the prevalence has been observed to be increasing in men. Cultural pressures to be lithe and slim are strong.

B. BODY COMPOSITION MISINFORMATION

Recreational athletes are frequently influenced by individuals who are not knowledgeable in the assessment of body fat percentages and the appropriate use of this information. Methods of assessing body fat have errors, and the most appropriate way to use the information is in monitoring progress over time. The association between a specific body fat percentage and performance has never been made, as all performance combines physiological and psychological attributes that are difficult to measure. A normal female body ranges between 18–33% body fat in the optimal health range with a minimal percentage of 14%, below which a female should not go.[87] Ideal fitness ranges between 16–25%. The media frequently focus on women with approximately 10% body fat, a level associated with eating disorders, amenorrhea and early osteoporosis. It is important for female recreational athletes to recognize that the lower body fats displayed in the media are unhealthy. Disordered eating becomes a reality when cultural influences outweigh education.

C. FEMALE ATHLETE TRIAD

It has been observed that the dietary practices of female athletes show seasonal variation related to exercise patterns and dieting may occur when activity levels decrease.[88] Some have suggested that disordered eating is confined to the season of athletic participation[86] and that problems are readily reversible with termination of athletic activity. This is not necessarily true, if the female recreational athlete progresses to amenorrhea and restricts calcium intake. There has been recognition of a combination of disorders designated as the female athlete triad that are found in adolescent and young adult female athletes.[89] The triad is composed of disordered eating, amenorrhea and osteoporosis. Disordered eating, which may then progress to amenorrhea (although menstrual irregularities can occur in the absence of an eating disorder) is usually the first observed difficulty in the exercising female. Amenorrhea, which can lead to bone loss seen in postmenopausal women, is a sign of decreased estrogen production. The bone loss may not be reversible. It is important that recreational female athletes be aware of this syndrome. The American College of Sports Medicine continues to provide a leadership role in disseminating current information concerning this issue.[90]

VII. MENSTRUAL CYCLE

A. GENERAL CONSIDERATIONS

Reviews have presented effects of exercise training on the menstrual cycle.[91–93] Athletic amenorrhea seems to be related to abrupt initiation of high-volume aerobic conditioning in some women who are predisposed by a yet-to-be-identified mechanism. Luteal suppression and lack of ovulation in regularly menstruating athletes may represent an endpoint of successful acclimatization to training in robust individuals. Temperature regulation during endurance exercise done at the luteal phase is adversely affected as elevated core temperatures have been observed.[94] Mechanisms are currently obscure. This research area is of interest to exercise physiologists because disruption of the menstrual cycle may have an adverse affect on the maintenance of bone density.[91]

B. DIET AND EXERCISE EFFECTS

It has been recognized that menstrual cycle function can be affected by diet and exercise habits.[95] Dietary habits of women are concomitantly affected by phases of the menstrual cycle.[96] Observations of 14 women over a period of 1 year showed regulatory and behavioral phenomena relating phases of the menstrual cycle to food selection and consumption.[97] Energy intake was elevated in the 10 days prior to menses, with a preference shown for fat; protein and carbohydrate intakes were nonsignificantly elevated. Basal metabolic rate was also elevated during this time. Postmenses energy intake and basal metabolic rate dropped for 10 days and began to reverse upward to repeat the cycle. Activity patterns may reflect similar changes, as women have been noted to be more active during the periods of increased food intake.[98] These observations have implications for treating eating disorders, obesity and premenstrual syndrome.

Menarche can be delayed with high levels of physical activity, but the reasons are not currently clear. Certain categories of females whose difficulties may begin early in life, such as those who participate in ballet, may become predisposed to eating disorders and early osteoporotic changes leading to increased bone injuries at early ages.[99] Menstrual disturbances that can persist into adult life are seen in these groups. Eating problems are an important consideration in the pathogenesis of amenorrhea in athletes, while it is clear that this is a multidimensional problem.[90,100] The pattern of increased musculoskeletal injuries is seen in adult premenopausal women who have menstrual irregulatities.[101]

The normal hormonal patterns of the menstrual cycle can be altered by reproductive status, prior menstrual and exercise history, stress, nutrition and body composition changes, all of which can be influenced by exercise.[90,102–108] Menstrual dysfunction secondary to active exercise participation is well documented, but not all who exercise are affected. Low resting metabolic rate that may be the result of caloric restriction is implicated.[109,110] In the past, it has been reported that the average adult woman consumes approximately 1700 kcals per day with a 20-year trend toward an increase of total energy intake;[111–113] women who exercise are known to consume less. Dieting alone can produce menstrual cycle disturbances.[114]

In one study of female recreational athletes, menstrual function and eating behavior were evaluated in recreational weight lifters and competitive body builders.[114] A control sample of 92 women who did not weight train was compared with 103 female weight lifters. All subjects were classified by menstrual cycle (eumenorrheic, oligomenorrheic, amenorrheic) and a subgroup of women who weight lifted were classified as competitive. The average percent body fat for all lifters was 20%, while for competitive lifters it was 17.7%. Two percent were amenorrheic and 18% were oligomenorrheic, which was considered high and an indication of menstrual dysfunction; the combined percentage is similar to that found in runners. Although there appeared to be an excessive concern with food and weight loss, the behaviors were not those of disordered eating. The authors expressed concern that these women were at risk due to their preoccupation with weight; close to a third of weight lifters and the majority of competitive body builders self-reported menstrual dysfunction. Thus, recreational athletes may have problems similar to competitive athletes, so it is important for recreational female athletes to consume adequate energy in their diets and to notice changes in menstrual cycle activity that may be associated with abrupt changes in volume of aerobic conditioning. The resulting changes in menstrual function are not just gynecological concerns, but should be thoroughly evaluated for nutritional status as well.

VIII. CONCLUSIONS

It has been shown that the female recreational athlete leads a healthier lifestyle than her inactive counterpart. However, there are many issues that must be addressed with respect to physical activity.

The female recreational athlete should become educated in energy delivery systems and should plan her diet to enhance her type of activity, be it nonaerobic, aerobic, anaerobic or various combinations of the three. Her diet should be planned to support and enhance her activity. Specificity of diet to activity is important.

She should pay particular attention to her caloric intake to ensure that it is adequate to meet her additional needs for activity. The consumption of iron, calcium, magnesium, zinc, vitamin B_6, vitamin A and folacin are of particular concern. If supplements are taken, labels should be read so that overconsumption of a particular nutrient does not occur. Fat, carbohydrate, dietary fiber and protein intakes should be appropriate for her activity level, while hydration is of paramount importance at all times.

Current recommendations made by the Institute of Medicine should be reviewed and incorporated into her diet. At least 30 min/day of activity should be a goal for her continued health. Macro- and micronutrient intakes should follow the recommendations of sport nutritionists.[115]

Weight control is usually a major concern of female recreational athletes. They should become educated in safe weight gain and weight loss recommendations made by national organizations such as the American College of Sports Medicine. If weight loss is desired, it is imperative that it be done safely so that bone density is not compromised. Should she experience menstrual difficulties, she should seek professional advice from those educated in the care of the female athlete.

It is wise for the female recreational athlete to become attuned to her body and pay attention to signs that exercise levels may be too intense. She should become educated in sound nutritional practices and eat a varied diet based on current recommendations put forth in the chapters of this book. The quality of her life will be greatly enhanced by her becoming educated in sound exercise and nutritional practices.

REFERENCES

1. U.S. Bureau of the Census, Statistical Abstract of the United States: 2000, Washington, D.C., 2001.
2. Van Dinter, N.R., Introduction: Competitive versus recreational athletes: An American recreational and cultural perspective, in *Nutrition for the Recreational Athlete*, C.G.R. Jackson, Ed., CRC Press, Boca Raton, FL, 1995.
3. Guyton, A.C., Sports Physiology, in *Textbook of Medical Physiology*, W.B. Saunders, Philadelphia, 1991, 940.
4. Jackson, C.G.R., Ed., *Nutrition for the Recreational Athlete*. CRC Press, Boca Raton, FL, 1995.
5. Jackson, C.G.R. and Simonson, S., The relationships between human energy transfer and nutrition, in *Nutrition for the Recreational Athlete*, Jackson, C.G.R., Ed., CRC Press, Inc., Boca Raton, FL, 1995.
6. Mertz, W., Tsui, J.C., Judd, J.T., Reiser, S., Hallfrisch, J., Morris, E.R., Steele, P.D. and Lashley, E., What are people really eating? The relationship between energy intake derived from estimated diet records and intake determined to maintain body weight, *Am. J. Clin. Nutr.*, 54, 291, 1991.
7. Welsh, S. and Guthrie, J.F., Changing American diets, in *Micronutrients in Health and in Disease Prevention*, Bendich A. and Butterworth, C.E., Eds., Marcel Dekker, New York, 1991.
8. *Dietary Reference Intakes for Energy, Carbohydrate, Fiber, Fat, Fatty Acids, Cholesterol, Protein and Amino Acids,* National Academy Press, Washington, D.C., 2002.
9. U.S. Department of Health and Human Services, Physical Activity and Health: A Report of the Surgeon General, Atlanta, GA: U.S. Department of Health and Human Services, Centers for Disease Control and Prevention, National Center for Chronic Disease Prevention and Health Promotion, 1996.
10. Pollock, M.L., Gaesser, G.A., Butcher, J.D., Despres, J-P, Dishman, R.K., Franklin, B.A. and Garber, C.E., The Recommended Quantity and Quality of Exercise for Developing and Maintaining Cardiorespiratory and Muscular Fitness and Flexibility in Healthy Adults: A Position Stand of the American College of Sports Medicine, *Med. Sci. Sports Exerc.*, 30, 975, 1998.
11. U.S. Department of Health and Human Services at a Glance 2002, Physical Activity and Good Nutrition: Essential Elements to Prevent Chronic Diseases and Obesity 2002, Atlanta, GA: U.S. Department of Health and Human Services, Centers for Disease Control and Prevention, National Center for Chronic Disease Prevention and Health Promotion, 2002.
12. Physical activity and cardiovascular health. NIH Consensus Development Panel on Physical Activity and Cardiovascular Health, *JAMA*, 276, 241, 1996.

13. Brownell, K.D., Nelson Steen, S. and Wilmore, J.H., Weight regulation practices in athletes: Analysis of metabolic and health effects, *Med. Sci. Sports Exerc.,* 19, 546, 1987.
14. Chen, J.D., Wang, J.F., Li, K.J., Zhao, Y.W., Wang, S.W., Jiao, Y. and Hou, X.Y., Nutritional problems and measures in elite and amateur athletes, *Am. J. Clin. Nutr.,* 49, 1084, 1989.
15. Manore, M.M., Dietary recommendations and athletic menstrual dysfunction, *Sports Med.,* 32(14), 887, 2002.
16. Pate, R.R., Sargent, R.G., Baldwin, C. and Burgess, M.L., Dietary intake of women runners, *Int. J. Sports Med.,* 11, 461, 1990.
17. Lewis, R.D. and Medlesky, C.M., Nutrition, physical activity and bone health in women, *Int. J. Sport Nutr.,* 8, 250, 1998.
18. Voss, L.A., Fadale, P.D. and Hulstyn, M.J., Exercise-induced loss of bone density in athletes, *J. Am. Acad. Orthop. Surg.,* 6(6), 349, 1998.
19. Nativ, A., Stress fractures and bone health in track and field athletes, *J. Sci. Med. Sport,* 3, 268, 2000.
20. Grandjean, A.C, Macronutrient intake of U.S. athletes compared with the general population and recommendations made for athletes, *Am. J. Clin. Nutr.,* 49, 1070, 1989.
21. Position of Dietitians of Canada, the American Dietetic Association and the American College of Sports Medicine: Nutrition and Athletic Performance, *Can. J. Diet. Pract. Res.,* 61, 176, 2000.
22. Grandjean, A.C., Nutrition for Swimmers, *Clin. Sport Med.,* 5, 65, 1986.
23. Frye, S., Fluids, hydration and performance concerns of all recreational athletes. in *Nutrition for the Recreational Athlete,* Jackson, C.G.R., Ed., CRC Press, Boca Raton, FL., 1995.
24. Convertino, V.A., Armstrong, L.E., Coyle, E.F., Mack, G.W., Waska, M.N., Senay, L.C., Jr. and Sherman W.M., American College of Sports Medicine position stand. Exercise and fluid replacement, *Med. Sci. Sports Exerc.,* 28, i, 1996.
25. Grandjean, A.C., Reimers, K.J. and Ruud, J.S., Nutritional concerns of female athletes, in *Nutrition in Exercise and Sport,* 3rd ed. I. Wolinsky, Ed., CRC Press, Boca Raton, FL., 1998, 421.
26. Somer, E., *Nutrition for Women, The Complete Guide,* Henry Holt, New York, 1993.
27. Maughan, R.J., McArthur, M. and Shirreffs, S.M., Influence of menstrual status on fluid replacement after exercise induced dehydration in healthy young women, *Br. J. Sports Med.,* 30, 41, 1996.
28. Congeni, J. and Miller S., Supplements and drugs used to enhance athletic performance, *Pediatr. Clin. North Am.,* 49, 435, 2002.
29. Haymes, E.M., Vitamin and mineral supplementation of athletes, *Int. J. Sport Nutr.,* 1, 146, 1991.
30. Manore, M.M., Nutritional needs of the female athlete, *Clin. Sports Med.,* 18, 549, 1999.
31. Cerny, L. and Cerny, K., Can carrots be addictive: An extraordinary form of drug dependence, *Brit. J. Addict.,* 87, 1195, 1992.
32. Hathcock, J.N., Safety of vitamin and mineral supplements, in *Micronutrients in Health and in Disease Prevention,* Bendich, A. and Butterworth, C.E., Eds., Marcel Dekker, New York, 1991.
33. Hathcock, J.N., Hattan, D.G., Jenkins, M.Y., McDonald, J.T., Sundaresan, P.R. and Wilkening, V.L., Evaluation of vitamin A toxicity, *Am. J. Clin. Nutr.,* 52, 183, 1990.
34. van Dam, M.A., The recognition and treatment of hypervitaminosis A., *Nurse Pract.,* 14, 28, 1989.

35. Deuster, P.A., Day, B.A., Singh, A., Douglass, L. and Moser-Veiflon, P.B., Zinc status of highly trained women runners and untrained women, *Am. J. Clin. Nutr.*, 49, 1295, 1989.

36. Lukaski, H.C., Magnesium, zinc and chromium nutriture and physical activity, *Am. J. Clin. Nutr.,* 72(2 Suppl), 585S, 2000.

37. Micheletti, A., Rossi, R. and Rufini, S., Zinc status in athletes: Relation to diet and exercise, *Sports Med.,* 31, 577, 2001.

38. Miller, W.C., Niederpruem, M.G., Wallace, J.P. and Lindeman, A.K., Dietary fat, sugar and fiber predict body fat content, *J. Am. Diet. Assoc.*, 94, 612, 1994.

39. Manore, M.M. and Leklem, J.E., Effect of carbohydrate and vitamin B6 on fuel substrates during exercise in women, *Med. Sci. Sports Exerc.*, 20, 233, 1988.

40. Clarkson, P.M. and Haymes, E.M., Exercise and mineral status of athletes: Calcium, magnesium, phosphorus and iron, *Med. Sci. Sports Exerc.,* 27, 831, 1995.

41. Yost, T.J. and Eckel, R.H., Fat calories may be preferentially stored in reduced-obese women: A permissive pathway for resumption of the obese state, *J. Clin. Endocrinol. Metab.*, 67, 259, 1988.

42. Miller, W.C., Lindeman, A.K., Wallace, J. and Niederpruem, M., Diet composition, energy intake and exercise in relation to body fat in men and women, *Am. J. Clin. Nutr.*, 52, 426, 1990.

43. Goldberg, L. and Elliot, D.L., The effect of exercise on lipid metabolism in men and women, *Sports Med.*, 4, 307, 1987.

44. Campaigne, B.N., Body fat distribution in females: Metabolic consequences and implications for weight loss, *Med. Sci. Sports Exerc.*, 22, 291, 1990.

45. Jakicic, J.M., Clark, K., Coleman, E., Donnelly, J.E., Foreyt, J., Melanson, E., Volek, J. and Volpe, S.L., American College of Sports Medicine position stand. Appropriate intervention strategies for weight loss and prevention of weight regain for adults, *Med. Sci. Sports Exerc.,* 33, 2145, 2001.

46. Angotti, C.M. and Levine, M.S., Review of five years of a combined dietary and physical fitness intervention for control of serum cholesterol, *J. Am. Diet. Assoc.*,94, 634, 1994.

47. Hagan, R.D., Upton, S.J., Wong, L. and Whittam, J., The effects of aerobic conditioning and/or caloric restriction in overweight men and women, *Med. Sci. Sports Exerc.*, 18, 87, 1986.

48. Haus, G., Hoerr, S.L., Mavis, B. and Robison, J., Key modifiable factors in weight maintenance: Fat intake, exercise and weight cycling, *J. Am. Diet. Assoc.*, 94, 409, 1994.

49. Grubbs, L., The critical role of exercise in weight control, *Nurse Pract.*, 18, 20, 1993.

50. Staten, M.A., The effect of exercise on food intake in men and women, *Am. J. Clin. Nutr.*, 53, 27, 1991.

51. Ponka, P., Schulman, H.M. and Woodworth, R.C., *Iron Transport and Storage*, CRC Press, Boca Raton, FL, 1990.

52. Haymes, E.M., Trace minerals and exercise, in *Nutrition in Exercise and Sport*, Wolinsky, I., Ed., CRC Press, Boca Raton, FL, 1998, 187.

53. Dietary Reference Intakes for Vitamin A, Vitamin K, Arsenic, Boron, Chromium, Copper, Iodine, Iron, Manganese, Molybdenum, Nickel, Silicon, Vanadium and Zinc, Food and Nutrition Board, Institute of Medicine, National Academies Press, 2002.

54. Hallberg, L. and Rossander-Hulten, L., Iron requirements in menstruating women, *Am. J. Clin. Nutr.*, 54, 1047, 1991.

55. Manore, M.M., Besenfelder, P.D., Wells, C.L., Carroll, S.S. and Hooker, S.P., Nutrient intakes and iron status in female long-distance runners during training, *J. Am. Diet. Assoc.*, 89, 257, 1989.

56. Newhouse, I.J., Clement, D.B. and Lai, C., Effects of iron supplementation and discontinuation on serum copper, zinc, calcium and magnesium levels in women, *Med. Sci. Sports Exerc.*, 25, 562, 1993.
57. Risser, W.L., Lee, E. J., Poindexter, H.B.W., West, M.S., Pivarnik, J.M., Risser, J.M.H. and Hickson, J.F., Iron deficiency in female athletes: Its prevalence and impact on performance, *Med. Sci. Sports Exerc.*, 20, 116, 1988.
58. Diehl, D.M., Lohman, T.G., Smith, S.C. and Kertzer, R., Effects of physical training and competition on the iron status of female field hockey players, *Int. J. Sports Med.*, 7, 264, 1986.
59. Lukaski, H.C., Hoverson, B.S., Gallagher, S.K. and Bolonchuk, W.W., Physical training and copper, iron and zinc status of swimmers, *Am. J. Clin. Nutr.*, 51, 1093, 1990.
60. Clarkson, P.M., Vitamins and trace minerals, in *Perspectives in Exercise Science and Sports Medicine, Ergogenics*, Lamb, D.R. and Williams, M.H., Eds, Brown & Benchmark, Dubuque, IA, 1991.
61. Newhouse, I.J., Clement, D.B., Taunton, J.E. and McKenzie, D.C., The effects of prelatent/latent iron deficiency on physical work capacity, *Med. Sci. Sports Exerc.*, 21, 263, 1989.
62. Lukaski, H.C., Hall, C.B. and Nielsen, F.H., Thermogenesis and thermoregulatory function of iron-deficient women without anemia, *Aviat. Space Environ. Med.*, 61, 913, 1990.
63. Lampe, J.W., Slavin, J.L. and Apple, F.S., Iron status of active women and the effect of running a marathon on bowel function and gastrointestinal blood loss, *Int. J. Sports Med.*, 12, 173, 1991.
64. Telford, R.D., Cunningham, R.B., Deakin, V. and Kerr, D.A., Iron status and diet in athletes, *Med. Sci. Sports Exerc.*, 25, 796, 1993.
65. Lamanca, J.J., Haymes, E.M., Daly, J.A., Moffatt, R.J. and Waller, M.F., Sweat iron loss of male and female runners during exercise, *Int. J. Sports Med.*, 9, 52, 1988.
66. Beard, J. and Tobin, B., Iron status and exercise, *Am. J. Clin. Nutr.*, 72, 694S, 2000.
67. Block, J.E., Genant, H.K. and Black, D., Greater vertebral bone mineral mass in exercising young men, *West. J. Med.*, 145, 39, 1986.
68. Heinrich, C., Going, S.B., Pamenter, R.W., Perry C.D., Boyden, T.W. and Lohman, T.G., Bone mineral content of cyclically menstruating female resistance and endurance trained athletes, *Med. Sci. Sports Exerc.*, 22, 558, 1990.
69. Snow-Harter, C. and Marcus, R., Exercise, bone mineral density and osteoporosis, in *Exerc. Sport Sci. Rev.*, 19, 351, 1991.
70. Meema, H.E. and Meema, S., Cortical bone mineral density versus cortical thickness in the diagnosis of osteoporosis: A roentgenological-densitometric study, *J. Am. Geriatric Soc.*, 17, 120, 1969.
71. Drinkwater, B.D., Nelson, K.L., Chesnutt, C.S., Bremner, Q.J., Shainholtz, S. and Southworth, M.B., Bone mineral content of amenorrheic and eumenorrheic athletes, *N. Engl. J. Med.*, 311, 277, 1984.
72. Drinkwater, B., Nilson, K., Ott, S. and Chesnut, C.H., III, Bone mineral density after resumption of menses in amenorrheic athletes, *JAMA*, 256, 380, 1986.
73. Frusztajer, N.T., Dhuper, S., Warren, M.P., Brooks-Gunn, J. and Fox, R.P., Nutrition and the incidence of stress fractures in ballet dancers, *Am. J. Clin. Nutr.*, 51, 779, 1990.
74. *Dietary Reference Intakes for Calcium, Phosphorus, Magnesium, Vitamin D and Fluoride*, Food and Nutrition Board, Institute of Medicine, National Academies Press, 1999.
75. Shea, B., Wells, G., Cranney, A., Zytaruk, N., Robinson, V., Griffith, L., Ortiz, Z., Peterson, J., Adachi, J., Tugwell, P. and Guyatt, G., Meta-analyses of therapies for postmenopausal osteoporosis. VII. Meta-analysis of calcium supplementation for prevention of postmenopausal osteoporosis, *Endocr. Rev.,* 23, 552, 2002.

76. Cook, J.D., Dassenko, S.A. and Whittaker, P., Calcium supplementation: Effect on iron absorption, *Am. J. Clin. Nutr.*, 53, 106, 1991.

77. Strand, S.M., Clarke, B.A., Slavin, J.L. and Kelly, J.M., Effects of physical training and iron supplementation on iron status of female athletes, *Med. Sci. Sports Exerc.*, 16, 161, 1984.

78. Monsen, E.R., Hallberg, L., Layrisse, M., Hegsted, D.M., Cook, J.D., Mertz, W. and Finch, C.A., Estimation of available dietary iron, *Am. J. Clin. Nutr.*, 31, 134, 1978.

79. Layrisse, M., Martinez-Torres, C. and Roche., M., Effect of interaction of various foods on iron absorption, *Am. J. Clin. Nutr.*, 21, 1175, 1968.

80. Fairburn, C.G., Phil M. and Beglin, S.J., Studies of the epidemiology of bulimia nervosa, *Am. J. Psychiatry*, 147, 401, 1990.

81. DiGioacchino DeBate, R., Wethington, H. and Sargent, R., Sub-clinical eating disorder characteristics among male and female triathletes, *Eat. Weight Disord.*, 7, 210, 2002.

82. Holdemess, C.C., Brooks-Gunn, J. and Warren, M.P., Eating disorders and substance use: A dancing vs. a nondancing population, *Med. Sci. Sports Exerc.*, 26, 297, 1994.

83. Loosli, A.R., Benson, J., Gillien, D.M., and Bourdet, K., Nutrition habits and knowledge in competitive adolescent female gymnasts, *Phys. Sportsmed.*, 14, 118, 1986.

84. Rosen, L.W., McKeag, D.B., Hough, D.O. and Curley, V., Pathogenic weight control behavior in female athletes, *Phys. Sportsmed.*, 14, 79, 1986.

85. Kurtzman, F.D., Yager, J., Landsverk, J., Wiesmeier, E. and Bodurka, D.C., Eating disorders among selected female student populations at UCLA, *J. Am. Diet. Assoc.*, 89, 45, 1989.

86. Wilson, G.T. and Eldredge, K.L., Pathology and development of eating disorders: Implications for athletes, in *Eating, Body Weight and Performance in Athletes, Disorders of Modern Society*, Brownell, K.D., Rodin, J. and Wilmore, J.H., Eds., Lea & Febiger, Philadelphia, 1992, p. 115.

87. Lohman, T.G., ACSM Tutorial: *Body Composition Assessment*, presented at the ACSM annual meeting, June, 1989, Unpublished Results.

88. Nutter, J., Seasonal changes in female athletes' diets, *Int. J. Sport Nutr.*, 1, 395, 1991.

89. Yeager, K.K., Agostini, R., Nattiv, A. and Drinkwater, B., The female athlete triad: Disordered eating, amenorrhea, osteoporosis, *Med. Sci. Sports Exerc.*, 25, 775, 1993.

90. Otis, C.L., Drinkwater, B., Johnson, M., Loucks, A. and Wilmore, J., American College of Sports Medicine position stand. The female athlete triad, *Med. Sci. Sports Exerc.*, 29, 1669, 1997.

91. Loucks, A.B., Effects of exercise training on the menstrual cycle: existence and mechanisms, *Med. Sci. Sports Exerc.*, 22, 275, 1990.

92. De Souza, M.J. and Metzger, D.A., reproductive dysfunction in amenorrheic athletes and anorexic patients: A review, *Med. Sci. Sports Exerc.*, 23(9), 995, 1991.

93. Warren, M.P. and Perlroth, N.E., The effects of intense exercise on the female reproductive system, *J. Endocrinol.*, 170, 3, 2001.

94. Pivarnik, J.M., Marichal, C.J., Spillman, H.T. and Morrow, J.R., Menstrual cycle phase affects temperature regulation during endurance exercise, *Med. Sci. Sports Exerc.*, 22, S119, 1990.

95. Puhl, J.L. and Brown, C.H., *The Menstrual Cycle and Physical Activity*, Human Kinetics Publishers, Inc., Champaign, Illinois, 1986.

96. Gong, E.J., Garrel, D. and Calloway, D.H., Menstrual cycle and voluntary food intake, *Am. J. Clin. Nutr.*, 49, 252, 1989.

97. Tarasuk, V. and Beaton, G.H, Menstrual-cycle patterns in energy and macronutrient intake, *Am. J. Clin. Nutr.*, 53, 442, 1991.

98. Webb, P., 24-hour energy expenditure and the menstrual cycle, *Am. J. Clin. Nutr.*, 44, 614, 1986.

99. Benson, J.E., Geiger, C.J., Eiserman, P.A. and Wardlaw, G.M., Relationship between nutrient intake, body mass index, menstrual function and ballet injury, *J. Am. Diet. Assoc.*, 89, 58, 1989.

100. Brooks-Gunn, J., Warren. M,P. and Hamilton, L.H., The relation of eating problems and amenorrhea in ballet dancers, *Med. Sci. Sports Exerc.*, 19, 41, 1987.

101. Lloyd, T., Triantafllou, S.J., Baker, E.R., Houts, P.S., Whiteside, J.A., Kalenak, A. and Stumpf, P.G., Women athletes with menstrual irregularity have increased musculoskeletal injuries, *Med. Sci. Sports Exerc.*, 18, 374, 1986.

102. Baker, E.R., Mathurl, R.S., Kirk., R.F. and Williamson, H.O., Female runners and secondary amenorrhea: Correlation with age, parity, mileage and plasma hormonal and sex-hormone-binding globulin concentrations, *Fertil. Seril.*, 36, 183, 1981.

103. Brooks, S.M., Sanborn, C.F., Albrecht, B.H. and Wagner, W.W., Diet in athletic amenorrhea, *Lancet*, 3, 559, 1984.

104. Carlberg, K.A., Buckman, M.T., Peake, G.T. and Riedesel, M.L., Body composition of oligo/amenorrheic athletes, *Med. Sci. Sports Exerc.*, 15, 215, 1983.

105. Dale, E. and Goldberg, D.L., Implications of nutrition in athletes with menstrual cycle irregularities, *Can. J. Appl. Sport Sci.*, 7, 74, 1982.

106. Loucks, A.B. and Horvath, S.M., Exercise induced stress responses of amenorrheic and eumenorrheic runners, *J. Clin. Endocrinol. Metab.*, 59, 1109, 1984.

107. Schwartz, B., Cumming, D.C., Biordan, E., Selye, M., Yen, S.C. and Rebar, R.W., Exercise associated amenorrhea: A distinct entity, *Am. J. Obstet. Gynecol.*, 141, 622, 1981.

108. Warren, M.P., Effect of undernutrition on reproductive function in the human, *Endocr. Rev.*, 4, 363, 1983.

109. Shetty, P.S., Adaptive changes in basal metabolic rate and lean body mass in chronic undernutrition, *Hum. Nutr. Clin. Nutr*, 38C, 443, 1984.

110. Myerson, M., Gutin, B., Warren, M.P., May, M.R., Contento, I., Lee, M., Pi-Sunyer, F.X., Pierson, Jr., R.N. and Brooks-Gunn, J., Resting metabolic rate and energy balance in amenorrheic and eumenorrheic runners, *Med. Sci. Sports Exerc.*, 23, 15, 1991.

111. Nationwide food consumption survey continuing survey of food intakes by individuals. Women 19–50 years and their children 1–5 years, 1 day, United States Dept. of Agriculture, NFCS CSFII Report No.85, 1985.

112. Haines, P.S., Hungerford, D.W., Popkin, B.M. and Gulkey, D.K., Eating patterns and energy and nutrient intakes of U.S. women, *J. Am. Diet. Assoc.*,92, 698, 1992.

113. Nielsen, S.J., Siega-Riz, A.M. and Popkin, B.M., Trends in energy intake in U.S. between 1997 and 1996: Similar shifts seen across age groups, *Obes. Res.*, 10, 370, 2002.

114. Walberg, J.L. and Johnston, C.S., Menstrual function and eating behavior in female recreational weightlifters and competitive body builders, *Med. Sci. Sports Exerc.*, 23, 30, 1991.

115. Manore, M.M., Nutritional needs of the female athlete, *Clin. Sports Med.*, 18, 549, 1999.

20 Nutrition and Vegetarianism

Sujatha Rajaram, Patricia A. Dyett and Joan Sabaté

CONTENTS

I. INTRODUCTION

Over the past few decades, the number of women adopting vegetarian diets[1-3] has increased significantly.[1,2] Professionals in the health care industry are seeking

knowledge on vegetarian dietary practices to better counsel their expanding vegetarian clientele.[2] Parallel to this trend, there has been an increase in published
scientific literature on the various aspects of vegetarian diets.[3] In the broadest context,
a vegetarian diet is one that contains no meat, poultry or fish, but in practice, there
are several variations of this. The American Dietetic Association issued a position
statement saying that appropriately planned vegetarian diets are healthful, nutritionally adequate and provide health benefits in the prevention and treatment of certain
diseases.[4] However, because of the different vegetarian dietary practices that exist,
the nutritional adequacy and the potential risks and benefits may vary. This chapter
will focus primarily on the adequacy of a vegetarian diet for women through different
stages of the life-cycle, discuss the role of plant foods in the prevention of chronic
diseases in women and present some practical guidelines for planning an optimal
vegetarian diet.

II. VEGETARIAN DIETARY PRACTICES

A. Types of Vegetarian Diets

While all vegetarian diets are primarily plant based, there are specific differences
among the various types of vegetarian diets.[5] Most vegetarians are lacto-ovo-vegetarians (LOV) who, besides plant foods, also include dairy and eggs in their diet,
but no flesh foods. Within this group, those that include dairy products but not eggs
are lacto-vegetarians. Strict vegetarian or vegan diets are exclusively plant based
with complete elimination of flesh foods, dairy and eggs. The pure macrobiotic diet
is based on rice and is rather restrictive. This diet also includes sea vegetables, grains,
soy and legumes, fruits, nuts and seeds and sometimes limited amounts of fish.
Fruitarian diets are based primarily on fruits, but they also include some nuts, seeds
and certain vegetables. Another variation of vegetarian diet is the raw-food diet,
which consists of fruits, vegetables, nuts, seeds, sprouted beans and grains, all eaten
uncooked. Although eating certain foods raw increases nutrient availability, for
certain other foods, cooking helps destroy microorganisms or inactivate enzyme
inhibitors. The final category is the semi-vegetarian diet, which is primarily a plant-
based diet, with the occasional inclusion of meat. Some of the more restrictive
vegetarian diets can be lacking or limiting in essential nutrients and therefore are
not advised for children unless suitably modified.[6,7]

B. Prevalence of Vegetarianism

In 1985, an estimated 6.5 million people in the United States were vegetarians and,
by 1995, this number had grown to about 12.4 million.[2] Of this number, 68% are
women,[8] with a greater percentage over 40 years of age and college educated,
compared with the general population. A weighted version of the Continuing Survey
of Food Intake (CSFII) data from 1322 respondents aged 12 and above was used to
estimate the number of self-defined and *de facto* (ate < 10g/d red meat, poultry, fish)
vegetarians. From this estimation, it was found that of the self-defined vegetarians

(2.6 ±0.4% of U.S. population), 74 ± 5% were women and of the *de facto* vegetarians (4.2 ± 0.5% of U.S. population), 67 ±4% were women.

Some of the reasons women choose to be vegetarian include health aspects, animal-rights issues, ethical and environmental concerns.[1] In some developing countries, vegetarianism is also practiced for economical reasons. A growing number of people who are not vegetarians are increasingly seeking vegetarian choices when they eat out.[10] Health care professionals are dealing with a greater percent of vegetarians than before,[3] which requires that they be better educated about the risks and benefits of the various types of vegetarian diets. Knowledge of vegetarian nutrition has expanded from nutritional adequacy issues to planning an optimum vegetarian diet to help reduce chronic disease risk. Research has moved from investigating the classical nutrients such as minerals and vitamins to nonnutrients such as phytochemicals. Adequate scientific publications and resources are available to support and provide information to any woman who decides to follow a vegetarian diet.

Since a greater percent of women follow either the LOV or vegan dietary practice, in this chapter we will discuss the nutritional adequacy and disease prevention aspects of only these two types of vegetarian diets. Wherever appropriate, mention will also be made of the macrobiotic diet. Other types of vegetarian diets are not considered here.

III. NUTRITIONAL ADEQUACY OF VEGETARIAN DIETS FOR WOMEN

A well-balanced vegetarian diet can adequately maintain normal nutritional status and promote health and reduce chronic disease risk.[4,11] However, a few nutrients are of concern either because the concentrations of these nutrients in plant foods is low or their bioavailability is low. This calls for careful planning of vegetarian diets to achieve optimum nutrition. In this section, the nutrients including protein, essential fatty acids, iron, zinc, calcium and vitamin B_{12} are discussed, with appropriate recommendations for increasing these nutrients from vegetarian diets.

A. PROTEIN

In a vegan diet, protein is primarily obtained from legumes, grains, soy and nuts. LOV diets include one or more servings of eggs and dairy in addition to plant proteins. Although vegetarians generally have lower protein intake than nonvegetarians, it tends to be adequate.[12] The percent energy from protein in an omnivore diet is about 14–18% compared with 12–14% and 10–12% from LOV and vegan diets, respectively.[5] Besides protein quantity, its quality as determined by digestibility and the amino acid content is also important to consider. Plant-based diets, such as the vegan diet, consisting mainly of whole grains and beans, have a digestibility of 85% compared with 95% digestibility of diets based on refined grains and meat, such as the omnivore diet.[13] Since plant proteins have lower digestibility, it has been suggested that the protein requirements from vegan diets be increased to 0.9 gram/kg body weight compared with the current recommended daily allowance of 0.8 gram/kg body weight of protein for adults consuming a mixed diet.[5,14]

Besides having a low digestibility, plant proteins are also limiting in one or more essential amino acids. For example, most legumes contain isoleucine and lysine, but are limiting in methionine and tryptophan, while cereal grains provide methionine and tryptophan, but are poor sources of lysine and isoleucine.[13] To achieve positive nitrogen balance, one will need more of the plant proteins than animal proteins since the latter tend to have all the essential amino acids in the recommended amounts. Unlike other plant proteins, the amount of soy protein that is needed to maintain positive nitrogen balance is the same as the amount of milk proteins[15] making soy an excellent source of protein for vegetarians, especially vegans. Protein complementation, a method of combining one or more foods, ensures intake of all essential amino acids and is thus a recommended practice for vegetarians. Unlike previously thought, protein foods need not be combined in the same meal, but can be consumed within a 24-hour period to be complementary with each other.[11] Overall, vegetarians should focus on obtaining adequate calories from proteins by including a variety of plant foods consumed throughout the day.

B. Essential Fatty Acids

Linoleic (18:2 n-6) and α-linolenic (18:3 n-3) acids are the two essential fatty acids that should be provided through the diet. They are both converted in the body by elongase and desaturase enzymes to long-chain polyunsaturated fatty acids (LCPUFA) that have important physiological functions. Linoleic acid is converted to arachidonic acid, an n-6 LCPUFA, while α-linolenic acid is converted to eicosapentaenoic acid (EPA) and docosahexaenoic acid (DHA), which are n-3 LCPUFAs. The conversion of the n-6 and n-3 essential fatty acids to the LCPUFA is a competitive process such that an excess of linoleic acid can inhibit the conversion of the α-linolenic acid and vice versa.[16] While plant foods provide both linoleic and α-linolenic acids, preformed arachidonic acid is obtained mainly from meat and dairy products and preformed EPA and DHA are obtained from marine sources. Vegans consume negligible amounts of EPA and DHA, and LOV consume less than 5 mg/day of EPA and varying amounts of DHA depending on the egg consumption. Omnivores consuming fish have an average intake of 100–150 mg/day of EPA and DHA.[17]

The LCPUFAs predominantly incorporated into membrane phospholipid is a reflection of the dietary fatty acid composition. When compared with omnivores, vegetarians tend to consume higher amounts of linoleic acid but similar amounts of α-linolenic acid. When we assess the membrane phospholipids, the arachidonic acid content in the vegetarian diet varies considerably,[18–21] while the concentration of EPA and DHA is lower in vegetarians than in omnivores.[22] Increased incorporation of n-3 LCPUFA in cell membrane phospholipids has important implications in the prevention of cardiovascular disease since they are converted to eicosanoids that are antithrombotic.[23]

Since vegetarians rely on the endogenous conversion of α-linolenic acid to EPA and DHA, they need to increase the absolute amount of α-linolenic acid intake from their diet. Table 20.1 provides a list of plant foods rich in α-linolenic acid and the ratio of n-6:n-3 of each of these foods. Vegetarians should strive to achieve an n-6:n-3 ratio of 5:1, for which at least 1.5–2% of the calories should come from

TABLE 20.1
Total Fat, Total Polyunsaturated Fat and a-Linolenic Acid Content of Selected Plant Foods (g/100 g Edible Portion)

Food	Total Fat	Polyunsaturated (PUFA)	α-Linolenic Acid
Nuts and Seeds			
Butternuts (Dried)	57.0	42.7	8.7
Flaxseed	34.0	22.4	18.1
Walnuts (English)	62.0	39.1	6.8
Legumes			
Soybeans (Dry)	21.3	12.3	1.6
Vegetables (Raw)			
Leeks	2.1	1.2	0.7
Kale	0.7	0.3	0.2
Broccoli	0.4	0.2	0.1
Fats and Oils			
Soybean oil	100	57.9	6.8
Soybean oil (hydrogenated)	100	37.6	2.6
Wheat germ oil	100	61.7	6.9
Canola oil	100	29.6	9.3
Linseed oil	100	66.0	53.3

Source: United States Department of Agriculture Nutrient Database for Standard Reference, August 15, 2002

α-linolenic acid. Besides including foods from this list, limiting n-6-rich vegetable oils such as safflower, sunflower, corn oils and replacing them with oils rich in monounsaturated and n-3 fatty acids such as canola, soy and flaxseed oils and limiting the intake of processed foods containing hard margarine may be beneficial.

C. IRON

The amount of iron that one can obtain from a plant-based diet is as much or more than what can be obtained through an omnivore diet. Some populations[24,25] that are vegans consume 20–34 mg of iron/day, which is much greater than the recommended daily intake (15 mg) of iron for adult women. Much of the concern with respect to the iron status of vegetarians is therefore due to the low bioavailability of iron from plant foods. The majority of the iron found in meat, fish and poultry is heme iron, the absorption of which is not affected by dietary factors. In contrast, all of plant iron is nonheme, the absorption of which is greatly influenced by other dietary factors. While 15–35% of the heme iron is absorbed, only 5–10% of the nonheme iron is absorbed.[26] Nonheme iron absorption is primarily influenced by the iron status and total amount of iron ingested. Individuals with low iron status absorb more nonheme than heme iron. However, the percent absorption of nonheme iron decreases with increasing amount in the diet. In contrast, the percent absorption of heme iron remains the same with increasing amounts in the diet such that the absolute amount is increased.[27]

Plant foods that primarily contribute to iron in the diet are whole grains, legumes, dark green leafy vegetables, dried fruits and nuts. Table 20.2 provides the iron content of some of these foods. Whole grains and legumes contain phytic acid, a potent inhibitor of nonheme iron absorption.[28] Vegan diets contain 2–3 times more phytates than omnivore diets and LOV diets contain an intermediate amount of phytates. Processing of grains can remove the phytates, but the iron content is also simultaneously reduced. Although consuming a whole-grain-based diet provides more iron than a diet based on refined grains, the overall iron status remains the same because of low iron bioavailability of the whole-grain diet.[29] Coffee, tea and some East Indian spices contain polyphenols and tannins that can also reduce nonheme iron absorption by 40–60%.[26,28] Dairy products included by

TABLE 20.2
Iron Content of Plant Foods

	Iron (mg)
Legumes, 1/2 cup (90 g) cooked	
Soybeans, 1/2 cup cooked (90 g)	2.3
Red kidney beans. 1/2 cup cooked (89g)	2.6
Lentils, 1/2 cup cooked (99g)	3.3
Peas, 1/2 cup cooked (80 g)	1.3
Grains and pasta	
Oatmeal, 1 cup (234 g)	1.6
Pasta, enriched, 1 cup (200 g)	2.3
Brown rice, 1 cup (195 g)	0.82
Whole-wheat bread, 1 slice (28 g)	0.92
Vegetables	
Brussel Sprouts, 1/2 cup (78 g)	0.9
Broccoli, 1/2 cup (78 g)	0.65
Pumpkin, 1/2 cup (122 g)	0.7
Nuts and seeds, 1 oz (28.4)	
Almonds	1.2
Peanuts	0.64
Fruits and dried fruits	
Prunes, 5 large (42 g)	1.0
Dates, 5 medium (42 g)	0.5
Strawberries, 10 large (180 g)	0.7
Raisins, 1.5 oz (43 g)	0.9
Orange juice, 1 cup (248 g)	0.5
Figs, 3 medium (150 g)	0.57

Source: United States Department of Agriculture Nutrient Database for Standard Reference, August 15, 2002.

LOV are poor sources of iron and, in fact, the calcium in these products can inhibit iron absorption. This effect of calcium on iron is, however, acute and no long-term implication on iron status has been observed.

One of the factors that enhance nonheme iron absorption is ascorbic acid. 75 mg of ascorbic acid (vitamin C) increases nonheme iron absorption by 3–4 fold.[26] This effect of vitamin C is partly due to its ability to counteract the inhibition of phytates and impair the formation of unavailable iron complexes with ligands normally present in the gastrointestinal lumen. It is thus considered a physiological factor essential for nonheme iron absorption.

Although the availability of iron from plant foods is lower than from animal products, the iron status of vegetarians seems to be similar to that of omnivores. In fact, the American Dietetic Association stated that Caucasian vegetarians in developed countries are no more prone to nutritional anemia than the general population.[4] Most studies[29–31] indicate that, while the iron intake and iron stores measured by serum ferritin are lower among adult vegetarians than among omnivores, the prevalence of anemia indicated by hemoglobin is similar in both groups. Iron stores can vary over a wide range without adversely affecting functional iron, but it does pose a slightly greater risk for developing iron deficiency. In fact, there is some indication that low iron stores may be protective of heart disease that might put vegetarians at a decreased risk for the same.[32] Hunt et al.[31] demonstrated that when individuals are on an LOV diet they tend to have lower iron absorption but this may be partially compensated for by a reduced excretion of ferritin in the feces. Among children, a balanced LOV or vegan diet helps maintain normal iron status similar to that seen in children on omnivore diets. But children on macrobiotic diets exhibit iron deficiency more frequently.[33]

Vegans and LOVs should plan their diet carefully and ensure adequate intake of vitamin C; avoid dietary factors that contain inhibitors of iron absorption; practice cooking methods that will increase iron absorption such as fermentation, soaking, germination and thermal processing of plant foods; avoid consumption of calcium or mineral supplements with iron-rich foods and avoid drinking coffee and tea with meals. All women, whether vegetarian or nonvegetarian, experience significant iron loss during their menstrual cycle and reproductive years. Hence, they should all seek to maintain adequate iron status and follow relevant dietary practices that enhance iron absorption. The use of iron-fortified food products and, in some cases, even supplementation, may be a prudent recommendation.

D. ZINC

Adult vegetarians tend to have lower intakes of zinc than omnivores but the zinc status is comparable.[34] Although several plant foods contain zinc in reasonable amounts, zinc bioavailability from some of these foods is low due to the high phytate content. This especially is a concern among children consuming a vegetarian diet since it can compromise growth and reproductive development.[35] When we compare the serum zinc levels of vegetarians with nonvegetarians, the former group tends to have lower levels but still fall within the normal range. Changes in food selection patterns such as reducing red meat intake and increasing cereal intake have been associated with lower serum zinc status in women.[36] This may be due to lower zinc intake among vegetarians, but it could also be that the cereals used were not fortified. Serum zinc is not considered the best indicator of zinc status and this makes it difficult to clarify the effects of marginal zinc status on overall health. However, it is important that vegetarian women focus on obtaining at least the recommended daily intake of zinc by selecting plant foods rich in zinc such as whole grains, peas, beans and nuts.

E.   CALCIUM AND VITAMIN D

One of the physiological roles of calcium is in maximizing peak bone mass until young adulthood and minimizing bone loss during the subsequent years. Of the different types of vegetarian diets, the LOV diet includes dairy products and is therefore the least restrictive for obtaining adequate calcium.[37] About 75% of the calcium in the American diet is from milk and other dairy products[38] and few other foods contain naturally occurring calcium in amounts similar to that in cow's milk. Vegans do not use dairy products and hence rely on plant foods, as well as fortified foods and beverages. Table 20.3 provides a list of calcium-rich plant foods and the total absorbable calcium from each of these foods. Calcium bioavailability from plant foods is affected by the content of oxalates and phytates, which are inhibitors of calcium absorption.[37] Calcium bioavailability is low from high-oxalate foods such as spinach and rhubarb, while it is high from low-oxalate vegetables like kale and broccoli. Legumes and soybeans also contain high amounts of phytates and oxalates, but the calcium from soybeans is highly available in contrast to the low availability from legumes.

Many individuals use calcium-fortified soymilk in place of cow's milk. The calcium content of these fortified soy products ranges from 80–500 mg/serving. In a recent study, Heaney et al.[39] demonstrated that the calcium absorption efficiency from fortified soymilk was only 75% of that of cow's milk. Since the calcium content of plant sources is either low or contains inhibitory factors that reduce absorption, individuals following a vegan diet should carefully plan their diet or consider including calcium supplements or fortified foods to ensure adequate intake. The fractional absorption rate of calcium supplements is similar to that of milk, with the exception of calcium citrate, which has a slightly higher absorption rate than calcium from cow's milk.[40]

Calcium absorption and balance are also affected by other dietary factors such as protein, sodium and vitamin D intakes. Sodium and calcium share the same transport systems in the kidney tubules and, for every gram of sodium ingested, 25 mg calcium is excreted in the urine.[41] The sodium intake of LOV is similar to omnivores while those of vegans seem somewhat lower than these two groups. This may be due to the lower amounts of processed foods in the diet of vegans, since they tend to be more health conscious.

Calcium balance is affected by both total and type of protein in the diet. An increase in protein intake by 50 g results in the urinary loss of 60 mg calcium.[42] For every gram increase in protein the calcium loss is increased by 1 mg. Over a period of time, the calcium loss can become significant enough to increase the risk of

TABLE 20.3
Comparison of Sources Of Absorbable Calcium With Milk

Food	Serving size[1] g	Calcium content mg	Estimated absorbable calcium[2] mg	Servings needed to equal 240 mL milk n
Milk	240	300	96.3	1.0
Beans				
Pinto	86	44.7	11.9	8.1
Red	172	40.5	9.9	9.7
White	110	113	24.7	3.9
Bok choy	85	79	42.5	2.3
Broccoli	71	35	21.5	4.5
Cheddar cheese	42	303	97.2	1.0
Chinese cabbage	85	239	94.7	1.0
Chinese mustard greens	85	212	85.3	1.1
Chinese spinach	85	347	29	3.3
Fruit punch with calcium citrate malate	240	300	156	0.62
Kale	85	61	30.1	3.2
Spinach	85	115	5.9	16.3
Sweet potatoes	164	44	9.8	9.8
Rhubarb	120	174	10.1	9.5
Tofu with calcium	126	258	80.0	1.2
Yogurt	240	300	96.3	1.0

[*]Based on half-cup serving size (Å 85 g for green leafy vegetables) except for milk and fruit punch (1 cup or 240 mL) and cheese (1.5 oz, 42 g).

[**]Calculated as calcium content fractional absorption.

Source: Weaver, C.M., Proulx, W.R., Heaney, R., Choices for achieving adequate dietary calcium with a vegetarian diet, *Am J Clin Nutr,* 70[3 Suppl], 543S, 1999. With permission.

osteoporosis. Vegetarians tend to have lower protein intake than omnivores. Of the total calories of nonvegetarians, 14–18% come from protein, while only 10–14% of the calories of vegetarians are derived from proteins.[5] Animal proteins contain sulfur amino acids that can increase the acid production, resulting in higher loss of urinary calcium.[43] Meat-containing diets produce the most acid, followed by the LOV diet and then the vegan diet. Besides the total calcium and protein content of the diet, the calcium:protein ratio is considered a better predictor of bone health.[44] The ideal ratio is 16:1, based on the recommended daily requirements for calcium and protein for adults. The ratio of meat-based diets is typically 10:1–12:1 compared with LOV diets that have a more favorable ratio of 15:1–17:1. Vegan diets tend to have lower protein and calcium content but their ratio is much better, ranging from 9:1–12:1.[5]

Vitamin D is essential for calcium absorption and for maintaining optimal bone health. Sufficient vitamin D can be manufactured when exposed to adequate sunlight. Several vitamin D-fortified foods are also available for inclusion in the diet such as cow's milk, some cereals and soymilk. Vegetarians tend to have lower mean intake of vitamin D and lower serum 25-hydroxyvitamin D levels than omnivores.[45] Therefore, vegetarians, especially vegans, are recommended to include vitamin D-fortified foods and a 5–10 μg supplement of vitamin D during the winter and early spring months when the sun exposure is limited.[45,46] This is critical to avoid long-term negative implications on bone health.

F.   VITAMIN B$_{12}$

A diet devoid of meats, fish, eggs and dairy contains no vitamin B$_{12}$ and thus increases the risk of developing vitamin B$_{12}$ deficiency. Since the overt symptoms of vitamin B$_{12}$ take years to develop, short-term studies on vegetarians do not show a higher incidence of macrocytic anemia or neurological disorders among vegetarians compared with nonvegetarians.[47] Very few studies have looked at the vitamin B$_{12}$ status of long-term vegetarians and vegans. Most demonstrate that serum vitamin B$_{12}$ levels are lower in vegans and LOV than in nonvegetarians.[47,48] In a study of 78 vegans, 60% had vitamin B$_{12}$ levels below 200 pg/ml (normal values are above 200 pg/ml) and 40% had levels below 160 pg/ml.[49] In contrast, vegans who used soymilk fortified with vitamin B$_{12}$ had serum values over 350 pg/ml. Macrobiotic diets that restrict dairy products also pose an increased risk for vitamin B$_{12}$ deficiency. A study on adult men and women residing in a macrobiotic community in New England showed that 51% had low serum vitamin B$_{12}$ and the levels correlated inversely with years on the macrobiotic diet.[47]

When clinical signs of vitamin B$_{12}$ deficiency manifest, the macrocytic anemia can be reversed by oral vitamin B$_{12}$ supplementation, but sometimes the neurological damage is not completely reversed.[50] One of the major concerns of low-serum vitamin B$_{12}$ is elevated homocysteine level, an independent risk factor for heart disease. Researchers have shown that vegetarians tend to have elevated plasma homocysteine levels, which corresponds to a lower intake of vitamin B$_{12}$.[51] Apart from vitamin B$_{12}$ deficiency, inadequate intake of folate can also contribute to hyper homocysteinemia. On the other hand, excess folate intake can mask vitamin B$_{12}$ deficiency. Vegetarians can easily obtain surplus amounts of folate from their diet. Folate can correct the anemia but without correcting the underlying B$_{12}$ deficiency. This results in permanent nerve damage if left untreated. Thus, folic acid intake should not exceed 1000 μg/d.[52]

Vitamin B$_{12}$ is found in animal products (milk, eggs and meat) as a result of microbial synthesis that occurs in the gut. Therefore, vegetarians who consume neither eggs nor dairy foods should consider using vitamin B$_{12}$ supplements or fortified foods such as cereals, soy beverages and yeast. Fermented soy products (tempeh, miso) and algae (spirulina, nori) are not good sources of vitamin B$_{12}$ since they contain analogs of vitamin B$_{12}$ that hinder absorption.[53] A listing for vegetarians of foods that contain vitamin B$_{12}$ is provided in Table 20.4.

TABLE 20.4
Vitamin B$_{12}$ Content of Foods

Food	Vitamin B$_{12}$ (µg)
Animal Products	
Milk, low fat 1% (1 cup, 244 g)	0.9
Yogurt, plain, low fat (1 cup, 227 g)	1.27
Cottage cheese (1 cup, 210 g)	1.3
Egg (1 large, 50 g)	0.6
Non-Dairy milk	
Eden Soy, extra (1 cup, 245 g)	3.0
Soy Dream, original enriched (1 cup, 245 g)	3.0
Rice Dream, original enriched (1 cup, 245 g)	1.5
Ready-to-Eat Cereals	
Kellogg's Wheat Bran Flakes (3/4 cup, 29 g)	6.0
Kellogg's Special K (1 cup, 31 g)	0.65
Kellogg's Product 19 (1 cup, 30 g)	6.0
General Mills Total Corn Flakes (1/3 cup, 30 g)	6.0
General Mills Raisin Bran (1 cup, 55 g)	6.0
Meat Substitute (1 serving)	
Worthington Foods, Morning Star patty (1, 38 g)	1.5
Worthington Foods, Big Franks (1 serving, 51 g)	2.9
Other	
Nutritional yeast, Red Star brand (1 tblsp, 12 g)	4.0

Source: United States Department of Agriculture Nutrient Database for Standard Reference, August 15, 2002.

IV. VEGETARIAN DIETS IN A WOMAN'S LIFE CYCLE

The nutritional need of a woman varies throughout her life cycle. There are certain stages of exponential growth and development such as pregnancy, infancy and adolescence, that place a greater demand on certain nutrients. As a woman goes through early adulthood and enters the menopausal years, there is also a greater emphasis placed on the role of nutrition and diet in health promotion and disease prevention. These special needs throughout the stages of her life in the context of vegetarian diets are discussed in the following section.

A. PREGNANCY

Pregnancy is a time when nutrition plays a vital role in the health and well-being of both the mother and her developing fetus. It is important that dietary regimens undertaken by women of childbearing age and during pregnancy provide adequate nourishment. Weight gain during pregnancy and infant birth weight is similar in both vegetarian and nonvegetarian women.[54,55] However, women on restrictive macrobiotic diets tend to have less weight gain during pregnancy and give birth to lower birth weight infants.[56] Inadequate energy and other critical nutrient intake seen among some macrobiotics may explain the low infant birth weight. Typically, vegetarian diets are higher in fiber and low in fat, hence low in energy density, compared with an omnivore diet. Inadequate gain is most likely to occur when caloric density is low, as is typical of diet regimens that exclude all animal foods.[56,57] Hence, vegetarians should choose energy-dense foods such as nuts and seeds to meet the increased caloric demands of pregnancy. Protein synthesis is increased by 20% during pregnancy and both vegans and LOV can easily meet this by consuming adequate calories and including a variety of plant protein sources.[4,58] A discussion on the quality of plant vs. animal protein is provided elsewhere in this chapter.

Maternal essential fatty acid status determines the essential fatty acid status of the infant and therefore becomes an important nutrient during pregnancy. During the last trimester of pregnancy, arachidonic acid and DHA are selectively transported via the placenta to the developing fetus, accumulating in the fetal brain and retina, which makes them essential for normal brain functions and visual development.[59] Vegetarian mothers do not consume a direct source of arachidonic acid and DHA but are able to convert the linoleic and α-linolenic acids to the respective LCPUFAs, although the efficiency of this conversion has been questioned. Total LCPUFAs in fetal plasma and cord artery phospholipid are similar among infants born to vegetarian and nonvegetarian mothers, but the proportion of DHA is lower and that of arachidonic acid higher.[60] Since DHA has an important role in brain and visual functions of the newborn and vegetarians do not include a direct supply of DHA in their diet, it is important for them to consume adequate α-linolenic acid and limit the intake of linoleic acid.[61]

To meet the demands of the expanding blood volume during pregnancy, vegetarian mothers should ensure adequate intakes of the two B-vitamins — folic acid and vitamin B_{12}.[62] Adequate folate is specially noted for preventing the development during pregnancy of neural tube defects in the fetus. Since plant foods are typically good sources of folate, vegetarians are able to easily meet the increased requirement for folate during pregnancy (400 µg compared with 180 µg that is required during the nonpregnant condition).[52] A prospective study on pregnant women showed that women who had a higher consumption of vegetables for over 8 years and followed a predominantly LOV diet had higher plasma and red blood cell folate status than women who followed an omnivore diet with low intake of vegetables.[63] Thus, following a well-planned vegetarian diet actually bestows an advantage in terms of improved folate status. In addition to folate, pregnant vegetarian women should also obtain sufficient vitamin B_{12} from their diet by including eggs and dairy. Vegans should consume fortified foods or take supplements.

During pregnancy, recommended intakes of minerals such as iron and zinc are increased[55] for placental nutrient transfer to the infant and development of various fetal systems, as well as for maintaining adequate maternal status. Infants born to women with low iron stores also tend to have low iron stores. This can increase the risk of iron deficiency in the infant, especially when the maternal iron status does not improve while she is breastfeeding the infant.[64] The incidence of iron deficiency, although common in pregnant women in general, is the same in both vegetarian and nonvegetarian pregnant women.[65] It is, however, important for vegetarian women to include iron-rich foods in their diet whether they use iron supplements or not. During pregnancy, the zinc requirements increase by 50%, which means that vegetarians need to plan their diets carefully to get sufficient zinc. Poor zinc status of the mother is associated with low birth weight.[66] Studies show that zinc intake of pregnant LOVs is less than their omnivore counterparts, which correlated with plasma zinc concentration.[55] During pregnancy it is important to include zinc-rich plant foods such as nuts, legumes, soy and whole grains to ensure adequate intake.

The recommended dietary allowance for calcium for pregnant women is not increased above that for a nonpregnant woman, but, because of skeletal system development and the need to ensure maternal bone integrity, calcium intakes should not be compromised in any way during pregnancy. Pregnant vegetarian women are recommended to include calcium-fortified foods, calcium-rich plant foods that have high bioavailable calcium or calcium supplements to meet the needs during pregnancy.

B. Lactation and Infancy

Suitable nutrition immediately following birth is dependent primarily on breastfeeding or, in those unable or unwilling breastfeed, on formula feeding. Well-nourished vegetarian women produce milk that is nutritionally adequate to sustain normal growth and development of infants.[58] Maternal diet influences the nutritional composition of breast milk, although the impact varies greatly with the nutrients.

The total fat content of breast milk from vegetarians is similar to that of omnivores,[67] although the specific fatty acid composition may vary with the maternal dietary fat intake. Typically, the breast milk from vegetarian women tends to be lower in saturated fat, higher in linoleic and α-linolenic acids and similar in the arachidonic acid content compared with nonvegetarian women.[20,67] Since vegetarian diets do not provide preformed DHA, the amount of DHA in breast milk is a reflection of the conversion from α-linolenic acid. The breast milk DHA content of vegan women is lower than omnivore women,[68] but it is still higher than that found in infant formulas in the United States. Only recently are changes being made to encourage manufacturers to incorporate DHA into infant formulas. Breast milk or DHA-supplemented formula fed to term infants increased DHA accumulation and improved visual acuity compared with nonsupplemented formula.[69–72] How much DHA is required to promote visual and brain development or how much α-linolenic acid should be provided in the maternal diet of vegetarians to increase DHA in breast milk remains to be determined.

One of the nutrients sensitive to maternal diet is vitamin B_{12}.[5,73] Increased urinary excretion of methylmalonic acid observed in vitamin B_{12} deficiency was noted in vegetarian and macrobiotic mothers and their infants.[33,74] Since low vitamin B_{12} status can cause developmental and neurological disorders in the growing infant, it is essential for vegan women to consider using vitamin B_{12} supplements or fortified foods during lactation.

The mineral content of breast milk is not typically influenced by maternal diet. Calcium concentrations in the milk of vegetarians are similar to that of omnivores.[75] However, a study on lactating macrobiotic women showed an increase in 1,25-dihydroxy-vitamin D over lactating and nonlactating omnivore women.[76] This may be due to the low calcium intake reported among macrobiotics, since they avoid dairy foods. However, the impact of increased concentrations of 1,25-dihydroxy-vitamin D on bone status is not clear. A well-planned vegan diet can be used to adequately nourish infants when they are introduced to solid foods.[77]

The American Academy of Pediatrics Committee on Nutrition has concluded that healthy infants who get sufficient amounts of either breast milk from the mother on an adequate vegan diet or soy-based infant formulas, do thrive during infancy.[78] Breast milk taken from well-nourished mothers during the first or second month of lactation is the standard developed by the American Academy of Pediatrics for manufacturers to use in formulating infant formulas. While most infant formulas meet this standard in terms of total nutrient composition, some differ with respect to protein type and specific nutrients. For example, the three main proteins used in the different types of formulas sold in the United States are casein, whey and soy isolates.

Recently, due to the potential exposure of infants to high levels of phytoestrogens, there has been some concern about the use of soy-based infant formulas. An animal study comparing casein, whey and soy protein isolate demonstrated that the soy isolates accelerated puberty in female rats, while whey protein delayed puberty in females compared with casein.[79] There is lack of evidence linking isoflavone consumption with altered steroid-dependent developmental process in human infants. However, there may be a delayed effect that might manifest after puberty. Thus, more studies are warranted to understand the long-term implications of using soy-based formulas. For infants who have lactase deficiency, milk allergies or are from vegan families, soy-based infant formulas remain the most feasible alternative since there are no other plant-based commercial infant formula options available.

For the first 4 to 6 months, breast milk or, alternatively, soy-based infant formula, should be the sole food of vegetarian neonates. Commercial soymilk should not be used as the primary beverage until the infant is 1 year or older. Typically, the first solid foods introduced to infants are cereals, fruits and vegetables, and the recommendations for vegetarian and nonvegetarian infants are the same. Protein foods such as well-mashed tofu and pureed legumes can be introduced around 7–8 months as part of the weaning process.

Around the time of weaning, some mothers become concerned about foods that may cause allergic reactions in their infants. The leading cause of food allergies in infants is cows' milk.[80] However, plant foods such as soy products, citrus fruits, peas, corn products, nut butters and wheat can also cause allergies and are of concern among vegan children.[81] The main recommendations for dealing with infant allergies are to introduce solid foods after 9 months of age, one at a time, at weekly intervals, in order to identify specific sources of food allergens.

C. Childhood

Most studies on the growth of vegetarian children show that it is comparable to that of omnivore children.[82–84] Vegetarian children tend to be leaner and shorter during the preschool years than omnivore children but they catch up with their peers during late childhood.[82] Poor growth has been observed in macrobiotic children as a result of calorie restriction.[85]

Vegetarian diets typically contain less fat than mixed diets. This is particularly true for vegans, but not necessarily for LOVs. For adults, a well-planned low-fat dietary pattern such as is seen with vegan diets may be a healthy practice. Children should not use fat-restricted diets since fat is an important source of energy at this stage of development and is necessary for normal growth and physical activity.[86] A diet containing 30% or fewer calories from fat should not be considered for children below 2 years of age.[86] A step-wise reduction of total fat and saturated fat intake among primary school children should be considered in order to improve long-term health. Vegetarian children (> 2 years of age) who consume diets lower in fat and cholesterol also have lower blood cholesterol levels than the nonvegetarian children.[87] LOV children should start choosing low-fat dairy foods as a way to reduce fat, especially saturated fat intake, after 2 years of age.

Since vegetarian meals tend to be low in fat and high in fiber, they may fill up the children with bulk without providing sufficient calories. Too much fiber and too few calories can compromise growth and brain function in young children, because protein from food is used for energy and not for growth.[88] Age of the child plus 5 grams fiber is a good estimate of the total amount of fiber required for children.[89] Thus, vegan diets that are well planned[90] can be nutritionally adequate for children.

D. Adolescence and Adulthood

A recent study demonstrated that adolescent vegetarians have a dietary pattern that is more likely than nonvegetarians to meet the Healthy People 2010 objectives.[91] Many teenage girls and young female adults are opting to become vegetarians. Although health is one reason for this choice, the more common reasons seem to pertain to body image, body size and weight.[92] This phenomenon is particularly observed in vegetarian women involved in sports and athletics.

Some women who already have eating disorders like anorexia nervosa, bulimia nervosa and athletica nervosa, seek to disguise their disordered eating practices by adopting a vegetarian diet pattern.[93] Vegetarian diet practices that are very restrictive or faddish may serve as a marker for eating disorders in young women, indicating a need for preventive intervention.[94] While vegetarianism may not always cause or increase the risk of developing eating disorders, in some instances, the adoption of restrictive vegetarian regimens can, in fact, promote increased risk of nutrient inadequacies and disordered eating behaviors.

While some young girls choose vegetarianism as a way to restrict calories, vegetarian diets that are appropriately planned and adopted for health reasons are

TABLE 20.5
Estimated Effect of Vegetarian Diet on Attained Height in Adolescent Girls

Term	Regression coefficient	Standard Error	P
Vegetarian status*	2.03 cm	(0.161)	0.001
Age (years)	10.30 cm	(0.607)	<0.001
Age cubed (years ³)	-0.013 cm	(-0.0012)	<0.001
Constant	45.62 cm	(5.01)	<0.001

* Vegetarian status defined as meat consumption of less than once a week, compared with meat consumers.

Source: Adapted with permission from Sabaté, J., Lindstead, K., Harris, R.D., Sanchez, A., *Eur J Clin Nutr*, 45, 51, 1991.

known to sustain adequate physical growth.[95] In fact, among Seventh-day Adventist adolescent girls, vegetarian diet was associated with taller stature compared with meat eaters. Table 20.5 reports the estimated effect of vegetarian diet on attained height from this study.[96] The effect of vegetarian diet on height stature remained even after adjusting for differences in food groups and socioeconomic status. Although this study does not suggest that vegetarian children will be taller, it does show that meat intake is not essential for normal growth of older children and adolescents.

Vegetarianism is also frequently associated with menstrual cycle disturbances, one of the three aspects of a female triad.[97] Age at menarche is similar in vegetarian and nonvegetarians when energy intake is the same in the two groups.[98] Studies that showed that vegetarians had delayed menarche compared with nonvegetarians[99] did not account for confounders such as height, body weight and socioeconomic status. Also, late menarche does not pose any health risks to the individual. On the contrary, it reduces the risk for breast cancer later in life.[100]

Both inadequate and excess energy intake can lead to menstrual cycle disturbances. Dieting or short-term weight changes can cause missed cycles, while significant weight loss can cause amenorrhea.[101] Hence, in long-term, weight-stable vegetarians with normal body mass index (BMI), there is no association with menstrual cycle disturbances. However, among women who choose vegetarian diet as a way to control weight, this association is possible. About 10% of women in their teen and early adult years experience severe dysmenorrhea.[102] Plant-based diets tend to increase sex hormone-binding globulin in the serum that binds estrogen and inactivates it. This effect can alter the production of prostaglandins, decrease intensity and duration of dysmenorrhea and reduce premenstrual symptoms.[103]

E. MENOPAUSE

Very limited data that compare the age at menopause between vegetarians and nonvegetarians are available. Among Seventh-Day Adventists, the median age at menopause was 48 years in LOVs and 50 years among omnivores.[104] However, this study did not discuss the differences in the use of oral contraceptives between these two groups, which might have confounded the results. At the time of menopause, some women choose to take hormone replacement therapy (HRT) to reduce the severity of menopausal symptoms such as vaginal dryness, mood swings and hot flashes.[105] However, because of the associated risk of HRT to breast cancer, plant phytoestrogens are being studied as an alternate therapy. It has been observed that menopausal symptoms are less intense in women from countries such as Japan who consume more soy foods than in Western countries.[106] Several trials with soy intervention on menopausal symptoms have been carried out but the results are not conclusive.[107,108] Some studies showed a decrease in hot flashes but no significant effect on other menopausal symptoms. It is possible that the duration of feeding soy phytoestrogens needs to be longer to experience beneficial effects or it may be that phytoestrogens are not as potent as estrogen in alleviating menopausal symptoms. Further studies will answer these more clearly.

V. VEGETARIAN DIETS AND CHRONIC DISEASE PREVENTION

Scientific data suggest a positive relationship between a vegetarian diet and reduced risk for several chronic diseases including coronary heart disease, several types of cancer, diabetes and obesity.[4] This section discusses the role of plant foods in the prevention of some of the chronic diseases specific to, or commonly seen, in women. More detailed discussions of these chronic diseases in women are presented elsewhere in this book.

A. CORONARY HEART DISEASE

Coronary heart disease (CHD) is the most frequent cause of death among women in the United States.[109] Vegetarians in the Western countries have lower serum cholesterol levels and 24% reduction in mortality from CHD compared with nonvegetarians.[110] Total fat and saturated fat consumption is lower among vegetarians than nonvegetarians and may be the reason for the associated decrease in serum cholesterol. Although one would expect that avoidance of meat, a major source of saturated fat in an omnivore diet, would lower the risk of CHD, no significant relationship between meat consumption and CHD was noted among women in the Adventist Health Study and Nurses' Health Study cohorts.[111,112] It is possible that, in premenopausal women, iron losses via menstrual cycle may offer some protection from CHD risk in the omnivore group as well as the vegetarian groups. Although red meat intake was not associated with an increased risk of CHD from these epidemiological studies, it is possible that other aspects of vegetarian diet such as increased consumption of fruits and vegetables, intake of whole grains and legumes and nuts may play a role in reducing serum cholesterol and low density lipoprotein cholesterol (LDL-C), which are both independent risk factors for CHD.

Vegetarian diets are higher in fiber, which is associated with reduced mortality from heart disease in older women.[113] A follow-up of 9632 subjects from the NHANES I prospective cohort[114] indicated a significant inverse relationship between legume intake and risk of CHD. The soluble fiber and protein in the legumes may have provided the cardioprotective effects. Legumes and nuts are also rich in arginine, the amino acid that is involved in regulating vascular functions via vasodilation and endothelial relaxation. These mechanisms also contribute in part to the lowering of CHD risk.

Until menopause, circulating estrogen protects women from heart disease by keeping the HDL-C elevated and LDL-C within desirable range. However, during menopause, the estrogen levels decrease and this protection is no longer there.[115] HRT is chosen by many to keep the benefit of estrogen, but the potential increase in the risk of breast cancer has caused some to turn toward alternate therapies, one of which is the use of phytoestrogen. A Japanese study found that risk of myocardial infarction among women eating tofu four or more times a week was reduced by 50% compared with those eating it two or fewer times per week.[116] Meta-analyses of several soy intervention trials report a dose-dependent inverse relationship between soy consumption and serum cholesterol levels.[117,118] Soy protein also reduces CHD risk via other mechanisms such as protecting LDL from oxidation[119] and inhibiting smooth muscle cell proliferation.[120]

Nuts such as almonds, pecans and walnuts have been shown to reduce total serum and LDL cholesterol and triglyceride while maintaining or increasing HDL-C in women.[121–123] The unsaturated fatty acids in nuts are partly responsible for this lipid lowering effect. Frequent consumption of nuts has been shown to reduce CHD mortality by 40% in women.[124] Incorporating an ounce of nuts in the daily diet will help in favorably modifying blood lipids and reducing CHD risk. Besides healthy fats, nuts also provide fiber, folate, calcium, iron, arginine, copper and magnesium, along with several phytochemicals. Monounsaturated fat from nuts and plant oils such as olive oil also have favorable impact on hemostatic and thrombotic factors, further contributing to the lowering of CHD risk. Olive oil-enriched diet was associated with lower factor VIIa than a diet enriched with sunflower oil.[125] Similarly, 8 weeks on an olive oil-enriched diet decreased the tendency of whole blood to agonist-induced aggregation.[126]

Fruits and vegetables are good sources of soluble fiber but they also contain a plethora of phytochemicals that have antioxidant functions. Fruit and vegetable intake, especially green leafy vegetable and vitamin C-rich fruits, is associated with reduced risk for CHD.[127] One of the mechanisms is the lowering of LDL oxidation that in turn reduces the inflammatory response and prevents or decreases the formation of foam cells and atherosclerotic plaques. Some vegetables are good sources of folate, a vitamin important in lowering homocysteine levels. Elevated homocysteine is an independent risk factor for CHD, and frequent consumption of fruits and vegetables tends to lower homocysteine levels.[128]

Certain phytochemicals have antithrombotic and anticoagulation properties that also help in reducing the risk for CHD. Organosulfur compounds found in garlic lowers blood coagulability by reducing fibrinogen and increasing fibrinolysis and inhibiting platelet aggregation.[129] Polyphenols found in cocoa and grape juice inhibit platelet aggregation,[130] and frequent consumption of polyphenol-rich foods decreases mortality from thrombosis and CHD.[131] Thus, including a variety of fruits and vegetables provides the antioxidants and other phytochemicals that reduce CHD risk beyond lowering blood lipids.

The type of fatty acid predominant in the diet also determines the susceptibility of LDL to oxidation. Vegetarian diets decrease susceptibility of LDL to oxidation,[132] despite their higher dietary PUFA intake. This could be because of the higher amount of antioxidants present in vegetarian diets compared with omnivore diet. Eating fish increases susceptibility of LDL to oxidation perhaps due to the high amounts of EPA in the fish and lower antioxidant in the diet.[133]

B. BREAST CANCER

Breast cancer is the second leading cause of cancer deaths among women, with 27.9 deaths per 100,000 women occurring per year.[8] According to the American Cancer Society, populations consuming primarily plant-based diets have a lower incidence of breast cancer than populations eating a Western-type diet. For instance, mortality from breast cancer in the U.S. is five times greater than in China, four times greater than in Japan and three times greater than in Mexico.[134] However, the Adventist Health Study did not find a strong association between intake of animal products and the risk of breast cancer.[135] Comparing current use of meat, poultry and fish, those that used these foods more than 3 times a week had a nonsignificant relative risk of 1.33 compared with those who never ate these foods. This showed that breast cancer risk was only weakly associated with meat consumption.

Aromatic amines such as heterocyclic amines are formed during thermal processing of protein foods, primarily meats, and have proven to be potent mutagens.[136] A cohort of the Iowa Women's Health Study was evaluated for the potential role of heterocyclic amines and risk of breast cancer.[137] A dose–response relationship was found between the consumption of well-done meat and breast cancer risk. Women who consumed meats very well done had 4.62 times higher risk of breast cancer than women who consumed the meats rare or medium done. In contrast, the consumption of red meats with concentrated sources of heterocyclic amines was not associated with increased breast cancer risk.[138] Based on potential mutagenic effects of heterocyclic amines on mammary cells, further studies are warranted to clarify the risk associated with the consumption of well-done red meats.

The role of total amount of fat consumed by an individual in modifying the risk of breast cancer is still debated. Meta-analyses of about 13 studies suggest that reducing total fat consumption to 20% of energy or lower significantly reduces circulating levels of estradiol, which may help lower the risk of breast cancer.[139] In fact, it has been shown that a reduction in total fat consumption reduces circulatory estradiol levels by 7% in premenopausal women and 23% in postmenopausal women in Western populations. Others,[140,141] however, have found no association between total fat intake and risk of breast cancer. The type of fatty acid may influence breast cancer risk more than the total amount of fat.

There is substantial evidence that n-6 PUFA enhances the risk for breast cancer and metastasis while n-3 PUFA and monounsaturated fatty acids reduce the risk.[142] Rat studies on mammary carcinogenesis indicate that n-6 PUFA such as arachidonic acid upregulates COX-2 enzyme expression.[143] This increases prostaglandin synthesis in the mammary glands, which in part may explain the tumor-promoting effects of n-6 PUFA. A study *in vitro* further provides evidence that arachidonic acid may be involved in inducing cell cycle progression and unregulated gene expression.[144] Fatty acids derived from fish such as EPA and DHA and also vegetarian diets that include oils rich in n-3 PUFA and monounsaturated fatty acids will be able to reduce the production of tumor-promoting eicosanoids.

A case-control study on 451 women with breast cancer and controls showed that women with high fiber intakes had less than half the risk of breast cancer than women with lower fiber intakes.[145] A review of 40 case-control studies found an odds ratio of less than 1 for breast cancer incidence when comparing high vs. low intake of whole grains.[146] Supplementing wheat bran to increase fiber intake from 15 g to 30 g/day significantly reduced serum estradiol levels in 62 premenopausal women.[147] This may be a mechanism by which fiber reduces the risk for breast cancer.

Breast cancer incidence is relatively rare in Japan and China compared with Western countries, suggesting that some component of the Asian diet may offer protection against breast cancer. One such dietary component is soy. Soy isoflavone genistein exhibits weak estrogenic properties by binding to estrogen receptor sites and competing with the much more potent estrogen.[148] Regular consumption of soyfoods was associated with a marked decrease in breast cancer risk in premenopausal women, with an odds ratio of 0.39 for the highest fifth compared with the lowest fifth of intake of total soy foods.[149] However, the Iowa Women's Study cohort showed that comparing women who consumed any soy with those who ate no soy had a relative risk of 0.76, but this was not significant. Preliminary evidence suggests that consumption of soy early in life may reduce breast cancer risk later in life,[150,151] but this has to be substantiated with more studies. On the other hand, isoflavones in soy may stimulate existing tumors in the breast and thus, women with current or past breast cancer should be aware of the potential risks when taking soy products.[152]

Urinary excretion of total isoflavones was significantly less in patients with breast cancer compared with controls, suggesting that high consumption of soy foods may decrease risk of breast cancer.[153] One of the mechanisms by which isoflavones seem to reduce the risk is by regulating expression of apoptosis-related genes and inhibiting growth of breast cancer cells.154 Another mechanism is via modifying menstrual cycle length in premenopausal women. Longer menstrual cycle is associated with a lowered risk of breast cancer and an average isoflavone intake of 32–200 mg/d increased cycle length by 1.1 days.[155] The evidence supporting the use of soy in reducing breast cancer risk is inconsistent or weak and further studies are needed before recommendations can be made.

C. Ovarian Cancer

Ovarian cancer is another female-specific disease that may be positively affected by a vegetarian diet. Animal product consumption was strongly associated with ovarian cancer death, with significant increases in risk with egg more than meat consumption.[156] It has been suggested that women might lower their risk of ovarian cancer by reducing the intake of saturated fats and eating more fruits and vegetables.[157,158] Significantly reduced risk of ovarian cancer was associated specifically with higher intakes of dietary fiber, carotenoids, β-carotene and vitamins A and E.

Various studies show beneficial effects of plant foods in relation to ovarian cancer. For instance, Zhang et al.[157] showed that ovarian cancer incidence appeared to increase for women who preferred fat, fried, cured and smoked foods. Meats tend to be the foods that are mostly prepared by such processes. Another case-control study[159] demonstrated significant trends of increasing risk of ovarian cancer with red meat consumption (odds ratio = 1.53 for the highest vs. lowest quintile of consumption). Inverse relationships were, however, observed for fish, vegetables and pulses.

A meta-analysis of 3782 subjects from five observational studies[160] reported that a high vs. low dietary intake of beta-carotene is associated with a 16% reduction in the risk of ovarian cancer. Carotenoids such as lutein and zeaxanthin seem to be especially protective with respect to ovarian cancer. In a population-based study,[161] participants with the highest intakes of carotenoids experienced a 40% lower risk of ovarian cancer. One of the highest sources of carotenoids and lutein is green leafy vegetables, higher intakes of which were more strongly associated with a decreased risk of ovarian cancer than total vegetable intake.[159] Intake of lycopene was significantly and inversely related to risk of ovarian cancer, especially in premenopausal women. Food items most strongly related to decreased risk were raw carrots and tomato sauce. Consumption of carotenoid- and lycopene-rich fruits and vegetables may be important in reducing risk of ovarian cancer.

D. Osteoporosis

A major concern among women, particularly during the postmenopausal years and primarily among those of Caucasian and Asian origin, is osteoporosis. Osteoporosis is characterized by loss of bone density, making particular bones like the hip, spine and wrist susceptible to fractures. In the United States, almost 34 million individuals are estimated to have low bone mass, thus placing them at increased risk for osteoporosis.[162] Many different factors ,including gender, physical activity, age, ethnicity, smoking, alcohol use, body weight/frame, estrogen level, calcium, vitamin D status and dietary protein quality, influence bone density.

Several cross-sectional studies have compared the bone health of vegetarians with omnivores and these are summarized in Table 20.6. A more in-depth review is published elsewhere.[163] Age-related bone loss is slower in LOVs than in omnivores. However, vegans consuming an exclusively plant-based diet may be at higher risk of exceeding lumbar spine fracture threshold and of being classified as having osteopenia of the femoral neck. Vegans have lower protein and a lower calcium: protein ratio than LOVs and omnivores, suggesting that total protein intake may be an important predictor of bone density. Others have observed no differences in bone mineral density among vegetarians and nonvegetarians after matching for age, height, weight, menarche and medical histories.[164] In spite of dietary differences in the two groups, no differences were observed in bone mineral density or other aspects of bone physiology. These studies, however, did not separate LOVs from vegans, which may have altered the findings on risk of osteoporosis differently. Further studies, with a more systematic approach including larger sample sizes of vegans, LOVs and omnivores, needs to be considered in the future.

TABLE 20.6

Summary of Studies on Vegetarian Population and BMD

Subjects	Diet practice	Outcome variable	Result
Postmenopausal	LOV/Omnivore (n = 25)	BMD of third metacarpal	LOV > Omnivore
Premenopausal	LOV/Omnivore (n = 51)	BMC of cortical site	LOV > Omnivore
Postmenopausal	LOV/Omnivore (n = 10)	Bone loss by 80 yrs of age	18% LOV vs. 36% Omnivore
Postmenopausal	Vegan/LOV/Omnivore (n = 258)	BMD at lumbar spine	Vegans at highest risk of spine fracture, osteopenia of femoral neck
Premenopausal	Vegan/LOV/Omnivore	BMD at lumbar spine	Vegan < LOV, Ominvore
Premenopausal	Vegetarian*/Omnivore (n = 15/20)	BMD	Vegetarian < Omnivore
Postmenopausal	Vegetarian*/Omnivore (n = 109)	BMD at hip	Vegetarian < Omnivore
Premenopausal	Vegetarian*/Omnivore (n = 27/37)	BMD of spine	No difference
Postmenopausal	Vegetarian*/Omnivore (n = 28)	BMD of trabecula and cortical bone	No difference
Postmenopausal	LOV/Omnivore (n = 88/287)	BMC and BMD of mid and distal radius	No difference
Postmenopausal	LOV/Omnivore (n = 49/140)	BMD of radius	No difference
Postmenopausal	LOV/Omnivore (n = 144/106)	BMC	No difference

*Vegetarians include both vegan and LOV; BMC is bone mineral content; BMD is bone mineral density.

Source: From Sabaté, J (Ed); *Vegetarian Nutrition.* CRC Press, 2001.

Animal protein increases risk of bone loss and urinary excretion of calcium, while plant proteins seem to reduce such risks.[165,166] Sellmeyer et al.[165] demonstrated that an increase in vegetable protein intake and a decrease in animal protein intake reduces bone loss and the risk of hip fracture. Similar findings were observed in the Nurses Health Study. The relative risk of forearm fracture was higher in women who consumed red meat five or more times a week compared with those who consumed meat less than once a week.[167]

Animal proteins contain high amounts of sulfur-containing amino acids, which are highly correlated with renal net acid excretion.[168–170] This has a negative effect on calcium balance since acidosis tends to stimulate osteoclastic activity and inhibit osteoblastic activity. Ball and Maughan[169] showed that, although dietary calcium intakes were no different between vegetarians and omnivores, urinary calcium excretion of the omnivores was significantly higher than that of the vegetarians. Although the endogenous acid production explains to some extent the increased loss of calcium in the urine with animal protein intake, the effects of acid load on the incidence of osteoporotic fracture are unclear.

One of the main differences between vegan and LOV diets is the inclusion of dairy products in the latter group. Calcium intervention trials using dairy as the source of calcium have shown that dairy consumption causes greater bone gain, decreased bone loss or decreased fracture risk.[171] Adequate intake of calcium through the consumption of dairy products in childhood and adolescence was an important marker for attaining peak bone mass and for the prevention of osteoporosis later in life.[172,173] The vast majority of studies lend support to the inclusion of dairy products to maintain bone mineral density (BMD) and reduce osteoporosis in women.

Differences in BMD between LOV and vegans may also be due to the differences in the calcium:protein ratio.[174] Since LOVs consume dairy, their calcium intake would be higher than that of vegans, who rely mostly on green vegetables from which calcium bioavailability is low. Those following a vegan diet are advised to identify calcium-fortified foods and plant foods containing highly bioavailable calcium or use appropriate calcium supplements to meet this need.

Vegetarians typically tend to consume more servings of fruits and vegetables compared with omnivores. Cross-sectional assessment of BMD at hip and forearm in women from the Framingham Heart Study showed that fruit and vegetable consumption was positively associated with BMD in women.[175] Minerals such as magnesium, potassium and boron, which are found in fruits and vegetables, also have a positive impact on bone health. They provide an alkaline milieu that best preserves BMD.[176] Although the evidence is limited at this time to link fruit and vegetable consumption to improved bone health, it is still prudent to encourage increased consumption of these foods to obtain other health benefits they offer.

A prospective study on Japanese women[177] demonstrated a positive association between soybean intake and BMD even after adjusting for confounders. An increase in bone mineral content and BMD in lumbar spine was noted in a group of women who received isoflavone (2.25 mg/g protein) compared with women who received casein supplement.[178] The soy isoflavone has a bone sparing effect that is mediated via stimulating bone formation rather than slowing bone resorption.[179] Also soy proteins are low in sulfur-containing amino acids and thus decrease calcium excretion. Since long-term studies are sparse, future studies have to look at how much soy and how long it needs to be consumed to derive benefits that are significant to bone health.

E. OBESITY AND OVERWEIGHT

Obesity and overweight in the U.S. are at an all-time high and the prevalence of overweight in females aged 20–74 has increased from 27% in the period 1976–1980 to 37% in the period 1988–94.[8] About 50.7% of women in the U.S. have a BMI score greater than or equal to 25.0.[180] Addressing obesity and overweight requires a comprehensive approach to exercise, dietary adjustment and behavior modification. Usually, males tend to address weight problems by exercising, while females concentrate more on dieting.

Various diet patterns have been researched to determine efficacy in weight loss or management. These include low-carbohydrate diets ($\leq 20\%$ energy from CHO), very-low-fat diets ($\leq 10\%$ energy from total fat), moderate-fat/high-carbohydrate diets (20–30% energy from fat and $> 55\%$ energy from CHO) and high-protein diets.[181]

Overall, any diet with an energy deficit will promote weight loss. Kennedy et al.[181] found that energy intakes were lowest for subjects eating low-fat diets, including a vegetarian diet, and BMI was lowest for women who were in the vegetarian group and the high-carbohydrate/low-fat group as opposed to all other dietary group assignments. In fact, the highest BMIs were noted for those on low-carbohydrate diets.

There are other studies that also show that long-term vegetarians tend to be leaner than their omnivore counterparts. For instance, in the study by Hebbelinck et al.,[182] it was observed that vegetarian subjects had lower relative body weights and skinfold thickness during adolescence than did nonvegetarians. Apparently, nonmeat eaters tend to be thinner than meat eaters, partly because of their higher intakes of dietary fiber and lower intake of animal fat.

However, between similarly health-conscious vegetarian and nonvegetarian women, there is no real difference in relative weight and weight loss efforts.[183] Furthermore, a well-planned LOV diet is not necessarily more beneficial for weight control and skinfold thickness than a balanced mixed diet.[184] In fact, one of the studies showed that subjects on the mixed diet experienced more weight loss (10.4 kg) and maintenance over a 1-year period than their LOV counterparts (9.2 kg).

Clearly, addressing obesity or overweight by dietary measures must involve a calorie deficit. Well-balanced vegetarian diets can typically provide such deficits due to lower intakes of high-saturated-fat foods and higher intakes of fruits, vegetables, legumes and grains. This does not mean that vegetarian diets in general promote weight loss since some vegetarian diets may be high in total and saturated fat. A "vegetarian advantage" will be realized if a well-planned vegetarian diet is used in conjunction with physical activity.

VI. PRACTICAL CONSIDERATIONS FOR VEGETARIAN WOMEN

There are different types of vegetarian diets and several motivating factors for choosing a vegetarian lifestyle. Careful planning is essential to achieve optimum nutrition; a practical approach to accomplish this is to follow a food guide. Food guides provide a foundation for choosing the type and amounts of foods that are needed to provide adequate nutrition. Each food group in the guide has a range for recommended servings/day. This is because the energy and nutrient requirement of individuals differ and those with a lower energy need can select the minimum servings while those with higher energy needs can select the higher servings of the foods in each group. Counseling with a registered dietitian can also provide tailor-made recommendations while addressing the individual's likes and dislikes.

According to Healthy People 2000 guidelines,[8] all diet planning should focus on three objectives:

1. Maintaining a healthy body weight by selecting the appropriate calorie level
2. Including regular physical activity
3. Including a variety of fruits, vegetables, legumes and whole grains and choosing sensibly the amount and type of fat, sugar and salt to be included in the daily diet

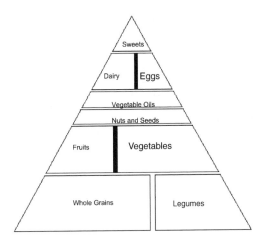

FIGURE 20.1 Loma Linda University Vegetarian Food Guide Pyramid. *Note*: A reliable source of vitamin B_{12} should be included if no dairy or eggs are consumed.

A healthy vegetarian diet should include a variety of plant foods. When different food items are selected from each food group there is greater variety, and such diets are more likely to meet nutritional needs than one that is limited to just a few foods.

Several food guides are available to vegetarians but they are typically adapted from guides developed for nonvegetarians, such as the USDA's food guide pyramid.[185] This may not be appropriate because there are differences in the emphasis of food groups in a vegetarian diet compared with an omnivore diet. Figure 20.1 is the Vegetarian Food Guide that was developed and presented at the Third International Congress on Vegetarian Nutrition at Loma Linda University.[186] Table 20.7 provides the serving sizes and number of servings of each food group depicted in the food pyramid for planning a nutritionally adequate vegetarian diet.

Whole grains and legumes form the base of the pyramid because these foods are energy dense and provide significant amounts of calories and plant proteins. The emphasis is to include more of the whole grains and less of the refined products to allow for adequate fiber intake. Also, whole grains provide more phytochemicals that might otherwise be lost during the refining and processing of grains. Commonly used grains include whole wheat, rice and corn, although oats, rye, sorghum and other millets are recommended for inclusion in the diet for variety. Including grains in every meal will help meet the 5–12 servings that are recommended.

Consumption of legumes in the Western countries is limited compared with some Asian and Mediterranean populations.[187] However, in vegetarian diets, legumes, soy and meat substitutes play an important role in providing proteins. Legumes include beans (pinto, kidney, lima, mung) and peas (garbanzo, split peas, black-eyed peas and lentils) and, besides protein, they also provide fiber, folate, calcium and iron. They contain oligosaccharides, which promote the growth of the beneficial bifido bacteria in the colon.[188] Legumes can cause flatulence that can be minimized by using lentils that are less gas producing or use cooking methods such as soaking to reduce the gas-producing sugars.

TABLE 20.7
Vegetarian Food Guide Pyramid: Suggested Number of Servings and Serving Sizes

Food Group	Number of Servings	Suggested Serving Sizes
Whole Grains	5–12	1 slice bread, 28 g
		1/2 bun, bagel, muffin, 60 g
		1/2 cup cooked cereal, rice, pasta, 76 g
		1/2 cup flaked cereal, 22 g
		1 1/2 cup puffed cereal, 21 g
Legumes	1–3	1/2 cup cooked beans, lentils, peas, 80-88 g
		4 oz tofu or tempeh, 114 g
		1 cup soy beverage, 244 g
Vegetables	6–9	1 cup raw vegetable, 180 g
		1/2 cup cooked vegetable, 91 g
		3/4 cup vegetable juice, 181 g
Fruits	3–4	1 piece fresh fruit, 110 g
		1 cup cubed fresh fruit (melons, berries), 170 g
		3/4 cup 100% fruit juice, 185 g
		1/2 cup canned or cooked fruit, 80 g
Nuts and Seeds	1	1 ounce nuts, 28 g
		2 Tbsp ground nuts or seeds, 24 g
Vegetable Oils	4–7	1 tsp vegetable oil, 4.5 g
Dairy	0–2	1 cup milk or yogurt, 244 g
		1 ounce cheese, 28 g
		1/2 cup cottage cheese, 56 g
Eggs	0–1	1 egg, 50 g
		2 egg whites, 66 g
Sweets		Use sparingly

Source: From Sabaté, J. (Ed)., *Vegetarian Nutrition*. CRC Press, 2001.

Soybeans are an excellent source of proteins for vegetarians. Soy is used in a variety of ways such as soy beverages, soy-based meat substitutes, soy nuts and tofu. Soymilk is also used instead of cow's milk by strict vegetarians and those with lactose intolerance. Meat substitutes are mainly made from soybeans and whey proteins and are made to look and taste like meat. Some of these are plant foods, while others may contain egg or milk components. Meat substitutes add variety to vegan diets but are not essential for meeting protein needs.

The middle layer of the vegetarian food guide is made up of fruits and vegetables. Vegetables should be part of all diets since they provide fiber, antioxidants, micro-nutrients and phytochemicals. Green leafy vegetables provide calcium, an important source for vegans. Fruits are typically consumed fresh, dried, frozen or as juice. Although there is a place for fruit juices in the diet, eating fresh and dried fruits increases the variety of phytonutrients and amount of fiber that can be obtained. In children, consuming too much fruit juice may displace other nutrient-rich foods and should be included with caution. Typically, vegetarians consume the minimum recommended servings of fruits and vegetables. Efforts to increase this to the upper end of the recommendation should be made.

Vegetarians also consume more nuts and seeds than omnivores. Nuts provide healthy fats and are a concentrated source of energy, fiber, calcium, folate, arginine, B-vitamins and iron. Some, like peanuts and almonds, are also good sources of protein. Nuts and seeds provide α-linolenic acid, the essential n-3 fatty acid. Since vegetarians do not consume a direct source of EPA and DHA this becomes important. The vegetarian food guide also recommends four to seven servings of oils and fats. In Western diets, the fat primarily comes from meat and dairy, increasing the amount of saturated fat. In vegan diets, vegetable oils typically used include canola, olive and flaxseed oils, all of which provide either monounsaturated fats or n-3 PUFA or a combination of the two. Strict vegetarians also tend to avoid highly processed foods that may contain trans fatty acids. It is best to avoid hydrogenated fats and replace them with oils containing healthy fats or use soft margarine to reduce trans fatty acid intake.

Milk, cheese and yogurt are foods commonly used by LOVs. Individuals who drink milk consume 70–80% more calcium than those who do not. An LOV diet that includes dairy products should include low-fat or no-fat options so the saturated fat intake is kept minimal. Vegans have to pay more attention to their intake of calcium and vitamin B_{12} because they do not include foods from the milk food group. Soy beverages are used instead of cow's milk by vegans and can provide similar amounts of protein but varied amounts of calcium and vitamin B_{12}. One has to read the nutrient label to make sure they are getting adequate calcium and vitamin B_{12} and, if not, include other foods that can provide the same.

To successfully follow a healthy vegetarian diet, individuals opting for a vegetarian lifestyle should make gradual changes in their dietary habits so that the changes are long term. Planning is essential for both LOV and vegan diets and there are several resources available besides the food guide that one can use for this purpose. Table 20.8 lists some of the key resources on vegetarian diets that might help someone planning to be a vegetarian.

VII. CONCLUSION

Optimizing the diet to meet nutrient needs or to prevent disease and promote health comes from careful planning, whether the diet is nonvegetarian or vegetarian. Since there is some restriction with vegetarian diets and more so with vegan diets, they call for extra attention in planning for ensuring adequacy. LOV diets can provide all nutrients but they may increase intake of saturated fat if full-fat dairy foods are chosen. Vegan diets provide all nutrients except vitamin B_{12}. This can be obtained by including fortified foods or a supplement. Also, calcium may be difficult to obtain unless appropriate foods are selected and hence, for some women, a calcium supplement may be required. Overall, a well-planned vegetarian diet does provide adequate nutrition and also helps in promoting health.[189] In addition, vegetarian diets

---

TABLE 20.8
Available Vegetarian Nutrition Resources

Organizations

Vegetarian Nutrition Dietetic Practice Group of the American Dietetic Association	www.vegetariannutrition.net
Seventh-Day Adventist Dietetic Association	www.sdada.org
Vegetarian Resource Group	www.vrg.org
The American Vegan Society	www.americanvegan.org
North American Vegetarian Society	www.navs-online.org

Books

Vegetarian Nutrition	Joan Sabaté (Ed), CRC Press, 2001
The Dietitian's Guide to Vegetarian Nutrition	Messina, M and Messina V, Aspen Publishers, Gaithersburg, MD 1996.

Magazines

Vegetarian Times	www.vegetariantimes.com
Vegetarian Newsletter	www.llu.edu/llu/vegetarian/
Veggie Life	www.veggielife.com

---

that include significant servings of fruits, vegetables, legumes, whole grains and nuts do decrease the risk for several chronic diseases such as heart disease, some cancers, osteoporosis and obesity that are commonly seen in women. Even for those who eat an omnivore diet, it is prudent to increase the intake of these foods to derive the health benefits provided by these plant foods.

REFERENCES

1. Johnston, P.K., Vegetarians among us: Implications for health professionals, *Top Clin Nutr*, 10, 1, 1995.
2. Stahler, C., How many vegetarians are there?, *Vegetarian J*, 13, 6, 1994.
3. Sabaté J, Ratzin-Turner R.A., Brown J.E., Vegetarian diets: Descriptions and trends, in *Vegetarian Nutrition*, Sabaté, J. Ed., CRC Press, Boca Raton, FL 2001, chap. 2.
4. Messina, V., Burke, K., Position of the American Dietetic Association, Vegetarian Diets, *J Am Diet Assoc,* 97, 1317, 1997.
5. Messina, M., Messina, V., *The Dietitian's Guide to Vegetarian Diets*, Aspen Publishers, Gaithersburg, MD, 1996, chap. 1.
6. Burr, M.L., Butland, B.K., Heart disease in British vegetarians, *Am J Clin Nutr*, 48, 830, 1988.
7. Dwyer, J.T., Palombo, R., Valadian, I., Reed, R.B., Preschoolers on alternate lifestyle diets, *J Am Diet Assoc*, 72, 264, 1978.
8. Department of Health and Human Services, Public Health Service, Healthy People 2000 Progress Review: Women's Health, May 20, 1998.

9. Tanzman, J.S., Sabaté, J., Prevalence of vegetarianism in the United States, presented at the Fourth International Congress on Vegetarian Nutrition, Loma Linda University; Loma Linda, April 8–11, 2002.

10. Murray, J., Vegetarian growth continues, *Food Serv Director*, 6, 74, 1993.

11. Havala, S., Dwyer, J., Position of the American Dietetic Association: Vegetarian diets, *J Am Diet Assoc,* 93, 1317, 1993.

12. Hardinge, M., Nutritional studies of vegetarians, *Am J Clin Nutr*, 2, 73 1943.

13. Joint Food and Agricultural Organization/World Health Organization/United Nations University Expert Consultation, *World Health Organization Technical Report Series 724*, World Health Organization, Geneva, Switzerland, 1985.

14. Acosta, P.B., Availability of essential amino acids and nitrogen in vegan diets, *Am J Clin Nutr,* 48, 868, 1988.

15. Scrimshaw, N.S., Wayler, A.H., Murray, E., Steinke, F.H. Rand, W.M. Young, V.R., Nitrogen balance studies in young men to assess the protein quality of an isolated soy protein in relation to meat proteins, *J Nutr*, 113, 2485, 1983.

16. Emken, E.A., Adolf, R.O., Gulley, R.M., Dietary linoleic acid influences desaturation and acylation of deuterium-labeled linoleic and linolenic acids in young adult males, *Biochim Biophys Acta*, 1213, 277, 1994.

17. Conquer, J., Holub, B., Docosahexaenoic acid (omega-3) and vegetarian nutrition. *Veg Nutr*, 1, 42, 1997.

18. Melchert, H.U., Limsthayourat, N., Mihajlovic, H., Eichberg, J., Thefeld, W., Rottka, H., Fatty acid patterns in triglycerides, diglycerides, free fatty acids, cholesteryl esters and phosphotidylcholine in serum from vegetarians and nonvegetarians, *Atherosclerosis*, 65, 159, 1987.

19. Phinney, S.D., Odin, R.S., Johnson, S.B., Holman, R.T., Reduced arachidonate in serum phospholipids and cholesteryl esters associated with vegetarian diets in humans, *Am J Clin Nutr,* 51, 385, 1990.

20. Sanders, T.A.B., Roshanai, F., Platelet phospholipid fatty acid composition in vegans compared with age- and sex-matched omnivore controls, *Eur J Clin Nutr*, 46, 823, 1992.

21. Haddad, E.H., Berk, L.S., Ketterin, J.D., Hubbard, R.W., Peters, W.R., Dietary intake and biochemical, hematologic and immune status of vegans compared with nonvegetarians, *Am J Clin Nutr*, 70s, 586s, 1999.

22. Sanders, T.A.B., Ellis, F.R., Dickerson, J.W., Studies of vegans: The fatty acid composition of plasma choline phosphoglycerides, erythrocytes, adipose tissue and breast milk and some indicators of susceptibility to ischemic heart disease in vegans and omnivore controls, *Am J Clin Nutr*, 31, 805, 1978.

23. Fisher, M., Levine, P.H., Weiner, B., Ockene, I.S., Johhnson, B., Johnson, M.H., Natale, A.M., Vaudreuil, C.H., Hoogasian, J., The effects of vegetarian diets on plasma lipid and platelet levels, *Arch Intern Med*, 146, 1193, 1986.

24. Rosado, J.L., Lopez, P., Morales, M., Munoz, E., Allen, L.H., Bioavailability of energy, nitrogen, fat, zinc, iron and calcium from rural and urban Mexican diets, *Br J Nutr*, 68, 45, 1992.

25. Kramer, L. ., Osis, D., Coffey, J., Spencer, H., Mineral and trace element content of vegetarian diets, *J Am Coll Nutr,* 3, 3, 1984.

26. Monsen, E.R., Iron nutrition and absorption: Dietary factors which impact iron bioavailability, *J Am Diet Assoc*, 88, 786, 1988.

27. Charlton, R.W., Bothwell, T.H., Iron absorption, *Ann Rev Med*, 34, 55, 1983.

28. Hallberg, L., Bioavailability of dietary iron in man, *Ann Rev Nutr*, 1, 123, 1981.

29. Craig, W.J., Iron status of vegetarians, *Am J Clin Nutr,* 59[5 Suppl], 1233S, 1994.

30. Reddy, S. and Sanders, T.A., Haematological studies on premenopausal Indian and Caucasian vegetarians compared with Caucasian omnivores, *Br. J. Nutr*, 64, 331, 1990.
31. Hunt, J.R., Roughead, Z.K., Nonheme-iron absorption, fecal ferritin excretion and blood indexes of iron status in women consuming controlled lacto-ovo vegetarian diets for 8 wk, *Am J Clin Nutr*, 69, 944, 1999.
32. Salonen, J.T., Nyyssonen, K., Korpela, H., Tuomilehto, J., Seppanen, R., Salonen, R., High stored iron levels are associated with excess risk of myocardial infarction in eastern Finnish men, *Circulation*, 86, 803, 1992.
33. Dagnelie, P.C., van Staveren, W.A., Vergote, F.J., Dingjan, P.G., van den Berg, H., Hautvast, J.G., Increased risk of vitamin B_{12} and iron deficiency in infants on macrobiotic diets, *Am J Clin Nutr*, 50, 818, 1989.
34. Ball, M.J., Bartlett, M.A., Dietary intake and iron status of Australian vegetarian women, *Am J Clin Nutr*, 70, 353, 1999
35. Prasad, A., Nutritional zinc today, *Nutr Today*, 16, 4, 1981.
36. Gibson, R.S., Heath, A.L., Limbaga, M.L., Prosser, N., Skeaff, C.M., Are changes in food consumption patterns associated with lower biochemical zinc status among women from Dunedin, New Zealand? *British J Nutr*, 86, 71, 2001.
37. Weaver, C.M., Proulx, W.R., Heaney, R., Choices for achieving adequate dietary calcium with a vegetarian diet, *Am J Clin Nutr*, 70[3 Suppl], 543S, 1999.
38. Fleming, K.H. and Heimbach, J.T., Consumption of calcium in the U.S.: Food sources and intake levels, *J Nutr*, 124, 1426S, 1994.
39. Heaney, R.P., Dowell, M.S., Rafferty, K., Bierman, J., Bioavailability of the calcium in fortified soy imitation milk, with some observations on method, *Am J Clin Nutr*, 71, 1166, 2000.
40. Heller, H.J., Stewart, A., Haynes, S., Pak, C.Y., Pharmacokinetics of calcium absorption from two commercial calcium supplements, *J Clin Pharmacol*, 39, 1151, 1999.
41. McBean, L.D., Forgac T. and Finn, S.C., Osteoporosis: Visions for care and prevention — A conference report, *J Am Diet Assoc*, 94, 668, 1994.
42. Kerstetter, J.E., Allen, L.H., Dietary protein increases urinary calcium, *J Nutr*, 120, 134, 1990.
43. Barzel, U.S., Massey, L.K., Excess dietary protein can adversely affect bone, *J Nutr*, 128, 1051, 1998.
44. Recker, R.R., Davies, K.M., Hinders, S.M., Heaney, R.P., Stegman, M.R., Kimmel, D.B., Bone gain in young adult women, *J Am Med Assoc*, 268, 2403, 1992.
45. Outila, T.A., Karkkainen, M.U., Seppanen, R.H., Lamberg-Allardt, C.J., Dietary intake of vitamin D in premenopausal, healthy vegans was insufficient to maintain concentrations of serum 25-hydroxyvitamin D and intact parathyroid hormone within normal ranges during the winter in Finland, *J Am Diet Assoc*, 100, 434, 2000.
46. Haddad, J.G., Vitamin D — Solar rays, the milky way, or both, *N Engl J Med*, 326, 1213, 1992.
47. Miller, D.R., Specker, B.L., Ho, M.L., Norman, E.J., Vitamin B_{12} status in a macrobiotic community, *Am J Clin Nutr*, 53, 524, 1991.
48. Herrmann, W., Schorr, H., Purschwitz, K., Rassoul, F., Richter, V., Total homocysteine, vitamin B_{12} and total antioxidant status in vegetarians, *Clin Chem*, 47, 1094, 2001.
49. Crane, M.G., Vitamin B_{12} studies in total vegetarians [vegans], *J Nutr Med*, 4, 419, 1994.
50. Grahamn, S.M., Arvela, O.M. and Wise, G.A., Long-term neurologic consequences of nutritional vitamin B12 deficiency in infants, *J Pediatr*, 121, 710, 1992.

51. Hung, C.J., Huang, P.C., Lu, S.C., Li, Y.H., Huang, H.B., Lin, B.F., Chang, S.J., Chou, H.F., Plasma homocysteine levels in Taiwanese vegetarians are higher than those of omnivores, *J Nutr*, 132, 152, 2002.
52. Butterworth, Jr., C.E. and Bendich, A., Folic acid and the prevention of birth defects, *Ann Rev Nutr*, 16, 73, 1996.
53. Herbert, V. and Drivas, G., Spirulina and vitamin B_{12}, *J Am Med Assoc*, 248, 3096, 1982.
54. Ward, R.J., Abraham, R., McFadyen, I.R., Haines, A.D., North, W.R., Patel, M. Bhatt, R.V., Assessment of trace metal intake and status in a Gujarati pregnant Asian population and their influence on the outcome of pregnancy, *Br J Obstet Gynaecol*, 95, 676, 1988.
55. King, J.C., Stein, T. and Doyle, M., Effect of vegetarianism on the zinc status of pregnant women, *Am J Clin Nutr*, 34, 1049, 1981.
56. Shull, M.W., Reed, R.B., Valadian, I., Palombo, R., Thorne, H., Dwyer, J.T., Velocities of growth in vegetarian preschool children, *Pediatrics*, 60, 410, 1977.
57. Drake, R., Reddy, S. and Davis, J., Nutrient intake during pregnancy and pregnancy outcome of lacto-ovo-vegetarians, fish-eaters and nonvegetarians, *Veg Nutr*, 2, 45, 1998.
58. Finley, D.A., Lonnerdal, B., Dewey, K.G., Grivetti, L.E., Breast milk composition: Fat content and fatty acid composition in vegetarians and nonvegetarians, *Am J Clin Nutr*, 41, 787, 1985.
59. Sanders, T.A.B., Reddy, S., Infant brain lipids and diet, *Lancet*, 304, 1093, 1992.
60. Reddy, S., Sanders, T.A., Obeid, O., The influence of maternal vegetarian diet on essential fatty acid status of the newborn, *Eur J Clin Nutr*, 48, 358, 1994.
61. Sanders, T.A., Essential fatty acid requirements of vegetarians in pregnancy, lactation and infancy, *J Clin Nutr*, 70, 555S, 1999.
62. Kuhne, T., Bubl, R. and Baumgartner, R. Maternal vegan diet causing a serious infantile neurological disorder due to vitamin B_{12} deficiency, *Eur J Pediatr*, 150, 205, 1991.
63. Koebnick, C., Heins, U.A., Hoffmann, I., Dagnielie, P.C., Leitzmann, C., Folate status during pregnancy in women is improved by long-term high vegetable intake compared with the average western diet, *J Nutr*, 131, 733, 2001.
64. Sanders, T.A.B. and Reddy, S., Nutritional implications of a meatless diet, *Proc Nutr Soc*, 53, 297, 1994.
65. Hardinge, M.G. and Stare, F.J., Nutritional studies of vegetarians. I. Nutritional, physical and laboratory studies, *J Clin Nutr*, 2, 73, 1954.
66. Hunt, J.R., Matthys, L.A. and Johnson, L.K., Zinc absorption, mineral balance and blood lipids in women consuming controlled lacto-ovo-vegetarian and omnivorous diets for 8 wks, *Am J Clin Nutr*, 67, 421, 1998.
67. Specker, B.L., Wey, H.E. and Miller, D., Differences in fatty acid composition of human milk in vegetarian and nonvegetarian women: Long-term effect of diet, *J Pediatr Gastroent, Nutr*, 6, 764, 1987.
68. Willatts, P., Forsyth, J.S., DiModugno, M.D., Varma, S., Colvin, M., Effect of long-chain polyunsaturated fatty acids in infant formula on problem solving at 10 months of age, *Lancet*, 352, 688, 1998.
69. Uauy, R., Peirano, P., Hoffman, D., Mena, P., Birch, D., Birch, E., Role of essential fatty acids in the function of the developing nervous system, *Lipids*, 31, 167S, 1996.

70. Cunnane, S.C., Francescutti, V., Brenna, J.T., Crawford, M.A., Breast-fed infants achieve a higher rate of brain and whole body docosahexaenoate accumulation than formula-fed infants not consuming dietary docosahexaenoate, *Lipids*, 35[1], 105, 2000.

71. Specker, B. L., Nutritional concerns of lactating women consuming vegetarian diets, *Am J Clin Nutr*, 59[5 Suppl], 1182S, 1994.

72. Birch, E.E., Hoffman, D.R., Uauy, R., Birch, D.G., Prestidge, C., Visual acuity and the essentiality of docosahexaenoic acid and arachidonic acid in the diet of term infants, *Pediatr Res*, 44, 201, 1998.

73. Specker, B.L., Black, A., Allen, L., Morrow, F., Vitamin B_{12}: Low milk concentrations are related to low serum concentrations in vegetarian women and to methylmalonic aciduria in their infants, *Am J Clin Nutr*, 52, 1073, 1990.

74. Schneede, J., Dagneli.e.,P.C., van Staveren, W.A., Vollset, S.E., Refsum, H., Ueland, P.M., Methylmalonic acid and homocysteine in plasma as indicators of functional cobalamin deficiency in infants on macrobiotic diets, *Pediatr Res*, 36, 194, 1994.

75. Allen, L.H., Women's dietary calcium requirements are not increased by pregnancy or lactation, editorial, *Am J Clin Nutr*, 67, 591, 1998.

76. Specker, B.L., Tsang, R.C., Ho, M., Miller, D., Effect of vegetarian diet on serum 1,25-dihydroxy vitamin D concentrations during lactation, *Obstet Gynecol*, 70, 870, 1987.

77. Mangels, A.R., Messina, V., Consideration in planning vegan diets: Infants, *J Am Diet Assoc*, 101, 670, 2001.

78. American Academy of Pediatrics, Committee on Nutrition, Soy protein-based formulas: recommendations for use in infant feeding, *Pediatrics*, 101, 148, 1998.

79. Irvine, C.H., Fitzpatrick, M.G., Alexander, S.L., Phytoestrogens in soy-based infant foods: Concentrations, daily intake and possible biological effects, *Proc Soc Exp Biol Med*, 217, 247, 1998.

80. Gerrard, J.W.,MacKenzie, J.W., Golohoff, I.V. and Maningas, C.S., Cow's milk allergy: Prevalence and manifestations in an unselected series of newborns, *Acta Paediatr Scand*, 234[Suppl], 1, 1973.

81. Sampson, H.A. Food hypersensitivities. In: Grant, J.A., Ed. *Insights in Allergy*, Mosby, MO, 1986.

82. O'Connell, J.M., Dibley, M.J., Sierra, J., Wallace, B., Marks, J.S., Yip, R., Growth of vegetarian children: The farm study, *Pediatrics*, 84, 475, 1989.

83. Nathan, I., Hackett, A.F., Kirby, S., A longitudinal study of the growth of matched pairs of vegetarian and omnivorous children, aged 7–11 years, in the northwest of England, *Eur J Clin Nutr*, 51, 20, 1997.

84. Leung, S.S., Lee, R.H., Sung, R.Y., Luo, H.Y., Kam, C.W., Yuen, M.P., Hjelm, M., Lee, S.H., Growth and nutrition of Chinese vegetarian children in Hong Kong., J *Paediatr Child Hlth*, 37, 247, 2001.

85. Dagnelie, P.C., van Staveren, W.A., Vergote, F.J., Burema, J., van't, Hof, M.A., Van Klaveren, J.D., Hautvast, J.G., Nutritional status of infants aged 4 to 18 months on macrobiotic diets and matched omnivorous control infants: A population-based mixed longitudinal study. II Growth and psychomotor development, *Eur J Clin Nutr*, 43, 325, 1989.

86. Uauy, R., Mize, C.E., Castillo-Duran, C., Fat intake during childhood: Metabolic responses and effects on growth, *Am J Clin Nutr*, 72[5supp], 1354S, 2000.

87. Rogers, I.S., Emmett, P.M., Fat content of the diet among preschool children in southwest Britain: II. Relationship with growth, blood lipids and iron status, *Pediatrics*, 108, E49, 2001.

88. Nathan, I., Hackett, A.F., Kirby, S., The dietary intake of a group of vegetarian children aged 7–11 years compared with matched omnivores, *Br J Nutr,* 75, 533, 1996.

89. Dwyer, J.T., Dietary fiber for children: How much? *Pediatrics,* 96, 1019, 1995.

90. Messina, V., Considerations in planning vegan diets: Children, *J Am Diet Assoc,* 101, 661, 2001.

91. Perry, C.L., McGuire, M.T., Neumark-Sztainer, D., Story, M., Adolescent vegetarians: How well do their dietary patterns meet the healthy people 2010 objectives? *Arch Pediatr Adolesc Med,* 156, 431, 2002.

92. Worsley, A., Skrzypiec, G., Teenage vegetarianism: Prevalence, social and cognitive contexts, *Appetite,* 30, 151, 1998.

93. Martins, Y., Pliner, P., O'Connor, R., Restrained eating among vegetarians: Does a vegetarian eating style mask concerns about weight? *Appetite,* 32, 145, 1999.

94. Perry, C.L., McGuire, M.T., Neumark-Sztainer, D., Story, M., Characteristics of vegetarian adolescents in a multiethnic urban population, *J Adolesc Health,* 29, 406, 2001.

95. Sabaté, J., Lindstead, K., Harris, R., Johnston, P.K., Anthropometric parameters of children with different lifestyles, *Am J Dis Child,* 144, 1159, 1990.

96. Sabaté, J., Lindstead, K., Harris, R.D., Sanchez, A., Attained height of lacto-ovo vegetarian children and adolescents, *Eur J Clin Nutr,* 45, 51, 1991.

97. Barr, S.I., Vegetarianism and menstrual cycle disturbances: Is there an association? *Am J Clin Nutr,* 70, 549S, 1999.

98. American Academy of Pediatrics, Committee on Nutrition. Nutritional aspects of vegetarian diets. In: *Committee on Nutrition, Pediatric Nutrition Handbook,* 3rd ed., American Academy of Pediatrics, Illinois, 1993, 302.

99. Kissinger, D.G. and Sanchez, A., The association of dietary factors with the age of menarche, *Nutr Res,*7, 471, 1987.

100. De Waard, F. and Trichopoulos, D., A unifying concept of the aetiology of breast cancer, *Int J Cancer,* 41, 666, 1988.

101. Loucks, A.B. and Heath, E.M., Dietary restriction reduces luteinizing hormone (LH) pulse frequency during waking hours and increases LH pulse amplitude during sleep in young menstruating women, *J Clin Endocrinol Metab,* 78, 910, 1994.

102. Task force on Taxonomy of the International Association for the study of pain, diseases of the bladder, uterus, ovaries and adnexa. In: Merskey, H. and Bogduk, N., Eds., *Classification of Chronic Pain,* IASP Press, Seattle, WA, 164, 1994.

103. Barnard, N.D., Scialli, A.R., Hurlock, D., Bertron, P., Diet and sex-hormone binding globulin, dysmenorrhea and premenstrual symptoms, *Obstet Gynecol,* 95, 245, 2000.

104. Baird, D.D., Tylavsky, F.A. and Anderson, J.J.B., Do vegetarians have earlier menopause?, *Am J Epidemiol,* 128, 907, 1988.

105. Glazier, M.G., Bowman, M.A., A review of the evidence for the use of phytoestrogens as a replacement for traditional estrogen replacement therapy, *Arch Intern Med,* 161[9], 1161, 2001.

106. Somekawa, Y., Chiguchi, M., Ishibashi, T., Aso, T., Soy intake related to menopausal symptoms, serum lipids and BMD in postmenopausal Japanese women, *Obstet Gynecol,* 97, 109, 2001.

107. Vincent, A. and Fitzpatrick, L.A., Soy Isoflavones: Are they useful in menopause?, *Mayo Clin Proc,* 75, 1174, 2000.

108. Han, K.K., Soares, J.M. Jr., Haidar, M.A., de-Lima, G.R., Baracat, E.C., Benefits of soy isoflavone therapeutic regimen on menopausal symptoms, *Obstet Gynecol,* 99, 389, 2002.

109. American Heart Association, Heart and stroke facts. Dallas, TX, 1992.

110. Thorogood, M., Carter, R., Benfield, L., McPherson, K., Mann, J.I., Plasma lipids and lipoprotein cholesterol concentrations in people with different diets in Britain, *British Med J,* 295, 351, 1987.

111. Snowden, D.A., Phillips, R.L., Fraser, G.E., Meat consumption and fatal ischemic heart disease, *Prev Med*, 13, 490, 1984.

112. Willet, W.C., Stampfer, M.J., Manson, J.E., Colditz, G.A., Speizer, F.E., Rosner, B.A., Sampson, L.A., Hennekens, C.H., Intake of trans fatty acids and risk of coronary heart disease among women, *Lancet*, 341, 581, 1993.

113. Liu, S., Buring, J.E., Sesso, H.D., Rimm, E.B., Willett, W.C., Manson, J.E., A prospective study of dietary fiber intake and risk of cardiovascular disease among women, *J Am Coll Cardiol*, 39, 49, 2002.

114. Bazzano, L.A., He, J., Ogden, L.G., Loria, C., Vupputuri, S., Myers, L., Whelton, P.K., Legume consumption and risk of coronary heart disease in U.S. men and women: NHANES I Epidemiologic Follow-up Study, *Arch Intern Med*, 161, 573, 2001.

115. Barrett-Connor, E., Miller, V., Estrogens, lipids and heart disease, *Clin Geriatr Med,* 9, 57.

116. Dewell, A., Hollenbeck, C.B., Bruce, B., The effects of soy-derived phytoestrogens on serum lipids and lipoproteins in moderately hypercholesterolemic postmenopausal women, *J Clin Endocrinol Metab,* 87, 118, 2002.

117. de-Kleijn, M.J., van-der-Schouw, Y.T., Wilson, P.W.F., Grobbee, D.E., Jacques, P.F., Dietary intake of phytoestrogens is associated with a favorable metabolic cardiovascular risk profile in postmenopausal U.S. women: the Framingham study, *J Nutr,* 132, 276, 2002.

118. Anderson, J.W., Johnstone, B.M. and Cook-Newell, M.E., Meta-analysis of the effects of soy protein intake on serum lipids, *N Engl J Med*, 333, 276, 1995.

119. Jenkins, D.J., Kendall, C.W., Garsetti, M., Rosenberg-Zand, R.S., Jackson, C.J., Agarwal, S., Rao, A.V., Diamandis, E.P., Parker, T., Faulkner, D., Vuksan, V., Vidgen, E., Effect of soy protein foods on low-density lipoprotein oxidation and ex vivo sex hormone receptor activity--a controlled crossover trial, *Metabolism*, 49, 537, 2000.

120. Dubey, R.K., Gillespie, D.G., Imthurn, B., Rosselli, M., Jackson, E.K., Keller, P.J. Phytoestrogens inhibit growth and MAP kinase activity in human aortic smooth muscle cells. *Hypertension,* 33, 177, 1999.

121. Rajaram, S., Burke, K., Connell, B., Myint, T., Sabaté, J. A monounsaturated fatty acid-rich pecan-enriched diet favorably alters the serum lipid profile of healthy men and women, *J Nutr,* 131, 2275, 2001.

122. Spiller, G.A., Jenkins, D.J., Cragen, L.N., Gates, J.E., Bosello, O., Berra, K., Rudd, C., Stevenson, J., Superko, R., Effect of a diet high in monounsaturated fat from almonds on plasma cholesterol and lipoproteins, *J Am Coll Nutr*, 11, 126, 1992.

123. Sabate, J., Fraser, G.E., Burke, K., Knutsen, S.F., Bennett, H., Lindsted, K.D., Effects of walnuts on serum lipid levels and blood pressure in normal men, *N Engl J Med,* 328, 603, 1993.

124. Hu, F.B., Stampfer, M.J., Manson, J.E., Rimm, E.B., Colditz, G.A., Rosner, B.A., Speizer, F.E., Hennekens, C.H., Willett, W.C., Frequent nut consumption and risk of coronary heart disease in women: Prospective cohort study, *Br Med J*, 317, 1341, 1998.

125. Larsen, L.F., Jespersen, J. and Marckmann, P. Are olive oil diets antithrombotic? Diets enriched with olive, rapeseed, or sunflower oil affect postprandial factor VII differently, *Am J Clin Nutr,* 70, 976, 1999.

126. Junker, R., Kratz, M., Neufeld, M., Erren, M., Nofer, J.R., Schulte, H., Nowak-Gottl, U., Assmann, G., Wahrburg, U., Effects of diets containing olive oil, sunflower oil, or rapeseed oil on the hemostatic system, *Thromb Haemost,* 85, 280, 2001.

127. Joshipura, K.J., Hu, F.B., Manson, J.E., Stampfer, M.J., Rimm, E. B., Speizer, F.E., Colditz, G., Ascherio, A., Rosner, B., Spiegelman, D., Willett, W.C., The effect of fruit and vegetable intake on risk for coronary heart disease, *Ann Intern Med,* 134, 1106, 2001.

128. Lu, S.C., Wu, W.H., Lee, C.A., Chou, H.F., Lee, H.R., Huang, P.C., LDL of Taiwanese vegetarians are less oxidizable than those of omnivores, *J Nutr,* 130, 1591, 2000.

129. Steiner, M. and Li, W. Aged garlic extract a modulator of cardiovascular risk factors: A dose-finding study on the effects of AGE on platelet functions. *J. Nutr,* 131, 1980S, 2001.

130. Keevil, J.G., Osman, H.E., Reed, J.D., Folts, J.D., Grape juice, but not orange juice or grapefruit juice, inhibits human platelet aggregation, *J Nutr,* 130, 53, 2000.

131. Keli, S.O., Hertog, M.G., Feskens, E.J., Kromhout, D., Dietary flavonoids, antioxidant vitamins and incidence of stroke: The Zutphen Study, *Arch Intern Med,* 156, 637, 1996.

132. Korpela, R., Seppo, L., Laakso, J., Lilja, K., Lahteenmaki, T., Solatunturi, E., Dietary habits affect the susceptibility of low-density lipoprotein oxidation, *Eur J Clin Nutr,* 53, 802, 1999.

133. Palozza, P., Sgarlata, E., Luberto, C., Piccioni, E., Anti, M., Marra, G., Armelao, F., Franceschelli, P., Bartoli, G.M., n-3 fatty acids induce oxidative modifications in human erythrocytes depending on dose and duration of dietary supplementation, *Am J Clin Nutr,* 64, 297, 1996.

134. World Health Organization, World Health Statistics Annual 1996, Geneva, Switzerland, World Health Organization, 1997.

135. Mills, P.K., Beeson, W.L., Phillips, R.L., Fraser, G.E., Dietary habits and breast cancer incidence among Seventh-Day Adventists, *Cancer,* 64, 582, 1989.

136. Felton, J.S., Knize, M.G., Salmon, C.P., Malfatti, M.A., Kulp, K.S. Human exposure to heterocyclic amine food mutagens/carcinogens: Relevance to breast cancer. *Environ Mol Mutagen,* 39, 112, 2000.

137. Zheng, W., Gustafson, D.R., Sinha, R., Cerhan, J.R., Moore, D., Hong, C.P. Anderson, K.E., Kushi, L.H., Sellers, T.A., Folsom, A.R., Well-done meat intake and the risk of breast cancer, *J Natl Cancer Inst,* 90, 1724, 1998.

138. Ambrosone, C.B., Freudenheim, J.L., Sinha, R., Graham, S., Marshall, J.R., Vena, J.E., Laughlin, R., Menoto, T., Shields, P.G., Breast cancer risk, meat consumption and N-acetyltransferase [NAT2] genetic polymorphisms, *Int J Cancer,* 75, 825, 1998.

139. Wu, A.H., Pike, M.C., Stram, D.O., Meta-analysis: Dietary fat intake, serum estrogen levels and the risk of breast cancer, *J Natl Cancer Inst,* 91, 529, 1999.

140. Hunter, D.J., Spiegelman, D., Adami, H.O., Beeson, L., van den Brandt, P.A., Folsom, A.R., Fraser, G.E., Goldbohm, R.A., Graham, S., Howe, G.R., Cohort studies of fat intake and risk of breast cancer – A pooled analysis, *N Eng J Med,* 334, 356, 1996.

141. Willett, W.C., Hunter, D.J., Stampfer, M.J., Colditz, G., Manson, J.E., Spiegelman, D., Rosner, B., Hennekens, C.H., Speizer, F.E., Dietary fat and fiber in relation to risk of breast cancer, *J Am Med Assoc,* 268, 2037, 1992.

142. Bartsch, H., Nair, J., Owen, R.W., Dietary polyunsaturated fatty acids and cancers of the breast and colorectum: Emerging evidence for their role as risk modifiers, *Carcinogenesis,* 20, 2209, 1999.

143. Badawi, A.F., El-Sohemy, A., Stephen, L.L., Goshal, A.K., Archer, M.C., The effect of dietary n-3 and n-6 polyunsaturated fatty acids on the expression of cyclooxygenase 1 and 2 and levels of p21ras in rat mammary glands, *Carcinogenesis*, 19 ,903, 1998.

144. Razanamahefa, L., Prouff, S., Bardon, S., Stimulatory effect of arachidonic acid on T-47D human breast cancer cell growth is associated with enhancement of cyclin D1 mRNA expression, *Nutr Cancer*, 38, 274, 2000.

145. Rose, D.P., Goldman, M., Connolly, J.M., Strong, L.E., High-fiber diet reduces serum estrogen concentrations in premenopausal women, *Am J Clin Nutr*, 54, 520, 1991.

146. Jacobs, D.R., Jr., Marquart, L., Slavin, J., Kushi, L.H., Whole grain intake and cancer; An expanded review and meta-analysis, *Nutr. Cancer*, 30, 85, 1998.

147. Baghurst, P.A., Rohan, T.E., High-fiber diets and reduced risk of breast cancer, *Int J Cancer*, 56, 173, 1994.

148. Collins-Burrow, B.M., Burrow, M.E., Duong, B.N., McLachlan, J.A., Estrogenic and antiestrogenic activities of flavonoid phytochemicals through estrogen receptor binding-dependent and -independent mechanisms, *Nutr Cancer*, 38, 229, 2000.

149. Lee, H.P., Gourley, L., Duffy, S.W., Esteve, J., Lee, J., Day, N.E., Dietary effects on breast-cancer risk in Singapore, *Lancet,* 337, 1197, 1991.

150. Trock, B., Butler, W., Clarke, R., Hilakivi-Clarke, L., Meta-analysis of soy intake and breast cancer risk. *J Nutr*, 130, 690s, 2000.

151. Yuan, J.M., Wang, Q.S., Ross, R.K., Henderson, B.E., Yu, M.C., Diet and breast cancer in Shanghai and Tianjin, China. *Br J Cancer*, 71, 1353,1995.

152. de Lemos, M.L., Effects of soy phytoestrogens genistein and daidzein on breast cancer growth, *Ann. Pharmocother,* 35, 1118, 2001.

153. Zheng, W., Dai, Q., Custer, L.J., Shu, X.O., Wen, W.Q., Jin, F., Franke, A.A., Urinary excretion of isoflavonoids and the risk of breast cancer, *Cancer Epidemiol Biomarkers Prev*, 8, 35, 1999.

154. Constantinou, A., Krygiera, E., Mehta, R.R., Genistein induces maturation of cultured human breast cancer cells and prevents tumor growth in nude mice, *Am J Clin Nutr*, 68(6 suppl), 1426S, 1998.

155. den Tonkelaar, I., de Waard, F., Regularity and length of menstrual cycles in women aged 41–46 in relation to breast cancer risk: Results from the DOM-project. *Breast Cancer Res Treat*, 38, 253, 1996.

156. McCann, S.E., Moysich, K.B., Mettlin, C., Intakes of selected nutrients and food groups and risk of ovarian cancer, *Nutr Cancer,* 39, 19, 2001.

157. Zhang, M., Yang, Z.Y., Binns, C.W., Lee, A.H., Diet and ovarian cancer risk: A case-control study in China, *Br J Cancer,* 86, 712, 2002.

158. Kushi, L.H., Mink, P.J., Folsam, A.R. Anderson, K.E., Zheng, W., Lazovich, D., Sellers, T.A., Prospective study of diet and ovarian cancer, *Am J Epidemiology*; 149, 21, 1999.

159. Bosetti, C., Negri, E., Francheschi, S., Pelucchi, C., Talamini, R., Montella, M., Conti, E., Diet and ovarian cancer risk: A case-control study in Italy, *Int J Cancer*, 93, 911, 2001.

160. Huncharek, M., Klassen, H., Kupelnick, B., Dietary beta-carotene intake and the risk of epithelial ovarian cancer: A meta-analysis of 3782 subjects from five observational studies, *In Vivo,* 15, 339, 2001.

161. Bertone, E. R., Hankinson, S. E., Newcomb, P. A., Rosner, B., Willet, W. C., Stampfer, M. J., Egan, K. M., A population-based case-control study of carotenoid and vitamin A intake and ovarian cancer (United States)., *Cancer Causes Control*, 12, 83, 2001.

162. Riggs, B.L. and Melton, L.J., III., Involutional osteoporosis, *N Engl J Med*, 314, 1676, 1986.

163. Rajaram, S., Wien, M. Vegetarian diets in the prevention of osteoporosis, diabetes and neurological disorders, in *Vegetarian Nutrition*, Sabaté, J., Eds., CRC Press, Boca Raton, FL, 2001, chap. 6.

164. Tylavsky, F.A. Anderson, J.J.B., Dietary factors in bone health of elderly lacto-ovo vegetarian and omnivorous women, *Am J Clin Nutr*, 56, 669, 1992.

165. Sellmeyer, D.E., Stone, K.L., Sebastian, A., Cummings, S.R., A high ratio of dietary animal to vegetable protein increases the rate of bone loss and the risk of fracture in postmenopausal women, *Am J Clin Nutr*, 73, 118 2001.

166. Hu, J.F., Zhao, X.H., Parpia, B., Campbell, T.C., Dietary intakes and urinary excretion of calcium and acids: A cross-section study of women in China, *Am J Clin Nutr*, 58, 398, 1993.

167. Feskanich, D., Willett, W.C., Stampfer, M.J., Colditz, G.A., Protein consumption and bone fractures in women, *Am J Epidemiol*, 143, 472, 1996.

168. Frassetto, L.A., Todd, K.M., Morris, R.C., Jr, Sebastian, A., Estimation of net endogenous noncarbonic acid production in humans from diet potassium and protein contents, *Am J Clin Nutr*, 68, 576, 1998.

169. Ball, D., Maughan, J., Blood and urine acid-base status of premenopausal omnivorous and vegetarian women, *Br J Nutr*, 78, 683, 1997.

170. Lau, E.M., Kwok, T., Woo, J., Ho, S. C., BMD in Chinese elderly female vegetarians, vegans, lacto-vegetarians and omnivores, *Eur J Clin Nutr*, 52, 60, 1998.

171. Marsh, A.G., Sanchez, T.V., Chaffee, F.L., Mayor, G.H., Mickelsen, O., Bone mineral mass in adult lacto-ovo-vegetarian and omnivorous males, *Am J Clin Nutr*, 37, 453, 1983.

172. Renner, E., Dairy calcium, bone metabolism and prevention of osteoporosis, *J Dairy Sci,* 77, 3498, 1994.

173. Honkanen, R., Kroger, H., Alhava, E., Turpeinen, P., Tuppurainen, M., Saarikoski, S., Lactose intolerance associated with fractures of weight-bearing bones in Finnish women aged 38–57 years, *Bone,* 21, 473, 1997.

174. Nordin, B.E.C., International patterns of osteoporosis, *Clin. Orthop*, 45, 17, 1966.

175. Tucker, K.L., Hannan, M.T., Chen, H., Cupples, L.A., Wilson, P.W., Kiel, D.P., Potassium, magnesium and fruit and vegetable intakes are associated with greater BMD in elderly men and women, *Am J Clin Nutr,* 69, 727, 1999.

176. Lemann, J., Jr., Pleuss, J.A. and Gray, R.W., Potassium causes calcium retention in healthy adults, *J Nutr,* 123, 1623, 1993.

177. Tsuchida, K., Mizushima, S., Toba, M., Soda, K., Dietary soybean intake and BMD among 995 middle-aged women in Yokohama, *J Epidemiol,* 9, 14, 1999.

178. Potter, S.M., Baum, J.A., Teng, H., Stillman, R.J., Shay, N.F., Erdman, J.W., Jr., Soy protein and isoflavones: Their effects on blood lipids and bone density in postmenopausal women, *Am J Clin Nutr,* 68[Suppl.], 1375S, 1998.

179. Arjmandi, B.H., Getlinger, J.J., Goyal, N.V., Alekel, L., Hasler, C.M., Juma, S., Drum, M.L., Hollis, B.W., Kukreja, S.C., Role of soy protein with normal or reduced isoflavone content in reversing bone loss induced by ovarian hormone deficiency in rats, *Am J Clin Nutr,* 68[Suppl.], 1358S, 1998.

180. Kuczmarski, R.J., Carroll, M.D., Flegal, K.M., Troiano, R.P., Varying body mass index cutoff points to describe overweight prevalence among U.S. adults, NHANES III [1988 to 1994], *Obes Res,* 5, 542, 1997.

181. Kennedy, E.T., Bowman, S.A., Spence, J.T., Freedman, M., King, J., Popular diets: Correlation to health, nutrition and obesity, *J Am Diet Assoc,* 101, 411, 2001.

182. Hebblelinck, M., Clarys, P., De Malsche, A., Growth, development and physical fitness of Flemish vegetarian children, adolescents and young adults, *Am J Clin Nutr*, 70, 579S, 1999.

183. Barr, S.I., Broughton, T.M., Relative weight loss efforts and nutrient intakes among health-conscious vegetarian, past vegetarian and nonvegetarian women ages 18 to 50, *J Am Coll Nutr*, 19, 781, 2000.

184. Hakala, P., Karvetti, R.L., Weight reduction on lactovegetarian and mixed diets. Changes in weight, nutrient intake, skinfold thickness and blood pressure, *Eur J Clin Nutr*, 43, 421, 1989.

185. U.S. Department of Agriculture, The Food Guide Pyramid, Hyattsville, Maryland: Human Nutrition Information Service, 1992, [Publication HG252].

186. Haddad, E.H., Sabaté, J. and Whitten, C.G., Vegetarian food guide pyramid: A conceptual framework, *Am J Clin Nutr*, 70[Suppl.] 615S, 1999.

187. Kushi, L. H., Meyer, K. A. and Jacobs, D. R., Jr., Cereals, legumes and chronic disease risk: evidence from epidemiological studies, *Am J Clin Nutr*, 70[Suppl.] 452S, 1999.

188. Anderson, J.W., Smith, B.M. and Washnock, C.S., Cardiovascular and renal benefits of dry bean and soybean intake, *Am J Clin Nutr*, 70[Suppl.], 464S, 1999.

189. Rajaram, S. and Sabaté, J., Health benefits of a vegetarian diet, *Nutrition,* 16, 531, 2000.

21 Nutrition Issues of Women in the U.S. Army*

Nancy King, Carol J. Baker-Fulco and E. Wayne Askew

CONTENTS

I. INTRODUCTION

Although the stereotypical image of military life is that of soldiers eating in large mess halls, the majority of peacetime American soldiers have the option of consum-

---

* The views, opinions or findings in this report are those of the authors and should not be construed as an official Department of the Army position, policy or decision, unless so designated by other official documentation

ing their meals away from the military environment, at home or in public establishments. However, some soldiers (e.g., basic trainees) are required to subsist in military dining facilities for certain extended time periods during their training. Periodically, all soldiers eat military rations* while in a field environment during field training or deployments. The type of ration provided in the dining facility or the field is contingent upon the unit's missions, tactical scenarios and availability of cooks and rations. Although nutritionally adequate military rations are provided, the soldiers pick and choose the ration components they eat based on what is available, their food preferences and what they think is good for them. This fact underscores the important role played by nutritional surveys to determine actual food consumption and nutrient intakes.

A small number of female soldiers have been included in military nutrition studies.[1-9] The results from these studies suggest that the nutritional problems encountered by women in the U.S. Army are not greatly different from those of their civilian counterparts. However, the nutritional problems of female soldiers may be exacerbated by the need to meet weight-for-height and body-fat standards and may be more consequential because of the physical performance demands imposed by military training.

II. HISTORICAL PERSPECTIVE ON ACTIVE-DUTY MILITARY WOMEN

With almost 204,000 female members on active duty in the U.S. military services (14.9% of total force),[10] women have become an integral part of the U.S. Armed Forces. For some time, the quota of women serving in any of the military services was set at 2%. In 1967, Public Law 90-130 lifted this ceiling. In the U.S. Army alone, between 1970 and 1980, the percentage of women escalated from 1.46 to 9.85%, almost a sevenfold increase.[11] In 1993, women composed 12.3% of the U.S. Army active-duty personnel.[12] As of September 15, 2001, 15.5% of active-duty Army personnel were women.[13]

Most women serving in the U.S. military before World War II were nurses. During World War II, women's jobs consisted mainly of nursing, administration and clerical; a few had jobs in naval intelligence and communications. Shortly after the war, women's positions were returned to the "traditional female jobs" of clerks, secretaries and routine communications. Military positions available to women today are diverse and not as traditional.[14,15] Until 1993, women could serve in any officer or enlisted specialty or position provided that the specialty, position or unit was not assigned a routine direct combat mission or routinely collocated with units assigned direct combat missions. However, in the event of hostilities, female soldiers would remain with their assigned unit and continue to perform their assigned duties.[15] Since the lifting of the combat exclusion in 1993, women may serve in more than 9000

---

* Generally, a ration is the nutritionally adequate food to subsist one person for 1 d, while a meal is a specified quantity of food provided to one person during one scheduled serving period. Thus, a ration in the dining hall setting consists of three meals.

previously closed positions in combat aviation.[16] In 1994, when the Secretary of Defense announced a new assignment rule for women based on direct ground combat, an additional 32,000 positions opened for women.[16] For instance, female officers in the U.S. Army may now serve in executive positions, tactical operations, intelligence, engineering/maintenance, scientific/professional, medical, administrative and supply/logistics. Military Occupational Specialties for enlisted women include infantry gun crew/seamanship, electronic equipment repair, communications/intelligence, medical/dental, technical specialist, functional support/administration, electrical/mechanical equipment repair, crafts and service/supply.

III. PROFILE OF U.S. ARMY WOMEN

The ethnic distribution of the 73,865 women on active duty in the Army on September 2001 was 41% White, 43% Black, 8.7% Hispanic and 7.3% other.[13] The anthropometric characteristics of U.S. Army women are depicted in Table 21.1.[10,17] For the female soldier, body weight and composition (thinness) denotes more than just appearance (esthetics) and health, since retention in the service and continuation of her military career is contingent on meeting body-fat standards (Table 21.2 and Table 21.3).[18–21] Body composition is related to physical fitness in that a high percentage of body fat correlates negatively to aerobic capacity.[22] Thus, desirable body composition is an integral part of physical fitness and essential for maintaining physical readiness.

Based on the 1998 Department of Defense Survey of Health Related Behaviors Among Military Personnel,[23] 6.25% of female soldiers 20 to 25 years of age and 9.72% of female soldiers 26 to 34 years of age were overweight, compared with 22.1% of women 20 to 29 years of age reportedly overweight in the civilian popu-

---

TABLE 21.1
Anthropometric Data of U.S. Army Women

Age distribution	
≤ 20 years	20.7%
21–24 years	26.1%
25–29 years	20.6%
30–39 years	24.6%
≥ 40 years	8.0%
Height [a] (cm)	162.8 ± 64.2/141.3–187.0
Body weight [a] (kg)	62.3 ± 8.7/38.9–99.5

[a] mean ± sd/range

From Ferris, Z.M., personal communication, 2002; Gordon, C.C. U.S. Army Anthropometric Survey Database: Downsizing, Demographic Change and Validity of the 1988 Data in 1996, Technical Report NATICK/TR-97/003, U.S. Army Natick Research, Development and Engineering Center, Natick, MA, 1996.

TABLE 21.2
Height/Weight Standards for U.S. Army Women

Height (in.)	Maximum Allowable Weight (lb), by Age Category			
	17–20	21–27	28–39	40 and over
58	112	115	119	122
59	116	119	123	126
60	120	123	127	130
61	124	127	131	135
62	129	132	137	139
63	133	137	141	144
64	137	141	145	148
65	141	145	149	153
66	146	150	154	158
67	149	154	159	162
68	154	159	164	167
69	158	163	168	172
70	163	168	173	177
71	167	172	177	182
72	172	177	183	188
73	177	182	188	193
74	183	189	194	198
75	188	194	200	204
76	194	200	206	209
77	199	205	211	215
78	204	210	216	220
79	209	215	220	226
80	214	220	227	232

From The Army Weight Control Program, Army Regulation 600-9 (update change 1), Headquarters, Department of the Army, Washington, D.C., 1994; Friedl, K.E., in *Body Composition and Physical Performance,* Marriott, B.M. and Grumstrup-Scott, J., Eds., National Academy Press, Washington, D.C., 1992, chap. 3 and appendix E.

lation.[24] In both surveys, overweight was defined as having a body mass index (BMI) greater than 27.3 for women aged 20 or older and BMI was calculated from self-reported heights and weights.

Army soldiers are required to pass a semiannual physical fitness test, with passing scores adjusted for gender and age.[25] The physical fitness test consists of timed push-ups, timed sit-ups and a 2-mi run, thus assessing muscular strength and endurance, flexibility and cardiorespiratory fitness.[18,25,26] Because of this requirement, female soldiers may be more physically active than their civilian counterparts. In 1998, 81.8% of female soldiers reported engaging in vigorous physical activity at least 3 days per week for at least 20 minutes per occasion.[23] Women assigned to operational units or undergoing initial entry or specialty training are probably more physically active on average than other women in the U.S. Army. Civilian females 20 to 29 years of age

TABLE 21.3
Percent Body Fat Standards for U.S. Army Women

Age (years)	Percent Body Fat
17–20	≤ 30
21–27	≤ 32
28–39	≤ 34
≥ 40	≤ 36

From The Army Weight Control Program, Army Regulation 600-9 (Update Change 1), Headquarters, Department of the Army, Washington, D.C., 1994; Friedl, K.E., in *Body Composition and Physical Performance,* Marriott, B.M. and Grumstrup-Scott, J., Eds., National Academy Press, Washington, D.C., 1992, chap. 3 and appendix E.

reported vigorous exercise (defined as "enough to work up a sweat") at a rate of 27.1% of them for "2 to 4 times per week" and 6.2% for "5 to 6 times per week."[24]

Pregnant and postpartum soldiers are required to meet the body-weight and body-fat standards and pass the physical fitness test 180 days after delivery.[18,25–27] This requirement adds an additional amount of postpartum stress, which may be unique to military compared with most civilian women. At the time of the 1998 Department of Defense Survey of Health Related Behaviors Among Military Personnel, 16% of military women, excluding those in basic training or at a military academy, were pregnant or had been pregnant in the preceding year.[23] The requirement to meet weight and physical fitness standards may encourage some of these women to limit their food intake during pregnancy as well as during lactation.

Since Army women have different physical fitness demands and body weight concerns that differ from those of their civilian counterparts, a closer look at their dietary intakes and nutritional status is warranted.

IV. MILITARY NUTRITION STUDIES

A. DESCRIPTION OF MILITARY NUTRITION STUDIES

Of the nine military nutrition studies that included female soldiers, seven included soldiers of both genders,[1–6,9] whereas only two were specifically designed to determine the nutrient intake of female soldiers.[7,8] One of these two studies[7] was part of a larger research project that assessed the health, performance and nutritional status of Army women during their initial entry into the military (U.S. Army Basic Combat Training).[28] In three studies,[2,4,6] soldiers were fed solely at a field site. In four studies, soldiers mostly ate in a military dining facility, while in two studies,[8,9] the soldiers were not required to eat their meals in a military dining facility and purchased and prepared their own foods. A description of these nutrition studies is presented in Table 21.4.

When food intake was primarily from a military dining facility or when hot meals were served in the field, dietary intake data were determined by visual esti-

TABLE 21.4
Description of Military Nutrition Studies

Type	Location	When	Duration	Ration	Soldiers Total	Soldiers Females	Age[a]	Ref.
Field	Hawaii	August/85	44 d	MRE/T	240	40[b]	23	2
	Bolivia[c]	July/90	15 d	MRE/B[d]	80	13[e]	24	4
	Camp Mackall	May/97	7 d	MRE or Concept[f]	162	53[g]	30	6
Dining hall	West Point	October/79	5 d	A	190	54[h]	20	1
	Ft. Jackson	August/88	7 d[i]	A[j]	81	40[k]	20	3
	West Point	March/90	7 d	A	205	86[h]	20	5
	Ft. Jackson	April/93	7 d	A	49	49[k]	21	7
	Ft. Sam Houston	August/95	7 d	Own Source	50	50[l]	25	8
	Ft. Bliss	Sep/96–Mar/97	9 d[i]	Own Source	106	15[m]	42	9

[a] Mean age of female soldiers.
[b] Combat service support.
[c] Elevation 11,500 ft.
[d] Plus a carbohydrate supplement (125 g).
[e] 50% medical, 33% engineer, 17% other.
[f] Similar to MRE but with specific breakfast, lunch and dinner menus.
[g] 67% enlisted, 37% officers.
[h] Officer candidates.
[i] Nonconsecutive.
[j] MREs served 2 d of field exercise.
[k] Soldiers-in-training.
[l] Officers-in-training.
[m] 80% Sergeants Major Academy students, 20% faculty members.
Adapted from King, N., Fridlund, K.E. and Askew, E.W., *J. Am. Coll. Nutr.,* 12, 344, 1993. With permission.

mation. For this method, subjects presented their trays to trained data collectors before sitting down to eat. The data collectors recorded the food items and visually compared the amounts of foods on the subjects' trays to weighed standards of the same foods. The data collectors were trained to estimate food portions to within 10% of the preweighed standards. After the meal, the test subjects returned to the data collectors, who recorded the quantities of foods remaining on the tray. Subjects recorded any foods consumed outside the military dining facility on standardized food records, which were reviewed daily by trained dietary data collectors.

For studies of individual field rations, dietary intakes also were obtained by self-recorded food record. Using cards precoded and printed with the menu items, the subjects circled the proportion of a serving consumed next to the appropriate menu item. There were separate prompts for recording canteens or cups of water and other beverages. A food record is a fairly accurate method of collecting intake of field rations because ration items are individually packaged single-serving-sized pouches or bars. Data collectors reviewed the food records with the subjects daily.

B. MILITARY RATIONS

Military rations are planned according to nutritional standards to ensure that the Military Dietary Reference Intakes (MDRIs), formerly Military Recommended Dietary Allowances (MRDAs), can be met.[29] The MDRIs are presented in a triservice regulation governing nutrition standards and education[30] and are based on the expert scientific opinion of the Food and Nutrition Board, Institute of Medicine, National Research Council. The 2001 MDRIs, for most nutrients, are based on the Dietary Reference Intakes (DRIs)[31–33] published at the time the regulation was drafted. The DRIs for vitamins A and K, iodine, iron and zinc[34] were released after the regulation was drafted. For these nutrients, the 2001 MDRIs are based on the 1989 Recommended Dietary Allowances.[35] Table 21.5 lists the MDRIs for women. The MDRIs are intended for healthy military personnel ages 17 to 50 years old, excluding pregnant and lactating women. The MDRIs are identical to the DRIs, except when known differences in the military population require adjustment of a particular nutrient.[29]

Operational rations (i.e., combat field rations) are designed to contain adequate nutrients to meet the MDRIs within an energy provision of at least 3600 kcal, thus meeting the energy requirements of most male and female soldiers working in a field environment.[29,30] Because male soldiers require and consume high energy, the nutrient density of the rations (unit of nutrient per 1000 kcal) is usually adequate for men to meet or exceed the MDRIs. Female soldiers are usually smaller and hence do not require or consume as much as 3600 kcal; therefore, the nutrient density of military rations is not optimal for many female soldiers. Depending on energy consumption of female soldiers, intake of some nutrients may be inadequate. For instance, female soldiers would have to consume approximately 3600 kcal (157% of energy MDRI) to meet the folate MDRI of 400 mcg, the calcium MDRI of 1000 mg and the iron MDRI of 15 mg.

The A-ration consists of meals prepared by cooks using perishable foods. The A-ration is served in installation dining facilities or in the field when cooking and refrigeration equipment are available. The Heat & Serve Ration (formerly called Tray Ration or T-Ration) is used for group feeding in the field when neither cooking nor refrigeration is possible. The components of the Heat & Serve Ration are thermally processed shelf-stable foods, packaged in hermetically sealed half-size steam-table containers. With this ration, the entire meal is prepared by submerging prepared food trays in hot water or by adding hot water to reconstitute the product; thus few cooks are required to prepare and serve a meal. The B-Ration, consisting of canned and dehydrated foods, is used in the field when kitchen facilities and cooks, but not refrigeration equipment, are available. This group ration is now solely used by the U.S. Marine Corps. The Meal, Ready-to-Eat (MRE) is an individually packaged shelf-stable meal used in the field when the mission and tactical scenario prevent group

TABLE 21.5
MDRIs and Mean Nutrient Intake of Female Soldiers

Nutrient	MDRIs[a]	Field Hawaii 1985 (n = 36)	Field Bolivia 1990 (n = 13)	Field Camp Mackall 1997 MRE (n = 28)	Field Camp Mackall 1997 Concept (n = 26)	Dining hall West Point 1979 (n = 54)	Dining hall Ft. Jackson 1988 (n = 40)	Dining hall West Point 1990 (n = 86)	Dining hall Ft. Jackson 1993 (n = 49)	Dining hall Ft. Sam Houston 1995 (n = 50)	Dining hall Ft. Bliss[b] 1996-97 (n = 15)
Energy (kcal)	2300	1834	1668	1834	2093	2454[c]	2467	2314[d]	2592	2037	1773[c]
Protein (g)	72	67	68	59	54	84	96	79	82	75	69
Carbohydrate (g)	300[f]	235	218	272	325	284	318	325	365	289	224
Fat (g)	≤77[f]	70	57	60	68	107	94	81	94	63	66
Cholesterol (mg)	≤300[f]	—[g]	235	122	105	403	418	234	466	201	208
Vitamin A (mcg RE)	800	1602	1030	1000	789	—	1690	1250[h]	1390	1259	601[h]
Vitamin D (mcg)	5	—	—	—	—	—	—	—	—	—	—
Vitamin E (mg)	15[i]	—	4.9[j]	13.1	5.7	—	—	—	—	—	30.8[h]
Vitamin K (mcg)	65	—	—	—	—	—	—	—	—	—	—
Ascorbic acid (mg)	75	142	107	212	224	147	165	172[h]	89	115	116[h]
Thiamin (mg)	1.1	4.0	2.0	2.2	2.5	11.6[h]	2.0	2.8[h]	1.8	1.7	7.5[h]
Riboflavin (mg)	1.1	1.6	1.5	1.4	1.8	9.3[h]	2.2	3.0[h]	2.0	2.1	7.7[h]
Niacin (mg NE)	14	16.5	19.4	20.2	22	37.3[h]	27	30[h]	20	24	29.9[h]
Vitamin B$_6$ (mg)	1.3	—	1.5	2.3	1.8	2.29[k]	—	2.6[h]	1.5	2.0	23.0[h]
Folate (mcg)	400	—	178	147	243	339[h,k]	—	428[h]	261	342	351[h]
Vitamin B$_{12}$ (mcg)	2.4	—	2.1	2.3	1.7	4.7[h,k]	3.7	6.2[h]	5.6	4.6	10.8[h]
Calcium (mg)	1000	577	664	458	540	954	907	1001	728	918	804
Phosphorus (mg)	700	1065	1059	903	715	1347	1600	1391	1296	1333	1141
Magnesium (mg)	320	—	218	206	217	238[k]	—	315	267	285	297
Iron (mg)	15	11.9	11.7	11.9	14.2	16.2	18.4	28[h]	16.2	16.8	19.1

Zinc (mg)	12	—	5[j]	8.1	6.4	11[k]	—	14	11	11.2	14.3
Sodium (mg)	3600	3343	3819	3283	3326	2764[l]	4420	3703	3994	3439	2697
Iodine (mcg)	150	—	—	—	—	—	—	—	—	—	—
Selenium (mcg)	55	—	—	—	—	—	—	—	—	—	—
Fluoride (mg)	3.1	—	—	—	—	—	—	—	—	—	—
Potassium (mg)	2500	2075	—	1789	1681	2454	—	2791	2681	2666	2478
Reference number:	29,30	2	4	6	6	1	3	5	7	8	9

a MDRIs for moderately active military women ages 17–50 years.

b Preliminary data; unpublished.

c 3% of kilocalories provided by alcohol intake.

d 0.6% of kilocalories provided by alcohol intake.

e 2% of kilocalories provided by alcohol intake.

f No MDRI established for carbohydrates or fats; requirements estimated using 50-55% of kcal from carbohydrates, ≤ 30% of kcal from fat and ≤ 300 mg of cholesterol.

g "—" indicates data not calculated for the study.

h Data include intake from multivitamin preparations and/or iron supplements.

i MDRI based only on mg alpha-tocopherol. Vitamin E intakes include all tocopherols and tocotrienols and are in alpha-tocopherol equivalents.

j Not total intake. Value is intake from one MRE meal.

k Limited food composition data available at the time of the study; calculated value may be an underestimation.

l Does not include discretionary salt.

Adapted from King, N., Fridlund, K. E. and Askew, E. W., J. Am. Coll. Nutr., 12, 344, 1993. With permission feeding. The components are heat processed in retort pouches (flexible containers). More complete descriptions of each of the military rations is presented elsewhere.[36,37]

Adequate calcium provision of A-ration menus served at installation dining facilities is ensured by inclusion of low-fat milk and many other dairy products. To increase the calcium content of group rations for field feeding, ultra-high-temperature-treated (UHT) milk is served when fresh milk is unavailable. Commercial sliced bread or shelf-stable "pouch" bread also must be served at each meal when group rations are provided. These supplements were mandated because of results of early tests of the field feeding system, especially the Hawaii survey[2] noted in Table 21.4. The pouch bread also is available for issue with the MRE. One pouch bread (200 kcal, 5.8 g of protein, 28 g of carbohydrate and 7.4 g of fat) is relatively high in calcium (74 mg) and iron (1.9 mg).

The A-ration was served in most of the dining hall studies.[1,3,5,7] Soldiers participating in the field studies received either one or two MREs with either B-Ration or Tray Packs (T-Ration) or three MREs.[2,4,6] The Concept Ration was a developmental test ration similar to the MRE, except that it was meal-focused (i.e., specific breakfast, lunch and dinner menus) and included more "eat-on-the-go" food items.[6]

C. NUTRIENT INTAKES

Table 21.5 shows the mean nutrient intakes of the female soldiers participating in the nine* aforementioned military nutrition studies.[1–9] Data on these 400 women indicate a generally lower nutrient intake in the field than in dining halls. From the data available, it cannot be determined if the lower intake was due to field conditions that did not favor food consumption or to the type of rations served.

Mean energy intakes were less than the MDRI in all the field studies but only in two of the six dining hall studies. The lowest energy intake (72% MDRI) was by female soldiers on a field training exercise in Bolivia.[4] The low intakes in Bolivia were likely due, in part, to an altitude-induced anorexia. Camp Mackall is the only military study reported here in which both energy intake and energy expenditure were measured during a field training exercise.[6] Energy expenditure was measured using doubly labeled water in a subgroup of 17 women. Baker-Fulco et al. found a mean energy expenditure of 2745 ± 87 kcal/d (mean ± S.E.), with a range of 2025 to 3205 kcal, suggesting an energy deficit of around 700 kcal/d.[6]

The mean protein intake also was less than the MDRI in each of the field studies, but in only one of the dining hall studies. The lowest protein intake (75% MDRI) was for subjects consuming the Concept Ration in the Camp Mackall study.[6]

The mean intakes of vitamins were adequate with the exception of folate, vitamin B_{12} and possibly vitamin E (vitamin E data missing for most of the studies). Only one dining hall study reported a folate intake meeting the MDRI. Folate intake was less than 70% of the MDRI in each field study and in one of the dining hall studies (folate data missing for one field and one dining hall study). Except for the field study at Camp Mackall, the folate intakes portray dietary states prior to the manda-

---

* The Camp Mackall data are presented for two groups, each receiving one of the two rations (MRE and Concept) provided in the study.[6]

tory folate fortification of all grain products. Folate intakes likely would be higher if current intakes were measured. Vitamin B_{12} intakes were less than the DRI in all the field studies, but none had intakes less than 70% MDRI. All the dining hall studies had adequate vitamin B_{12} intake (vitamin B_{12} data are missing for one field study). Niacin intake in one of the dining hall studies was higher than the DRIs Tolerable Upper Intake Level (UL) of 35 mg/d.[32]

Mean intakes of minerals were variable and were frequently lower than desirable. Although only one dining hall study reported a mean calcium intake meeting the MDRI, calcium intakes in the dining hall studies were generally greater than those reported in national nutrition surveys (Table 21.6). However, in all the field studies, calcium and magnesium intakes were less than 70% of the MDRI (magnesium data missing for one field and one dining hall study). Compared with the MDRI of 15 mg, mean iron intakes were adequate in all the dining hall studies but were significantly less than this in all the field studies. Mean zinc intakes for the dining hall studies approached or exceeded the MDRI and in all cases exceeded the updated DRI guideline. However, zinc nutriture of women in the field studies was low to marginal (zinc data missing for one field and one dining hall study). Mean potassium intakes met or almost met the MDRI in the dining hall studies. Conversely, potassium intakes were less than desirable in all three of the field studies calculating intakes of this mineral (potassium data missing for one field and one dining hall study).

Energy intake studies of male soldiers (not shown) also found lower energy intakes of soldiers in the field than soldiers eating in military dining facilities.[1-6,9] However, despite marginal or low energy intakes in the field, men still consumed enough food to meet the MDRI for most nutrients.

Two of the national nutrition surveys, the Third National Health and Nutrition Examination Survey (NHANES III) and the Continuing Survey of Food Intakes by Individuals (CSFII), also have reported low intakes of folate, calcium, magnesium and iron in the general female population ages 20 to 29 years old in the U.S. (Table 21.6).[24,38] This suggests that most of the nutritional problems of female soldiers are similar to those of their civilian counterparts and, therefore, the military setting and the type of ration are not the exclusive determinants of low intakes.

The percentages of total energy intake from protein, carbohydrate, fat and alcohol found in the military nutrition studies are shown on Table 21.7.[1-9] Figure 21.1 compares the average caloric distribution of the dietary intakes in the military nutrition studies with the distribution found in the 1994–1996 CSFII[24] and with that of the formulation recommendations for field rations.[29,30] The average macronutrient distribution of energy intakes in the field studies was close to the national recommendations of 10–15% from protein, 55–60% from carbohydrate and no more than 30% from fat.[39] The average macronutrient distribution of intakes in the dining hall studies was modestly higher in total fat and protein and lower in carbohydrate than that of the field study intakes and was close to the intake distribution reported for the 1994–96 CSFII.[24] Averaging the caloric distribution from the dining hall studies that provided A-Ration (i.e., omitting the studies of women who provided their own diets), still shows a distribution similar to the national survey.

The energy intake distributions in the different studies generally paralleled those of the respective ration provision. As the ration or menu content of fat has been

TABLE 21.6
Nutrient Intake of U.S. Female Population

Nutrient	DRI[a]	NHANES II[b] 1976–1980 n=1366	CSFII[c] 1985–1986 n=1000	NHANES III[d] 1988–1991 n=838	CSFII[e] 1989–1991 n=1272	CSFII[f] 1994–1996 n=720
				Nutrition Monitoring Surveys		
Energy (kcal)	2200	1675	1674	1957	1655	1841
Protein (g)	46–50[g]	64	65	69	66	66
Carbohydrate (g)	—	195	198	241	206	242
Fat (g)	—	67	68	75	64	66
Cholesterol (mg)	—	270	302	244	250	219
Vitamin A (mcg RE)	700[h]	841	1048	786	5162[i]	855
Vitamin D (mcg)	5	—	—	—	—	—
Vitamin E (mg)	15	—	—	7.7	—	7.1
Vitamin K (mcg)	90	—	—	—	—	—
Ascorbic acid (mg)	75	95	86	87	89	93
Thiamin (mg)	1.1	1.09	1.17	1.43	1.32	1.37
Riboflavin (mg)	1.1	1.49	1.51	1.71	1.58	1.63
Niacin (mg NE)	14	16.2	17.3	19.6	18.3	19.3
Vitamin B_6 (mg)	1.3	—	—	1.5	—	1.53
Folate (mcg)	400	—	—	230	—	230
Vitamin B_{12} (mcg)	2.4	—	—	3.97	—	3.78
Pantothenic Acid (mg)	5	—	—	—	—	—
Biotin (mcg)	30	—	—	—	—	—
Choline (mg)	425	—	—	—	—	—
Calcium (mg)	1000	662	691	778	666	701
Phosphorus (mg)	700	1117	1065	1137	1048	1090
Magnesium (mg)	310–320[j]	—	—	240	—	229
Iron (mg)	18	10.7	11.1	12.4	12.5	13.5
Zinc (mg)	8	—	—	9.7	—	9.5
Sodium (mg)	—	2404	2593	3002	2639	3001

Iodine (mcg)	150	—	—	—	—	—
Selenium (mcg)	55	—	—	—	—	—
Fluoride (mg)	3	—	—	—	—	—
Potassium (mg)	—	2055	2143	2260	2129	2255
Chromium (mcg)	25	—	—	—	—	—
Copper (mcg)	900	—	—	1130	—	1100
Manganese (mg)	1.8	—	—	—	—	—
Molybdenum (mcg)	45	—	—	—	—	—
Reference number:	31-35	38	38	38	38	24

[a] DRI for women 19–50 years.

[b] Second National Health and Nutrition Examination Survey, women 20–29 years (1 d).

[c] Continuing Survey of Food Intakes by Individuals for 1985, women 20–29 years (1 d).

[d] Third National Health and Nutrition Examination Survey, women 20–29 years (1 d).

[e] Continuing Survey of Food Intakes by Individuals for 1989, women 20–29 years (1 d).

[f] Continuing Survey of Food Intakes by Individuals for 1994, women 20–29 years (1 d).

[g] 46 g for ages 19–24; 50 g for ages 25–50.

[h] DRI in mcg Retinol Activity Equivalents (RAE), which is based on new estimates for the conversion of pro-vitamin A carotenoids to vitamin A. The 1989 RDA for vitamin A was 800 mcg Retinol Equivalents (RE). Except for 1989–1991 CSFII, table values for vitamin A intakes are in RE.

[i] Vitamin A data in international units (IU). The 1989 RDA for vitamin A would have equated to approximately 4000 IU.

[j] 310 mg for ages 19–30; 320 mg for ages 31–50.

From Food and Nutrition Board, Recommended Dietary Allowances, 10th ed., National Academy of Sciences, Washington, D.C., 1989; Food and Nutrition Board, Institute of Medicine, *Dietary Reference Intakes for Calcium, Phosphorus, Magnesium, Vitamin D and Fluoride*, National Academy Press, Washington, D.C., 1997; Food and Nutrition Board, Institute of Medicine, *Dietary Reference Intakes for Thiamin, Riboflavin, Niacin, Vitamin B_6 Pantothenic Acid, Biotin and Choline*, National Academy Press, Washington, D.C., 1998; Food and Nutrition Board, Institute of Medicine, *Dietary Reference Intakes for Vitamin C, Vitamin E, Selenium and Carotenoids*, National Academy Press, Washington, D.C., 2000; Food and Nutrition Board, Institute of Medicine, *Dietary Reference Intakes for Vitamin A, Vitamin K, Arsenic, Boron, Chromium, Copper, Iodine, Iron, Manganese, Molybdenum, Nickel, Silicon, Vanadium and Zinc*, National Academy Press, Washington, D.C., 2001; Life Sciences Research Office, Federation of American Societies for Experimental Biology, Third Report on Nutrition Monitoring in the United States: Volume 2, prepared for the Interagency Board for Nutrition Monitoring and Related Research, U.S. Government Printing Office, Washington, D.C., 1995; U.S. Department of Agriculture, Agricultural Research Service, Data Table: Results from USDA's 1994–96 Continuing Survey of Food Intakes by Individuals and 1994–96 Diet and Health Knowledge Survey, on 1994–96 Continuing Survey of Food Intakes by Individuals and 1994–96 Diet and Health Knowledge Survey, CD-ROM, NTIS Accession Number PB98-500457, 1997.

TABLE 21.7
Percentages of Calories from Protein, Carbohydrate, Fat and Alcohol in Military Nutrition Studies

	Field					Dining hall				
			Camp Mackall 1997							
Nutrient	Hawaii 1985	Bolivia 1990	MRE	Concept	West Point 1979	Ft. Jackson 1988	West Point 1990	Ft. Jackson 1993	Ft. Sam Houston 1995	Ft. Bliss 1996-97
Energy[a] (kcal)	1834	1668	1834	2093	2454[b]	2467	2314[c]	2592	2037	1773[d]
Protein (%)	14.6	16.3	12.9	10.3	13.7	15.6	13.7	12.7	14.7	15.6
Carbohydrate (%)	51.0	52.8	57.7	60.5	44.1	50.1	54.2	54.7	57.5	48.9
Fat (%)	34.4	30.9	29.4	29.2	39.2	34.3	31.5	32.6	27.8	33.5

[a] Energy consumed during the study period.
[b] 3% of kilocalories provided by alcohol intake.
[c] 0.6% of kilocalories provided by alcohol intake.
[d] 2% of kilocalories provided by alcohol intake.

Adapted from King, N., Fridlund, K.E. and Askew, E.W., *J. Am. Coll. Nutr.*, 12, 344, 1993. With permission.

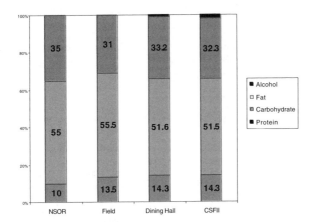

FIGURE 21.1 Percentages of calories from protein, carbohydrate, fat and alcohol in nutritional surveys. NSOR bar = macronutrient distribution established for operational rations; field bar = average from macronutrient distribution in military field surveys; dining hall bar = average from macronutrient distribution in military dining hall surveys; CSFII bar = calculated macronutrient distribution for the 1994–96 CSFII survey.

(Data from Nutrition Standards and Education, Army Regulation 40-25/Bureau of Medical Instruction 10110.6/Air Force Instruction 44-141, Headquarters, Departments of the Army, Navy and Air Force, Washington, D.C., 2001; Kretsch, M.J., Conforti, P.M. and Sauberlich, H.E., Nutrient Intake Evaluation of Male and Female Cadets at the U.S. Military Academy, West Point, New York, LAIR Report No. 218, Letterman Army Institute of Research, Presidio of San Francisco, 1986; Combat Field Feeding System — Force Development Test and Experimentation, Vol. 1, Basic Report No. CDEC-TR-85-006A, U.S. Army Research Institute of Environmental Medicine, Natick, MA and U.S. Army Combat Developments Experimentation Center, Fort Ord, CA, 1986; Rose, R.W., Baker, C.J., Salter, C., Wisnaskas, W., Edwards, J.S.A. and Rose, M.S., Dietary Assessment of U.S. Army Basic Trainees at Fort Jackson, S.C., Technical Report No. T6-89, U.S. Army Research Institute of Environmental Medicine, Natick, MA, 1989; Edwards, J.S.A., Askew, E.W., King, N., Fulco, C.S., Hoyt, R.W. and Delany, J.P., An Assessment of the Nutritional Intake and Energy Expenditure of Unacclimatized U.S. Army Soldiers Living and Working at High Altitude, Technical Report No. T10-91, U.S. Army Research Institute of Environmental Medicine, Natick, MA, 1991; Klicka, M. V., Sherman, D. E., King, N., Friedl, K. E. and Askew, E. W., Nutritional Assessment of Cadets at the U.S. Military Academy: Part 2. Assessment of Nutritional Intake, Technical Report No. T94-1, U.S. Army Research Institute of Environmental Medicine, Natick, MA, 1993; Baker-Fulco, C.J., Kramer, F.M., Johnson, J., Lesher, L.L., Merrill, E. and Delany, J., Dietary Intakes of Female and Male Combat Support Hospital Personnel Subsisting on Meal-Focused or Standard Versions of the Meal, Ready-to-Eat, Technical Report NOT-02/03, U.S. Army Research Institute of Environmental Medicine, Natick, MA, 2002; King, N., Arsenault, J.E., Mutter, S.H., Murphy, T.C., Champagne, C., Westphal, K.A. and Askew, E.W., Nutritional Intake of Female Soldiers During the U.S. Army Basic Combat Training, Technical Report No. T94-17, U.S. Army Research Institute of Environmental Medicine, Natick, MA, 1994; Cline, A.D., Patton, J.F., Tharion, W.J., Strowman, S.R., Champagne, C.M., Arsenault, J., Reynolds, K.L., Warber, J.P., Baker-Fulco, C., Rood, J., Tulley, R.T. and Lieberman, H.R., Assessment of the Relationship Between Iron Status, Dietary Intake, Performance and Mood State of Female Army Officers in a Basic Training Population, Technical Report No. T98-24, U.S. Army Research Institute of Environmental Medicine, Natick, MA, 1998; Karge, W.H., unpublished data, 1999; and U.S. Department of Agriculture, Agricultural Research Service, Data Table: Results from USDA's 1994–96 Continuing Survey of Food Intakes by Individuals and 1994–96 Diet and Health Knowledge Survey, on 1994–96 Continuing Survey of Food Intakes by Individuals and 1994–96 Diet and Health Knowledge Survey, CD-ROM, NTIS Accession Number PB98-500457, 1997.)

reduced and that of carbohydrate increased, dietary intakes have changed in the same direction. But, the greater proportional intake of protein compared with the ration provision in most of the field studies and the relative consistency in the proportion of energy from protein across field and dining hall studies suggest that food preferences also influenced which ration components the women chose to consume.

V. NUTRITION ISSUES

A. OVERVIEW

Although sporadic low nutrient intakes may be inconsequential, this is not the case when inadequate intake occurs repetitively due to participation in multiple field training exercises. This impact may be even greater if experienced for longer periods of time during extended deployments. Furthermore, since low intakes are observed in many women in the U.S.,[24,38] and, thus, are likely in free-living military women as well, low nutrient intakes in field feeding situations may exacerbate a marginal nutritional status.

In 1998, 31.8% of military women reported being under a "great deal" or a "fairly large amount" of stress attributed to being a woman in the military.[23] Greater than average proportions of U.S. Army women (36.1%) and Marine Corps women (38.5%) reported stress associated with being a woman in the military.[23] Part of the stress may be due to having to achieve and maintain body-weight standards, even after childbirth. The efforts of female soldiers to achieve or maintain their weight goals, combined with the demands of coordinating their work and family roles, surely have a negative impact on their diets.

The nutrient density of military rations is a concern because female soldiers may not want to or may not be able to eat as much as male soldiers. For example, in the 1993 Fort Jackson study, the two main reasons given for not finishing entire portions were (1) not being hungry and (2) being too full.[7] Furthermore, it would be difficult for most female soldiers to consume the amount of energy required to meet their MDRIs for most nutrients without gaining weight.

B. VITAMINS

1. FOLATE

Low intakes of folate in the civilian population have been associated with neural tube defects[40] and other adverse pregnancy outcomes.[41] Therefore, folate is of particular concern to pregnant women. It has been suggested that adequate folate intake is essential from at least 4 weeks before conception through the first 3 months of pregnancy.[42] Since most female soldiers are of childbearing age[17] and not all pregnancies are planned (many conceptions occur upon returning from field training exercises or deployments, when folate intake potentially has been poor for several days), inadequate intake of folate is an important issue for military women as well. An estimated 16% of military women, to include 20.1% of U.S. Army women, reported in 1998 that they had been pregnant within the previous year; approximately 36% of military women had been pregnant within the past 5 years.[23]

TABLE 21.8
Hematological Values[a] of Female Soldiers

	Normal Range	West Point 1979 (n = 30–72[b])	West Point 1990 (n = 22[c])	Ft. Jackson 1993 (n = 49[d])	Ft. Sam Houston 1995 (n = 45[e])
RCB folate (ng/ml)	169–707	431.0 ± 138.0	309.0 ± 65.0	157.2 ± 53.3	293.1 ±98.0
Serum folate (ng/ml)	2.2–17.3	11.7 ± 6.2	9.3 ± 3.7	3.6 ± 0.3	6.8 ± 2.9
Hemoglobin (g/dl)	12–16	13.3 ± 1.2	12.5 ± 1.0	12.6 ± 0.2	13.3 ± 0.8
Hematocrit (%)	37–47	39.1 ± 2.3	37.8 ± 2.4	37.4 ± 0.4	40.0 ± 2.2
Serum iron (mcg/dl)	65–175	80.0 ± 38.0	72.0 ± 41.0	69.2 ± 6.0	76.6 ± 39.4
TIBC (mcg/dl)	300–360	344.0 ± 44.0	326.0 ± 46.0	334.1 ± 6.8	380.5 ± 66.6
Iron saturation (%)	20–55	23.0 ± 11.2	22.1 ± 13.3	20.4 ± 1.8	21.5 ± 14.0
Ferritin (ng/ml)	22–447	25.0 ± 11.0	18.0 ± 13.0	10.6 ± 1.7	21.7 ± 15.4

[a] Mean ± SD.

[b] Reference 45.

[c] Females that did not donate blood the week prior to testing and did not use iron or general vitamin-mineral supplements.[43]

[d] Soldiers that participated on nutrition intake data only; blood drawn 10 d after nutrient intake data collection.[44]

[e] Reference 8.

Adapted from King, N., Fridlund, K.E. and Askew, E.W., *J. Am. Coll. Nutr.*, 12, 344, 1993. With permission.

Red blood cell and serum folate levels from the two West Point studies, the 1993 Fort Jackson study and the Fort Sam Houston study are shown in Table 21.8.[8,43–45] The relationship between low folate intake and biochemical markers of folate status has been assessed in few military studies. The 1993 Fort Jackson study data reveal a significant ($p < 0.05$) but weak (r = 0.37) correlation between folate intake and serum folate.[44] The Fort Sam Houston study found a significant ($p < 0.001$) decrease in both red blood cell and serum folate over the 8 weeks of training,[8] suggesting that marginally low folate intake results in negative folate balance.

C. Minerals

1. Calcium

Adequate calcium intake is important for bone health throughout life.[46,47] Although osteoporosis is a multifactorial disorder, it is generally recognized that low calcium intake during the first three decades of life may jeopardize the optimization of peak bone mass and increase the risk of osteoporosis later in life.[46–48] Optimizing and maintaining bone mineral density is of particular concern to the military because of the high incidence of stress fractures in young military women.[28,49–52] Furthermore, recent evidence, although inconclusive, suggests that increased intake of calcium-rich foods reduces fat mass, blood pressure and risk of colon cancer.[46,53]

In the Army Food and Nutrition Survey conducted in 1997,[54] female soldiers (n = 467) reported consuming a mean of 2.3 foods each day from the dairy group. In general, these female soldiers were slightly more aware than the general population of the relationship of dietary calcium to health. Seventy-nine percent of the Army women responding to the survey versus 67% of the civilian population correctly attributed inadequate calcium intake to a potential development of osteoporosis. Despite this awareness, 50% of the female soldiers believed their diets were low in calcium.

2. Magnesium

Magnesium affects the metabolism of calcium, sodium and potassium. Its deficiency is considered rare because hypocalcemia symptoms do not develop until the magnesium deficiency is moderate to severe. However, mild magnesium deficiency may cause a significant decrease in serum calcium.[31] Low intakes of magnesium have been associated with several chronic conditions such as osteoporosis and cardiovascular disease. Although these associations are weak at best and further investigation is warranted, the results from the Dietary Approaches to Stop Hypertension (DASH) trial suggest that increasing intake of magnesium-rich foods in conjunction with a diet that is adequate in potassium, calcium, and high fiber, and low in saturated fat, total fat and cholesterol significantly (p <0.001) reduces blood pressure.[55,56]

3. Iron

Negative iron balance has been associated with decrements in physical performance and has also been related to various neurological, cognitive and immunological problems.[57–59]Therefore, suboptimal intakes of dietary iron could impact job performance of military women. Hematological data from the two West Point studies, the 1993 Fort Jackson study and the Fort Sam Houston study are shown in Table 21.8.[8,43–45] The relationship between low iron intake and iron status markers has not been assessed extensively in military studies. Friedl and coauthors reported high prevalences of iron deficiency in the female cadets at West Point: 36.6% of the female cadets that did not donate blood (n = 41, include iron supplement users and nonusers) had ferritin levels less than 12 ng/ml (indicating low iron stores), 22% had iron saturation levels less than 16% and 4.9% had hemoglobin levels less than 12 g/dl.[43] Nevertheless, serum markers of iron status in cadets from the 1990 West Point study were not significantly related to dietary iron intakes.[5] Westphal and Friedl observed that 63.3% of the female soldiers in training (n = 49) had ferritin levels less than 12 ng/ml, 42.9% had iron saturation levels less than 16% and 24.5% had hemoglobin levels less than 12 g/dl.[44] Though these mean hematological values were lower than those reported in the West Point studies, the Fort Jackson study also found that serum markers of iron status were not significantly associated with iron intakes.[44] Cline et al. observed significant decreases in serum iron (p <0.001), ferritin (p <0.001) and transferrin (p <0.01) over the 8 weeks of officer training at Fort Sam Houston.[8] They reported that the prevalence of women with iron depletion increased from 33% to 64% and those with anemia increased from 7% to 13% over the 8 weeks of training. However, again, serum markers of iron status were not significantly related to dietary iron intake. Furthermore, there was no effect of iron depletion on any of the measures of physical or mental performance, which may be due to the short duration of the study.[8]

4. Zinc

The zinc intake of female soldiers was low in the field settings (Table 21.5).[4,6] Given that intakes of zinc seem to be adequate in the civilian population[24] and in military women who are not subsisting on field rations, low intakes may be tolerated during short-term field feeding situations. Nevertheless, cases of zinc deficiency exist. And, since zinc and iron are best absorbed from many of the same food sources and the same dietary components inhibit their absorption, it is not uncommon to have zinc and iron deficiency in tandem.[60] Zinc is a component of the body's antioxidant defenses[61] and plays a role in many biological systems including immune[62] and neuropsychological[60] functions. Recently, it has been reported that zinc plays a role in maintaining normal ocular function.[63]

VI. MILITARY NUTRITION INITIATIVES

Of the 15 leading causes of death in the U.S. (heart diseases, cancers, strokes, chronic obstructive lung diseases, unintentional injuries, pneumonia and influenza, diabetes mellitus, HIV infection, suicide, homicide, chronic liver disease and cirrhosis, kidney diseases, septicemia, atherosclerosis and perinatal complications), five have been associated with diet (coronary heart disease, some types of cancer, stroke, diabetes mellitus and atherosclerosis) and another four (accidents, suicide, homicide and cirrhosis of the liver) have been associated with excessive alcohol intake.[64] Furthermore, high blood pressure, obesity, dental caries, osteoporosis and gastrointestinal diseases are attributed to dietary excesses and imbalances.[65] The heightened awareness of nutrition-related health issues generated several Department of the Army Military Nutrition Initiatives in 1985[66] that were consistent with national health objectives. The Nutrition Initiatives led to changes in the Armed Forces Recipe Service,[67] the Army Master Menu (no longer produced)[68] and the Army Food Service Program[69] in an attempt to provide soldiers with a variety of nutritious menu alternatives lower in fat, cholesterol and sodium. Furthermore, the initiatives were designed to heighten soldiers' awareness of the importance of nutrition and to educate soldiers and their families to make appropriate food choices.

Between 1988 and 1993, there were significant improvements in Army menus, as evidenced by analyses of the menus provided at the military dining facility at Fort Jackson, S.C.[7] Energy provided by fat was reduced from 38% to 33% (energy from saturated fat in 1993 was 10%), while energy provided from carbohydrate was increased from 50% to 56%. These changes brought the menu closer to the recommendations of 55% or more from carbohydrate, 10% to 15% from protein and 30% or less from fat.[29] The 1993 menu also was lower in dietary cholesterol than the 1988 menu (928 mg vs. 1299 mg). However, 928 mg remains considerably higher than desirable to promote the cholesterol intake goal of 300 mg or less. The reduction in sodium content of the menu from 1731 mg/1000 kcal in 1988 to 1640 mg/1000 kcal brought the menu within the target of an average of 1400–1700 mg/1000 kcal of food served in military food service systems.

Table 21.9 presents nutrient intakes of female soldiers before introduction of the Nutrition Initiatives (West Point 1979), soon after their implementation (Ft. Jackson 1988) and after changes had been in place for some time (West Point 1990 and Ft. Jackson 1993). These data highlight the progress made as of 1993.[7] The higher dietary cholesterol intake at Ft. Jackson in 1993 was due to increased visible egg consumption. The number of female soldiers consuming more than three eggs per week increased from 50% in 1988 to 64% in 1993. In 1988, visible eggs contributed 39% of the total dietary cholesterol, while in 1993, visible eggs accounted for 43% of the total dietary cholesterol (the cholesterol value in the 1993 food composition data base was adjusted to the 1988 value). This finding is one illustration of the need for nutrition education programs.

The services continue to build on the foundation laid by the Military Nutrition Initiatives, although this term is no longer used. In their place, the military adopted the Dietary Guidelines for Americans and the Food Guide Pyramid, which is included in most nutrition education messages. The Department of Defense (DoD) Nutrition Committee incorporated specific Healthy People 2000 nutrition objectives into its first strategic plan in 1997. The goals targeted by the Committee were:

Reducing fat, sodium and alcohol consumption
  • Increasing carbohydrate, fiber, water and calcium intakes
  • Providing point of service nutrition information.

Although these goals remain, the 2002 strategic plan has placed primary emphasis on weight management and avoidance of risky or inappropriate nutritional supplements.

The DoD is a provider of the National 5-A-Day for Better Health Program (www.5aday.gov). This program is extensively marketed in military commissaries (grocery stores), which have demonstrated a significant increase in produce sales since the program was implemented. The U.S. Army Center for Health Promotion and Preventive Medicine (CHPPM) adapted 5-A-Day Program materials for a folate education campaign targeted to Army women. The folate brochure material is available, along with additional nutrition information, as part of the Hooah 4 Health program on the CHPPM website, www.hooah4health.com (visited July 16, 2002).

Nutrition education remains the cornerstone in motivating soldiers and their families to adopt healthy eating habits. During basic combat training, soldiers at Fort Jackson, South Carolina, receive general nutrition information as part of a mandated 90-minute class on health and hygiene. Nutrition education efforts in military dining facilities include information on the caloric value of each menu item plus nutrition posters, brochures and table tents. Nutrition Facts panels are now on almost all field ration food items and the protective cardboard packaging on a few items displays fortification information and relevant nutrition messages. Finally, during National Nutrition Month® (March) and throughout the year, Army dietitians provide nutrition education opportunities for soldiers and their families.

TABLE 21.9
Impact of Nutrition Initiatives on Female Soldiers' Nutrient Intakes:
From 1979 to 1993

	West Point 1979 (n = 54)	Ft. Jackson 1988 (n = 40)	West Point 1990 (n = 86)	Ft. Jackson 1993 (n = 49)
Energy/kg of body wt (kcal)	41.1	41.7	37.8	41.0
Mean energy intake (kcal)	2454	2467	2314	2592
Nutrients with mean intake <100% MDRIs	Ca, Fe Folate, Mg, Zn[a]	Ca[b]	Mg	Folate, Ca, Mg, Zn
Percent of total kcal (%)				
Protein	13.7	15.6	13.7	12.7
Fat	39.2	34.3	31.5	32.6
Carbohydrate	44.1	50.1	54.2	54.7
Proportion (percent) of soldiers with fat calories intake				
<25% fat	c	0	5	6
25%–29% fat	c	23	35	22
30%–34% fat	c	30	41	47
35%–39% fat	54	40	16	18
>40% fat	34	7	2	6
Mean cholesterol intake (mg)	403	418	234	466
Mean sodium intake (mg)	2764[d]	4420	3703	3994

[a] Limited food composition data available at the time of the study for folate, magnesium and zinc.

[b] Limitations of the 1988 nutrient data base precluded analyses of several nutrients, such as vitamin B_6, folate, magnesium, zinc and potassium.

[c] 11% of soldiers consumed <35% fat calories.

[d] Sodium from discretionary salt not included.

From Kretsch, M.J., Conforti, P.M. and Sauberlich, H.E., Nutrient Intake Evaluation of Male and Female Cadets at the U.S. Military Academy, West Point, New York, LAIR Report No. 218, Letterman Army Institute of Research, Presidio of San Francisco, 1986; Rose, R.W., Baker, C.J., Salter, C., Wisnaskas, W., Edwards, J.S.A. and Rose, M.S., Dietary Assessment of U.S. Army Basic Trainees at Fort Jackson, S.C., Technical Report No. T6-89, U.S. Army Research Institute of Environmental Medicine, Natick, MA, 1989; Klicka, M.V., Sherman, D.E., King, N., Friedl, K.E. and Askew, E.W., Nutritional Assessment of Cadets at the U.S. Military Academy: Part 2. Assessment of Nutritional Intake, Technical Report No. T94-1, U.S. Army Research Institute of Environmental Medicine, Natick, MA, 1993; King, N., Arsenault, J.E., Mutter, S.H., Murphy, T.C., Champagne, C., Westphal, K.A. and Askew, E.W., Nutritional Intake of Female Soldiers During the U.S. Army Basic Combat Training, Technical Report No. T94-17, U.S. Army Research Institute of Environmental Medicine, Natick, MA, 1994.

VII. SUMMARY AND CONCLUSIONS

It can be seen from the limited data collected on U.S. Army women that the nutrition issues relevant to servicewomen are similar to those faced by their counterparts in the civilian population. Optimal intakes of folate, calcium, magnesium and iron are difficult to achieve due to the density of these nutrients in the typical military and civilian diets. The emphasis the military places upon weight control further exacerbates this problem.

Paradoxically, within what can be a restrictive military environment, soldiers are free to choose what they want to eat from what is available. Their choices are influenced by a complex interaction of factors, including the circumstances faced at the moment of eating and their beliefs about nutrition. Nutrition education is an integral part of any viable solution to the nutritional problems of military women. With increased knowledge and awareness, some of the behaviors that influence food selection and consumption may change to promote a healthier diet.

VIII. RECOMMENDATIONS

In September 1996, the Committee on Body Composition, Nutrition and Health of Military Women (a subcommittee of the Committee on Military Nutrition Research of the Institute of Medicine) convened a panel of experts at a workshop to examine issues of body composition, fitness and appearance standards and their impact on the health, nutritional status and performance of military women.[70] The following recommendations concur with the committee's recommendations.

More research is needed to ascertain the short- and long-term effects of both sporadic and routine suboptimal nutrient intakes on nutritional status, health and performance of military women. Considering that approximately 53% of the women in the U.S. Army are older than 25 years of age,[17] particular emphasis should be given to including older military women in future studies. Also, research is needed on the effect of environmental extremes on the nutritional status of military women. With the increased popularity of nutritional supplements, nutritional surveys must capture these data and present nutrient intakes with and without nutritional supplements to accurately assess intake from military rations.

Implementation of nutrition education programs tailored for the military woman is crucial. These programs should feature the importance of eating nutritionally balanced varied diets and emphasize the relevance of dietary calcium, magnesium, iron and folate to women's health. Practical "how to" guidelines to assist military women in the selection of low-fat, nutrient-rich foods in the field and in the dining facilities would be essential parts of these programs. To this end, the nutrition facts panel of the rations must be accurate. In addition, nutrition facts as well calorie information should be posted for each menu item in the dining facilities.

Since it is neither realistic nor practical for military women to consume excess calories to achieve their vitamin and mineral intake goals, the nutrient-to-energy density of the field rations should be adjusted to provide for the nutritional needs of military women within an energy intake of no more than 2300 kcal. Augmenting ration fortification and promoting gender-specific supplements with iron, calcium and folate need to be further explored.

ACKNOWLEDGMENTS

The authors are grateful to the following individuals: LTC Kathleen A. Westphal and Dr. James A. Vogel for assistance in the preparation of the original manuscript when assigned to the U.S. Army Research Institute of Environmental Medicine; LTC (P) Michael H. Custer from the U.S. Army Center for Health Promotion and Preventive Medicine; Dr. Robert M. Bray and Ms. Kristine Rae from the Research Triangle Institute for facilitating and providing DoD Survey data; Dr. Betty D. Maxfield from the Office of the Deputy Chief of Staff for Personnel and Zietta M. Ferris from the Defense Manpower Data Center for providing U.S. Army demographics data. Their contribution is acknowledged and greatly appreciated.

REFERENCES

1. Kretsch, M.J., Conforti, P.M. and Sauberlich, H.E., Nutrient Intake Evaluation of Male and Female Cadets at the U.S. Military Academy, West Point, New York, LAIR Report No. 218, Letterman Army Institute of Research, Presidio of San Francisco, 1986.
2. Combat Field Feeding System — Force Development Test and Experimentation, Vol. 1, Basic Report No. CDEC-TR-85-006A, U.S. Army Research Institute of Environmental Medicine, Natick, MA and U.S. Army Combat Developments Experimentation Center, Fort Ord, CA, 1986.
3. Rose, R.W., Baker, C.J., Salter, C., Wisnaskas, W., Edwards, J.S.A. and Rose, M.S., Dietary Assessment of U.S. Army Basic Trainees at Fort Jackson, S.C., Technical Report No. T6-89, U.S. Army Research Institute of Environmental Medicine, Natick, MA, 1989.
4. Edwards, J.S.A., Askew, E.W., King, N., Fulco, C.S., Hoyt, R.W. and Delany, J.P., An Assessment of the Nutritional Intake and Energy Expenditure of Unacclimatized U.S. Army Soldiers Living and Working at High Altitude, Technical Report No. T10-91, U.S. Army Research Institute of Environmental Medicine, Natick, MA, 1991.
5. Klicka, M.V., Sherman, D.E., King, N., Friedl, K.E. and Askew, E.W., Nutritional Assessment of Cadets at the U.S. Military Academy: Part 2. Assessment of Nutritional Intake, Technical Report No. T94-1, U.S. Army Research Institute of Environmental Medicine, Natick, MA, 1993.
6. Baker-Fulco, C.J., Kramer, F.M., Johnson, J., Lesher, L.L., Merrill, E. and DeLany, J., Dietary Intakes of Female and Male Combat Support Hospital Personnel Subsisting on Meal-Focused or Standard Versions of the Meal, Ready-to-Eat, Technical Report, U.S. Army Research Institute of Environmental Medicine, Natick, MA., 2002.
7. King, N., Arsenault, J.E., Mutter, S.H., Murphy, T.C., Champagne, C., Westphal, K.A. and Askew, E.W., Nutritional Intake of Female Soldiers During the U.S. Army Basic Combat Training, Technical Report No. T94-17, U.S. Army Research Institute of Environmental Medicine, Natick, MA, 1994.

8. Cline, A.D., Patton, J.F., Tharion, W.J., Strowman, S.R., Champagne, C.M., Arsenault, J., Reynolds, K.L., Warber, J.P., Baker-Fulco, C., Rood, J., Tulley, R.T. and Lieberman, H.R., Assessment of the Relationship Between Iron Status, Dietary Intake, Performance and Mood State of Female Army Officers in a Basic Training Population, Technical Report No. T98-24, U.S. Army Research Institute of Environmental Medicine, Natick, MA, 1998.

9. Karge, W.H., unpublished data, 1999.

10. Ferris, Z.M., personal communication, 2002.

11. Army Demographic Data, Project No. M001443, Defense Manpower Data Center, Arlington, VA, 1988.

12. Department of Defense Military Manpower Statistics, June 30, 1993, Washington Headquarters Services, Directorate for Information Operations and Reports, Washington, D.C., 1993.

13. Army Demographics FY01, Headquarters, Department of Army, Office of the Deputy Chief of Staff for Personnel, Human Resources Directorate, Washington, D.C., 2001.

14. Military Women in the Department of Defense, Vol. 6, U.S. Department of Defense, Washington, D.C., 1988.

15. Army Policy for the Assignment of Female Soldiers, Army Regulation 600-13, Headquarters, Department of the Army, Washington, D.C., 1992.

16. Women in the Army – Historical Highlights, in Women in the Army Page of the Deputy Chief of Staff for Personnel, U.S. Army, Pentagon (visited June 4, 2002 http://odcsper.army.mil/directorates/hr/women_in_the_army/women-army.doc).

17. Gordon, C.C., U.S. Army Anthropometric Survey Database: Downsizing, Demographic Change and Validity of the 1988 Data in 1996, Technical Report NATICK/TR-97/003, U.S. Army Natick Research, Development and Engineering Center, Natick, MA, 1996.

18. DoD Physical Fitness and Body Fat Program, Department of Defense Directive 1308.1, Washington, D.C., 1995.

19. The Army Weight Control Program, Army Regulation 600-9(Update Change 1), Headquarters, Department of the Army, Washington, D.C., 1994.

20. ODCSPER Weight Control, in Page of the Deputy Chief of Staff for Personnel, U.S. Army, Pentagon (visited June 3, 2002 http://odcsper.army.mil/Directorates/hr/hr_pr_/ WeightControl/weight_control_faqs.asp).

21. Friedl, K.E., Body composition and military performance: Origins of the army standards, in *Body Composition and Physical Performance*, Marriott, B.M. and Grumstrup-Scott, J., Eds., National Academy Press, Washington, D.C., 1992, chap. 3 and appendix E.

22. Vogel, J.A., Patton, J.F., Mello, R.P. and Daniels, W.L., An analysis of aerobic capacity in a large U.S. population, *J. Appl. Physiol.*, 60, 494, 1986.

23. DoD Survey of Health Related Behaviors among Military Personnel, 1998 (special analyses provided by R. Bray and K. Rae at Research Triangle Institute).

24. U.S. Department of Agriculture, Agricultural Research Service, Data Table: Results from USDA's 1994–96 Continuing Survey of Food Intakes by Individuals and 1994–96 Diet and Health Knowledge Survey, on 1994-96 Continuing Survey of Food Intakes by Individuals and 1994-96 Diet and Health Knowledge Survey, CD-ROM, NTIS Accession Number PB98-500457, 1997.

25. Physical Fitness Training, Field Manual 21-20, Headquarters, Department of the Army, Washington, D.C., 1992.

26. Army Health Promotion, Army Regulation 600-63, Headquarters, Department of the Army, Washington, D.C., 1996.

27. Standards of Medical Fitness, Army Regulation 40-501, Headquarters, Department of the Army, Washington, D.C., 2002.

28. Westphal, K.A., King, N., Friedl, K.E., Sharp, M.A. and Reynolds, K.L., Health, Performance and Nutritional Status of U.S. Army Women During Basic Combat Training, Technical Report No. T96-2, U.S. Army Research Institute of Environmental Medicine, Natick, MA, 1996.

29. Baker-Fulco, C.J., Bathalon, G.P., Bovill, M.E. and Lieberman, H.R., Military Dietary Reference Intakes: Rationale for Table Values, Technical Note No. 00-10, U.S. Army Research Institute of Environmental Medicine, Natick, MA, 2001.

30. Nutrition Standards and Education, Army Regulation 40-25/Bureau of Medical Instruction 10110.6/Air Force Instruction 44-141, Headquarters, Departments of the Army, Navy and Air Force, Washington, D.C., 2001.

31. Food and Nutrition Board, Institute of Medicine, *Dietary Reference Intakes for Calcium, Phosphorus, Magnesium, Vitamin D and Fluoride*, National Academy Press, Washington, D.C., 1997.

32. Food and Nutrition Board, Institute of Medicine, *Dietary Reference Intakes for Thiamin, Riboflavin, Niacin, Vitamin B_6, Pantothenic Acid, Biotin and Choline*, National Academy Press, Washington, D.C., 1998.

33. Food and Nutrition Board, Institute of Medicine, *Dietary Reference Intakes for Vitamin C, Vitamin E, Selenium and Carotenoids*, National Academy Press, Washington, D.C., 2000.

34. Food and Nutrition Board, Institute of Medicine, *Dietary Reference Intakes for Vitamin A, Vitamin K, Arsenic, Boron, Chromium, Copper, Iodine, Iron, Manganese, Molybdenum, Nickel, Silicon, Vanadium and Zinc*, National Academy Press, Washington, D.C., 2001.

35. Food and Nutrition Board, Recommended Dietary Allowances, 10th ed., National Academy of Sciences, Washington, D.C., 1989.

36. Operational Rations of the Department of Defense, Natick Pamphlet 30-25 (5th ed), U.S. Army Soldier and Biological Chemical Command — Soldier Systems Center, Natick, MA, 2002. (Available online at: http://www.sbccom.army.mil/programs/food/index.htm.)

37. Baker-Fulco, C.J., Patton, B.D., Montain, S.J. and Lieberman, H.R., Nutrition for Health and Performance, 2001: Nutritional Guidance for Military Operations in Temperate and Extreme Environments, Technical Note No. 01-4, U.S. Army Research Institute of Environmental Medicine, Natick, MA, 2001.

38. Life Sciences Research Office, Federation of American Societies for Experimental Biology, Third Report on Nutrition Monitoring in the United States: Volume 2, prepared for the Interagency Board for Nutrition Monitoring and Related Research, U.S. Government Printing Office, Washington, D.C., 1995.

39. National Research Council, *Diet and Health: Implications for Reducing Chronic Disease Risk,* National Academy Press, Washington, D.C., 1989.

40. Scott, J. M., Kirke, P.N. and Weir, D.G., The role of nutrition in neural tube defects, *Annu. Rev. Nutr.,* 10, 277, 1990.

41. Scholl, T.O. and Johnson, W.G., Folic acid: Influence on the outcome of pregnancy, *Am. J. Clin. Nutr.,* 71, 1295S, 2000.

42. Rush, D. and Rosenberg, I.H., Folate supplements and neural tube defects, *Nutr. Rev.,* 50, 25, 1992.

43. Friedl, K.E., Marchitelli, L.J., Sherman, D.E. and Tulley, R., Nutritional Assessment of Cadets at the U.S. Military Academy: Part 1. Anthropometric & Biochemical Measures, Technical Report No. T4-91, U.S. Army Research Institute of Environmental Medicine, Natick, MA, 1990.

44. Westphal, K.A. and Friedl, K.E., unpublished data, 1994.

45. Sauberlich, H.E., Skala, J.H., Johnson, H.L. and Nelson, R.A., Hematological Parameters and Lipid Profiles Observed in Cadets at the U.S. Military Academy, West Point, New York, LAIR Report No. 126, Letterman Army Institute of Research, Presidio of San Francisco, 1982.

46. Gurr, M., *Calcium in Nutrition*, International Life Science Institute Press, Washington, D.C., 1999, 22–36.

47. Heaney, R.P., Calcium, dairy products and osteoporosis, *J. Am. Coll. Nutr.*, 19, 83S, 2000.

48. Heaney, R.P., Nutritional factors in causation of osteoporosis, *Ann. Chirur. Gynaecol.*, 77, 176, 1988.

49. Protzman, R.R. and Griffis, C.G., Stress fractures in men and women undergoing military training, *J. Bone Joint Surg.*, 59A, 825, 1977.

50. Schmidt Brudvig, T.J., Gudger, T.D. and Obermeyer, L., Stress fractures in 295 trainees: A one-year study of incidence as related to age, sex and race, *Milit. Med.*, 148, 666, 1983.

51. Zahger, D., Abramovitz, A., Zelikovsky, L., Israel, O. and Israel, P., Stress fractures in female soldiers: An epidemiological investigation of an outbreak, *Milit. Med.*, 153, 448, 1988.

52. Friedl, K.E., Nuovo, J.A., Patience, T.H. and Dettori, J.R., Factors associated with stress fractures in young army women: Indications for further research, *Milit. Med.*, 157, 334, 1992.

53. Zemel, M.B., Calcium modulation of hypertension and obesity: mechanisms and implications, *J. Am. Coll. Nutr.*, 20, 428S, 2001.

54. Warber, J.P., McGraw, S.M., Kramer, F.M., Lesher, L.L., Johnson, W. and Cline, A.D., The Army Food and Nutrition Survey, 1995–1997, Technical Report No. T00-6, U. S. Army Research Institute of Environmental Medicine, Natick, MA, 1999.

55. Vogt, T.M., Appel, L.J., Obarzanek, E., Moore, T.J., Vollmer, W.M., Svetkey, L.P., Sacks, F.M., Bray, G.A., Cutler, J.A., Windhauser, M.M., Lin, P. and Karanja, N.M., Dietary approaches to stop hypertension: Rationale, design and methods, *J. Am. Diet. Assoc.*, 99, S12, 1999.

56. Harsha, D.W., Lin, P., Obarzanek, E., Karanja, N.M., Moore, T.J. and Caballero, B., Dietary approaches to stop hypertension: A summary of study results, *J. Am. Diet. Assoc.*, 99, S35, 1999.

57. Gardner, G.W., Edgerton, V.R., Senewiratne, B., Barnard, R.J. and Ohira, Y., Physical work capacity and metabolic stress in subjects with iron deficiency anemia, *Am. J. Clin. Nutr.*, 30, 910, 1977.

58. Lukaski, H.C., Hall, C.B. and Siders, W.A., Altered metabolic response of iron-deficient women during graded maximal exercise, *Eur. J. Exerc. Physiol.*, 63, 140, 1991.

59. Brownlie, T., IV, Utermohlen, V., Hinton, P.S., Giordano, C. and Haas, J.D., Marginal iron deficiency without anemia impairs aerobic adaptation among previously untrained women, *Am. J. Clin. Nutr.*, 75, 734, 2002.

60. Sandstead, H.H., Causes of iron and zinc deficiencies and their effect on brain, *J. Nutr.*, 130, 347S, 2000.

61. Halliwell, B., Antioxidants in human health and disease, *Ann. Rev. Nutr.*, 16, 33, 1996.

62. Shankar, A.H. and Prasad, A.S., Zinc and immune function: The biological basis of altered resistance to infection, *Am. J. Clin. Nutr.*, 68, 447S, 1998.

63. Grahn, B.H., Paterson, P.G., Gottschall-Pass, K.T. and Zhang, Z., Zinc and the eye, *J. Am. Coll. Nutr.*, 20, 106, 2001.

64. National Center for Health Statistics, Monthly Vital Statistics Report, 42(13), 1994.

65. The Surgeon General's Report on Nutrition and Health, Publ. No. 88-50210, U.S. Department of Health and Human Services, Washington, D.C., 1988.

66. The Committee on Military Nutrition Research, Military Nutrition Initiatives, Publ. IOM-91-05, National Academy of Sciences, Washington, D.C., 1991.

67. Armed Forces Recipe Services, Technical Manual 10-412/NAVSUP Publ. 7/AFM 146-12, Vol. 1/MCOP 10110.42A, Headquarters, Departments of the Army, the Navy and the Air Force, Washington, D.C., 1992.

68. The Master Menu, Supply Bulletin No. 10-260, Headquarters, Department of the Army, Washington, D.C., published monthly.

69. The Army Food Service Program, Army Regulation 30-1, Headquarters, Department of the Army, Washington, D.C., 1989.

70. Committee on Body Composition, Nutrition and Health of Military Women, Institute of Medicine, *Assessing Readiness in Military Women: The Relationship of Body Composition, Nutrition and Health*, National Academy Press, Washington, D.C., 1998.

Appendix:
Dietary Reference Intakes:
RDA, AI and UL

DIETARY REFERENCE INTAKES: RDA, AI, AND UL

Recommended Dietary Allowances (RDA) and Adequate Intakes (AI)

Age (yr)	Thiamin RDA (mg/day)	Riboflavin RDA (mg/day)	Niacin RDA (mg/day)[a]	Biotin AI (µg/day)	Pantothenic acid AI (mg/day)	Vitamin B₆ RDA (mg/day)	Folate RDA (µg/day)[b]	Vitamin B₁₂ RDA (µg/day)	Choline AI (mg/day)	Vitamin C RDA (mg/day)[c]	Vitamin A RDA (µg/day)[d]	Vitamin D AI (µg/day)[e]
Infants												
0–0.5	0.2	0.3	2	5	1.7	0.1	65	0.4	125	40	400	5
0.5–1	0.3	0.4	4	6	1.8	0.3	80	0.5	150	50	500	5
Children												
1–3	0.5	0.5	6	8	2	0.5	150	0.9	200	15	300	5
4–8	0.6	0.6	8	12	3	0.6	200	1.2	250	25	400	5
Males												
9–13	0.9	0.9	12	20	4	1.0	300	1.8	375	45	600	5
14–18	1.2	1.3	16	25	5	1.3	400	2.4	550	75	900	5
19–30	1.2	1.3	16	30	5	1.3	400	2.4	550	90	900	5
31–50	1.2	1.3	16	30	5	1.3	400	2.4	550	90	900	5
51–70	1.2	1.3	16	30	5	1.7	400	2.4	550	90	900	10
>70	1.2	1.3	16	30	5	1.7	400	2.4	550	90	900	15
Females												
9–13	0.9	0.9	12	20	4	1.0	300	1.8	375	45	600	5
14–18	1.0	1.0	14	25	5	1.2	400	2.4	400	65	700	5
19–30	1.1	1.1	14	30	5	1.3	400	2.4	425	75	700	5
31–50	1.1	1.1	14	30	5	1.3	400	2.4	425	75	700	5
51–70	1.1	1.1	14	30	5	1.5	400	2.4	425	75	700	10
>70	1.1	1.1	14	30	5	1.5	400	2.4	425	75	700	15
Pregnancy												
≤18	1.4	1.4	18	30	6	1.9	600	2.6	450	80	750	5
19–30	1.4	1.4	18	30	6	1.9	600	2.6	450	85	770	5
31–50	1.4	1.4	18	30	6	1.9	600	2.6	450	85	770	5
Lactation												
≤18	1.4	1.6	17	35	7	2.0	500	2.8	550	115	1200	5
19–30	1.4	1.6	17	35	7	2.0	500	2.8	550	120	1300	5
31–50	1.4	1.6	17	35	7	2.0	500	2.8	550	120	1300	5

Note: For all nutrients, values for infants are AI.

[a] Niacin recommendations are expressed as niacin equivalents (NE), except for recommendations for infants younger than 6 months, which are expressed as preformed niacin.

[b] Folate recommendations are expressed as dietary folate equivalents (DFE).

[c] Values are for nonsmokers. Smokers require an additional 35 milligrams per day.

[d] Vitamin A recommendations are expressed as retinol activity equivalents (RAE).

[e] Vitamin D recommendations are expressed as cholecalciferol and assume an absence of adequate exposure to sunlight.

Recommended Dietary Allowances (RDA) and Adequate Intakes (AI) (continued)

Vitamins		Minerals											
Vitamin E RDA (mg/day)	Vitamin K AI (µg/day)	Calcium AI (mg/day)	Phosphorous RDA (mg/day)	Magnesium RDA (mg/day)	Iron RDA (mg/day)	Zinc RDA (mg/day)	Iodine RDA (µg/day)	Selenium RDA (µg/day)	Copper RDA (µg/day)	Manganese AI (mg/day)	Fluoride AI (mg/day)	Chromium AI (µg/day)	Molybdenum RDA (µg/day)
4	2.0	210	100	30	0.27	2	110	15	200	0.003	0.01	0.2	2
5	2.5	270	175	75	11	3	130	20	220	0.6	0.5	5.5	3
6	30	500	460	80	7	3	90	20	340	1.2	0.7	11	17
7	55	800	500	130	10	5	90	30	440	1.5	1.0	15	22
11	60	1300	1250	240	8	8	120	40	700	1.9	2	25	34
15	75	1300	1250	410	11	11	150	55	890	2.2	3	35	43
15	120	1000	700	400	8	11	150	55	900	2.3	4	35	45
15	120	1000	700	420	8	11	150	55	900	2.3	4	35	45
15	120	1200	700	420	8	11	150	55	900	2.3	4	30	45
15	120	1200	700	420	8	11	150	55	900	2.3	4	30	45
11	60	1300	1250	240	8	8	120	40	700	1.6	2	21	34
15	75	1300	1250	360	15	9	150	55	890	1.6	3	24	43
15	90	1000	700	310	18	8	150	55	900	1.8	3	25	45
15	90	1000	700	320	18	8	150	55	900	1.8	3	25	45
15	90	1200	700	320	8	8	150	55	900	1.8	3	20	45
15	90	1200	700	320	8	8	150	55	900	1.8	3	20	45
15	75	1300	1250	400	27	13	220	60	1000	2.0	3	29	50
15	90	1000	700	350	27	11	220	60	1000	2.0	3	30	50
15	90	1000	700	360	27	11	220	60	1000	2.0	3	30	50
19	75	1300	1250	360	10	14	290	70	1300	2.6	3	44	50
19	90	1000	700	310	9	12	290	70	1300	2.6	3	45	50
19	90	1000	700	320	9	12	290	70	1300	2.6	3	45	50

e Vitamin E recommendations are expressed as α-tocopherol.

Source: Adapted with permission from the Dietary Reference Intakes series, National Academy Press. Copyright 1997, 1998, 2000, 2001, 2002 by the National Academy of Sciences. Courtesy of the National Academy Press, Washington, D.C.

DIETARY REFERENCE INTAKES: RDA, AI, AND UL (continued)

Tolerable Upper Intake Levels (UL)

Age (yr)	Vitamins								Minerals			
	Niacin (mg/day)[a]	Vitamin B6 (mg/day)	Folate (µg/day)[a]	Choline (mg/day)	Vitamin C (mg/day)	Vitamin A RDA (µg/day)[b]	Vitamin D (µg/day)	Vitamin E (mg/day)[c]	Calcium (mg/day)	Phosphorous (mg/day)	Magnesium (mg/day)[d]	Iron (mg/day)
Infants												
0–0.5	—	—	—	—	—	600	25	—	—	—	—	40
0.5–1	—	—	—	—	—	600	25	—	—	—	—	40
Children												
1–3	10	30	300	1000	400	600	50	200	2500	3000	65	40
4–8	15	40	400	1000	650	900	50	300	2500	3000	110	40
9–13	20	60	600	2000	1200	1700	50	600	2500	4000	350	40
Adolescents												
14–18	30	80	800	3000	1800	2800	50	800	2500	4000	350	45
Adults												
19–70	35	100	1000	3500	2000	3000	50	1000	2500	4000	350	45
>70	35	100	1000	3500	2000	3000	50	1000	2500	4000	350	45
Pregnancy												
≤18	30	80	800	3000	1800	2800	50	800	2500	3500	350	45
19–50	35	100	1000	3500	2000	3000	50	1000	2500	3500	350	45
Lactation												
≤18	30	80	800	3000	1800	2800	50	800	2500	4000	350	45
19–50	35	100	1000	3500	2000	3000	50	1000	2500	4000	350	45

[a] The UL for niacin and folate apply to synthetic forms obtained from supplements, fortified foods, or a combination of the two.

[b] The UL for vitamin A applies to the preformed vitamin only.

[c] The UL for vitamin E applies to any form of supplemental α-tocopherol, fortified foods, or a combination of the two.

[d] The UL for magnesium applies to synthetic forms obtained from supplements or drugs only.

DIETARY REFERENCE INTAKES: RDA, AI, AND UL (continued)

Tolerable Upper Intake Levels (UL) (continued)

Minerals

Zinc (µg/day)	Iodine (µg/day)	Selenium (µg/day)	Copper (µg/day)	Manganese (µg/day)	Fluoride (µg/day)	Molybdenum (µg/day)	Boron (µg/day)	Nickel (µg/day)	Vanadium (µg/day)
4	—	45	—	—	0.7	—	—	—	—
5	—	60	—	—	0.9	—	—	—	—
7	200	90	1000	2	1.3	300	3	0.2	—
12	300	150	3000	3	2.2	600	6	0.3	—
93	600	280	5000	6	10	1100	11	0.6	—
34	900	400	8000	9	10	1700	17	1.0	—
40	1100	400	10,000	11	10	2000	20	1.0	1.8
40	1100	400	10,000	11	10	2000	20	1.0	1.8
34	900	400	8,000	9	10	1700	17	1.0	—
40	1100	400	10,000	11	10	2000	20	1.0	—
34	900	400	8,000	9	10	1700	17	1.0	—
40	1100	400	10,000	11	10	2000	20	1.0	—

Note: An upper level was not established for vitamins and minerals not listed and for those age groups listed with a dash (—) because of a lack of data, not because these nutrients are safe to consume at any level of intake. All nutrients can have adverse effects when intakes are excessive.

Source: Adapted with permission from the Dietary Reference Intakes series, National Academy Press. Copyright 1997, 1998, 2000, 2001, by the National Academy of Sciences. Courtesy of the National Academy Press, Washington, D.C.

Dietary Reference Intakes: Energy, Carbohydrate, Fiber, Essential Fatty Acids, and Protein

Age (yrs)	Energy EER[a] (cal/day[b])	Carbohydrate RDA (g/day)	Total Fiber AI (g/day)	α-Linoleic Acid AI (g/day)	a-Linolenic Acid AI (g/day)	Protein RDA (g/kg/day)
Males						
0–0.5	570	60	—	4.4	0.5	1.52
0.5–1	743	95	—	4.6	0.5	1.5
1–3[c]	1,046	130	19	7	0.7	1.1
4–8[c]	1,742	130	25	10	0.9	0.95
9–13	2,279	130	31	12	1.2	0.95
14–18	3,152	130	38	16	1.6	0.85
19–30	3,067[d]	130	38	17	1.6	0.8
31–50	3,067[d]	130	38	17	1.6	0.8
>51	3,067[d]	130	30	14	1.6	0.8
Females						
0–0.5	520	60	—	4.4	0.5	1.52
0.5–1	676	95	—	4.6	0.5	1.5
1–3[c]	992	130	19	7	0.7	1.1
4–8[c]	1,642	130	25	10	0.9	0.95
9–13	2,071	130	26	10	1.0	0.95
14–18	2,368	130	36	11	1.1	0.85
19–30	2,403[d]	130	25	12	1.1	0.8
31–50	2,403[d]	130	21	12	1.1	0.8
>51	2,403[d]	130	21	11	1.1	0.8
Pregnancy						
14–18, *1st trimester*	2,368	175	28	13	1.4	1.1
2nd trimester	2,708	175	28	13	1.4	1.1
3rd trimester	2,820	175	28	13	1.4	1.1
19–50, *1st trimester*	2,403[e]	175	28	13	1.4	1.1
2nd trimester	2,743[e]	175	28	13	1.4	1.1
3rd trimester	2,855[e]	175	28	13	1.4	1.1
Lactation						
14–18, *1st 6 months*	2,698	210	29	13	1.3	1.1
2nd 6 months	2,768	210	29	13	1.3	1.1
19–50, *1st 6 months*	2,733[e]	210	29	13	1.3	1.1
2nd 6 months	2,803[e]	210	29	13	1.3	1.1

Note: For all nutrients, values for infants are AI; AI is not equivalent to RDA.

Dashes indicate that values have not been determined.

[a] Estimated Energy Requirement (EER) is the average dietary energy intake predicted to maintain energy balance and is consistent with good health in healthy adults. EER values are determined at four physical activity levels; the values above are for the "active" person.

[b] Kilocalories per day.

[c] For energy, the age groups for young children are 1–2 years and 3–8 years.

[d] Subtract 10 calories per day for males and 7 calories per day for females for each year of age above 19.

[e] Subtract 7 calories per day for each year of age above 19.

Index

D

protein synthesis and, 56
requirements, 56
status
  biochemical status of, 473
  HPV infection and, 351
  impairment of, 110
  low, 162
Folic acid
  fortification program, initiation of, 39
  U.S. PHS recommendation for, 83
Follicle-stimulating hormone (FSH), 63, 193
Food
  advertising practices, 386
  assistance programs, 171
  aversions, during pregnancy, 87
  competing emotions about, 385
  consumption surveys, 458
  costs, 49
  cravings, 68
    during pregnancy, 87
    PMS and, 70
  insecurity, definition of, 171
  items, convenient, 16
  labels, 400
  marketing, 371
  products
    energy density of, 386
    iron-fortified, 425
  security, 34
  supply, changes in American, 371
  upsized portions of, 371
Food and Agricultural Organization (FAO), 267
Food and Drug Administration (FDA), 5, 6, 8, 167
Food Guide Pyramid, 50, 163, 164, 171, 444
Food and Nutrition Board, 401
Formiminoglutamic acid (FIGLU), 102, 110, 111, 234
Framingham Heart Study, 441
Framingham Knee Osteoarthritis Study, 311
Framingham Study, 20, 135, 259, 263
Fruit and vegetable consumption, breast cancer risk and, 345
FSH, *see* Follicle-stimulating hormone

G

Gallbladder disease, 186
GAO, *see* Government Accounting Office
Gastric ulcers, 186
Gastrointestinal distress, 402
GDM, *see* Gestational diabetes mellitus
Gender, culture and nutrition, 29–42
  American culture and nutrition, 38–39

cultural differences influencing income-generating opportunities, 33–35
cultural variation in good care practice for mothers and impact on child nutrition, 35–36
elements of culture, 29–30
food security, household power imbalances and gender, 37–38
nutrient problems across culture and gender, 31–33
  early childhood growth failure, 31–32
  iodine deficiency, 32–33
  iron deficiency anemia, 32
  low birthweight, 31
  vitamin A deficiency, 33
relationships, 30
role of mother's education in nutrition, 36–37
Gender-specific hypotheses, relevance of, 7
Gene
  expression
    role of thyroid hormone in, 334, 335
    stimulation of, 335
  mutations, 336
Genetics
  diabetes and, 297
  fatness and, 373
Genistein, 138, 272, 438
Gestational diabetes, 77, 298
Gestational diabetes mellitus (GDM), 88
Gestodene, 100, 101
GH, *see* Growth hormone
Ginkgo biloba, 167
Glossitis, 104
Glucocorticoid(s), 144
  secretion, 105
  therapy, thyroid hormone status and, 331
Glucosamine, 311, 312, 319
Glucose
  intolerance, CVD and, 264
  metabolism, deranged, 295
  tolerance
    cyclic variations in, 303
    impaired, 299
Glycogen depletion, 379
Glycolysis, 334
Goiter, 326
  disappearance of, 328
  nontoxic, 326
Good care practices, 35
Gout, 312
Government Accounting Office (GAO), 5
Grain products, iron-fortified, 218, 225
Growth hormone (GH), 194, 200

X

XA, *see* Xanthurenic acid

Xanthurenic acid (XA), 105,
        106, 118

Xerophthalmia, 104

Xerostomia, 169

Z

Zinc
    deficiency, 56, 402, 475
    levels
        during pregnancy, 81
        vegetarian, 452
    protein synthesis and, 56
    status, low birth weight and, 431